Jose Russo · Irma H. Russo

Molecular Basis of Breast Cancer

Prevention and Treatment

Springer

Berlin
Heidelberg
New York
Hong Kong
London
Milan
Paris
Tokyo

Jose Russo
Irma H. Russo

Molecular Basis of Breast Cancer

Prevention and Treatment

With 338 Figures and 63 Tables

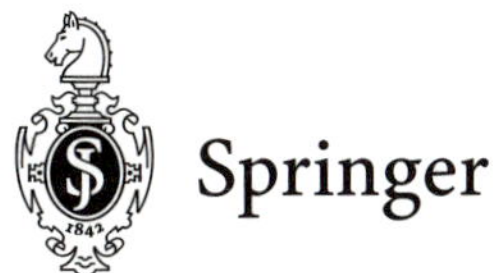

Springer

Jose Russo MD, FACP
Irma H. Russo, MD, FACP

Breast Cancer Research Laboratory
Fox Chase Cancer Center
333 Cottman Avenue
Philadelphia, PA 19111
USA

J_russo@fccc.edu
I_russo@fccc.edu

ISBN 3-540-00391-6
Springer-Verlag Berlin Heidelberg New York

Library of Congress Cataloging-in-Publication Data
Russo, Jose. Molecular basis of breast cancer: prevention and
treatment/J. Russo, Irma H. Russo. p.; cm. Includes biblio-
graphical references and index. ISBN 3-540-00391-6 (alk paper)
1. Breast–Cancer–Molecular aspects. 2. Breast–Cancer–Pathogenesis. I. Russo, Irma H. II. Title. [DNLM: 1. Breast Neoplasm–prevention & control. 2. Breast Neoplasms–therapy. WP
870 R969m 2004] RC280.B8R87 2004 616.99'449071–dc21

Springer-Verlag Berlin Heidelberg New York a member of
BertelsmannSpringer Science + Business Media GmbH

http://www.springer.de

Cover design: E. Kirchner, Heidelberg
Product management and layout: B. Wieland, Heidelberg
Reproduction and typesetting: AM-production, Wiesloch
Printing and bookbinding: Appl, Wemding

21/3150 – 5 4 3 2 1 0
Printed on acid-free paper

Preface

During the past 30 years we have witnessed the emergence of new disciplines whose contribution to the understanding of the biology of breast cancer have been enormous. Advances in the field of steroid hormone nuclear receptors, which control the expression of genetic programs involved in cellular processes that are essential for normal and aberrant cell growth, have been major contributors to the therapy and prevention of hormone-dependent cancers. The discoveries of the association of hereditary breast cancers with mutations in the BRCA1 and BRCA2 genes, and the concept that they essentially represent a continuum of mutations with different degrees of penetrance within given families, have added considerable understanding to the molecular basis of breast cancer. These advances have been hastened by the use of recombinant DNA technology, which has become a revolutionary tool for probing the human genome. This explosion in knowledge on the hormonal and genetic basis of breast cancer, and considerable advances in its early detection and therapeutic modalities have awakened great hopes for the conquest of this disease. However, they have not been fulfilled as yet, since the mortality caused by this disease has remained almost unchanged for the past five decades, a dismal picture worsened by the gradual increase in breast cancer incidence reported in most Western countries and in societies that are becoming westernized.

The realization that traditional developmental concepts need to provide the necessary framework for the interpretation of data generated by these modern techniques, in order to complete the still unfinished puzzle that the etiology, pathogenesis and progression of cancer represent, led us to design this book, whose goal is to comprehensively review in ten chapters the fundamental knowledge on breast cancer. The opening chapter links epidemiology, influence of geographic and environmental exposures on cancer incidence to the development of the organ and its role in cancer initiation. Central to this approach is the endocrine control of breast development, the relationship of cell proliferation with the presence of steroid hormone receptors in the breast epithelium, and finally the importance of full differentiation as a tool for protecting the breast from developing cancer. Reported are studies of the pathogenesis of breast cancer that have elucidated the site of origin of breast cancer and have been validated by in vitro experimentation. The utilization of these models for the analysis of molecular and genetic changes in the initiation and progression of breast cancer has uncovered key processes during the immortalization and transformation of human breast epithelial cells and genetic heterogeneity within single lesions. A chapter has been devoted to animal models for human breast cancer, pathological classification of rat mammary tumors, and genetically engineered mice model. These studies are complemented with in vitro models for human breast cancer, unifying various aspects of growth properties of normal and neoplastic breast epithelial cells in vitro, transformation of cells with carcinogens and oncogenes. This knowledge is essential for determining the functional relevance of genomic changes in cancer initiation and progression and for developing strategies for breast cancer prevention.

Jose Russo, MD, FCAP
Irma H. Russo, MD, FCAP

Acknowledgements

I am a part of all that I have met

ULYSSES Alfred, Lord Tennyson

We pay tribute to the visionaries that ignited our imagination and fed our hunger for knowledge: Dr. Julián Echave Llanos and Dr. Mario H. Burgos opened for us the magnificent doors of science and experimentation at the School of Medical Sciences in Mendoza, Argentina. Dr. Michael Brennan of the Michigan Cancer Foundation provided a fertile ground for developing seminal ideas. In the same institution a valued colleague, Dr. Herbert Soule, through the development of breast epithelial cell lines provided invaluable tools for the scientific community to advance the understanding of hormonal regulation of cell growth and cell transformation. And last, but not least, the expertise and support of the staff members of the Fox Chase Cancer Center is a continuous source of encouragement.

We are indebted to our postdoctoral associates who through the years have been contributors to the publications reported or referenced in this book, among them Drs. A. Adesina, M. E. V. Alvarado, F. Basolo, B. Bove, G. Calaf, D. Ciocca, G. Fontanini, S. Higa, T.-Y. Ho, Y. Huang, X. Jiang, F. Martinez, J. Ochieng, A. M. Salicione, I. D. C. Silva, N. Sohi, L. K. Tay, and P.-L. Zhang.

We acknowledge the special contribution of Drs. Hasan M. Lareef and Gabriela Balogh in providing data supporting the work presented in Chapter 4, Dr. Yun Fu Hu in writing and compiling the numerous references of Chapter 9, and Dr Pramod Srivastava for data presented in Chapter 10. We are also grateful for the assistance of Dr. Fathima Sheriff for performing literature searches, Ms. Joan Levin for typing tables and references for this book, and Ms. Patricia A. Russo for her artwork contribution in Chapter 2.

Contents

9 Preventive Strategies in Breast Cancer

10 The New Paradigm in Breast Cancer Prevention

Epidemiological Considerations in Breast Cancer

1.1 Introduction

Breast cancer incidence rates in the United States have increased at a rate of 1 % per year since 1940 [1]. Despite considerable advances in early detection and in therapeutic modalities, the mortality caused by this disease has remained almost unchanged for the past five decades [2, 3]. This already dismal picture is worsened by the gradual increase in breast cancer incidence in most Western countries and in societies that recently became westernized or that are in the process of westernization [2, 3]. Epidemiological observations that daughters of women who migrate from low-incidence to high-incidence countries acquire the breast cancer risk prevailing in the new country [4], suggest that aspects of lifestyle or the environment are major determinants of breast cancer risk. A study of population-attributable risks has estimated that at least 45 % to 55 % of breast cancer cases in the United States may be explained by the following factors: advanced age at the time of the first full-term pregnancy, nulliparity, family history of breast cancer, higher socioeconomic status, earlier age at menarche, and prior benign breast disease [5]. Other statistical models appear to explain an even higher proportion of breast cancer on the basis of known risk factors [6]. Studies of atomic bomb survivors have shown that environmental exposures, such as ionizing radiation, are a risk factor for breast cancer [7]. Exposure to radiation at a young age has been identified as a causative agent of breast cancer in selected populations [8, 9, 10, 11], but there is no definitive proof of what causes breast cancer in the population at large. The increased risk associated with exposure to environmental chemicals, such as alcohol [12] and cigarette smoke [13–19], makes these agents suspects for causing cancer in the human population.

1.2 Geographical Influences

In the United States, breast cancer rates among older women have been reported to be higher in the Northeast than in the South; they are also higher in urban than in rural areas [20, 21]. A population-based study in New York State found an increasing linear relationship between standardized incidence rates of breast cancer and population density [22]. Consistent with these findings, the Surveillance, Epidemiology, and End Results (SEER) Program of the National Cancer Institute reported higher breast cancer incidence in the San Francisco Bay Area when compared to the other seven registries located throughout the country [23]. Regional differences in the prevalence of known breast cancer risk factors, such as low parity, higher education, and higher income, seem to play an important role in the elevated rates of breast cancer reported in affluent communities, such as in Marin County, California [24].

Geographic variations in breast cancer incidence in USA and other countries, like Russia, have been attributed to differences in exposure to sunlight [25–27]. Sunlight is necessary for synthesis of vitamin D in the skin, and in vitro studies have suggested that vitamin D inhibits growth of breast cancer cells in culture [26].

1.3 Radiation as an Etiologic Agent

Radiation from natural sources is ubiquitous in the environment; it includes cosmic rays, terrestrial radiations influenced by the distribution of radioactive elements in the soil, and internally deposited radionuclides, such as radon [28]. However, up to now, only accidental or iatrogenic radiation has been demonstrated to exert a carcinogenic effect on the breast. High energy X- or γ rays from A bomb exposures in Hiroshima and Nagasaki in Japan [29], and chest radiation administered for the treatment of scoliosis, or repeated fluoroscopies for tuberculosis [30] have been well-documented causes of breast cancer For radiation to act as a carcinogen exposure has to occur at a young age. Only those women that were younger than 29 at the time of the bombing in Japan developed breast cancer [29], whereas older women developed benign breast diseases. Estimates of the effects of low doses of radiation have been extrapolated from the results of the atomic bomb and medical radiation studies [31, 32]. There is convincing evidence that age at exposure influences the relative risk. Excess risk decreases with increasing age at exposure; the highest relative risks are observed for women exposed between the ages of 10 and 20, and there is little risk for those greater than 40 [33]. Parity, in addition to age at exposure, modifies the risk of developing radiation-induced breast cancer, since the risk is greater in nulliparous women, but no carcinogenic effect has been reported in women treated with radiation for postpartum mastitis.

A new population of women at high-risk for breast cancer is emerging as young women are successfully treated with radiation for early-stage Hodgkin's disease [8–11]. Retrospective multicentric studies both in Europe and USA have consistently demonstrated that women in whom Hodgkin's disease is diagnosed at a median age of 21 to 24 years, subsequently develop breast cancers after a median interval of 15 years. The predominant tumor type is the infiltrating ductal carcinoma, with a large number of aggressive tumors with a very unfavorable prognosis. These women have an increased risk of developing additional cancers and significantly lower overall survival than women treated for sporadic breast cancer. While the risk of recurrent Hodgkin's disease decreases as time from treatment elapses, the risk of radiation-induced breast cancer rises. Women irradiated between the time of puberty and the age of 30 are at the highest risk of developing cancer. It would be of great interest to consider the possibility of preventing breast cancer in this patient population by administering a hormonal treatment that would differentiate their breast "before" or shortly after administering radiation, in order to reduce the susceptibility of the organ to be transformed by the treatment (see Chapter 10).

There is little reliable evidence of an increased risk of breast cancer due to occupational exposures to radiation [34–37]. In a Finnish study, an elevated risk of breast cancer in airline attendants was observed; but was demonstrated to be a residual confounding by socioeconomic status and parity [38]. Breast cancer risk in women employed as radiologic technologists, was not associated with personal exposure to radiation as defined by job history and length of employment [39, 40]. There has been no evidence of excess breast cancer mortality among the general population from low-dose environmental radiation exposures such as fallout from nuclear weapons testing and nuclear installations [32, 41, 42].

1.4 Electromagnetic Fields

The electrification of America began in 1880 with nighttime street lighting systems, and by the beginning of the 1930s, many electrical appliances had been introduced into the home [43]. Alternating currents from electric power facilities and household appliances produce electromagnetic fields (EMF) in the extremely low-frequency range. Exposure to environmental lighting in the visible range of the spectrum [44] and low-level EMF [45] have been hypothesized to increase the risk of breast cancer due to a decrease in the secretion of the hormone melatonin and a subsequent increase in circulating estrogens [46–48]. Although there is little experimental human evidence, in vitro and in vivo studies in animals have demonstrated a link among EMF, melatonin, and breast cancer [49–52].

The general population is exposed to EMF primarily from power lines, transformer substations, and electrical appliance use. Elevation in female breast cancer incidence has been associated with magnitude of exposure at the current residence [53]. Studies in Britain [54], Netherlands [55], and Taiwan [56], did not observe an association between female breast cancer deaths and residence in the vicinity of electricity transmission facilities. Studies on the use of electric blankets [57, 58] revealed a statistically nonsignificant increase in premenopausal or postmenopausal breast cancer in women using electric blankets continuously throughout the night [59, 60] compared to never users.

1.5 Environmental Pollutants

Epidemiological studies of breast cancer incidence in relation to exposures to environmental synthetic chemicals have focused on biologically persistent organochlorines. This class of compounds includes pesticides, e.g., 2,2-bis(p-chlorophenyl)-1,1,1-trichloromethane (DDT), chlordane, hexachloro-cyclohexane (HCH, lindane), hexachlorobenzene (HCB), Kepone, and mirex; industrial chemicals, e.g., polychlorinated biphenyls (PCBs); and dioxins (polychlorinated dibenzo-furans (PCDFs), and polychlorinated dibenzodioxin (PCDDs), produced as combustion byproducts of PCBs or contaminants of pesticides. Another industrial chemical group, polybrominated biphenyls (PBBs), has also been studied. Because many of these chemicals are weakly estrogenic and are excreted in breast milk, it has been hypothesized that they increase breast cancer risk by mimicking 17-β-estradiol and by a direct exposure of ductal and other cells in the breast to these compounds or their active metabolites [61]. Other compounds, specifically dioxins [62] and some PCB congeners [63], exhibit antiestrogenic activity; therefore, despite the established carcinogenicity of dioxin in animal tests [62], in women they might be protective from breast cancer. There is some evidence of an association of DDE levels with the estrogen-receptor (ER) status in breast tumors [64]. Most of the recent large studies, however, have not found evidence of increased breast cancer risk associated with blood levels of DDE or total PCBs. The possibility exists that a positive association might be limited to women with particular reproductive characteristics [65].

The organochlorines are highly lipophilic and resistant to metabolism. Thus, many of these compounds bioaccumulate in the food chain and persist in the body and in the environment. The concentrations of these chemicals can be measured in breast milk, adipose tissue, and blood. Most of the epidemiologic literature on organochlorines focuses on DDT, DDE [1,1-dichloro-2,2,-bis(p-dichlorophenyl)ethylene, the main metabolite of DDT], and PCBs because they are among the most persistent in humans [66]. Exposure of the general population to these compounds occurs predominantly through ingestion of fish, dairy products, and meat. Almost everyone in the United States has had some measurable exposure; however, the average body burden of some of these chemicals (e.g., DDT) has been decreasing with time since the cessation of their use in this country [67]. The experimental and epidemiological evidence of potential links to cancer has been reviewed in detail elsewhere by Adami et al. [68], Ahlborg et al. [69], and Wolff and associates [70].

1.6 Reproductive Factors

All women in the general population are exposed to similar environmental influences; yet, not all of them develop breast cancer. Among women with no family history of breast or breast/ovarian cancer [71, 72], or Li-Fraumeni Syndrome [73], the higher risk of developing breast cancer is associated with a history of early menarche [74], nulliparity [75–78], late first full-term pregnancy [75, 79], and late menopause [75], all conditions that are under the direct control of the ovary. The central role played by the ovary in breast cancer development is further confirmed by the marked reduction in cancer incidence after surgical or chemical ovariectomy [80]. The indirect evidence that depression of gonadal function, attributed to elevated melatonin levels in profoundly blind women, decreases the risk of breast and other cancers [81–84] suggests that light acts as an important environmental factor modulating breast cancer risk through endocrine disruption [85]. The paradox that ovarian stimulation such as that induced by pregnancy [71–75] or by treatment of women with the pregnancy hormone human chorionic gonadotropin (hCG) [86] exerts a protective effect, highlights the importance of induction of complete breast differentiation for protecting the breast from developing cancer. Differentiation, however, has to be induced during a specific period in the lifetime of a woman, as indicated by epidemiological observations that a full-term pregnancy that markedly reduces the lifetime breast cancer risk of a woman if it occurs before 24 years of age, increases the risk above that observed in nulliparous women when it is postponed beyond the 30th to 35th birthday [75–79].

1.7 Environmental Exposures at a Young Age that Increase the Risk of Breast Cancer

1.7.1 Endocrinological Milieu

The comparison of events influencing the initiation of cancer in humans and animals and of the factors that influence both led us to postulate that a common thread is starting to emerge. Central to this hypothesis is the initiation of puberty. Menarche, or the first menstruation that marks the initiation of puberty, is an objective manifestation of ovarian function [82, 87]. The age at menarche has been observed to decrease in the Western world, with no clear explanation for this phenomenon. It is of great importance to take into consideration the facts that pubertal development is modulated by ovarian function, which in turn is under the control of the hypothalamic-pituitary axis under the control of two interacting time-keeping mechanisms in the central nervous system (CNS): endogenous circadian rhythmicity and sleep-wake homeostasis [85]. Circadian rhythmicity is an endogenous, near 24-h oscillation, generated in the suprachiasmatic nuclei (SCN) of the hypothalamus (H) that generate pulses transmitted to the pituitary-gonadal (PG) axis via neural and humoral mechanisms. The SCN, under the light-dark cycle, controls the pineal gland and the levels of circulating melato-

nin. The photoperiod via melatonin secretion determines the timing of puberty in some species and delays reproductive maturity in both males and females. The production of melatonin is inhibited by visible light, which alters the circadian rhythm, disrupting the body's physiology and metabolism [85]. The stimulus of the ovary by pituitary follicle stimulating hormone (FSH) results in follicular maturation and estrogen secretion, followed by a mid-cycle peak of luteinizing hormone (LH) that triggers ovulation and subsequent progesterone secretion. Ovarian stimulation per se is insufficient for driving the breast to the completely differentiated condition that should be reached for achieving protection from cancer development. Additional hormonal supplementation, such as that provided by full-term pregnancy, or specific hormonal regimens, are required for that purpose [86].

1.7.2 Smoking

In the last two decades, approximately 3 million women have died prematurely from smoking-related diseases, including cancer. In 1998, 22 % of all women in the USA smoked cigarettes, with a higher percentage of high school senior girls smoking. Lung cancer surpassed breast cancer in 1987 as the leading cause of cancer death in women and it killed nearly 68,000 women in 2000 [14, 88]. Tobacco smoke is a complex mixture of several thousand chemicals that include carcinogens, namely polycyclic hydrocarbons (PAHs) such as benzo(a)pyrene (BP), which are metabolically activated, forming carcinogen-DNA adducts in human breast tissues. BP selectively binds to deoxyguanine at CpG dinucleotides within codons of the gene, making them mutational hotspots. The resultant G:C to T:A transversions in the p53 gene show a dose-response relationship in lung cancers of smokers [14, 88]. The need to determine whether tobacco smoking is a causative agent in breast cancer has stimulated numerous studies at both epidemiological and basic research levels. The fact that several studies support the hypothesis that "women are more susceptible than men to smoking-induced lung cancer," and that estradiol regulates activities that enhance lung carcinogenesis and tumor progression, as supported by the detection of ER and progesterone receptors (PR) in lung cancer [88], indicate that there similarities at least in hormone dependence between breast and lung cancer. The use of smokeless tobacco has been reported to elevate significantly the risk of developing younger-onset (<55 years) breast cancer (OR=7.79, 95% CI=1.05–66.0) for ever-users of smokeless tobacco [13]. Additional support to the etiologic role of chemical carcinogens in the initiation of breast cancer has been obtained from our experimental studies of in vitro transformation of human breast epithelial cells with BP [89] (see Chapter 7).

1.7.3 Alcohol as a Neuroendocrine Disruptor

A clear association has been found between breast cancer occurrence and drinking alcohol. Any history of drinking alcohol increases the risk of breast cancer 1.2-fold above that of women who never drank alcohol (95% confidence interval 0.7–1.8). A greater than average consumption of alcohol for 6 months or more increases the relative risk of breast cancer to 2.6 (95% confidence interval 1.1–5.8) [12]. Positive dose-response trends have been also reported in pooled analysis of large cohort studies and meta-analyses of a broader spectrum of studies. Although the ultimate mechanism through which alcohol increases breast cancer risk has not been clarified, it has been suggested that alcohol consumption alters hormonal levels by affecting the opioid hypothalamic activity, altering LH secretion [87]. These changes have been associated with an advance in the onset of sexual behavior when alcohol is consumed before puberty [87]. An effect of alcohol consumption on the hypothalamic-pituitary-gonadal axis is also supported by the reported observations that the nocturnal urinary concentration of 6-sulfatoxymelatonin, the primary metabolite of melatonin, decreases in a dose-dependent manner with increasing consumption of alcoholic beverages in the preceding 24-h period [90]. A categorical analysis revealed no effect of one drink, but a 9% reduction with two drinks, a 15% reduction with three drinks, and a 17% reduction with four or more drinks [90].

1.7.4 Effect of Light on Puberty and Breast Cancer Risk

A higher breast cancer incidence has been reported in women that work at night, whereas the risk is lower in profound bilateral blind women [82–84]. The rate of breast cancer risk reduction in blind women is proportional to the degree of blindness [85]. Experimental studies have demonstrated that exposure to constant light from birth enhances mammary carcinogenesis in rodents [83]. Pinealectomy, that suppress nocturnal melatonin production and increases prolactin levels, also stimulates tumor progression in rodents [84]. Exposure to constant light initiated at the age of 26 days in rat, on the other hand, induces lactational changes and inhibits rat mammary carcinogenesis. A suggested mechanism for the effect of light on mammary carcinogenesis is its suppressive effect on nocturnal melatonin, in association with increased levels of DNA synthesis and elevated circulating levels of prolactin [83–85]. Discrepancies in results obtained when constant light exposure is initiated at birth and those initiated at 26 days of age might reflect age-related differences in the maturation of the suprachiasmatic nucleus (SCN) and hypothalamic-pituitary-gonadal axis in response to environmental stimuli that deserve further investigation.

During the past 4 years, significant progress has been made in identifying the molecular components of the mammalian circadian clock system [91]. An autoregulatory transcriptional feedback loop similar to that described in Drosophila appears to form the core circadian rhythm generating mechanism in mammals. Two basic helix-loop-helix (bHLH) PAS (PER-ARNT-SIM) transcription factors, CLOCK and BMAL1, form the positive elements of the system and drive transcription of three Period and two Cryptochrome genes. The protein products of these genes are components of a negative feedback complex that inhibits CLOCK and BMAL1 to close the circadian loop. The novel findings that environmental carcinogens bind to epithelial cells through the aryl hydrocarbon receptor (AhR), which upon translocation to the nucleus it dimerizes with the co-factor AhR nuclear translocator (ARNT), a member of the Per-ARNT-Sim (PAS) protein-containing the same transcription factors CLOCK and BMAL1 found in the suprachiasmatic nucleus (SCN), suggest that in addition to being involved in the initiation of puberty, the SCN might be affected by environmental carcinogens that are traditionally considered to exert their carcinogenic effects on peripheral organs by acting directly on mammary epithelial receptors.

1.8 Conclusions

Current level of knowledge indicates that the higher breast cancer incidence observed in Westernized societies might be the consequence of modifications in the neuroendocrine profile induced during childhood by an industrialized lifestyle. Research strategies are being developed for determining whether these changes act synergistically with environmental physical and chemical carcinogens for increasing the susceptibility of the breast to undergo neoplastic transformation early in life, even though it will become clinically detectable 15 or 20 years later (see Chapters 2 and 5). The proof of these postulates will open new avenues for developing strategies for preventing breast cancer by modulating the factors that influence the initiation of puberty, and hence, breast development (see Chapters 2, 3, and 10). The identification of a "high risk window" for every individual will provide a physiological framework for minimizing exposures to environmental carcinogens during the high susceptibility periods (see Chapters 4, 5, and 6). The ultimate goal would be to narrow the "high risk window" by inducing full differentiation of the breast before it is "hit" by one or many of the known or suspected environmental carcinogens. These goals, however, are far from reach in the human population because our level of knowledge is insufficient for testing in young girls the neuroendocrine-environmental interactions postulated above.

References

1. Harris, J.R., Lippman, M.E., Veronesi, U., and Willett, W. Breast cancer. N. Engl. J. Med. 327:319–328, 1992.
2. Jemal, A., Murray, T., Samuels, A., Ghafoor, A., Ward, E., and Thun, M. J. Cancer Statistics, 2003. CA Cancer J. Clin. 53: 5–26, 2003.
3. Howe, H.L., Wingo, P.A., Thun, M.J., Ries, L.A., Rosenberg, H.M., Feigal, E.G., Edwards, B.K. Annual report to the nation on the status of cancer (1973 through 1998), featuring cancers with recent increasing trends. J. Natl. Cancer Inst. 93: 824–842, 2001.
4. Buell, P. Changing incidence of breast cancer in Japanese-American women. J. Natl. Cancer Inst. 51:1479–1383, 1973.
5. Madigan, M.P., Ziegler, R.G., Benichou, J., Byrne, C., Hooper, R.N. Proportion of breast cancer cases in the United States explained by well-established risk factors. J. Natl. Cancer Ist. 87:1681–1685, 1995.
6. Colditz, G.A., Frazier, A.L. Models of breast cancer show that risk is set of events of early life: Prevention efforts must shift focus. Cancer Epidemiol. Biomarkers Prev. 4:567–571, 1995.
7. Segaloff, A., Maxfield, W.S. The synergism between radiation and estrogen in the production of mammary cancer in the rat. Cancer Res. 31:166, 1971.
8. Hancock, S.L., Tucker, M.A., and Hoppe, R.T. Breast cancer after treatment of Hodgkin's disease. J. Natl. Cancer Inst. 85:25–31, 1993.
9. Cutuli, B., Borel, C., Dhermain, F., Magrini, S.M., Wasserman, T.H., Bogart, J.A., Provencio, M., de Lafontan, B., de la Rochefordiere, A., Cellai, E., Graic, Y., Kerbrat, P., Alzieu, C., Teissier, E., Dilhuydy, J., Mignotte, H., Velten, M. Breast cancer occurred after treatment for Hodgkin's disease: analysis of 133 cases. Radiother. Oncol. 59:247–255, 2001.
10. Gaffney, D.K., Hemmersmeier, J., Holden, J., Marshall, J., Smith, L.M., Avizonis, V., Tran, T., Neuhausen, S.L. Breast cancer after mantle irradiation for Hodgkin's disease: correlation of clinical, pathologic, and molecular features including loss of heterozygosity at BRCA1 and BRCA2. Int. J. Radiat. Oncol. Biol. Phys. 49:539–46, 2001.
11. Janov, A.J., Tulecke, M., O'Neill, A., Lester, S., Mauch, P.M., Harris, J., Schnitt, S.J., Shapiro, C.L. Clinical and Pathologic Features of Breast Cancers in Women Treated for Hodgkin's Disease: A Case-Control Study. Breast J. 7:46–52, 2001.
12. Lash, T.L., Aschengrau, A. Alcohol Drinking and Risk of Breast Cancer. Breast J. 6:396–399, 2000.
13. Spangler, J.G., Michielutte, R., Bell, R.A., Dignan, M.B. Association between smokeless tobacco use and breast cancer among Native-American women in North Carolina. Ethn. Dis. 11:36–43, 2001.
14. Satcher, D. Women and Health: A report of the Surgeon General-2001. U.S.Dept.Health and Human Serv., PHS Office of the Surgeon General, 1–4. 2001.

15. Russo, I. H., Tahin, Q., Huang, Y., and Russo, J. Cellular and molecular changes induced by the chemical carcinogen benzo(a)pyrene in human breast epithelial cells and its association with smoking and breast cancer. J.Women's Cancer 3:29–36, 2001.

16. Baron, J. A. Breast cancer, hormone-related disorders and cigarette smoking. J.Women's Cancer 3:23–28, 2001.

17. Phillips, D. H., Martin, F. L., Grover P.L., and Williams, J. A. Toxicological basis for a possible association of breast cancer with smoking and other sources of environmental carcinogens. J.Women's Cancer 3:9–16, 2001.

18. Ambrosone, C. B. Impact of genetics on the relationship between smoking and breast cancer risk. J.Women's Cancer 3:17–22, 2001.

19. Morabia, A., Ambrosone, C. B., Baron, J. A., Phillips, D. H., and Russo, I. H. What do we currently know about the epidemiological and biologic plausibility of the association of smoking and breast cancer? J.Women's Cancer 3:5–8, 2001.

20. Blot, W.J. Fraumeni, J.F., Stone, B.J. Geographic patterns of breast cancer in the United States. J. Natl. Cancer Inst. 59:14–07, 1977.

21. Sturgeon, S.R., Schairer, C., Gail, M., McAdams, M., Brinton, L.A., and Hoover, R.N. Geographic variation in mortality from breast cancer among white women in the United States. J. Natl. Cancer Inst. 87:1846–1853, 1995.

22. Nasca, P.C., Mahoney, M.C., Wolfgang, P.E. Population density and cancer incidence differentials in New York State. Cancer Causes Control 3:7–15, 1992.

23. Robbins, A.S., Brescianini, S., Kelsey, J.L. Regional differences in known risk factors and the higher incidence of breast cancer in San Francisco. J. Natl. Cancer Inst. 89:960–965, 1997.

24. Clarke, C.A., Glaser, S.L., West, D.W., Ereman, R.R., Erdmann, C.A., Barlow, J.M., and Wrensch, M.R. Breast cancer incidence and mortality trends in an affluent population: Marin County, California, USA, 1990–1996. Breast Cancer Res. 4: R13, 2002.

25. Garland, F.C., Garland, C.F., Gorham, E.D.,Young, J.F. Geographic variation in breast cancer mortality in the United States: a hypothesis involving exposure in solar radiation. Prev. Med. 19:614–622, 1990.

26. Eisman, J.A., Mcintyre, I., Marti, T.J., Frampton, R.J., King, R.J. Normal and malignant breast tissue is a target organ for 1,25-(OH)$_2$ vitamin D$_3$. Clin. Endocrinol. 13: 267–272, 1980.

27. Gorham, ED., Garland, F.C., Garland, C.F. Sunlight and breast cancer incidence in the USSR. Int. J. Epidemiol. 19: 820–824, 1990.

28. National Council on Radiation Protection and Measurements. Ionizing radiation exposures of the population of the United States. Rep. 93, Natl. Counc. Radiation. Prot. Meas., Washington, D.C., 1987.

29. McGregor, D.H., Land, C.E., Choi, K., Tokuoka, S., Liu, P.I., Wakabayashi, I., Beebe, G.W. Breast cancer incidence among atomic bomb survivors, Hiroshima and Nagasaki 1950–1989. J Natl Cancer Inst 59:799–811, 1977.

30. Boice, J.D. Jr., Preston, D., Davis, F.G., Monson, R.R. Frequent chest X-ray fluoroscopy and breast cancer incidence among tuberculosis patients in Massachusetts. Radiation Research. 125: 214–222, 1991.

31. Boice, J.D. Jr., Land, C.E., Preston, D.L. Ionizing radiation. In Cancer Epidemiology and Prevention, ed D.l Scottenfeld, J.F. Fraumedni, Jr. pp. 319–372. New York: Oxford Univ. Press. 2nd ed., 1996.

32. National Academy Press. Health Effects of Exposure to Low Levels of Ionizing Radiation (BIER V). Washington, D.C.: Natl. Acad. Press. 421 pp., 1990.

33. Brenner, D.J., Sawant, S.G., Hande, M.P., Miller, R.C., Elliston, C.D., Fu, Z., Randers-Pehrson, G., Marino, S.A. Routine screening mammography: how important is the radiation-risk side of the benefit-risk equation? Int. J. Radiat. Biol. 78:1065–1067, 2002.

34. Vaughn, T.L., Lee, J.A.H., Strader, C.H. Breast cancer incidence at a nuclear facility: demonstration of a morbidity surveillance system. Health Phys. 64:349–354, 1992.

35. Adams, E.E., Brues, A.M. Breast cancer in female radium dial workers first employed before 1930. J. Occup. Ed. 22:583–587, 1980.

36. Stebbings, J.H. Lucas, H.F., Stehney, A.F. Mortality from cancers of major sites in female radium dial workers. A. J. Ind. Med. 5:435–459, 1984.

37. Braverstock, K.F., Papworth, D., Vennart, J. Risk of radiation at low dose rates. Lancet 1:430–433, 1981.

38. Pukkala, E. Auvinen, A., Wahlberg, G. Incidence of cancer among Finnish airline cabin attendants. 1967–92, Br. Med. J. 311:649–652, 1995.

39. Boice, J.D. Mandel, J.S., Doody, M.M. Breast cancer among radiologic technologists. JAMA 274:394–401, 1995.

40. Doody, M.M., Mandel, J.S., Boice, J.D. Employment practices and breast cancer among radiologic technologists. J. Occup. Environ. Med. 37:321–327, 1995.

41. Berkheiser, S.W. Breast cancer incidence and the TMI accident. Pa. Med. 80:40–42, 1987.

42. Neuberger, J.S., Field, R.W. Radon and breast cancer. Risk Anal. 16:729–730, 1996.

43. U.S. Department of Energy. Energy Information Administration. The changing structure of the Electric Power Industry; An Updata Rep. DOE/EIA-0562(96). U. S. Dept. Energy, Washington, D.C., 1996.

44. Cohen, M., Lippman, M., Chabner, B. Role of pineal gland in etiology and treatment of breast cancer. Lancet 2:814–816, 1978.

45. Stevens, R.G. Electric power use and breast cancer: a hypothesis. Am. J. Epidemiol. 125:556–561, 1987.

46. Tamarkin, L., Baird, C.J., Almeida, O.F. Melatonin: a coordinating signal for mammalian reproduction? Science 227: 714–720, 1985.

47. Wurtman, R.J., Axelrod, J. The pineal gland. Sci. Am. 213: 50–60, 1965.

48. Reiter, R.J. Melatonin suppression by static and extremely low frequency electromagnetic fields: relationship to the re-

ported increased incidence of cancer. Rev. Environ. Health. 10:1711–186, 1994.

49. Baum A., Mevissen, M., Kamino, K., Mohr, U., Loscher, W. A histopathological study on alterations in DMBA-induced mammary carcinogenesis in rats with 50 Hz, 100 muT magnetic field exposure. Carcinogenesis 16:119–125, 1995.

50. Liburdy, R.P., Loscher, W. Laboratory studies on extremely low frequency (50/60-Hz) magnetic fields and carcinogenesis. In: The Melatonin Hypothesis, breast Cancer and Use of Electric Power, ed. R. G Stevens. BW Wilson, Le Anderson, Columbus: Batelle Press. pp. 585–668, 1997.

51. Liburdy, R.P., Sloma, T.R., Sokolic, R., Yaswen, P. ELF magnetic fields, breast cancer, and melatonin: 60 Hz fields block melatonin's oncostatic action on ER + breast cancer cell proliferation. J. Pineal Res. 14:84–97, 1993.

52. Loscher, W., Mevissen, M. Mini-review: animal studies on the role of 50/60-Hertz magnetic fields in carcinogenesis. Life Sci. 54:1531–1543, 1994.

53. Wertheimer, N., Leeper, E. Magnetic Field exposure related to cancer subtypes. Ann. NY Acad. Sci. 502:43–54, 1987.

54. McDowall, M.E. Mortality of persons resident in the vicinity of electricity transmission facilities. Br. J. Cancer 53:271–279, 1986.

55. Schreiber, G.H., Swaen, G.M.H., Meijers, J.M.M., Slangen, J.J.M., Sturmans, F. Cancer mortality and residence near electricity transmission equipment: a retrospective cohort study. Int. J. Epidemiol. 22:9–15, 1993.

56. Li, C-Y, Theriault, G., Link R.S. Residential exposure to 60-Hertz magnetic fields and adult cancers in Taiwan. Epidemiology 8:25–30, 1997.

57. Florig, H.K., Hoburg, J.F. Power-frequency magnetic fields from electric blankets. Health Phys. 58:493–502, 1990.

58. Preston-Martin, S., Peters, J.M., Yu, M.C., Garabrant, D.H., Bowman, J.D. Myelogenous leukemia and electric blanket use. Bioelectromagnetics 9:207–213, 1988.

59. Vena, J.E., Freudenheim, J.L., Marshall, Jr.R., Laughlin, R., Swanson, M., Graham, S. Risk of premenopausal breast cancer and use of electric blankets. Am. J. Epidemiol. 140:974–979, 1994.

60. Vena, J.E., Graham, S., Hellmann, R., Swanson, M., Graham, S. Risk of premenopausal breast cancer and use of electric blankets. Am. J. Epidemiol. 140:974–979, 1994.

61. Davis, D.L., Bradlow, H.L., Wolff, M., Woodruff, T., Hoel, D.G., Anton-Culver, H. Medical hypothesis: xenoestrogens as preventable causes of breast cancer. Environ. Health Perspect. 101:372–377, 1993.

62. Holcomb, M., Safe, S. Inhibition of 7,12-dimethylbenzanthracene-induced rat mammary tumor growth by 2,3,-7,8-tetrachlorodibenzo-p-dioxin. Cancer Lett. 82:43–47, 1994.

63. Wolff, M.S., Toniolo, P.G. Environmental organochlorine exposure as a potential etiologic factor in breast cancer. Environ. Health Perspect. 103 (Suppl 7):141–145, 1995.

64. Dewailly, E., Dodin, S., Verreault, R., Ayotte, P., Sauve, L., Morin, J. High organochlorine body burden in women with estrogen receptor-positive breast cancer. J. Natl. Cancer Inst. 86:232–234, 1994.

65. Moysich, K.B., Ambrosone, C.B., Vena, J.E. Kostyniak, P., Shields, P.G., et al. Serum polychlorinated biphenyls (PCBs) and postmenopausal breast cancer risk. Proc. Am. Assoc. Cancer Res. 38:627a, 1997.

66. Longnecker, M.P., Rogan, W.J., Lucier, G. The human health effects of DTT (dichlorodiphenyl- trichloroethane) and PCBs (polychlorinated biphenyls) and an overview of organochlorines in public health. Annu. Rev. Public Health 18:211–44, 1997.

67. Kutz, F.W, Wood, P.H., Bottimore, D.P. Organochlorine pesticides and polychlorinated biphenyls in human adipose tissue. Rev. Environ. Contam. Toxicol. 120:1–82, 1991.

68. Adami, H-O., Lipworth, L., Titus-Ernstoff, L., Hsieh, C-C., Hanberg, A. et al. Organo-chlorine compounds and estrogen-related cancers in women. Cancer Causes Control 6:551–566, 1995.

69. Ahlborg, U.G., Lipworth, L., Titus-Ernstoff, L., Hsieh, C-C., Hanberg, A., et al. Organo-chlorine compounds in relation to breast cancer, endometrial cancer, and endometriosis: an assessment of the biological and epidemiological evidence. Crit. Rev. Toxicol. 25:463–531, 1995.

70. Wolff, M.S., Collman, G.W., Barrett, J.C., Huff, J. Breast cancer and environmental risk factors: epidemiological and experimental findings. Annu. Rev. Pharmacol. Toxicol. 36:573–596, 1996.

71. Bergthorsson, JT, Ejlertsen, B., Olsen, J.H., Borg, A., Nielsen, K.V., Barkardottir, R,B, Klausen, S., Mouridsen, H.T., Winther, K, Fenger, K., Niebuhr, A., Harboe, T.L., Niebuhr, E. BRCA1 and BRCA2 mutation status and cancer family history of Danish women affected with multifocal or bilateral breast cancer at a young age. J. Med. Genet. 38: 361–368, 2001.

72. Greenblatt, M.S., Chappuis, P.O., Bond, J.P., Hamel, N., Foulkes, W.D. TP53 Mutations in Breast Cancer Associated with BRCA1 or BRCA2 Germ-line Mutations: Distinctive Spectrum and Structural Distribution. Cancer Res., 61:4092–4097, 2001.

73. Lehman, T.A., Haffty, B.G., Carbone, C.J., Bishop, L.R., Gumbs, A.A., Krishnan, S., Shields P.G., Modali, R., Turner, B.C. Elevated frequency and functional activity of a specific germ-line p53 intron mutation in familial breast cancer. Cancer Res., 60: 1062–1069, 2000.

74. Kelsey, J.L, Horn-Ross, P.L. Breast Cancer: Magnitude of the problem and descriptive epidemiology. Epidemiologic Reviews 15:7–16,1993.

75. MacMahon, B., Cole, P., Lin, T.M. et al. Age at first birth and breast cancer risk. Bull. Nat'l. Hlth. Org. 43:209–217,1970

76. Vessey, M.D., McPherson, K., Roberts, M.M., Neil, A. and Jones, L. Fertility and the risk of breast cancer. Br. J. Cancer 52:625–628, 1985.

77. Trapido, E.J. Age at first birth, parity and breast cancer risk Cancer 51:946–948, 1983.

78. De Waard, F. and Trichopoulos, D. A unifying concept of the etiology of breast cancer. Int. J. Cancer 41:666–669,1988.

79. Lambe, M., Hsieh, H.-W., Chan, A., Ekbom, D. Trichopoulos and H. O. Adami Parity, age at first and last birth, and risk of breast cancer: A population-based study in Sweden. Breast Cancer Res. Treat. 38: 305–311, 1996.

80. Meiser, B., Butow, P., Barratt, A., Friedlander, M., Gattas, M., Kirk, J., Suthers, G., Walpole, I., Tucker, K. Attitudes toward prophylactic oophorectomy and screening utilization in women at increased risk of developing hereditary breast/ovarian cancer. Gynecol. Oncol., 75:122–129, 1999.

81. Feychting, M., Osterlund, B., Ahlbom, A. Reduced cancer incidence among the blind. Epidemiology, 9: 490–494, 1998.

82. Wurtman, R.J. Fall of nocturnal melatonin during puberty and prepubescence. Lancet, 362:85, 1984.

83. Dauchy, R.T., Blask, D.E., Sauer, L.A., Brainard, G.C., Krause, J.A. Dim light during darkness stimulates tumor progression by enhancing tumor fatty acid uptake and metabolism. Cancer Letters, 144: 131–136, 1999.

84. Tamarkin, L., Cohen, M., Roselle, D., Reichert, C., Lippman, M, Chabner, B. Melatonin inhibition and pinealectomy enhancement of 7,12-dimethylbenz(a)anthracene-induced mammary tumors in the rat. Cancer Res. 44: 4432–4436, 1981.

85. Pillittere, D., Miller, M. Researchers search for link between circadian rhythms, breast cancer. J. Natl. Cancer Inst., 92:686–689, 2000.

86. Bernstein, L., Hanisch, R., Sullivan-Halley,J., Ross, R.K. Treatment with human chorionic gonadotropin and risk of breast cancer. Cancer Epidemiol. Biomarkers & Prevention, 4: 437–440, 1995.

87. Hernandez-Gonzalez, M., Juarez, J. Alcohol before puberty produces an advance in the onset of sexual behavior in male rats. Alcohol 21(2):133–140, 2000.

88. Harris, C. Tobacco smoking and cancer risk in women. J. Women's Cancer, 3:1–4, 2001.

89. Russo, J., Barnabas, N., Higgy, N., Salicioni, A.M., Wu, Y.L. and Russo, I.H. Molecular Basis of Human Breast Cell Transformation. In: Advances in Breast Cancer Research, (Calvo, F., Crepin, M. and Magdelenat, H., Eds.). Eurotext,, Paris, 1996, pp 33–43.

90. Stevens, R.G., Davis, S., Mirick, D.K., Kheifets, L., Kaune, W. Alcohol consumption and urinary concentration of 6-sulfatoxymelatonin in healthy women. Epidemiology 11(6):660–665, 2000.

91. Falcon, J. Cellular circadian clocks in the pineal. [Review] Progress in Neurobiology. 58:121–162, 1999.

The Breast as a Developing Organ

2.1 Introduction

The breast is a bilateral organ that in the female undergoes dramatic changes in size, shape, and function in association with infantile growth, puberty, pregnancy, lactation, and post-menopausal regression [1–4]. The fact that the breast is the source of the most frequently diagnosed malignancy in the female population [5, 6] requires to fully understand how the various phases of development are influenced by endocrinological and reproductive events, because they will ultimately determine the risk of developing breast cancer [3, 4, 7].

The development of the human breast is a lifelong process initiated during embryonic life. While the main growth spurt occurs with lobule formation at puberty, the development and differentiation of the breast are completed only by the end of the first full-term pregnancy [3]. It has long been known that the risk of breast cancer shows an inverse relationship with early parity [3, 4, 7–12]. Case control studies have demonstrated that breast cancer risk increases with the age at which a woman bears her first child. The important factor in this protection seems to be related to the interval of time between menarche and the first pregnancy, since increased risk has been reported when this interval is lengthened over 14 years [12]. In order to be protective, however, pregnancy has to occur before age 30. In fact, evidence indicates that women who first become pregnant after that age appear to have a risk above that of nulliparous women [12]. Although multiparity appears to confer additional protection, the protective effect remains largely limited to the first birth. The protection conveyed by an early reproductive event persists at all subsequent ages, even in women older than 75 years of age [7, 12]. Although the ultimate mechanisms through which an early first full-term pregnancy protects the breast from cancer development are not known, a likely explanation has been provided by studies performed in experimental animal models: that completion of full-term pregnancy prior to the administration of a chemical carcinogen inhibits rat mammary cancer initiation through the induction of differentiation. The fact that mammary gland differentiation activates specific genes such as inhibin [13], mammary derived growth factor inhibitor [14], a serpin-like gene [15] and others whose function remains to be determined [15, 16], led us to postulate that these genomic changes prime the breast epithelium to subsequent hormonal milieu, and that this is also responsible for the protection that an early full-term pregnancy confers to women. Currently there is no explanation for the higher risk to develop malignancies exhibited by nulliparous and late parous women. The fact that experimentally induced rat mammary carcinomas develop only when the carcinogen interacts with the undifferentiated and highly proliferating mammary epithelium of young nulliparous rats [3, 4, 17–21], suggests that the breast of late parous and of nulliparous women might exhibit some of the undifferentiated and/or cell proliferative characteristics that predispose the tissue to undergo neoplastic transformation [3, 19–22]

2.2 Prenatal and Perinatal Development

The mammary gland parenchyma arises from a single epithelial ectodermal bud. Most authors agree on the successive stages of development of the mammary gland during the embryonic and fetal stages. However, there are variations in nomenclature, and in the exact time of appearance of each structure, depending upon whether the authors choose to express the age of the embryo based on the estimated time of conception, the last missed menstrual period, or the length of the embryo. Because of difficulties in precisely establishing the day of conception, we consider that embryonic or fetal length is more accurate for assessing the intrauterine phases of mammary gland development. These phases have been divided into the following stages: Ridge, milk hill, mammary disc, G lobule type, cone, budding, indentation, branching, canalization, and end-vesicle stages (Fig. 2.1, Table 2.1). It is important to emphasize that the last stage or end vesicle stage (Fig. 2.1), which characterized by the production of colostrums, does not represent a fully differentiated stage, because it lacks of fully de-veloped lobules, which only become apparent in the postnatal life at the end of pregnancy.

In the newborn the breast consists of very primitive structures (Fig. 2.2 a–e), composed of ducts ending in short ductules lined by one to two layers of epithelial and one of myoepithelial cells (Fig. 2.2 d, e). Epithelial cells have a finely vacuolated eosinophilic cytoplasm, with typical apocrine secretion. The fine vacuolization is caused by the presence of lipid droplets (Fig. 2.2 e), as confirmed by electron microscopy. However, secretory activity does not seem to be confined to the primitive alveolar structures, since the entire ductal system appears dilated, secretion filled, and lined by a secretory-type epithelium (Fig. 2.2 f–h). These observations suggest that secretory activity is a generalized response of all the mammary epithelium to maternal hormonal levels. The secretory activity of the newborn gland subsides after 3 to 4 weeks of birth [3, 23].

Table 2.1. Stages of prenatal development of the human breast. CR crown rump

Stage	Mammary gland developmental stage	Developmental period/ gestational age		CR length
1	Ridge stage	Embryonic period	Week 4 (day 27–28)	4–5 mm
2	Milk hill stage		Week 4–5 (day 28–30)	6–7 mm
3	Mammary disc stage		Week 5 (day 29–35)	5–12 mm
4	Globule stage		Week 6 (day 36–42)	14–22 mm
5	Cone stage		Week 7 (day 43–49)	28–30 mm
6	Budding stage		Week 8 (day 50–56)	31–42 mm
7	Indentation stage	Fetal period	Week 10–13 (day 64–91)	60–98 mm
8	Branching stage		Week 14 (day 92–98)	105–120 mm
9	Canalization stage		Week 20–32 (day 134–224)	185–300 mm
10	End-vesicle stage – ductal end vesicles lined by a monolayered epithelium contain colostrum	Newborn	Week 40 (day 274–280)	>360 mm

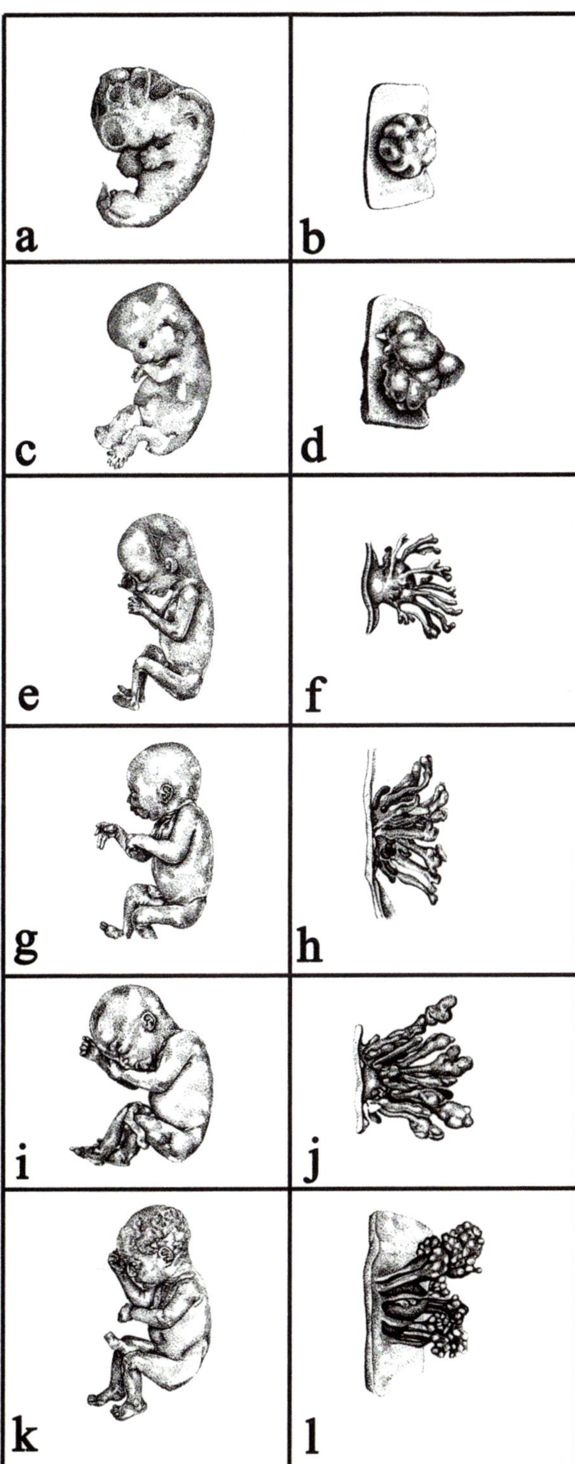

Figure 2.1 a–l

Stages of breast prenatal development. **a** Week 5 embryo (12 mm crown-rump [CR]). **b** Mammary disc stage. **c** Week 6 embryo (22 mm CR). **d** Globule stage. **e** Week 8 embryo (42 mm CR). **f** Budding stage. **g** Week 14 fetus (120 mm CR). **h** Branching stage. **i** Week 30 fetus (200 mm CR). **j** Canalization stage. **k** Week 34 fetus (380 mm CR). **l** End vesicle stage. (Original drawings by Patricia A. Russo, B.A.)

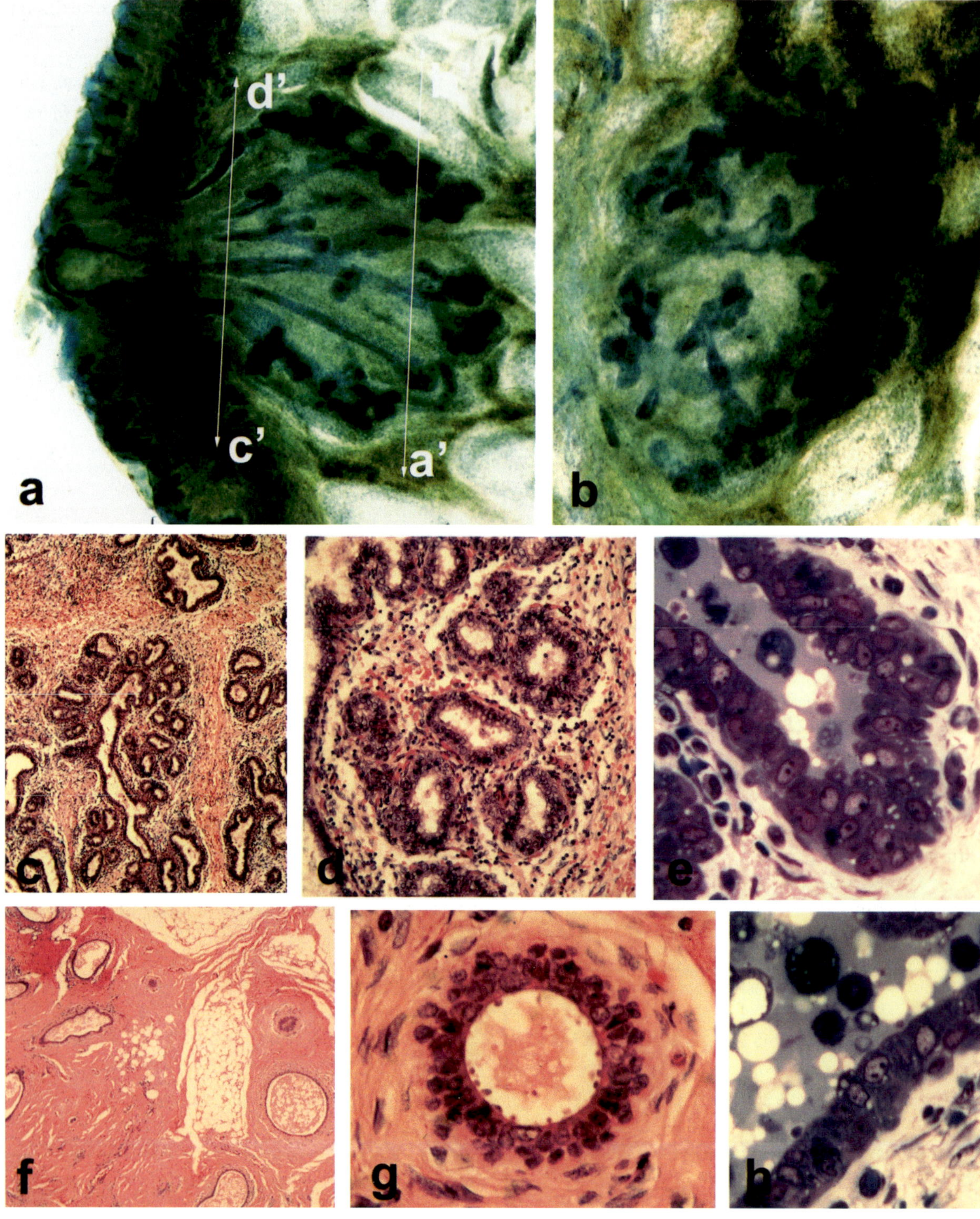

◀ **Figure 2.2 a–h**

a Mammary gland of a 2-week-old girl is composed of ductal structures that from the galactophorous sinus under the nipple branch and end in primitive alveolar bud (AB). **b** Cross-section taken at the *a'–b'* level shown in **a** (**a** and **b**, whole mount stained with toluidine blue, ×2.5). **c** Cross section taken from **a** at the *a'–b'* level. The lumen of all ducts and AB is dilated and filled with proteinaceous fluid (hematoxylin and eosin [H&E], ×4.0). **d** The ducts are lined by two layers of epithelial cells. Proliferation takes place chiefly in the basal cells. The inner or luminal cells have secretory properties from which the 'witches milk' is formed (H&E, ×10. **e** Terminal duct in the breast of a 2-week-old girl. The lumen contains proteinaceous and lipidic secretion. (One-micron section of plastic embedded tissue; toluidine blue, ×40). **f** Cross section of major lactiferous ducts taken at level *c'–d'* of **a** (H&E, ×2.5). **g** The cross section of a duct reveals a luminal layer of epithelial cells projecting snouts into the protein-containing lumen (H&E, ×40). **h** A thin section of plastic embedded breast tissue shows a pseudostratified epithelium lining the secretion filled lumen (toluidine blue, ×40)

2.3 Postnatal Development

Mammary gland development during childhood does little more than keep pace with the general growth of the body until the approach of puberty. Although the main changes occurring in the mammary gland are initiated at puberty, ulterior development of the gland varies greatly from woman to woman. Mammary gland development can be assessed from the external appearance of the breast [1] or by evaluation of mammary gland area, volume, degree of branching, or degree of structures whose appearance indicates the level of differentiation of the gland, such as the formation of lobules in various stages of development [2, 3, 21].

The adolescent period begins with the first signs of sexual change at puberty and terminates with sexual maturity [1, 2]. Puberty in the female sets in between the ages of 10 and 12 years. With the approach of puberty, the rudimentary *mammae* begin to show growth activity both in the glandular tissue and in the surrounding stroma. Glandular increase is due to the growth and division of small bundles of primary and secondary ducts (Fig. 2.3). They grow and divide partly dichotomously (from the Greek word *dichotomos*, or repeated bifurcation) and partly sympodially (from Greek *syn* + *podion* base, involving the formation of an apparent main axis from successive secondary axes), on a dichotomous basis. The ducts grow and divide, ending in club-shaped bulbous structures, the terminal end buds (TEBs). Each TEB cleaves into two smaller structures or alveolar buds (AB) (Fig. 2.3 c). We have coined the term AB for identifying that transitional structure that morphologically appears more developed than the TEB and will either progress to form new branches or will further sprout into ductules, which are smaller terminal structures that cluster around a terminal duct. The structural unit composed by the terminal duct and the 4 to 11 ductules that sprouted from it represent the first identifiable lobule, the lobule type 1 (Lob 1), or terminal ductal lobular unit (TDLU), or virginal lobule (Fig. 2.4). Lobule formation in the female breast, which is the hallmark of differentiation, usually starts 1 to 2 years after the first menstrual period. Ovarian hormones play a significant role in breast development. However, the effect of estrogen and progesterone fluctuations during the menstrual cycle on parenchymal cell proliferation has not been definitively elucidated. The normal breast epithelium undergoes cyclic variations in DNA synthesis, as determined in normal breast samples cultured in the presence of ^{3}H-thymidine. Even though cell proliferation and cell death seem balanced to maintain the equilibrium of the resting breast, mammary development induced by ovarian hormones during a menstrual cycle never fully returns to the starting point of the preceding cycle. Accordingly, each ovulatory cycle fosters slightly more mammary development with new budding of structures that continues until about age 35 [3].

The breast tissue of normally cycling non-pregnant adult women contains three identifiable types of lobules, the already described Lob 1 and the more developed lobules type 2 (Lob 2) (Fig. 2.5) and type 3 (Lob 3) (Fig. 2.6). The gradual sprouting of new ductules determines the transition from Lob 1 to Lob 2 when their number reaches an average of 47 per lob-

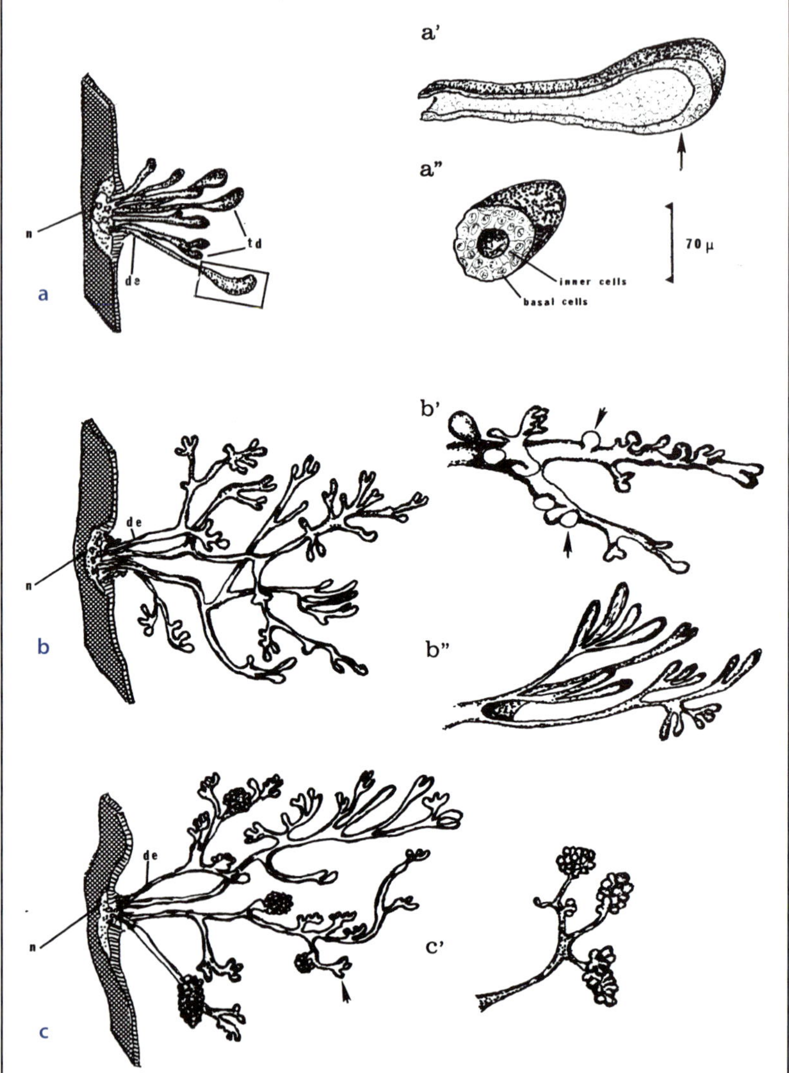

Figure 2.4 a–d ▶

a Breast tissue of an 18-year-old nulliparous woman composed of lobules type 1 (Lob 1). (Whole mount, toluidine blue, ×2.5). **b**, **c**, **d** Histological sections of the Lob 1 shown in **a** stained with H&E. Photographs taken at ×2.5, ×10 and ×40, respectively

Figure 2.3 a–c

a Mammary gland at birth formed by several excretory ducts (*de*) ending in terminal ducts (*td*). **a'** detail of the inset showing the club-shaped terminal end buds from which lengthening and further divisions of the virginal duct originate; **a"** cross section at the level shown in a'; the duct is lined by the two layers of cells. Proliferation takes place chiefly in the basal cells, whereas the inner (luminal) cells have secretory properties from which the 'witches milk' is formed (*n* nipple). **b** Before the onset of puberty, the ducts grow and divide in a dichotomous or sympodial manner. **b'** Ball-shaped lateral buds sprout from the duct; **b"** new branches and twigs develop from the terminal and lateral buds. **c** Mammary gland at puberty; lobule formation occurs after menarche. The number of lobules progressively increases with age. Some portions of the gland remain as undifferentiated terminal ducts or alveolar buds and do not undergo further development if pregnancy does not supervene (*arrow*); **c'** virginal lobule or lobule type 1 (Lob 1). (Reprinted with permission from: Russo J. et al. Breast Cancer Res. Treat. 2:2, 1982)

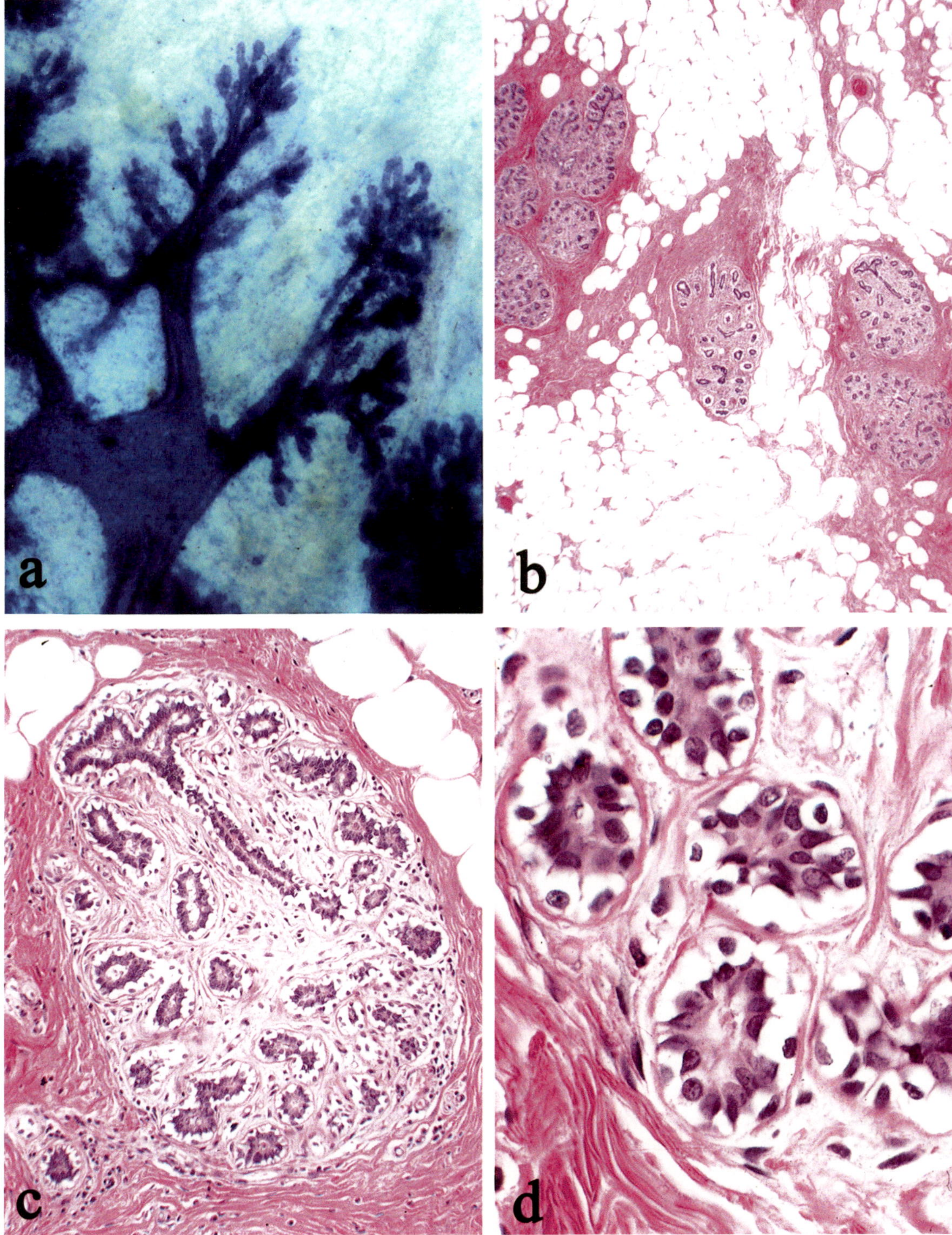

Table 2.2. Characteristics of the lobular structures of the human breast. *Lob 1* lobule type 1, *Lob 2* lobule type 2, *Lob 3* lobule type 3

Structure	Lobular area* (μm^2)	Number of ductules/lobules**	Number of cells/cross section***
Lob 1	48±44	11.2±6.3	32.4±14.1
Lob 2	60±26	47.0±11.7	13.1±4.8
Lob 3	129±49	81.0±16.6	11.0±2.0

   * Student's *t*-tests were done for all possible comparisons. Lobular areas showed significant differences between Lob 1 vs. Lob 3 and Lob 2 vs. Lob 3 ($p < 0.005$)

  ** The number of ductules per lobule was different ($p < 0.01$) in all the comparisons

 *** The number of cells per cross section was significantly different in ductules of Lob 1 vs. Lob 2 and Lob 3 ($p < 0.01$)

ule, and to Lob 3 when a minimum of 80 ductules are identified around the terminal duct (Table 2.2). Although with progressive branching individual ductules become smaller, the increase in their number results in a concomitant increase in overall size of the more developed lobules (Figs. 2.4–2.6). In Lob 1 each ductule is composed of approximately 32 epithelial cells per cross section and measures an average of $0.232 \times 10^{-2} mm^2$, practically twice the size of the ductules composing the Lob 2. Although individual ductules are further reduced in size in Lob 3, this reduction is less dramatic, although still significant (Table 2.2).

The lobular composition of the breast of sexually mature women is determined by numerous endogenous and exogenous factors. Principal among them are age, and hence, number and regularity of menstrual cycles, endocrine imbalances, use of exogenous hormones, environmental exposures that could act as endocrine disruptors, and pregnancy. In nulliparous women the breast contains a moderate number of undifferentiated structures such as terminal ducts and Lob 1 (Fig. 2.7), although occasional Lob 2 and Lob 3 are also present. The percentage of Lob 1 remains almost constant throughout the lifespan of nulliparous women. The facts that Lob 2 are present in moderate numbers during the early reproductive years, and sharply decrease after age 23, while the number of Lob 1 remains significantly higher (Fig. 2.7), and Lob 3 are almost totally absent, suggest that a certain percentage of Lob 1 might have progressed to Lob 2, but very few or no Lob 2 have pro-

Figure 2.5 a–d ▶

a Breast tissue of a 24-year-old nulliparous woman composed of lobules type 2 (Lob 2). (Whole mount preparation, toluidine blue, ×2.5). **b, c, d** Histological sections of the Lob 2 shown in **a** stained with H&E, and photographed at ×2.5, ×10, and ×40, respectively

gressed to Lob 3. In parous women, on the other hand, a history of one or more full-term pregnancies between the ages of 14 to 20 years correlates with a significant increase in the number of Lob 3. This type of lobules remains present as the predominant structure until a woman reaches the age of 40 (Fig. 2.8). Their percentage decreases after the fourth decade of life, the time at which a decrease in the number of Lob 3 occurs, probably due to their involution to predominantly Lob 1 (Fig. 2.8) [3].

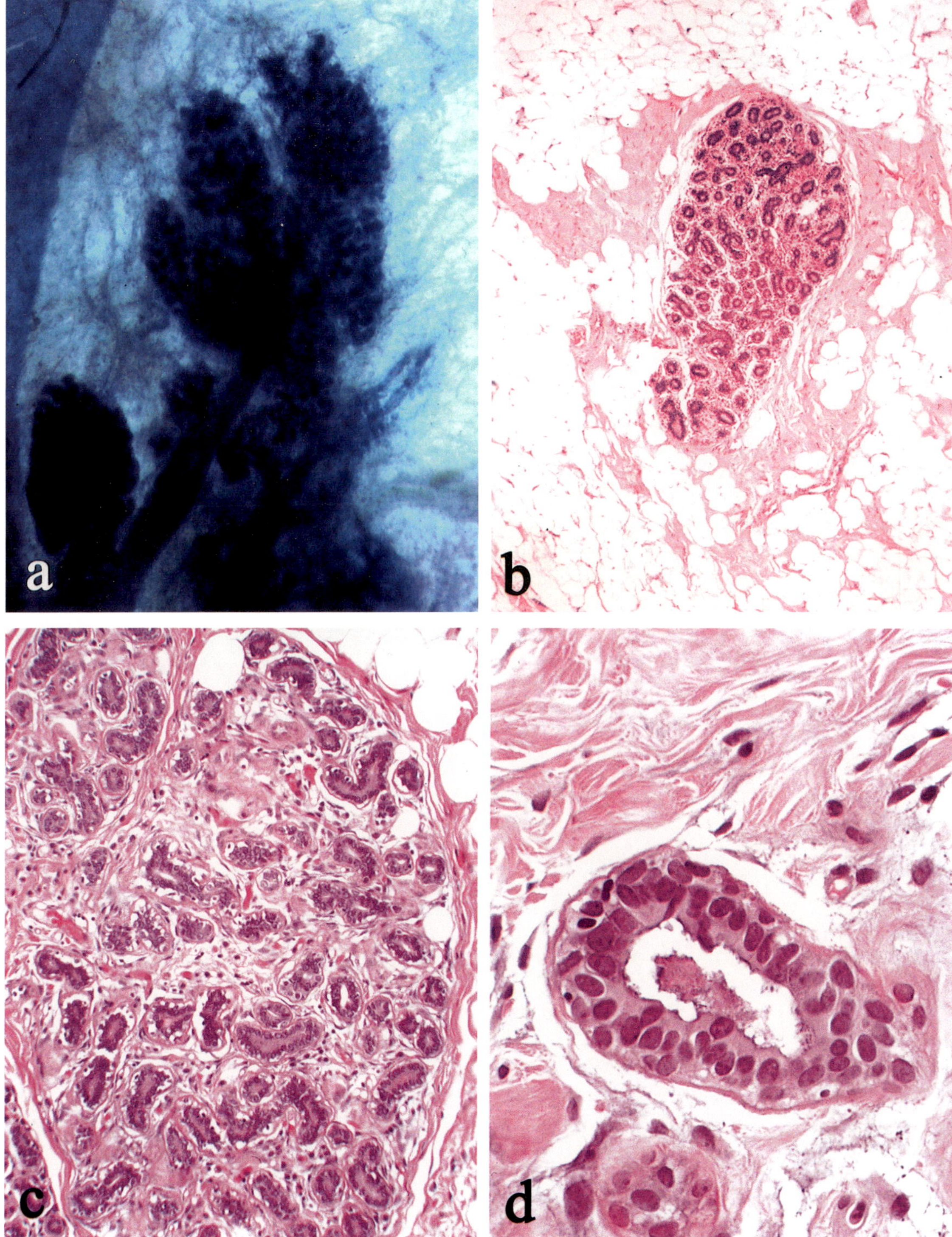
a
b
c
d

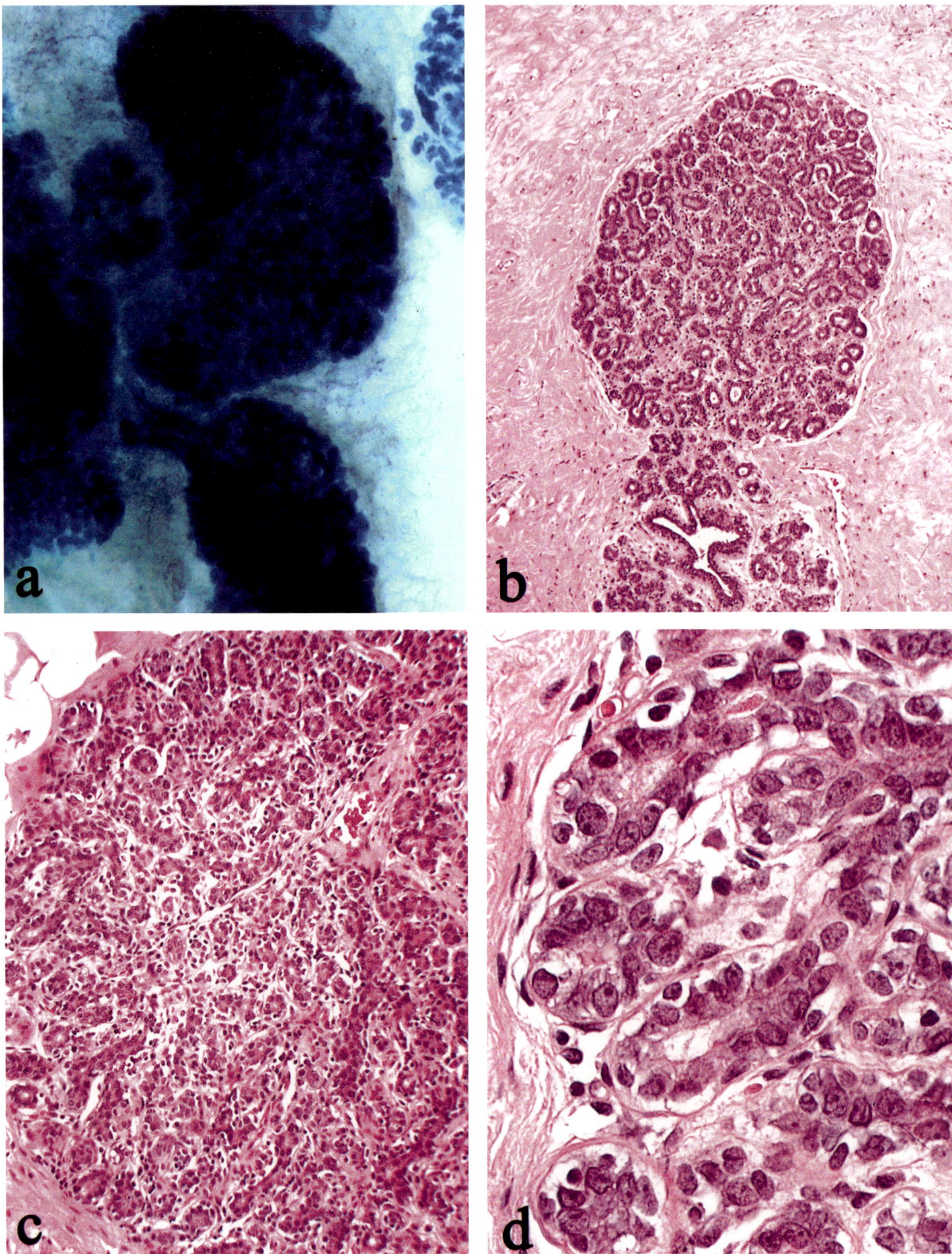

Figure 2.7

Percentage of terminal ductal structures (*TS*), lobules type 1 (Lob 1), 2 (Lob 2) and 3 (Lob 3) in the breasts of nulliparous women between the ages of 14–58 years. Values represent the mean ± SE of 3 samples (14–18); 4 samples (19–23); 1 sample (24–28); 2 samples (34, 38), and 1 sample (54–58). No samples were available for the groups 29–33, 39–43, 44–48, and 49–53. The curves were therefore traced connecting the points available. (Reprinted with permission from: Russo J. et al, Breast Cancer Res. Treat. 23:211–218, 1992)

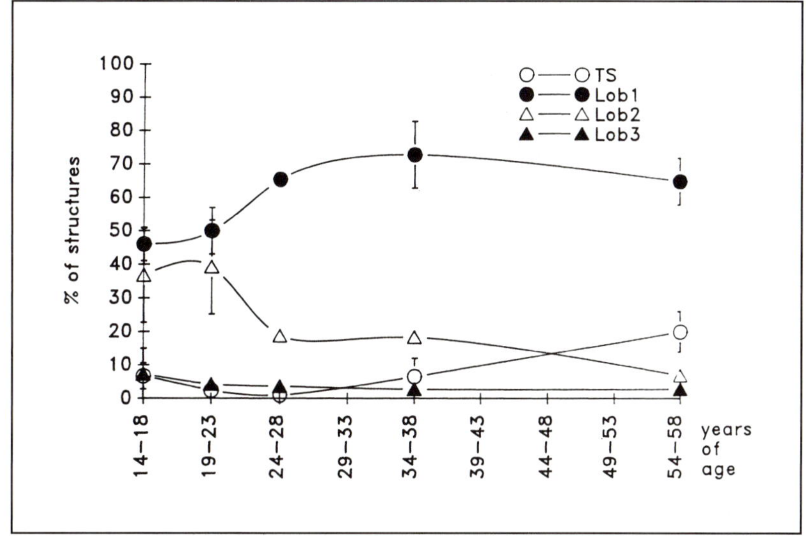

Figure 2.8

Percentage of TS. Lobules type I (Lob 1), 2 (Lob 2) and 3 (Lob 3) in the breasts of parous women between the ages of 14–58 years. Values represent the mean ± SE of 1 sample (14–18); 5 samples (19–23); 6 samples (24–28); 6 samples (29–33); 5 samples (34–38); 7 samples (44–48); 2 samples 49–53); and 3 samples (54–58). (Reprinted with permission from: Russo J. et al, Breast Cancer Res. Treat. 23:211–218, 1992)

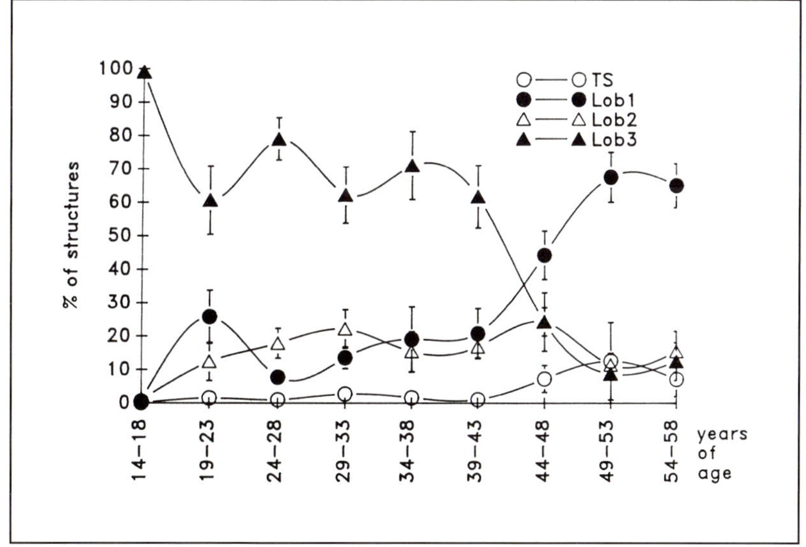

◀ **Figure 2.6 a–d**

a Breast tissue of a 35-year-old parous woman composed of lobules type 3 (Lob 3). (Whole mount preparation, toluidine blue, × 2.5). b, c, d Histological sections of the Lob 3, shown in a stained with H&E and photographed at × 2.5, × 10, and × 40, respectively

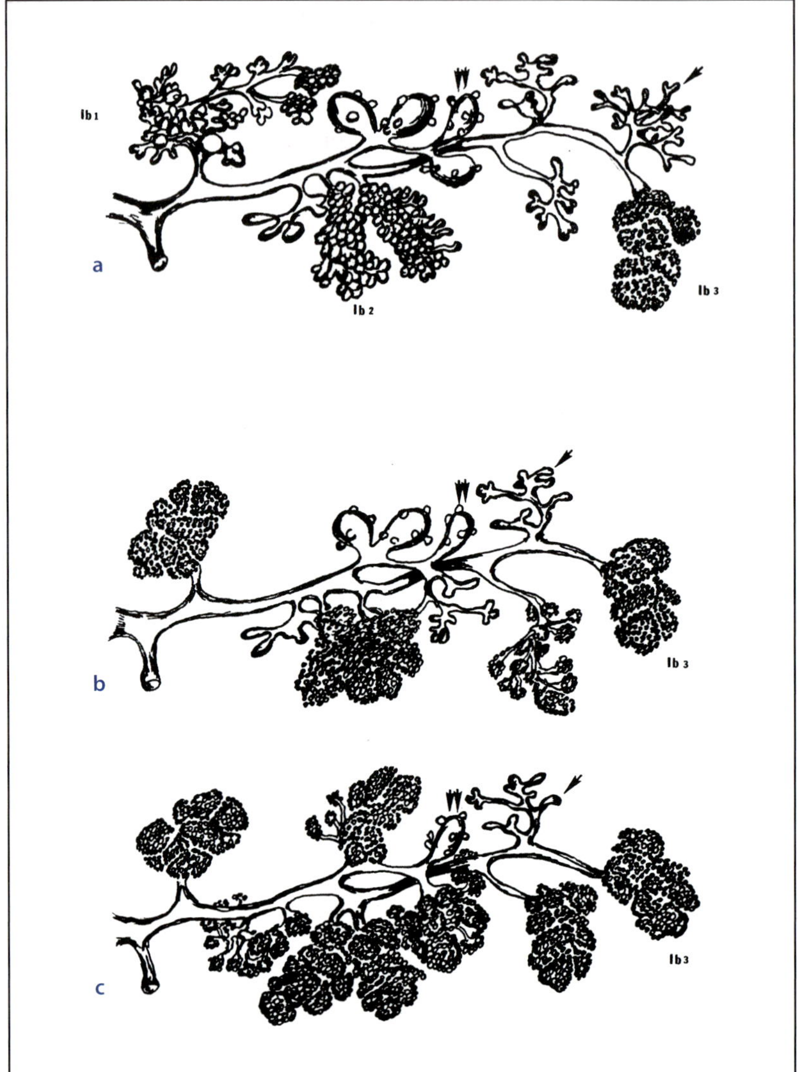

Figure 2.9 a–c

a Diagram of the architecture of the human mammary parenchyma during the first month of pregnancy, **b** at the third month of pregnancy, and **c** at the middle of pregnancy. Terminal end buds, *double arrows*; alveolar buds, *single arrow*; *lb1* lobule type 1; *lb2* lobule type 2; *lb3* lobule type 3. (Reprinted with permission from: Russo J. et al. Breast Cancer Res. Treat. 2:2, 1982)

2.4 Pregnancy

The breast attains its maximum development during pregnancy; it occurs in two distinctly dominant phases (Fig. 2.9): an early stage, characterized by ductal lengthening and profuse branching, sustained by active cell proliferation at the distal end of the ductal tree; the rapid increase in number of newly formed ductules results in the progression of Lob 2 to Lob 3 (Fig. 2.6). The intensity of budding and degree of lobule formation goes beyond what has been observed in the virginal breast. By the third month of pregnancy the number of well-formed lobules exceeds the number of primitive budding stages; however, TEBs are still found (Fig. 2.9 c). The beginning of secretory activity is indicative of the progression from ductules to secretory acini, which are characteristics of the fully differentiated Lob 4 (Fig. 2.10). In newly formed lobules, the epithelial cells composing each acinus in-

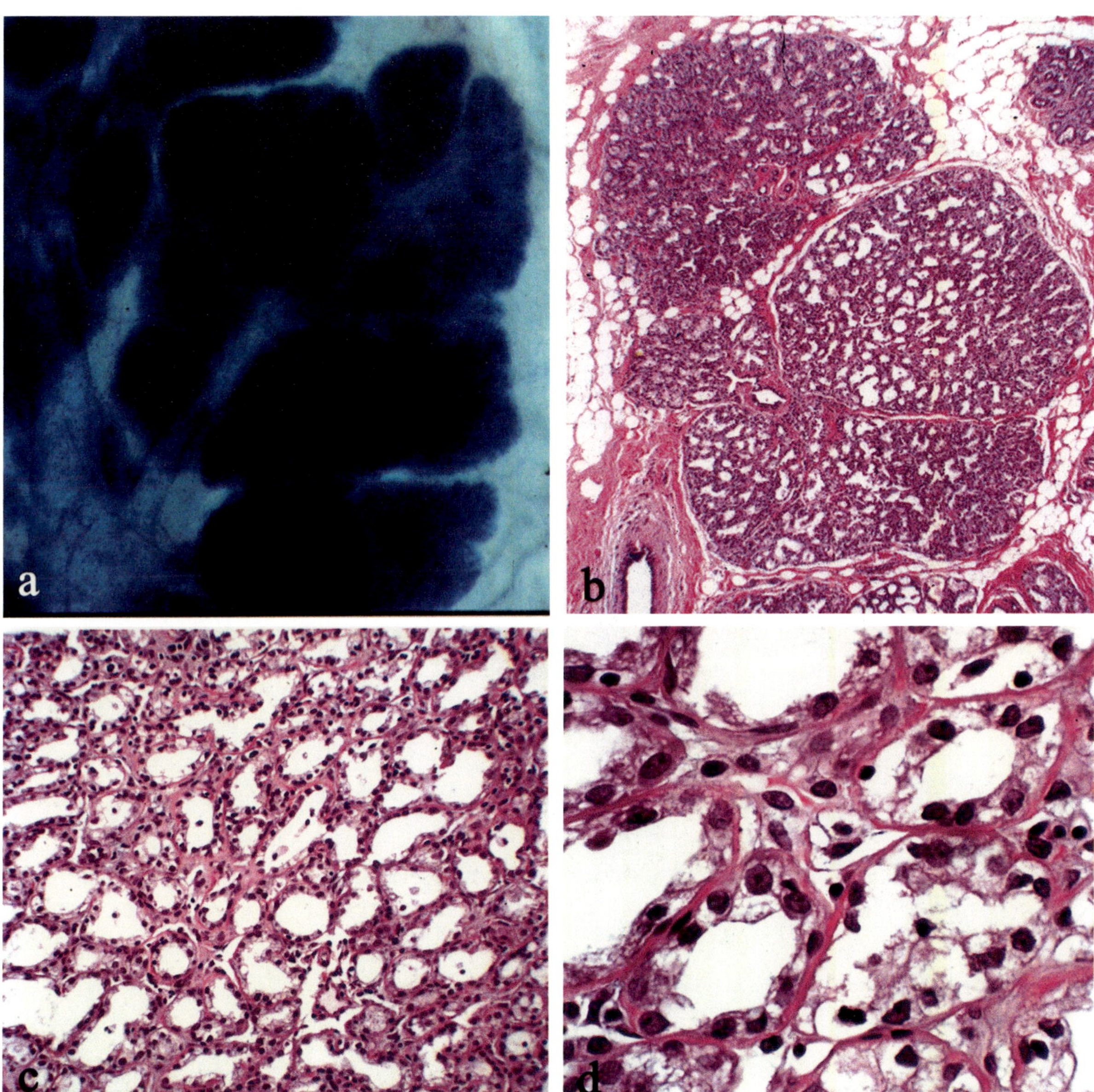

Figure 2.10 a–d

a Lactating breast of a 25-year-old woman showing lobules type 4 (Lob 4). (Whole mount preparation, toluidine blue, ×2.5). **b**, **c**, **d** Histological sections of the Lob 4 shown in **a** stained with H&E and photographed at ×2.5, ×10, and ×40, respectively

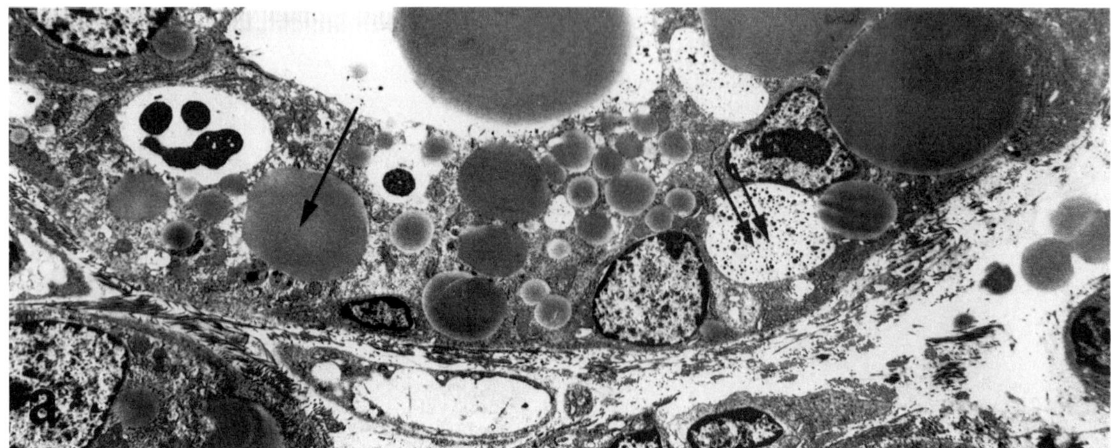

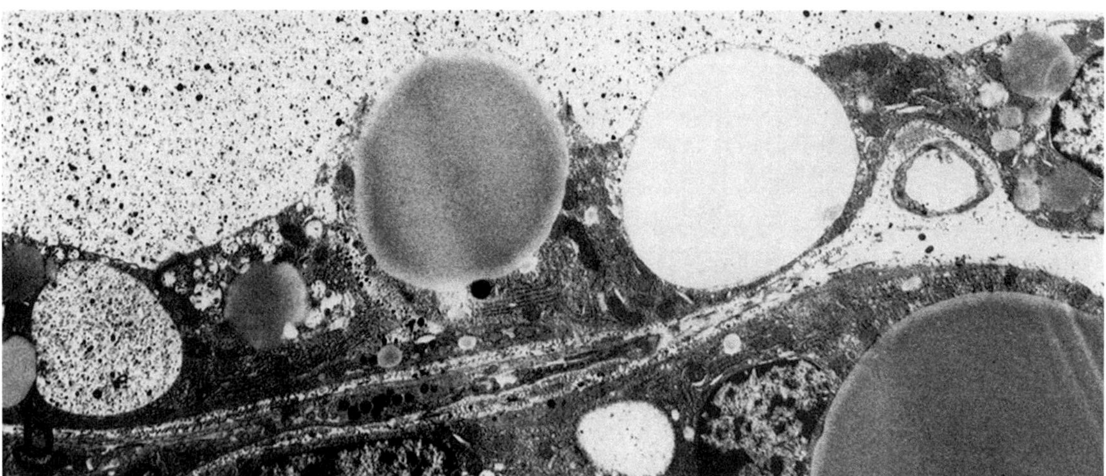

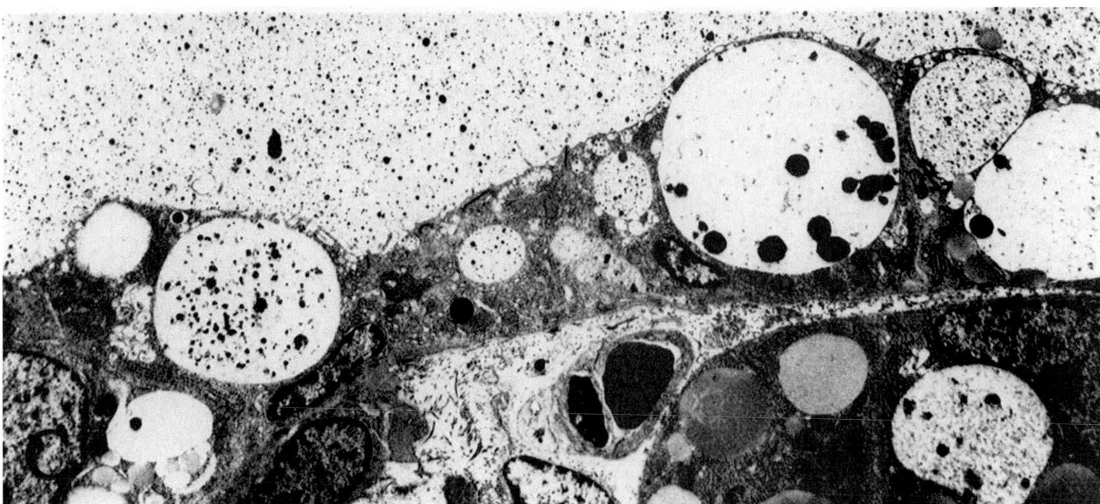

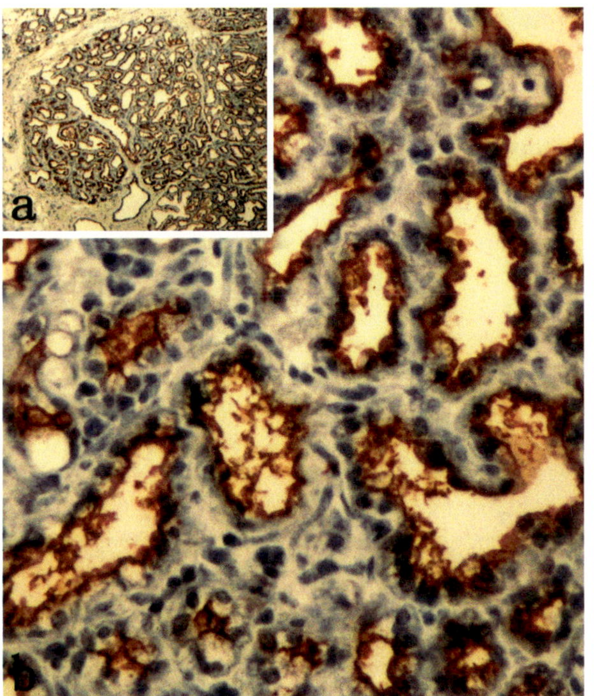

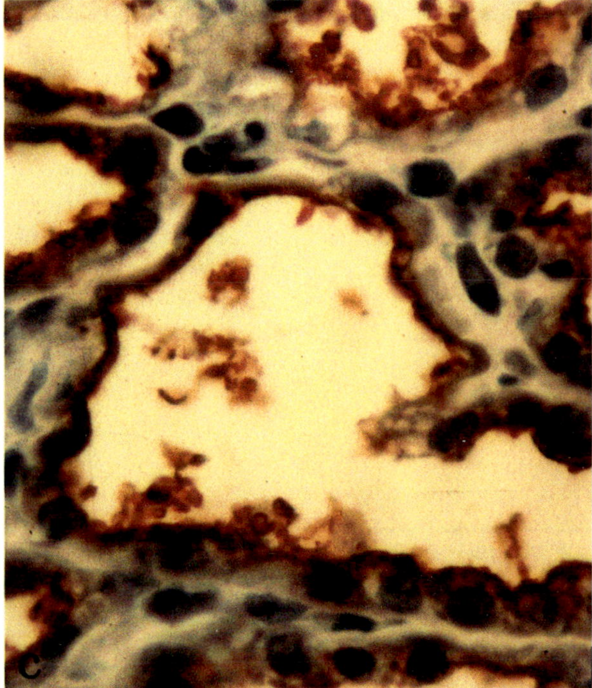

Figure 2.12 a–c ▲

a Immunohistochemical reaction with milk fat globule membrane antigen antibody in Lobule type 4 (Lob 4) (× 2.5). b Lumen of Lob 4 alveolar structures decorated with a positive reaction against milk fat globule membrane protein (× 10). c Milk fat globule membrane is a mucoprotein that covers the apical border of the luminal epithelial cells (× 40) (a–c, 3′, 5′ diaminobenzidine [DAB] counterstained with hematoxylin)

◄ **Figure 2.11 a–c**

Electron micrographs of the normal lactating breast epithelium. a A single layer of epithelial cells containing lipid droplets in the cytoplasm (*one arrow*) and small granular material with dense core structures (*two arrows*) (× 2,500). b Lipid droplets being released into the lumen (× 3,500). c Dense core of proteinaceous material being released into the lumen (× 4,000). (a–c stained with uranyl acetate and lead nitrate)

crease in number due to active cell division and in addition their size becomes larger mainly due to cytoplasmic enlargement [3]. By mid-pregnancy, the acini composing each lobule are further enlarged and more numerous. They surround the duct from which their central branch proceeds so thickly that the chief duct, the terminal or intra lobular terminal duct, cannot longer be recognized. The transition between the terminal ducts and the budding acini is gradual, making the histological distinction between the two of them difficult, since both show evidence of early secretory activity. The definitive structure of the ductal tree is essentially settled by the end of the first half of pregnancy; the mammary changes that characterize the second half of pregnancy are chiefly continuation and accentuation of secretory activity. Further progressive branching continues with less prominent bud formation. At this time, the formation of true secreting units or acini, the differentiated structures, becomes increasingly evident. Proliferation of new acini is reduced to a minimum, and the lumina of those already formed become distended by accumulation of secretory material or colostrum (Figs. 2.10–2.12). The epithelium is vacuolated due to the accumulation of lipids (Fig. 2.10d). Under the electron microscope the mammary epithelium shows numerous lipid droplets and proteinaceous material (Fig. 2.11). In Lob 4 reactivity against milk fat globule protein is highly expressed (Fig. 2.12). The secretory acinus formed during pregnancy is a terminal outgrowth that marks the end of glandular differentiation. However, just before and during parturition, there is a new wave of mitotic activity with an increase in the total DNA of the gland. During lactation, the process of growth and differentiation may be observed in the same lobule type, side by side with the process of milk secretion [3, 4, 13, 23].

2.5 Postlactational Changes

From mid-pregnancy onwards, a yellowish fluid containing a high concentration of protein is secreted into the mammary alveoli and may be expelled from the nipple. Lactation starts after postpartum withdrawal of placental lactogen and sex steroids, which appear to prevent the action of prolactin on the mammary epithelium. Colostrum is secreted during the first week postpartum, followed by a 2- to 3-week period of transitional milk secretion, leading to the secretion of mature milk [3, 21].

No major morphological changes of the mammary gland are observed during lactation. The mammary lobules are enlarged and the acini have a dilated lumen filled with granular, slightly basophilic material admixed with fat. There is a significant variation in lobule size throughout the gland, suggestive of a variation in lactogenic activity from lobule to lobule. Milk is continuously synthesized and released into the mammary acini and ductal system as long as it is removed regularly from the mammary gland [3, 21]. It can be stored in the ductal system for up to 48 h, but thereafter the rates of synthesis and secretion begin to decrease. The accumulation of milk in the ducto-acinar lumina and within the cytoplasm of the lactogenic epithelial cells that occurs after weaning has an inhibitory effect on further milk synthesis. This effect is followed by a series of involutional changes in the

mammary gland consisting of a multifocal asynchronous process of reduction in volume of the secretory epithelial cells and further inhibition of their secretory activity.

It is considered that post-lactational regression is due to two complementary mechanisms, cell autolysis, with collapse of acinar structures and narrowing of the tubules, and appearance of round cell infiltration and phagocytes in and about the disintegrating lobules, and finally, regeneration of the periductal and perilobular connective tissue with renewed budding and proliferation in the terminal tubules. Until menopausal involution sets in, the parous organ contains more glandular tissue than if pregnancy or pregnancy and lactation had never occurred [3, 21].

2.6 The Menopausal Breast

Menopause supervenes when more than 99% of the 400,000 follicles that were present in the ovaries when the fetus had a gestational age of 5 months become exhausted through ovulation or atresia. The lack of endometrial stimulation caused by the reduced or absent levels of ovarian estrogen and progesterone leads to the cessation of menses, or amenorrhea, the most characteristic sign of menopause. Gonadotropin-releasing hormone secretion is implicated in this phenomenon, indicating that the hypothalamus is also involved in the development of menopause. The years leading up to the final menstrual period, until menopause sets in, generally at around the age of 51 years, constitute the perimenopause. During this period many women ovulate irregularly, either because the rise in estrogen during the follicular phase is insufficient for triggering a surge of pituitary luteinizing hormone (LH), or because the existing follicles are resistant to the ovulatory stimulus. The increase in human longevity occurring in our society has caused a considerable increment in the number of women that will live one third or more of their lives in the menopausal period, namely without natural estrogen and progesterone. After menopause, the breast undergoes a regressive phenomenon both in nulliparous and parous women. This regression is manifested in the breast as an increase in the number

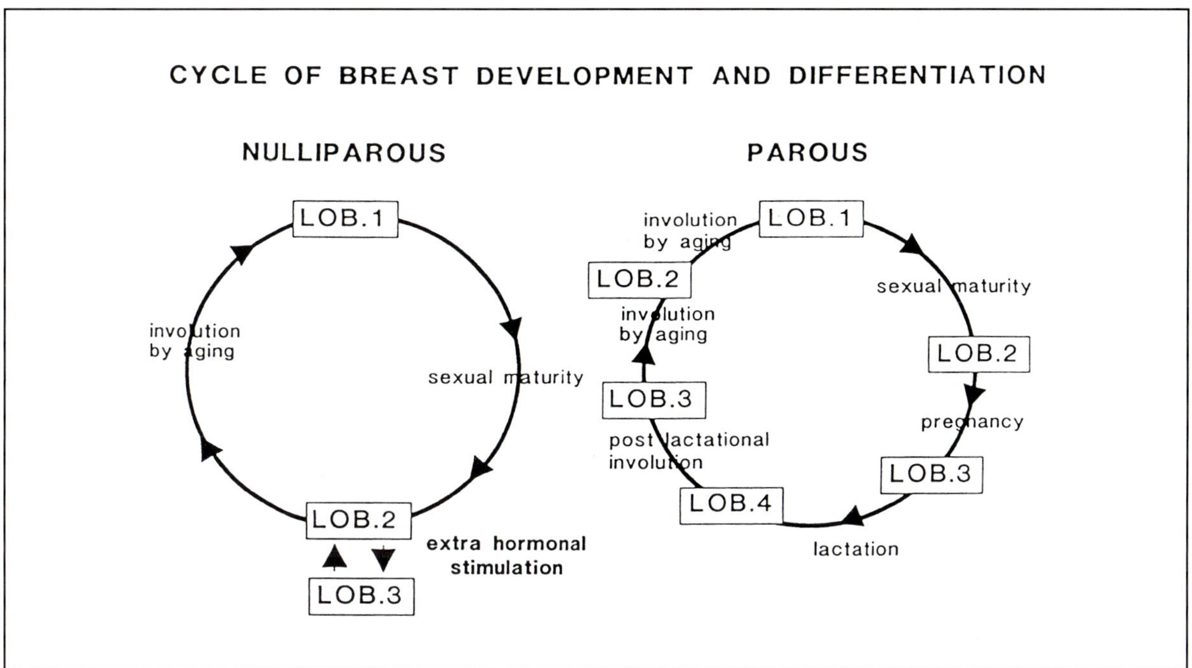

of Lob 1, and a concomitant decline in the number of Lob 2 and Lob 3. At the end of the fifth decade of life, the breast of both nulliparous and parous women contains predominantly Lob 1 [3, 21]. These observations led us to conclude that the understanding of breast development requires a horizontal study in which all the different phases of growth are taken into consideration. For example, the analysis of breast structures at a single given point, i. e., age 50 years, would lead us to conclude that the breast of both nulliparous and parous women appears identical. However, the phenomena occurring in prior years might have imprinted permanent changes in the breast biology that affect the potential of this organ to develop neoplasms, even though they are no longer morphologically identifiable. Thus, from a biological and quantitative point of view, the regression of the breast at menopause differs in nulliparous and parous women. In nulliparous women, the predominant breast structure is the Lob 1, which comprises 65 to 80% of the total lobular components and their relative percentage is independent of age (Fig. 2.7). Second, in frequency is the Lob 2 that represents 10 to

Influence of parity on lifetime breast development. Diagrammatic representation based on the relative percentage of lobules present. In nulliparous women the breast contains primarily lobules type 1 (*Lob 1*) with some progression to type 2 (*Lob 2*), and only minimal formation of lobules type 3 (*Lob 3*). In parous women, pregnancy and lactation complete the cycle of lobular development through the formation of lobules type 4 (*Lob 4*), which regress to Lob 3 at post-weaning and to Lob 2 and Lob 1 after menopause. (Reprinted with permission from: Russo, J. et al. Breast Cancer Res. Treat. 23:211, 1992)

35% of the total. The least frequent is the Lob 3, which represent only 0 to 5% of the total lobular population. In premenopausal parous women, on the other hand, the predominant lobular structure is the Lob 3, which comprises 70 to 90% of the total lobular component (Fig. 2.8). Only after menopause Lob 3 decline in number, and the relative proportion of the three lobular types present approach that observed in nulliparous women (Figs. 2.7, 2.8, 2.13). These observa-

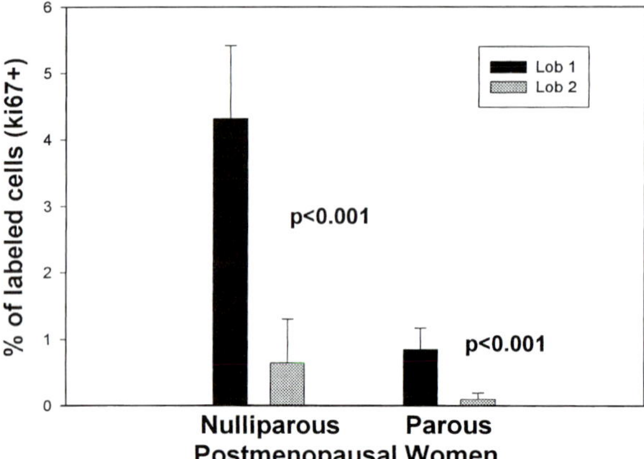

Figure 2.14

Comparison of proliferative activity (Ki67 Index) in the breast of parous and nulliparous post-menopausal women, determined in lobules type 1 (*Lob 1*) and type 2 (*Lob 2*). Breast tissues from three nulliparous women, 59, 60 and 61 years old, and from three parous, 58, 61 and 62 years old, were immunoreacted with anti-K67 antibody. The percentage of positive cells was determined in Lob 1 and Lob 2, and the values are expressed as a mean ± standard deviation

tions led us to conclude that early parous women truly underwent lobular differentiation, which was evident at a younger age, whereas nulliparous women seldom reached the Lob 3 stage, and never the Lob 4 stages (Figs. 2.13, 2.14) [21].

Even though during the post-menopausal years in the breast of both parous and nulliparous women the preponderant structure is the Lob 1, only the nulliparous women are at high risk of developing breast cancer, whereas parous women remain protected [21]. Since ductal breast cancer originates in Lob 1 (TDLU) [19], the epidemiological observation that nulliparous women exhibit a higher incidence of breast cancer than parous women [3, 4] indicates that Lob 1 in these two groups of women might be biologically different, or exhibit different susceptibility to carcinogenesis [17, 24–26]. The presence of Lob 1 in the breasts of parous women has also been interpreted as a failure of the mammary parenchyma to respond to the influences of pregnancy and lactation [21, 22]. It

is possible to postulate that unresponsive lobules that fail to undergo full differentiation under the stimuli of pregnancy and lactation are responsible of cancer development despite the parity history of a woman. If this were the case, then this unresponsive Lob 1 would be as sensitive to carcinogenesis as the lobules found in the breasts of nulliparous women. We have reported the presence of intralobular hyalinization and lower proliferative activity in the Lob 1 of the parous woman's breast, whereas hyalinization is absent and cell proliferation is higher in the Lob 1 of the nulliparous woman's breast. We have also shown that during the fourth and fifth decades of life there is a decrease in the number of Lob 2. We postulate that this type of lobule is the site of origin of both lobular hyperplasia and carcinoma in situ [19, 21, 27]. Since it has been reported that the incidence of atypical lobular hyperplasia decreases significantly with advancing age, it is possible to postulate that the observed diminution in Lob 2 is responsible for the decreased incidence of this type of preneoplastic lesions.

In addition to the differences in proliferative activity the three types of lobules exhibit variations in their in vitro growth characteristics. Lob 1 and Lob 2 grow faster; have a higher DNA labeling index, and a shorter doubling time than Lob 3 [18]. They also exhibit different susceptibility to carcinogenesis [15, 17]. Cells obtained from Lob 1 and Lob 2 express in vitro phenotypes indicative of neoplastic transformation when treated with chemical carcinogens, whereas cells obtained from Lob 3 do not manifest those changes [15, 17]. Collectively, our data establish a baseline for understanding the evolution of glandular development, and how it is influenced by age and parity. This knowledge is of utmost importance for understanding the role of differentiation in the protection of the mammary gland against carcinogenesis [27–30]. In addition, these data establish well-defined endpoints for studying the response of the mammary gland to hormonal or chemopreventive agents, which could be utilized in modulating the susceptibility of the breast to carcinogenesis.

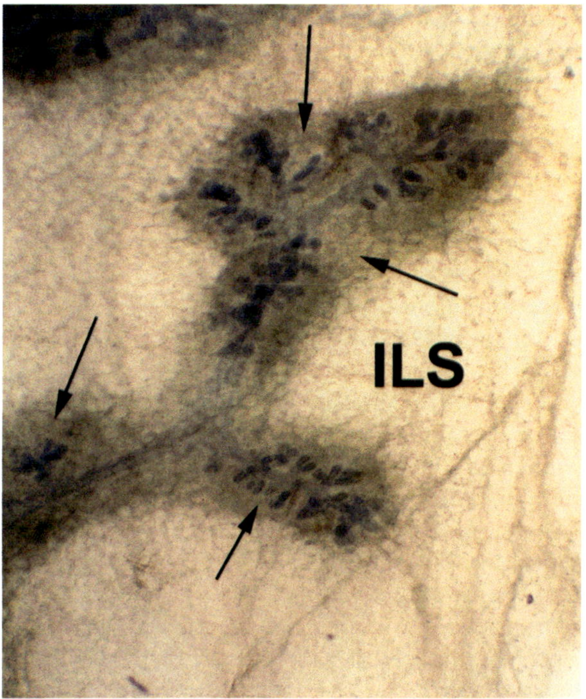

Figure 2.15

Fig. 2.15. Breast tissue of a 19-year-old woman in which individual ductules of a lobule type 1 (Lob 1) are surrounded by the intra-lobular stroma (*arrows*). Lobules are separated from each other by the inter-lobular stroma (*ILS*) (Whole mount preparation, toluidine blue, ×2.5)

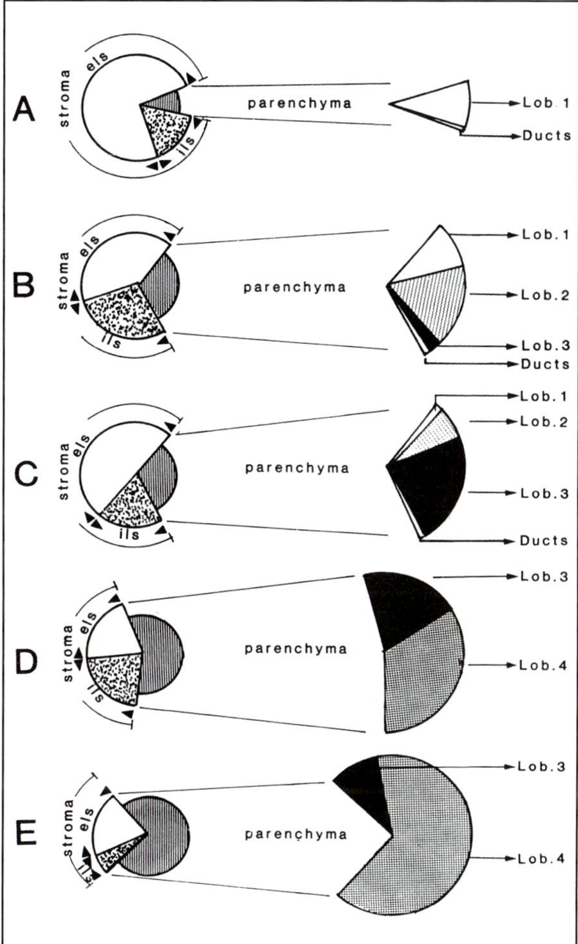

Figure 2.16 a–e

Proportion of parenchymal and stromal components of the breast: intralobular (*ils*) and interlobular (*els*) stroma (*left hand pie charts*). The *right-hand pie charts* represent the average of the proportion of parenchyma occupied by ducts and Lob 1, Lob 2, Lob 3, and Lob 4 in breast tissues of: **a** two pubertal age girls; **b** two post-pubertal women; **c** six parous women; **d** three women in their first half of pregnancy; and **e** two women at the end of pregnancy. (Reprinted with permission from: Russo, J. and Russo, I.H. In: The mammary gland (Neville and Daniel, Eds.). Plenum Publishing, 1987)

2.7 Parenchyma-Stroma Relationship

Breast development occurs through a process of ductal elongation, branching and sprouting of ductules or acini, a process that requires extensive cell proliferation and penetration of the ductal epithelium into the stroma [3]. Both the intralobular and the inter-lobular stroma are affected simultaneously during development, pregnancy, lactation, and involution (Figs. 2.15, 2.16). These processes occur, in turn, in a synchronous manner in response to specific hormonal and growth factor stimuli [27]. Two major mechanisms are considered to be involved in the interaction of the stroma with epithelial cells, the production of soluble growth factors and a modification of the composition of the extracellular matrix. This interaction seems to be bi-directional, such that epithelial cells are also capable of influencing stromal cell behavior and governing gene expression [31, 32]. The study of the stroma-parenchyma ratio in 14 breasts of pubertal, post-pubertal, parous, and pregnant women, showed that the relationship between parenchyma and stroma is a dynamic process. At puberty, almost 90% of the mammary gland is made up of stroma: the intralobular stroma, that represents 17% of the total, consists of the loose connective tissue that surrounds each individual ductule, and the interlobular stroma, composed of fat and connective tissue, that separates one lobule from another (Fig. 2.15). The parenchyma of the pubertal breast comprises 10% of the mammary area; it is made up almost exclusively of Lob 1 and ductal structures. In post-pubertal and young nulliparous women's breast, the parenchyma increases from 10 to 30% of the total area of the gland (0–10% is composed of Lob 1, 10–18% of Lob 2, and 1–3% of Lob 3) (Fig. 2.16). The intralobular stroma represents about 28% of the total breast area [21]. Parity induces significant differences in mammary gland development. The breast of non-pregnant parous women is mostly composed of Lob 3 with a markedly reduced proportion of Lob 1 (Fig. 2.16).

2.8 Genetic Influences in Breast Development

Genetic influences are responsible of at least 5% of the breast cancer cases; they also seem to influence the pattern of breast development and differentiation, as evidenced by the study of prophylactic mastectomy specimens obtained from women with familial breast and breast/ovarian cancer, or proven to be carriers of the BRCA1 gene, as determined by linkage analysis [33]. Morphological and architectural analysis of prophylactic mastectomy specimens revealed that these characteristics were similar in breasts obtained from either nulliparous or parous women. In both groups of women the breast tissues were predominantly composed of Lob 1, and only a few specimens contained Lob 2 and Lob 3, in frank contrast with the predominance of Lob 3 found in parous women without familial history of breast cancer (Fig. 2.17) [33]. We concluded that the developmental pattern of the breast of parous women of the familial breast cancer group was similar to that of nulliparous women, and less developed than the breast of parous women without history of familial breast cancer. The breast of women belonging to the familial breast cancer group also presented differences in the branching pattern of the ductal tree, observations that suggested that the genes that control lobular development might have been affected in women carrying breast cancer predisposing genes [33].

Table 2.3. Influence of parity on the lobular composition and proliferative activity of the breast. *Lob 4* lobule type 4

Group	Number of cases	Donor's age	Lob 1		Lob 2	
			Lobular structures[a]	Ki 67 index[b]	Lobular structures[a]	Ki 67 index[b]
Nulliparous	7	40.85±10.93	81.13±6.90	4.97±2.51*	18.87±6.89	0.62±0.30
Parous	25	48.76±11.00	66.84±7.55	1.56±0.29*	23.10±6.37	0.85±0.31

[a] Percentage of each type of lobular structures over total number of structures present
[b] Ki67 index, proliferative activity determined as the percentage of Ki67 positive cells
* Proliferative activity of Lob 1 nulliparous vs. Lob 1 parous, t = 2.44, p = <0.02

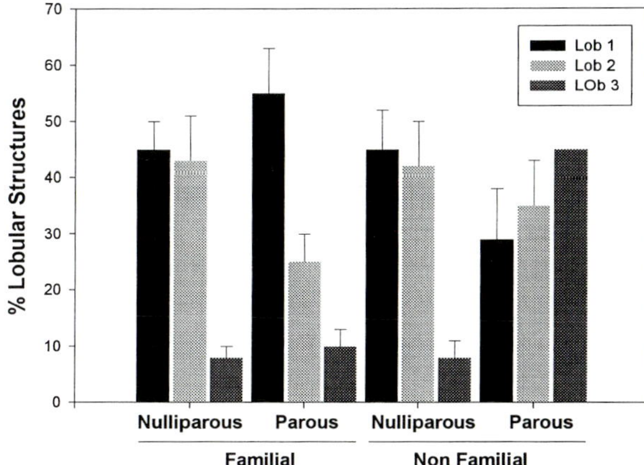

Figure 2.17

Relative percentage of lobules type 1, 2, and 3 (Lob 1, Lob 2 and Lob 3) (ordinate) in the breast of nulliparous and parous women with history of familial breast cancer in comparison with that of women with no family history. (Adapted from: Russo, J. and Russo, I.H. Prog. Clin. Biol. Res. 396:1–16, 1997)

2.9 Cell Proliferation and Hormone Receptors in Relation to Breast Structure

The determination of the breast proliferative activity, expressed as the percentage of cells that react positively with the antibody Ki67 (Ki67 or Proliferative Index) revealed that it is maximal in those Lob 1 present in the breast of nulliparous women (Table 2.3). It is two-fold lower in Lob 1 of parous women ($p < 0.02$) (Table 2.3), but in both groups cell proliferation decreases progressively and proportionally as the lobules mature to Lob 2 and Lob 3 (Table 2.3). These differences are not abrogated when the phases of the menstrual cycle are taken into consideration [25]. Parity, in addition to exerting an important influence in the lobular composition of the breast, as described above, profoundly influences the proliferative activity of the mammary epithelium. Lob 1 and Lob 2 present in the breast of premenopausal nulliparous women exhibit a significantly higher proliferative activity than the same type of lobules found in the breast of parous women. Even though in the breast of menopausal women the proliferative activity of the mammary epithelium decreases, the differences in Proliferation Index between nulliparous and parous women still persist.

Estrogens and progesterone are known to promote proliferation and differentiation in the normal breast epithelium. Both steroids act intracellularly through a receptor which, when activated by its binding with the hormone, regulates the expression of specific genes [34]. However, the mechanism by

Lob 3		Lob 4		Ducts
Lobular structures[a]	Ki 67 index[b]	Lobular structures[a]	Ki 67 index[b]	Ki 67 index[b]
00.00	00.00	0.0	0.0	2.00±0.75
8.03±4.67	0.22±0.18	0.0	0.0	1.47±0.19

which these molecules exert their mitogenic and differentiation effects has not been clearly established [35–45]. One of the accepted mechanisms of action of steroid hormones postulates that the proliferation of cells is the response to direct stimulation, as the result of the interaction of the estradiol bound to the classical estrogen receptor alpha (ER α) with the DNA [35]. Measurements of the levels of ERα and progesterone receptor (PgR) in normal breast in the cytosol fraction, using standard biochemical techniques, is inaccurate because of the low cellularity of the tissue. The use of monoclonal antibodies that specifically recognize ERα and PgR makes it possible to identify and to quantify the cells expressing these receptors [45]. Both ERα and PgR are present in the nucleus of epithelial cells. The percentage of cells expressing these receptors, however, varies as a function of the degree of lobular development of the breast, and therefore of the type of lobular structure analyzed. Lob 1 are the structures more consistently containing a higher percentage of ERα and PgR positive cells than Lob 2, 3 and 4, an observation that indicates that a progressive decrease in the percentage of cells exhibiting an immunocytochemically positive reaction for these markers occurs as the structures become more differentiated. These data allowed us to conclude that degree of differentiation of the breast is an important determinant in the expression of both ERα and PgR, in addition to modulate the proliferative activity of the breast epithelium. Age and parity history do not affect the percentage of cells reacting with these receptors except through their influence on the lobular composition of the breast [45].

2.10 Extracellular Matrix Protein Expression in the Normal Breast

The molecular organization of the extracellular matrix consists of multifunctional proteins, which play an important role in cell growth, adhesion, migration and differentiation. It cannot be seen as a simple amorphous gel anymore. Indeed we know today that, besides its mechanical properties, the extracellular matrix can show a variety of biochemical changes in response to minimal variations in the parenchyma's metabolism [46, 47]. We have identified by immunohistochemistry tenascin and elastin, two proteins of the extracellular matrix that might have been produced or repressed during the differentiation process of the breast. These proteins play an important role in the cell-cell, cell-substratum interactions and malignant transformation. Studies of tenascin's structure, tissue distribution and in vitro models have indicated that this is a multifunctional glycoprotein participating in cell adhesion, motility and migration pathways, shedding of epithelial cells from surfaces, promotion of cell growth, demarcation of tissue boundaries, angiogenesis, tissue remodeling and immune modulation. Tenascin is also largely confined to areas of epithelial-mesenchymal interactions during the process of development of the embryo [48] suggesting an important role during the differentiation process.

2.10.1 Angiogenic Index in the Lobular Structures

Using factor VIII as a marker of endothelial cells for identifying blood vessels, we determined the angiogenic index (AI), based on a count of the number of identifiable vascular spaces are counted in the intralobular stroma of Lob 1, Lob 2 and Lob 3 (Fig. 2.18, Table 2.4). AI was 1.64 in Lob 1, which was significantly higher ($p < 0.00000$) than in Lob 2 and Lob 3, in which AI was 0.84 and 0.55, respectively. There were no differences in AI between nulliparous and parous women when comparisons were done between similar lobular types (Table 2.4), and the same phenomenon was observed with aging (Table 2.5) [22].

Table 2.4. Angiogenic index in the normal breast

Group	Number of cases	Age[a]	Lob 1	Lob 2	Lob 3
All women	48	43.36±7.59	1.64±0.40	0.84±0.28	0.55±0.11
Nulliparous	13	40.16±8.32	1.66±0.35	0.82±0.19	0.57±0.09
Parous	35	44.36±7.29	1.63±0.42	0.84±0.31	0.55±0.13

[a] Age in years, mean ± standard deviation

Table 2.5. Effect of age on parous women's breast angiogenic index

Number of cases	Donors' age	Angiogenic index		
		Lob 1	Lob 2	Lob 3
4	30–39	1.54±0.30	0.75±0.03	0.59±0.11
10	40–50	1.42±0.41	0.76±0.	0.44±0.14
4	>50	1.88±0.58	0.97±0.02	0.47±0.02

Table 2.6. Influence of parity on elastin reactivity. *NA* no Lob 4 available for examination

Number of cases	Group	Percentage of elastin-positive lobules			
		Lob 1	Lob 2	Lob 3	Lob 4
44	All Women	10.35±1.55[a,b,c]	19.82±2.37[a]	36.64±4.63[b,d]	33.80±20.75[c,d]
11	Nulliparous	7 37±174[e,f]	19.36±5.92[f,g]	28.71±7 74[f,g]	NA
33	Parous	11.50±2.03[h,i,j]	19.92±2.64[h,k,l]	40.60±5.61[h,k,m]	84.52±452[j,l,m]

[a] Lob 1 vs. Lob 2; $t=3.47, p<0.0009$
[b] Lob 1 vs. Lob 3; $t=6.58, p<0.00000001$
[c] Lob 1 vs. Lob 4; $t=2.89, p<0.005$
[d] Lob 3 vs. Lob 4; $t=3.47, p<0.001$
[e] Lob 1 vs. Lob 2; $t=2.58, p<0.02$
[f] Lob 1 vs. Lob 3; $t=3.30, p<0.004$
[g] Lob 2 vs. Lob 3; not significant

[h] Lob 1 vs. Lob 2; $t=2.87, p<0.006$
[i] Lob 1 vs. Lob 3; $t=7.91, p<0.000000$
[j] Lob 1 vs. Lob 4; $t=9.75, p<0.0000000$
[k] Lob 2 vs. Lob 3; $t=5.66, p<0.000004$
[l] Lob 2 vs. Lob 4; $t=8.68, p<0.000000$
[m] Lob 3 vs. Lob 4; $t=3.74, p<0.002$

Table 2.7. Influence of age on elastin reactivity

Donor's age	Number of cases	Percentage of elastin-positive lobules			
		Lob 1	Lob 2	Lob 3	Lob 4
20–40	17	14.53±3.57	20.02±3.73	40.91±5.76	84.52±4.52
41–50	18	8.21±1.83	20.47±3.46	34.61±7.26	NA
51–80	9	7.70±2.65	12.25±5.90	54.15±20.85	NA

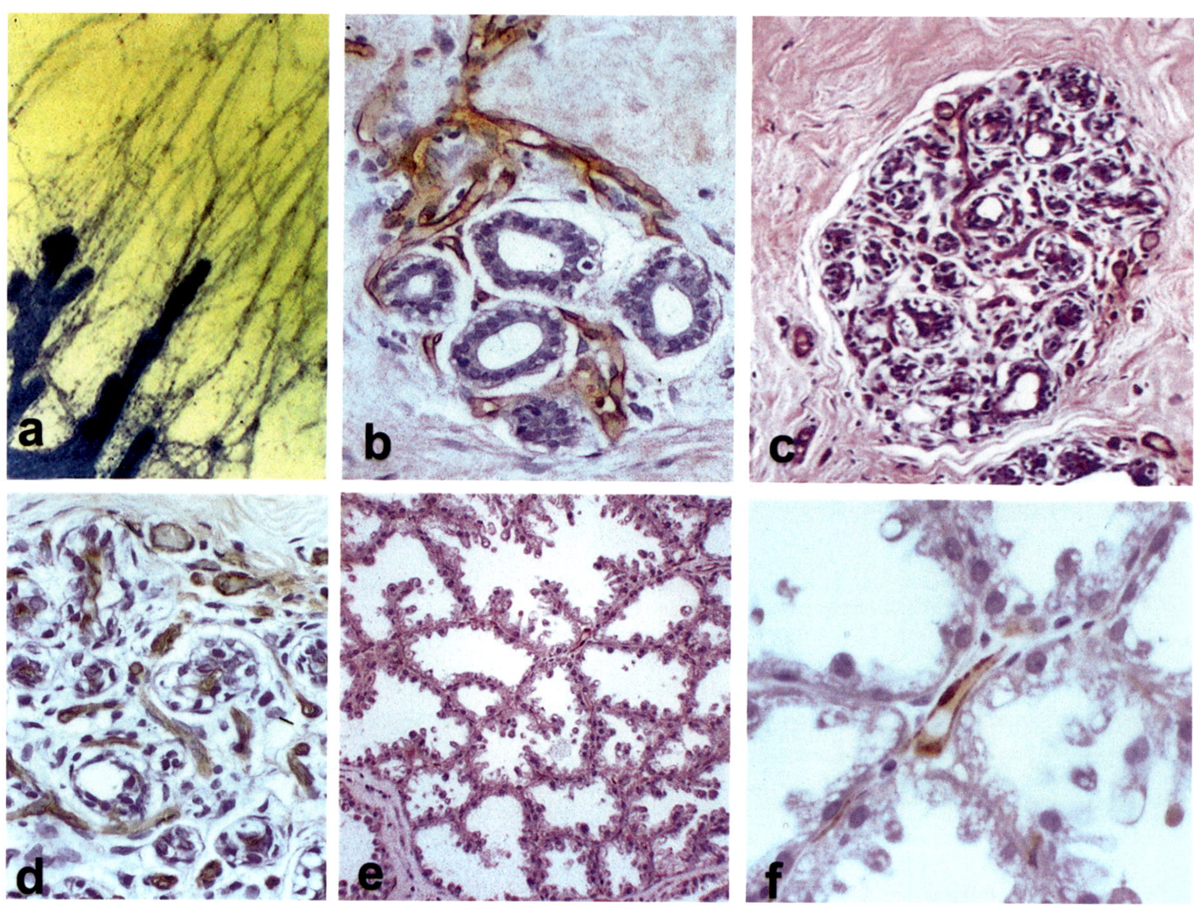

Figure 2.18 a–f

a Breast tissue of a 19-year-old nulliparous woman showing a network of capillaries surrounding terminal ductal structures and extending into the adjacent stroma. (Whole mount preparation, toluidine blue, ×2.0). **b** Cross section the terminal ductal structures shown in **a**, showing the endothelial cells of blood vessels reacting positively with anti-factor VIII antibody used for determining the angiogenic index (AI), based on a count of the number of identifiable vascular spaces in the intralobular stroma (DAB counterstained with hematoxylin [H] (×20); **c–f** endothelial cells of blood vessels reacting positively with anti-factor VIII antibody (DAB counterstained with H). Lob 1 **c** (×4), and **d** (×10); Lob 4 **e** (×20), **f** (×40), showing progressive reduction in the ratio of ductule/acinus to intralobular blood vessels with lobular differentiation

2.10.2 Elastin in the Lobular Structures

Elastin interacts with microfibrillar proteins; it has also been demonstrated that peptide segments of elastin elicit a chemotactic response by fibroblast and monocytes, suggesting that this protein has domains with biologically important activities other than those related to its mechanical properties [49].

Immunocytochemical reactivity reveals elastin to surround each individual ductule as a continuous layer (Fig. 2.19a). Although the intensity of the reaction was similar in all the ductules and acini that were positive, the number of structures positive varied depending upon the type of lobules. Lob 1 had the lowest percentage of positive ductules (10.35%), which increased to 19.82% in Lob 2, and to 36.64% and

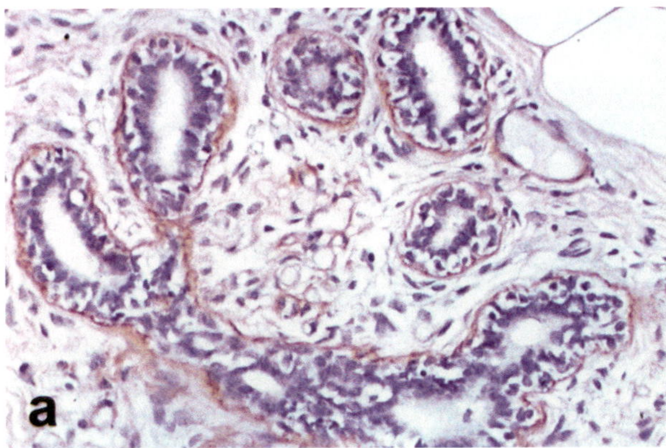

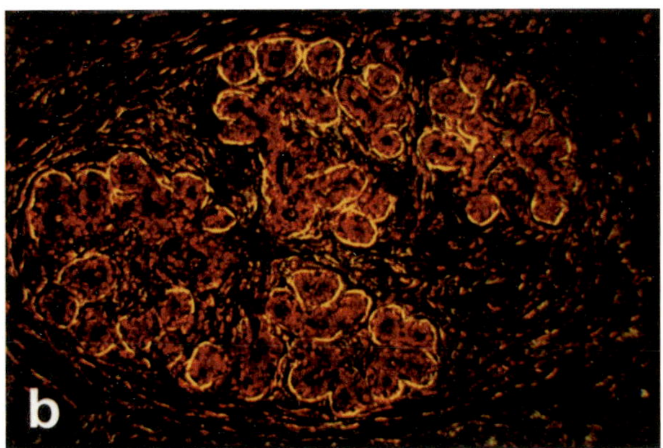

Figure 2.19 a, b

a Lobule type 1 stained with anti elastin antibody, (DAB-H&E, ×10). **b** Lobule type 2 stained with anti-tenascin antibody (DAB-H&E, ×4)

33.80% in Lob 3 and Lob 4, respectively (Table 2.6). Whereas parity slightly increases the percentage of elastin positive Lob 1 and Lob 3 the differences were not statistically significant (Table 2.6). Aging did not affect the percentage of lobules presenting positive elastin reactivity (Table 2.7) [22].

2.10.3 Tenascin in the Lobular Structures

Tenascin is identified in the intralobular stroma of all the lobular structures of the human breast (Fig. 2.19b). The percentage of lobules reacting with tenascin is varies from 44% and 41% in Lob 1 and Lob 2, respectively, to 30% in Lob 3, with Lob 4 exhib-

iting the highest percentage of reactivity, 89.25% (Table 2.8). Parity and aging did not affect the percentage of structures reacting for tenascin [20].

In conclusion, there is a direct relationship between proliferative activity and angiogenic index, which is, in turn, inversely proportional to the degree of differentiation of the lobular structures. Thus, Lob 1, that are the less differentiated ones, have the highest proliferative index and AI. Elastin, on the other hand, follows an inverse pattern, being expressed more highly in the more differentiated Lob 3 and Lob 4. Tenascin is moderately expressed in the less differentiated Lob 1 and Lob 2, and highly expressed in the stroma of Lob 4, with the lowest level of expression in Lob 3, and indication that its expression is not linear with the degree of differentiation of the lobules. Overall, age and parity do not affect the expression of elastin and tenascin independently of the degree of lobular development. The only significant difference induced by pregnancy is the proliferative activity of Lob 1, which is two fold lower in the breast of parous women than in those of nulliparous women.

Table 2.8. Tenascin expression in lobular structures

Number of cases	Lob 1	Lob 2	Lob 3	Lob 4
43	44.43±16.28[a,b,c]	41.53±18.22[b,d]	30.67±22.87[b,d]	89.25±0.91[c,d]

[a] Lob 1 vs. Lob 2; not significant
[b] Lob 1 vs. Lob 3; $t=2.35, p<0.02$
[c] Lob 1 vs. Lob 4; $t=3.84, p<0.00003$
[d] Lob 3 vs. Lob 4; $t=3.50, p<0.0004$

2.11 Genomic Profile of Lobular Structures in Nulliparous and Parous Women's Breasts

For assessing whether the differentiation of the breast induced by pregnancy imprints permanent genomic changes in the mammary epithelium, we compared the genomic profile of the well differentiated Lob 3 from he breast of parous women with that of the undifferentiated Lob 1 from the breast of nulliparous women. Reduction mammoplasty specimens free from pathological lesions were obtained from three parous and in three nulliparous premenopausal women. Epithelial cells from Lob 3 and Lob 1 of the parous and nulliparous women's breasts respectively were microdissected by laser capture microdissection (LCM). Total RNA was extracted and 20–25 µg were hybridized to cDNA array membranes that contained 1,176 human genes (Clontech Human Cancer 1,2 array). Microarrays were hybridized to fluorescent cDNA probes that were synthesized with control total or poly(A)+RNA through indirect incorporation of Cy3/Cy5 fluorescent label using aminoallyl-dNTP incorporation and chemical coupling of the dyes. cDNA expression microarrays and gene clustering analysis performed utilizing BioDiscovery's ImaGene and GeneSight software applications reveal that the level of reproducibility between replicate microarray hybridizations was >90%; the average coefficient of covariance per gene between replicate array data sets was ~14%; and the level of falsely detected genes as differentially expressed when the cut-off range was a 2-fold change in expression) was less than 1%.

The genomic signature of Lob 3 of parous women differed by 82 genes from that of Lob 1 of nulliparous women (Fig. 2.20). We have clustered these genes according to functional properties (Table 2.9). With this array, it is clear that Lob 3 have a gene expression profile significantly different from that of Lob 1 of the nulliparous breast. Of interest is the Rho-E gene, which is amplified 14 folds in the Lob 3 of the parous breast (Table 2.9). This gene belongs to a small G protein superfamily that includes the Ras, Rho, Rab, Arf, Sarl, and Ran families. Members of the Rho family of small guanosine triphosphatases (GTP) have

emerged as key regulators of the actin cytoskeleton, and furthermore, through their interaction with multiple target proteins, they ensure coordinated control of other cellular activities such as gene transcription and adhesion [50]. Rho-E is a Rho protein that binds GTP but lacks intrinsic GTPase activity and is resistant to Rho-specific GTPase-activating proteins. Within a region that is highly conserved among small GTPases, RhoE contains amino acid differences specifically at three positions that confer oncogenicity to Ras. Replacing all three positions in Rho-E with conventional amino acids completely restores GTPase activity [51, 52]. Rho-E may act to inhibit signaling downstream of Rho-A, altering some Rho-A-regulated responses, such as stress fiber formation, but not affecting others, such as peripheral actin bundle formation. In vivo, Rho-E is found exclusively in the GTP-bound form, suggesting that unlike previously characterized small GTPases, RhoE may be normally maintained in an activated state [51, 52]. This might be of importance in maintaining this gene activated in Lob 3, even after its involution Lob 1 in the postmenopausal state. Another gene that is significantly overexpressed (five-fold) in Lob 3 is the protein tyrosine phosphatase (HPTPCAAX1 or PRL-1) (Table 2.9). This gene encodes a unique nuclear protein-tyrosine phosphatase that is regulated by a mechanism different from those of other immediate early genes such as *c-fos* and *c-jun* [53]. Importantly, this gene has been shown to be upregulated in villus enterocytes and in confluent differentiated colon carcinoma cells, but not in crypt enterocytes or undifferentiated proliferating Caco-2 colon carcinoma cells, respectively. In other systems this gene has been found to be related to differentiation, development and regeneration [54–57]. Therefore in the breast epithelial cells of Lob 3 its function may be related to differentiation rather than to proliferation, since Lob 3 have a lower proliferative activity than Lob 1 (Table 2.9).

Insulin-like growth factor binding protein-3 (IGFBP-3) is significantly overexpressed in the Lob 3 over the Lob 1 of the breast of premenopausal women. This gene codes a specific binding protein for the insulin-like growth factors (IGFs). Insulin-like growth factor binding protein 3 (IGFBP-3) modulates the mitogenic and metabolic effects of IGFs [58]. IG-

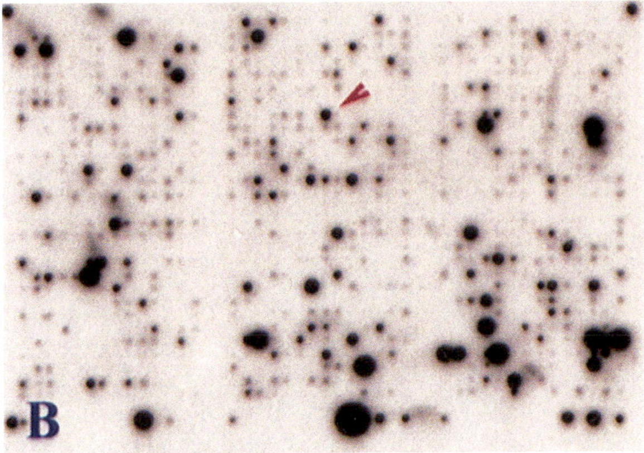
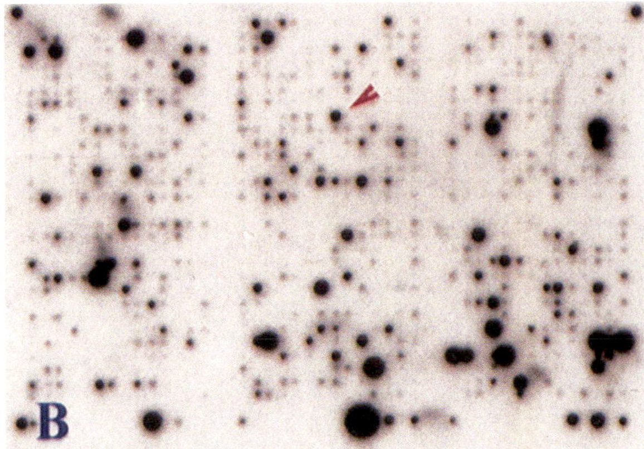

Figure 2.20 a, b

Gene expression analysis of the human breast. For Panel **a** RNA was extracted from Lob 1 of a 28-year-old nulliparous woman, and for Panel **b** from Lob 3 of a 26-year-old parous woman. RNAs were hybridized to Atlas Human cDNA Expression Array membranes. The *arrow* points to the amplification spot for the IGFBP-3 gene

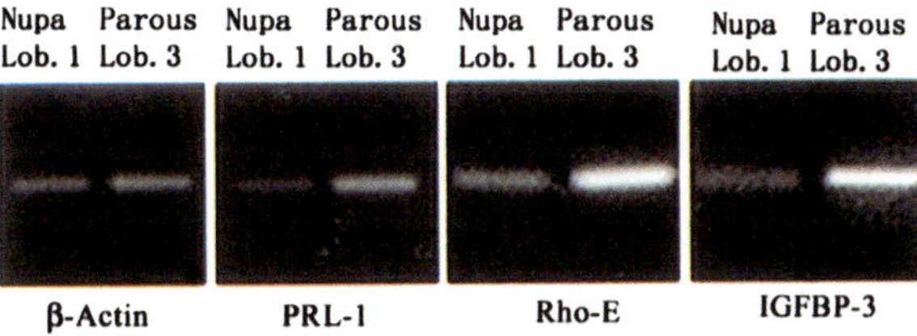

Figure 2.21 ▲

Verification of cDNA microarray results with semi-quantitative RT-PCR. Genes PRL-1, Rho-E and IGFBP-3, which were overexpressed in Lob 3 show a more intense band, whereas beta actin, that was not modified, gives two equally intense bands in Lob 1 and Lob 3. *Nu-Pa* nulliparous

FBP-3 forms a ternary complex with IGF-I or IGF-II and an 85 kDa glycoprotein acid-labile subunit ALS. IGFBP-3 may also play more active, IGF-independent, roles in growth regulation of cancer cells [59]. IGFBP-3 protein levels are developmentally regulated and influenced by a number of hormonal stimuli both in vitro and in vivo. p53 may regulate apoptosis in tumor cells via transactivation of the IGFBP3 gene [59–61]. It has been shown that IGFBP-3 can be modulated by hCG, and this could represent an important pathway in the differentiating effect of this hormone on the mammary gland. IGFBP-3 expression in the Lob 3 is a new finding that requires further investigation.

The final biological significance of changes in gene expression in relation to the process of breast differentiation, post-menopausal involution, and how they are influenced by a reproductive event in women, is not known. Neither there is a clear understanding of the role of these known or still unidentified genes play for conferring protection to the breast through pregnancy. It was of interest the observation that the expression of cytoskeletal proteins, such as cytokeratins 18, 19, and 8, did not differ between Lob 1 and Lob 3, even though they are overexpressed in tumor cells [62]. Known genes that are overexpressed in breast cancer, such as HER-2/neu [63] and mucin [64, 65], were not expressed in any of the lobular structures. The levels of expression of other genes, such as fibroblast-like growth factor 1 (FGF-1), insulin-like growth factor-1 (IGF-1) binding protein-2, and Zinc-a-2-glycoprotein [66], which are generally up or down regulated in neoplastic lesions, did not differ between Lob 3 and Lob 1. The fact that cells derived from the undifferentiated Lob 1 express transforma-

Table 2.9. Gene expression in Lob 3 of parous women versus Lob 1 of nulliparous women

Gene category/name[a]	Fold increase (- decrease) Mean ± SD[b]	Gene category/name[a]	Fold increase (- decrease) Mean ± SD[b]
Intracellular kinase network		**Oncogenes, tumor suppressor genes, transcription activators and repressors, intracellular transducers, effectors and modulators**	
– CDC7-related kinase	2.4±0.8	– c-jun proto-oncogene; transcription factor AP-1	2.8±0.5
– c-jun N-terminal kinase 2 (JNK2)	4.5±1.2	– Interferon-inducible protein 9–27	2.0±0.3
– Ribosomal protein S6 kinase II	1.6±0.4	– Neurogenic locus notch protein (N)	3.0±0.7
Caspases		– c-myc oncogene	−1.5±0.4
– Caspase-4 (CASP4)	2.3±0.5	– c-myc binding protein MM-1	9.5±1.2
Protein turnover		– Cyclin-dependent kinase 4 inhibitor, p16	−2.0±0.4
– Ubiquitin-conjugating enzyme E2	−2.0±0.5	– Epidermal growth factor receptor (EGFR)	1.6±0.3
– Basigin precursor (BSG)	−2.0±0.4	– Fos-related antigen (FRA1)	5.0±0.9
– Heterogen nuclear ribonucleoprot K	3.2±0.8	– Active breakpoint cluster region-related protein	2.5±1.0
Calcium binding proteins		– ETS-related protein	1.6±0.4
– Calmodulin 1	7.0±1.6	– ETS domain protein elk-3, NET	3.0±0.8
– Guanine nucleotide-binding protein	10.5±2.5	– Purine-rich single-stranded DNA-binding protein	−1.6±0.4
Metabolism		– Early growth response protein 1 (hEGR1)	2.0±0.2
– Cytosolic superoxide dismutase 1 (SOD1)	1.6±0.3	– Neutrophil gelatinase-associated lipocalin precursor	2.0±0.5
– Glutathione-S-transferase (GST) homolog	2.0±0.5	**Extracellular matrix, cell adhesion, cellular matrix**	
– L-lactate dehydrogenase M subunit (LDHA)	6.5±1.5	– Cadherin 3 (CDH3); placental cadherin precursor	−2.0±0.7
– L-lactate dehydrogenase H subunit (HDHB)	3.2±0.8	– Integrin beta 6 precursor (ITGB6)	4.5±0.9
Replication factors, DNA damage and repair		– Integrin beta 4 (ITGB4); CD104 antigen	−1.8±0.5
– G/T mismatch-specific thymine DNA glycosylase	3.5±0.9	– Integrin beta 8 precursor (ITGB8)	4.0±1.2
– MutL protein homolog, DNA mismatch repair	−3±−0.8	– Paxillin	1.6±0.3
– Proliferating cyclic nuclear antigen (PCNA); cyclin	3±0.8	– Alpha catenin (CTNNA1)	2.2±0.6
Cell cycle and proliferation related		– Desmoplakin I & II (DSP, DPI & DPII)	−2.0±0.2
– G1/S-specific cyclin D1 (CCND1)	3.5±1.6	– Polycystin precursor	−3.3±1.8
– Cell cycle protein P38–2G4 homolog, HG4–1	3.0±1.1	– Wnt-8B	−2.3±0.9
– Cyclin-dependent kinase inhibitor 1 (CDKN1A)	−1.5±0.9	– Vimentin (VIM)	1.6±0.8
– Btg protein precursor	−3.6±1.1	– Type I cytoskeletal 13 keratin	−2.4±1.2
– Cdc2-related protein kinase PISSLRE	−2±0.6	– Nm23-H4; nucleoside-diphosphate kinase	−2.5±0.5
– PTPCAAX1 nuclear tyrosine phosphatase (PRL-1)	5.0±0.0	– Type II cytoskeletal 2 epidermal keratin (KRT2E)	−2.0±0.5
DNA binding nuclear proteins		– BIGH3	3.0±0.8
– DNA-binding protein CPBP	2.2±0.4	– Fibronectin precursor (FN)	5.2±1.6
Undefined		**Receptors**	
– Interferon-induced 56-kDa protein (IFI-56 K)	1.6±0.5	– Arylhydrocarbon receptor (AH receptor)	5.0±1.1
– TRAM protein	13.0±1.9	– Signaling lymphocytic activation molecule	−3.0±0.6
– BENE	4.0±0.8	– Bone morphogenetic protein 4 type II receptor precursor	1.8±0.4
Metalloproteinases and protease inhibitors		– Oncostatin M-specific receptor beta subunit	1.6±0.5
– PRSM1 metallopeptidase	−2.0±0.7	– IgG receptor FC large subunit P51 precursor	−3.0±1.0
– Matrix metalloproteinase 3 (MMP3)	16.0±1.9	– CD59 glycoprotein precursor	2.0±0.4
– Matrix metalloproteinase 7 (MMP7); matrilysin	4.0±1.3		

		Intracellular transducers, effector modulators, symporters and antiporters	
– Metalloproteinase inhibitor 3 precursor	3.2±1.0	– 14–3-3-protein sigma, stratifin;	–2.0±0.4
– Leukocyte elastase inhibitor (LEI)	3.0±0.5	epithelial cell marker protein	–1.5±0.7
– Bikunin; hepatocyte growth factor	–1.5±0.7	– T3 receptor-associating cofactor 1	–2.0±0.4
activator inhibitor 2		– Growth factor receptor-bound protein 2 (GRB2) isoform	2.5±0.7
– Metalloproteinase inhibitor 1 precursor (TIMP1)	2.9±1.0	– Elongation factor 1 alpha (EF1 alpha)	1.6±1.3
Growth factors and hormones		– ADP/ATP carrier protein	3.0±0.2
– Vascular endothelial growth factor precursor (VEGF)	2.6±0.6	– ATP synthase coupling factor 6 mitochondrial precursor	1.6±1.7
– Macrophage inhibitory cytokine 1 (MIVI)	2.1±0.4		
– Insulin-like growth factor binding protein 3	9.5±1.8		
precursor (IGF-bind)			
– Interleukin-1 beta precursor (I)	1.5±0.3		

[a] Genes classified according to function

[b] Mean fold increase (- decrease) of gene expression in Lob 3 in three parous women compared with Lob 1 of three nulliparous women ± SD, standard deviation of the mean

tion phenotypes upon in vitro carcinogen treatment indicates that genomic changes detected in tumors are a late event in the process of cancer progression [13, 15, 67].

The differential expression of some of those genes that were detected to be overexpressed in the Lob 3 by microarray analysis were quite consistently confirmed by semiquantitative RT-PCR (Fig. 2.21).

2.12 Novel Differentiation-Associated Serpin is Upregulated During Lobular Development

For understanding the molecular basis of biological differences between Lob 1 and Lob 3 we used differential display technique for comparing gene expression in breast epithelial cells of the more differentiated Lob 3 with that of cells from the undifferentiated Lob 1; two cDNA fragments, identified as L342C and L346C, which were preferentially expressed in the breast epithelial cells of Lob 3 (Fig. 2.22). The differential expression of these genes was then confirmed by reverse Northern blot analyses, which showed that plasmid DNA containing either L342C or L346C cDNA hybridized to the labeled cDNA synthesized from Lob 3 RNA, but not to that from Lob 1 RNA.

Sequence analysis indicated that L342C and L346C consisted of 665 and 416 nucleotides (nt), respectively. Remarkably, the sequence of L346C was identical to L342C, except that a stretch of 249 nucleotides in L342C was missing in L346C. Search for homology in the gene bank databases revealed that L342C and L346C each were nearly identical to two stretches of two sequences, accession Nos. K01500 [68] and J05176 [69] of a human α1-antichymotrypsin (α1-ACT), a serine protease inhibitor or serpin [68, 69].). When the three sequences were aligned, it became apparent that L342C and L346C contained 327-nt and 576-nt deletions, missing nucleotides 1041–1367 and 783–1367 of the α1-ACT, respectively. These results suggested that these two differentially expressed genes represented potentially alternatively spliced transcripts of a novel serpin. For differentiating this novel serpin from human α1-ACT and for detecting its isoforms, an antisense riboprobe was synthesized using the RSA-linearized L342C plasmid DNA. The

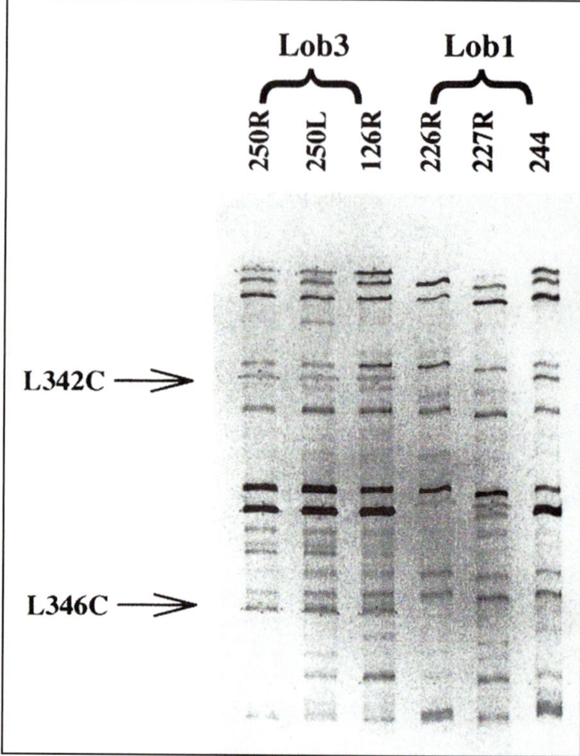

Figure 2.22

Differential display between mRNA from human breast epithelial cells (HBEC) obtained from Lob 3 of breast samples 250R, 250L, and 126R and from Lob 1 of samples 226R, 227A, and 244). cDNA bands that were preferentially expressed in HBEC from Lob 3 were identified as L342C and L346C. (Reprinted with permission from: Russo J. et al., Microsc. Res. Tech. 52:204, 2001)

antisense riboprobe was approximately 464 bp in full length and contained 68 bp of vector sequences and covered the entire region that was missing in L346C (Fig. 2.23). The riboprobe was predicted to protect two fragments in human α1-ACT transcripts, a 228-bp fragment protected by its 3'-end and a 168-bp fragment protected by its 5'-end. These two fragments were expected to be protected equally well. In addition, if the novel serpin was present as two isoforms in human breast cells, the riboprobe was predicted also to protect two fragments, a full-length

Figure 2.23

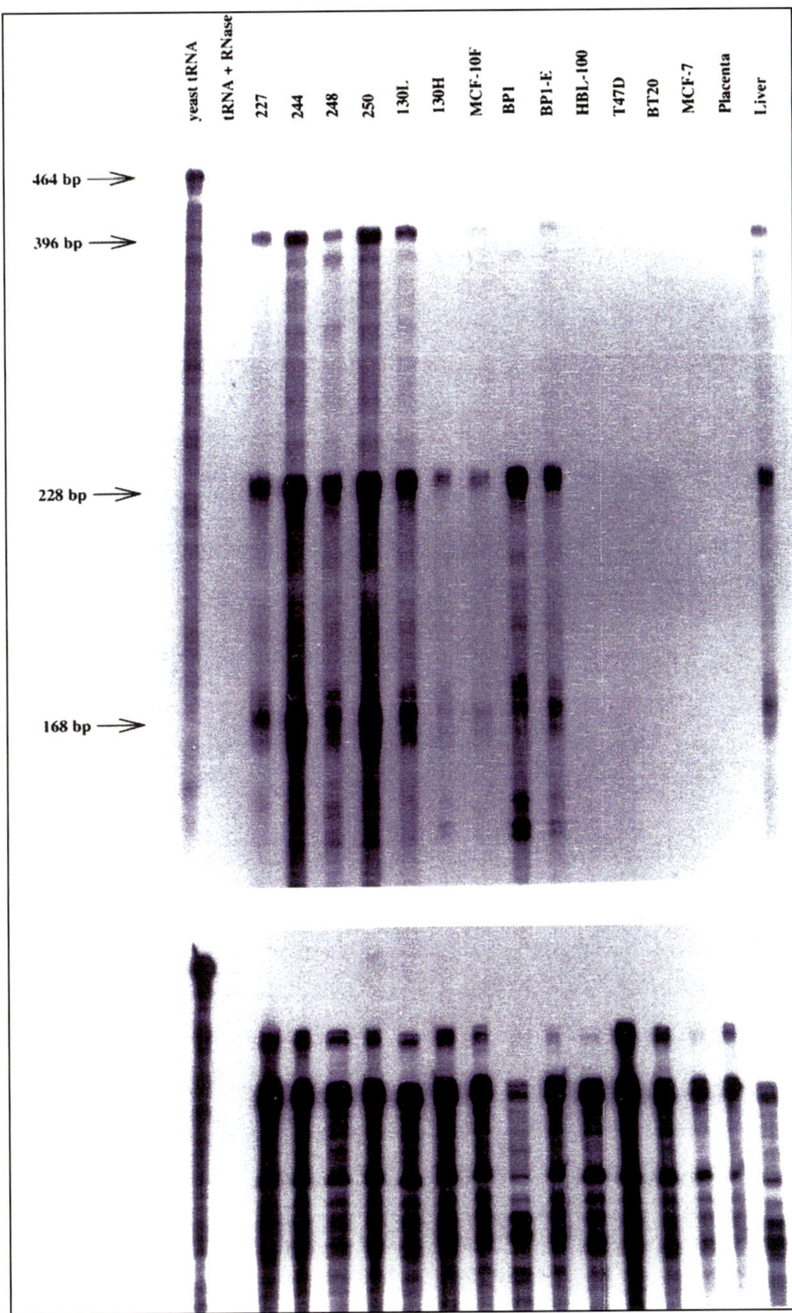

RNase protection assays of the novel serpin L342C (*top*) and, β-actin (*bottom*) in cultured human breast epithelial cells (HBECs), placenta and liver tissues. The sizes of the protected fragments are indicated by *arrows* on the left side of yeast tRNA band; samples used for analysis are listed on top of the lanes. The samples include four primary cultures of HBECs obtained from normal human breast tissues, samples number 227, 244, 248, and 250; a mortal HBEC line cultured in low calcium medium, 130, and the same cell line cultured in high (*H*) calcium medium, sample 130H; the normal immortalized HBEC line MCF-10F and transformed cells derived from BP treated MCF-10F cellsBP1 and BP1E. HBL-100, another normal HBEC line and T47D, BT20, and MCF-7, three breast carcinoma cell lines, were also tested. Yeast tRNA with or without RNase digestion was used as control. RNase protection analysis of β-actin expression served as controls of equal sampling. (Reprinted with permission from: Russo J. et al, Microsc. Res. Tech. 52:204, 2001)

396-bp fragment found in L342C and a 168-bp fragment found in L346C. Results from the RNase protection assay showed that the antisense riboprobe protected three fragments in human breast cells, namely, the full-length 396-bp fragment found in L342C and the 168-bp fragment expected for its isoform as well as the 228-bp fragments apparently from α1-ACT. Similarly, the same antisense riboprobe protected three differently sized transcripts in liver, but not in full-term human placenta (Fig. 2.23). Yeast tRNA, used as control, did not protect any fragments from RNase digestion (compare lanes yeast tRNA versus yeast tRNA + RNase in Fig. 2.23), and a sense riboprobe did not protect any of the RNA fragments from the same panel of cells (data not shown). The amount of various transcripts protected by the antisense riboprobe varied with the status of immortalization and neoplastic transformation in the panel of cells we studied. Protection of the full-length 396-bp fragments indicative of expression of the long transcripts of the novel serpin was highest in primary cultures of human breast epithelial cells (HBECs) obtained from normal human breast tissues containing well differentiated Lob 3, samples number 244 and 250, and less intense in samples 227, 248, and in the mortal HBEC line 130L, cultured in 0.04 M calcium concentration, or low (L). Protection was low in line 130H, cultured in high (H) calcium medium, in MCF-10F cell line, and in BP1 and BP1-E, two transformed cell lines derived from benzo(a)pyrene (BP)-treated MCF-10F cells,. It was completely absent in HBL-100, a normal HBEC line, and in T47D, BT20, and MCF-7, three breast carcinoma cell lines. In contrast, expression of the human α1-ACT, determined as the 228-bp fragments, was evident in the four primary cell lines tested, the mortal HBECs 130L and 130H, in MCF-10F cells and in BP-transformed cell lines. A similar pattern of expression was also observed for the 168-bp fragment (Fig. 2.23). β-actin gene expression, used as control of equal sampling, appeared to be similar in all the samples tested by RNase protection analysis (Fig. 2.23). These results, confirmed by Northern blot analysis, indicated that we have cloned a novel serpin different from human α1-ACT that was present as two isoforms in differentiated human breast epithelial cells and in liver tissue [22].

The physiological function of this novel serpin in human breast is completely unknown. It is clearly a biomarker of lobular differentiation because of its preferential expression in the more differentiated HBEC obtained from Lob 3 as compared to those obtained from Lob 1, as determined by differential display and reverse Northern analyses. In fact, it is of interest to note that expression of the novel serpin, as determined by RNase protection analyses, was higher in primary cultures established from breast tissues containing more of the well-differentiated structures than those containing a lower amount of the more differentiated structures. Since degree of mammary lobular differentiation is a critical determinant of mammary susceptibility to carcinogenesis [30], the preferential expression of the novel serpin in more differentiated epithelium may confer protection against breast cancer development, as has been proposed for other differentiation-associated genes [15, 24]. Thus, it is reasonable to speculate that silencing of the serpin in the normal undifferentiated Lob 1, which is known to be the site of origin of ductal carcinomas [19, 70], may render the mammary cells susceptible to events leading to carcinogenesis [15, 24]. This notion is supported by our evidence that the full-length transcription of the novel serpin is indeed down regulated during the process of immortalization and neoplastic transformation of human breast epithelial cells in vitro. We have evaluated the expression of the differently sized transcripts of the novel serpin in relation to lobular differentiation and found that the Lob 1 has no expression, whereas the Lob 3 has sufficient expression of this serpin (Fig. 2.24) [22].

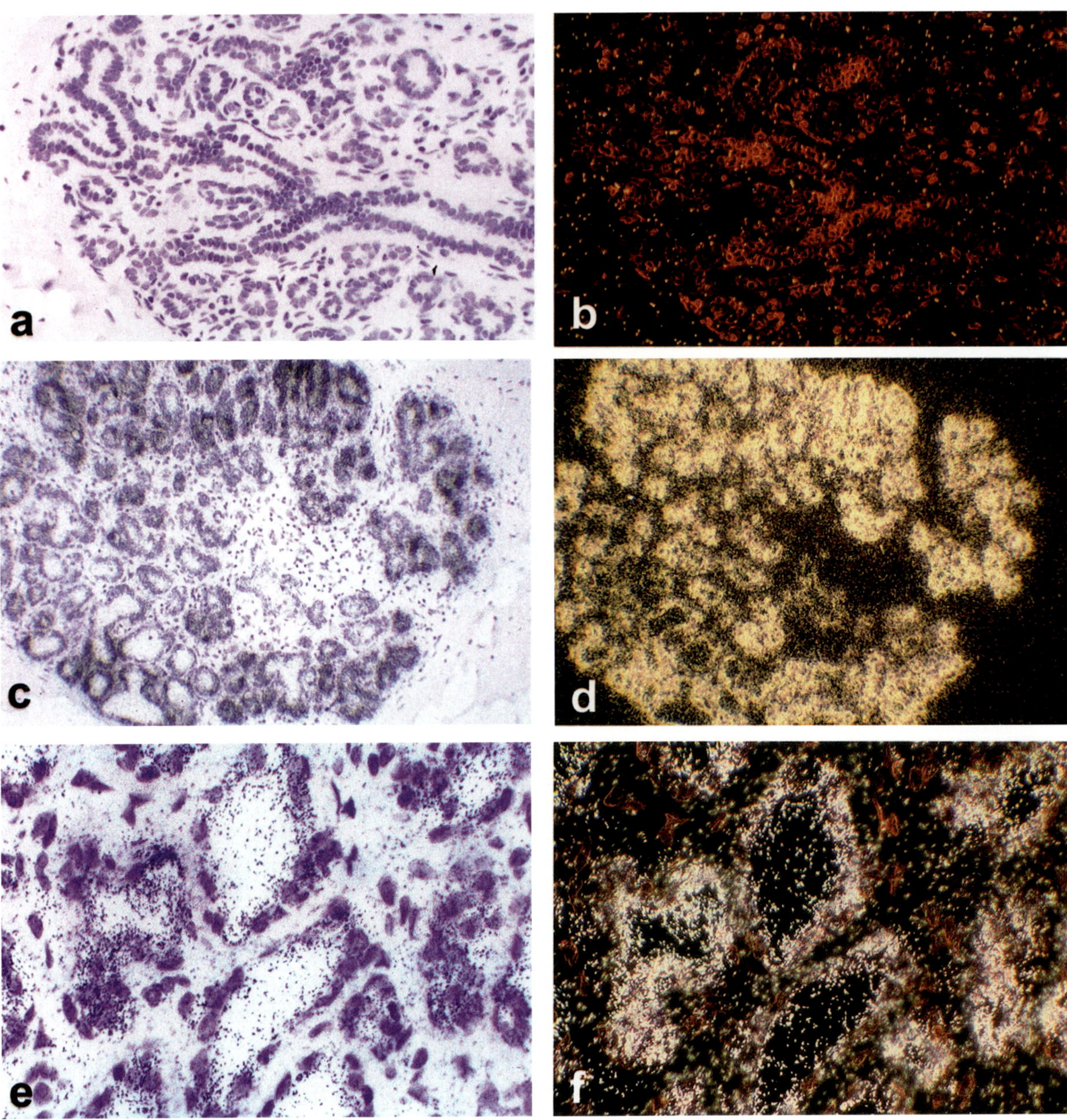

Figure 2.24a–f

Histological characteristics and localization of a serpin-like mRNA by in situ hybridization in normal breast tissues with varying degree of lobular differentiation. **a** Low level of expression in lobule type 1 (Lob 1) (bright field, ×2.5). **b** Lob 1 shown in **a** in dark field (×2.5). **c** intense reactivity in Lob 4 (bright field, ×2.5). **d** Lob 4 shown in **c** in dark field (×2.5). **e** Acini of Lob 4 showing intense reactivity in luminal epithelial cells (bright field, ×40), and **f** same as acini shown in **e** in dark field (×40)

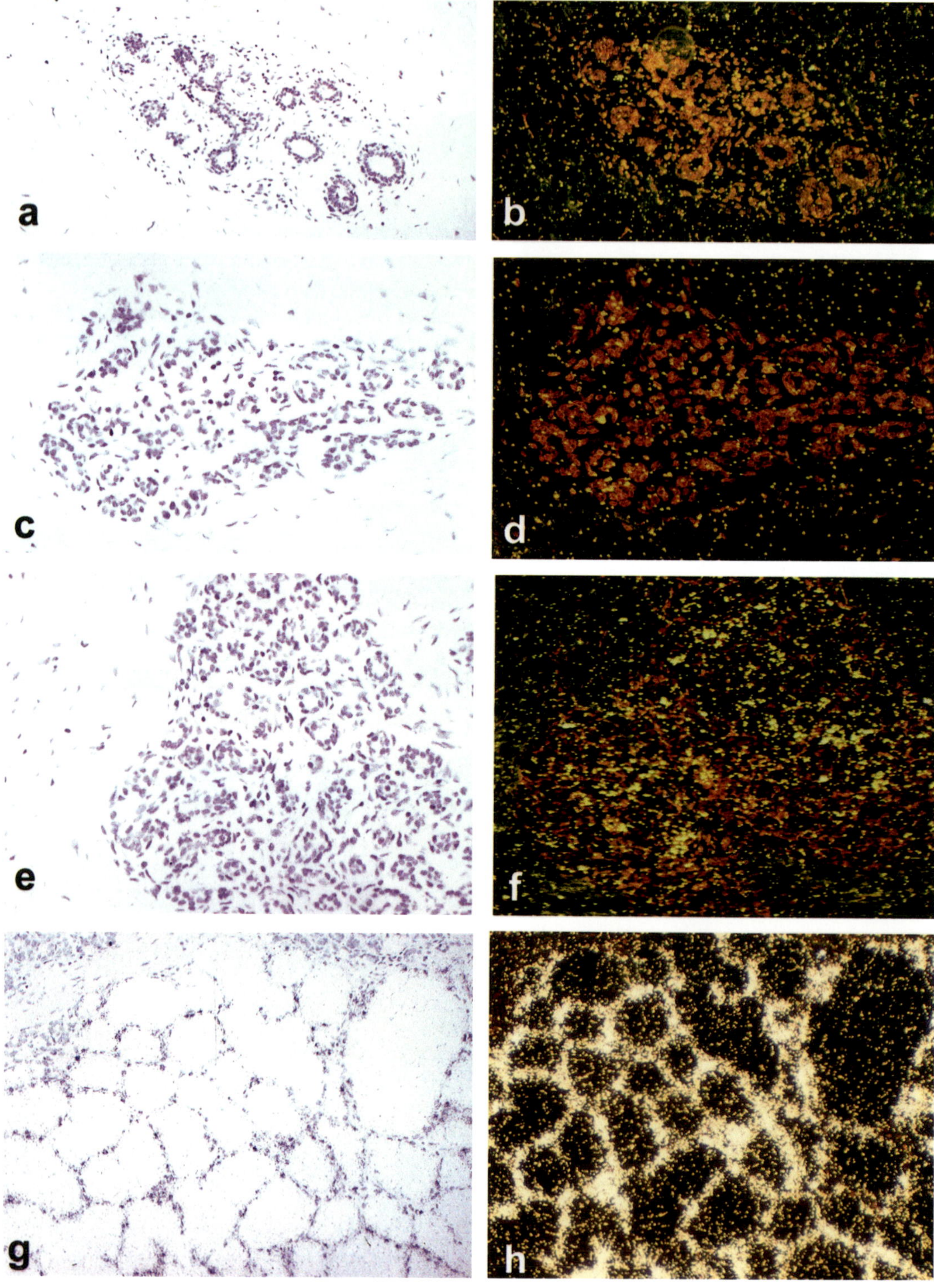

◄ Figure 2.25 a–h

Histological characteristics and expression of MDGI in normal breast tissues with varying degree of lobular differentiation. Progressively increasing level of expression from the least differentiated lobules type 1 **a, b** Lob 1, to **c, d** Lob 2; and **e, f** moderately differentiated Lob 3, to **g, h** maximal expression in the fully differentiated Lob 4. **a, c, e,** and **g**: bright field, H & E, × 2.5; **b, d, f,** and **h**: dark field, × 2.5

2.13 Mammary-Derived Growth Inhibitor

Mammary-derived growth inhibitor (MDGI) has been shown to induce rodent mammary gland differentiation, to suppress human breast cancer cell growth in vitro, and carcinogenesis in transfected human breast cancer cells [71]. It was first detected in ascitic fluid; where it inhibited the growth of Ehrlich ascites carcinoma cells [72]. MDGI belongs to a multigene family of fatty acid-binding proteins (FABP) known to bind long-chain fatty acids, retinoids, and eicosanoids [73]. The amino-acid sequence of MDGI and/or the gene encoding it have been sequenced in cattle [74], rat [75] mouse [76], and human heart [71]. The human heart FABP3, which is considered to be an identical homologue to the bovine MDGI, covers an 8-kb region of genomic DNA [77]. This gene has been localized to chromosome 1p32–35 [71], a locus that has been associated with frequent loss of heterozygosity in sporadic breast cancer [78–80], suggesting that MDGI serves as a tumor suppressor gene.

We have cloned MDGI from cultured HBECs as a 640-bp fragment that contained a single open reading frame encoding a protein of 133 amino acids identical to MDGI/FABP3. In situ hybridization analysis of paraffin-embedded normal human breast tissues revealed that HBEC-MDGI was highly expressed in the most differentiated Lob 4, poorly expressed in moderately differentiated Lob 3, and absent in the least differentiated Lob 1 and Lob 2 (Fig. 2.25). In addition, HBEC-MDGI was not expressed in breast tissues that contained ductal hyperplasia, carcinoma in situ or invasive carcinomas. Our results suggest that HBEC-

MDGI is a biomarker of lobular differentiation in the human breast, and its expression is silenced in poorly differentiated lobules as well as in the early and late stages of breast cancer progression [15, 24]. In light of a strong correlation between MDGI expression and lobular differentiation, and the fact that the degree of mammary differentiation is a critical determinant of mammary susceptibility to carcinogenesis [17], it is tempting to speculate that the protective effects of pregnancy against breast cancer may result from expression of MDGI, which might be in turn responsible for pregnancy-associated mammary differentiation, however, more studies in this direction are necessary.

2.14 Conclusions

The human breast undergoes a complete series of changes from intrauterine life to senescence. These changes can be divided into two distinct phases; the developmental phase and the differentiation phase. The developmental phase includes the early stages of gland morphogenesis, from nipple epithelium to lobule formation. In lobule formation, both processes, development and differentiation, take place almost simultaneously. For example, the progressive transition of Lob 1 to Lob 2, Lob 3, and Lob 4 requires active cell proliferation, to acquire the cell mass necessary for the function of milk secretion. This latter process implies differentiation of the mammary epithelium. Therefore, the presence of Lob 4 is the maximal expression of development and differentiation in the adult gland. It is important to point out that even though the presence of proteins that are indicative of milk product synthesis, such as α-lactalbumin, casein, or milk fat globule type membrane protein, are indicators of breast epithelial cellular differentiation, only when all the milk components are coordinately synthesized within the appropriate structure can full differentiation of the mammary gland be acknowledged.

References

1. Tanner, J.M. (Ed) The development of the reproductive system. In: Growth at Adolescence, Blackwell Scientific, Oxford, UK, pp 28–39, 1962.
2. Vorherr, H. (Ed) Development of the female breast. In: The Breast, Academic Press, New York, pp.1–18, 1974.
3. Russo, J. and Russo, I.H. In: The Mammary Gland (Neville, M.C. and Daniel, C.W. Eds), Plenum Publishing Corporation, New York, NY. pp 67–93, 1987.
4. Russo, I.H., and Russo, J. Mammary gland neoplasia in long-term rodent studies. Environ. Health Perspect. 104: 938–967, 1996.
5. Jemal, A., Murray, T., Samuels, A., Ghafoor, A., Ward, E., and Thun, M. J. Cancer Statistics, 2003. CA Cancer J. Clin. 53: 5–26, 2003.
6. Chu, K.C., Tarone, R.E., Brawley, O.W. Breast cancer trends of black women compared with white women. Archives of Family Medicine 8:521–528, 1999.
7. MacMahon, B., Cole, P., Liu, M., Lowe, C.R., Mirra, A.P., Ravin, I., Har, B., Salber, E.J., Valaoras, V.G. and Yuasa, S. Age at first birth and breast cancer risk. Bull. World Health Organ. 34:209–221, 1970.
8. McGregor, D.H., Land, C.E., Choi, K., Tokuoka, S., Liu, P.I., Wakabayashi, I., Beebe, G.W. Breast cancer incidence among atomic bomb survivors, Hiroshima and Nagasaki 1950–1989. J. Natl. Cancer Inst. 59:799–811, 1977.
9. De Waard, F. and Trichopoulos, D. A unifying concept of the etiology of breast cancer. Int. J. Cancer 41:666–669, 1988.
10. Henderson, B.E., Ross, R.K. and Pike, M.C. Hormonal chemoprevention of cancer in women. Science 9:633–638, 1993.
11. Briand, P., Petersen, O.W., van Dews, B. A new diploid nontumorigenic human breast epithelial cell line isolated and propagated in chemically defined medium. In vitro Cell Dev. Biol. 23:181–188, 1987.
12. Rosner, B., Colditz, G.A. and Willett, W.C. Reproductive risk factors in a prospective study of breast cancer: The nurses health study. Am. J. Epidemiol. 139:819–835, 1994.
13. Russo, I.H., and Russo, J. Role of hCG and inhibin in breast cancer. Int. J. Oncol. 4:297–306, 1994.
14. Hu, Y.F., Russo, I.H., Ao, X., and Russo, J. Mammary derived growth inhibitor (MDGI) cloned from human breast epithelial cells is expressed in fully differentiated lobular structures. Int. J. Oncol. 11:5–11, 1997.
15. Hu, Y.F., Silva, I.D.C.G., Russo, I.H. Ao, X. and Russo, J. A novel serpin gene cloned from differentiated human breast epithelial cells is a potential tumor suppressor. Proc. Am. Assoc. Cancer Res., 39: 775, 1998.
16. Mailo, D., Russo, J., Sheriff, F., Hu, Y.F., Tahin, Q., Mihaila, D., Balogh, G. and Russo, I.H. Genomic signature induced my differentiation in the rat mammary gland. Proc. Am. Assoc. Cancer Res. 43:2002.
17. Russo, J., Reina, D., Frederick, J. and Russo, I.H. Expression of phenotypical changes by human breast epithelial cells treated with carcinogens in vitro. Cancer Res. 48:2837–2857, 1988.
18. Russo, J., Mills, M.J, Moussalli, M.J. and Russo, I.H. Influence of breast development and growth properties in vitro. In vitro Cell Develop. Biol. 25:643–649, 1989.
19. Russo, J., Gusterson, B.A., Rogers, A.E., Russo, I.H., Wellings, S.R. and Van Zwieten, M.J. Comparative study of human and rat mammary tumorigenesis. Lab. Invest. 62:1–32, 1991.
20. Russo, J., Romero, A.L. and Russo, I.H. Architectural pattern of the normal and cancerous breast under the influence of parity. J. Cancer Epidemiol., Biomarkers & Prevention 3:219–224, 1994.
21. Russo, J., Rivera, R. and Russo, I.H. Influence of age and parity on the development of the human breast. Breast Cancer Res. Treat. 23:211–218, 1992.
22. Russo, J. Hu, Y-F., Silva, I.D.C.G., and Russo, I.H. Cancer risk related to mammary gland structure and development. Microsc. Res Tech. 52:204–223, 2001.
23. Russo J, Tay, L.K. and Russo IH. Differentiation of the mammary gland and susceptibility to carcinogenesis. Breast Cancer Res. Treat. 2:5–73, 1982.
24. Hu, Y.F., Russo, I.H., Zalipsky, U., and Russo, J. Lack of involvement of bcl2 and cyclin D1 in the early phases of human breast epithelial cell transformation by environmental chemical carcinogens. Proc. Am. Assoc. Cancer Res. 37:1005a, 1996.
25. Russo, J. and Russo, I.H. Role of differentiation in the pathogenesis and prevention of breast cancer. Endocrine-Related Cancer 4:1–15, 1997.
26. Russo, J., Hu, Y-F., Yang, X. and Russo, I.H. Developmental, cellular, and molecular basis of human breast cancer: J. Natl. Cancer Inst. Monograph 27, pp 17–38, 2000.
27. Russo, J. and Russo, I.H. Development of the Human Breast. In: Encyclopedia of Reproduction, (E. Knobil and J. D. Neill, Eds.) Academic Press, New York, Vol. 3, pp 71–80, 1998.
28. Russo, J. and Russo, I.H. The cellular basis of breast cancer susceptibility. Oncol. Res., 11:169–178, 1999.
29. Russo, J. and Russo, I.H. Development pattern of human breast and susceptibility to carcinogenesis. European J. Cancer Prevent. 2:85–100, 1993.
30. Russo, J. and Russo, I.H. Toward a physiological approach to breast cancer prevention. Cancer Epidemiology, Biomarkers & Prev. 3:353–364, 1994.
31. Xie, J., Haslam, S.Z. Extracellular matrix regulates ovarian hormone-dependent proliferation of mouse mammary epithelial cells. Endocrinology. 138:2466–73, 1997
32. Petersen, O.W., Ronnov-Jessen, L., Weaver, V.M., Bissell, M.J. Differentiation and cancer in the mammary gland: shedding light on an old dichotomy. Adv. Cancer Res. 75:135–61, 1998.
33. Russo, J., Lynch, H., and Russo, I.H. Mammary gland architecture as a determining factor in the susceptibility of the human breast to cancer. Breast Journal 7:278–291, 2001.

34. Kumar, V., Stack, G.S., Berry, M., Jin, J.R. and Chambon, P. Functional domains of the human estrogen receptor. Cell 51:941–951, 1987.

35. King, R.J.B. Effects of steroid hormones and related compounds on gene transcription. Clin. Endocrinol. 36:1–14, 1992.

36. Soto, A.M. and Sonnenschein, C. Cell proliferation of estrogen-sensitive cells: the case for negative control. Endocr. Rev. 48:52–58, 1987.

37. Huseby, R.A., Maloney, T.M. and McGrath, C.M. Evidence for a direct growth-stimulating effect of estradiol on human MCF-7 cells in vitro. Cancer Res. 144:2654–2659, 1987.

38. Huff, K.K., Knabbe, C., Lindsey, R., Kaufman, D., Bronzert, D., Lippman, M.E., Dickson, R.B. Multi hormonal regulation of insulin-like growth factor-1 -related protein in MCF-7 human breast cancer cells. Mol. Endocrinol. 2:200–208, 1988.

39. Dickson, R.B., Huff, K.K., Spencer, E.M. and Lippman, M.E. Introduction of epidermal growth factor related polypeptides by 17β-estradiol in MCF-7 human breast cancer cells. Endocrinol. 118:138–142, 1986.

40. Page, M.J., Field, J.K., Everett, P and Green, C.D. Serum regulation of the estrogen responsiveness of the human breast cancer cell line MCF-7. Cancer Res. 43:1244–1250, 1983.

41. Katzenellenbogen, B.S., Kendra, K.L., Norman, M.J. and Berthois, Y. Proliferation, hormonal responsiveness and estrogen receptor content of MCF-7 human breast cancer cells growth in the short-term and long-term absence of estrogens. Cancer Res. 47:4355–4360, 1987.

42. Aakvaag, A., Utaacker, E., Thorsen, T., Lea, O.A. and Lahooti, H. Growth control of human mammary cancer cells MCF-7 cells in culture: Effect of estradiol and growth factors in serum containing medium. Cancer Res. 50:7806–810, 1991.

43. Dell'aquilla, M.L., Pigott, D.A., Bonaquist, D.L. and Gaffney, E.V. A factor from plasma derived human serum that inhibits the growth of the mammary cell line MCF-7: characterization and purification. J. Natl. Cancer Inst. 72:291–298, 1984.

44. Markaverich, B.M., Gregory, R.R., Alejandro, M.A., Clark, J.H., Johnson, G.A. and Middleditch, B.S. Methyl p-hydroxphenyllactate. An inhibitor of cell growth and proliferation and an endogenous ligand for nuclear type-11 binding sites. J. Biol. Chem. 263:7203–7210, 1988.

45. Russo, J., Ao, X., Grill, C. and Russo, I.H. Pattern of distribution of cells positive for estrogen receptor α and progesterone receptor in relation to proliferating cells in the mammary gland. Breast Cancer Res. Treat. 53–217-227, 1999.

46. Bonte, F. Constitution de la matrice extracellulaire normal et pathologique. Arch. Anat. Cytol. Path. 433:170–172, 1995.

47. Shrevestha, P., Kusakabe, M., Mori, M. Tenascin in human neoplasia: Immuno-histochemical observations using seven different clones of monoclonal antibodies. Int. J. Oncol. 8:741–755, 1996.

48. Chiquet-Ehrisman, R., Mackie, E.J., Pearson, C.A., Sakakura, T. Tenascin: An extracellular matrix protein involved in tissue interactions during fetal development and oncogenesis. Cell 47:131–139, 1986.

49. Wrenn, D.S., Griffin, G.L., Senior, R.M., Mechan, R.P. Characterization of biologically active domain on elastin: Identification of monoclonal antibody to a cell recognition site. Biochemistry 25:5172–5176, 1986.

50. Hall, A. Rho GTPases and the actin cytoskeleton. Science 279:509–514, 1998.

51. Foster, R., Hu, K.Q., Lu, Y., Nolan, K.M., Thissen, J., Settleman, J. Identification of a novel human Rho protein with unusual properties: GTPase deficiency and in vivo farnesylation. Mol. Cell Biol. 6:2689–2699, 1996.

52. Guasch, R.M., Scambler, P., Jones, G.E., Ridley, A.J. RhoE regulates actin cytoskeleton organization and cell migration. Mol. Cell. Biol. 18:4761–4771, 1998.

53. Peng, Y., Du, K., Ramirez, S., Diamond, R.H., Taub, R. Mitogenic up-regulation of the PRL-1 protein-tyrosine phosphatase gene by Egr-1. Egr-1 activation is an early event in liver regeneration. J. Biol. Chem. 274:4513–4520, 1999.

54. Takano, S., Fukuyama, H., Fukumoto, M., Kimura, J., Xue, J.H., Ohashi, H., Fujita, J. PRL-1, a protein tyrosine phosphatase is expressed in neurons and oligodendrocytes in the brain and induced in the cerebral cortex following transient forebrain ischemia. Mol. Brain Res. 40:105–115, 1996.

55. Diamond, R.H., Peters, C., Jung, S.P., Greenbaum, L.E., Haber, B.A., Silberg, D.G., Traber, P.G., Taub, R. Expression of PRL-1 nuclear PTPase is associated with proliferation in liver but with differentiation in intestine. Am. J. Physiol. 271:121–129, 1996.

56. Rundle, C.H., Kappen, C. Developmental expression of the murine Prl-1 protein tyrosine phosphatase gene. J. Exp. Zool. 283:612–617, 1999.

57. Peng, Y., Genin, A., Spinner, N.B., Diamond, R.H., Taub, R. The gene encoding human nuclear protein tyrosine phosphatase, PRL-1. Cloning, chromosomal localization, and identification of an intron enhancer. J. Biol. Chem. 273: 17286–17295, 1998.

58. Phillips, L.S., Pao, C.I., Villafuerte, B.C. Molecular regulation of insulin-like growth factor-I and its principal binding protein, IGFBP-3. Prog Nucleic Acid Res. Mol. Biol. 60:195–265, 1998.

59. Oh, Y. IGFBPs and neoplastic models. New concepts for roles of IGFBPs in regulation of cancer cell growth. Endocrine 71:111–113, 1997.

60. Cubbage, M.L., Suwanichkul, A., Powell, D.R. Insulin-like growth factor binding protein-3. Organization of the human chromosomal gene and demonstration of promoter activity. J Biol. Chem. 265:21:12642–12649, 1990.

61. Coverley JA, Baxter RC. Phosphorylation of insulin-like growth factor binding proteins. Mol Cell Endocrinol 128:1–5, 1997.

62. Brotherick, I., Robson, C.N., Bronell, D.A. et al. Cytokeratin expression in breast cancer: phenotypic changes associated with disease progression. Cytometry 32:301–308, 1998.

63. Welch, D.R., and Wei, L.L. Genetic and epigenetic regulation of human breast cancer progression and metastasis. Endocrine Related Cancer 5:155–197, 1998.

64. Aoki, R., Tanaka, S., Haruma, K., Yoshihara, M., Sumii, K., et al. MUC-1 expression as a predictor of the curative endoscopic treatment of submucosally invasive colorectal carcinoma. Dis. Colon Rectum 41:1262–1272, 1998.

65. Segal Eiras, A., and Croce, M.V. Breast cancer associated mucin: a review. Allergol. Immunopathol. 25:176–181, 1997.

66. Manni, A., Badger, B., Wei, L. et al. Hormonal regulation of insulin-growth factor II and insulin growth factor binding protein expression by breast cancer cells in vivo. Evidence for epithelial stromal interactions. Cancer Research 54:2934–2942, 1994.

67. Russo, J., Calaf, G. and Russo, I.H. A critical approach to the malignant transformation of human breast epithelial cells. CRC Critical Reviews in Oncogenesis 4:403–417, 1993.

68. Chandra, T., Stackhouse, R., Kidd, V.J., Robson, K.J. and Woo, S.L. Sequence homology between human alpha 1-antichymotrypsin, alpha 1-antitrypsin and antibrombin III. Biochemistry 22:5055–5061, 1983.

69. Rubin, H., Wang, Z.M., Nickbarg, E.B., McLarney, S., Naidoo, N., Schoenberger, O.L., Johnson, J.L. and Cooperman, B.S. Cloning expression, purification and biological activity of recombinant native and variant human a1-antichymotrypsin. J. Biol. Chem. 265:1199–1207, 1990.

70. Wellings, S.R., Jansen, M.M. and Marcum, R.G. An atlas of sub-gross pathology of the human breast with special reference to possible pre-cancerous lesions. J.N.C.I. 55:231–275,1975.

71. Huynh, H.T., Larsson, C., Narod, S. and Pollak, M. Tumor suppressor activity of the gene encoding mammary-derive growth inhibitor. Cancer Res. 55:2225–2231, 1995.

72. Lehmann, W., Graetz, H., Schutt, M. and Langen, P. Chalone-like inhibition of Ehrlich ascites cell proliferation in vitro by an ultra-filtrate obtained from the ascetic fluid. Acta Biol. Med. Germ. 36:K43-K52, 1977.

73. Veerkamp, J.H., Peeters, R.A. and Maatman, R.G. Structural and functional features of different types of cytoplasmic fatty acid-binding proteins. Biochim. Biophys. Acta 1081: 1–24, 1991.

74. Bohmer, F.D., Kraft, R., Otto, A., Wernstedt, C., Hellman, U., Kurtz, A., Muller, T., Rohde, K., Etzold, G., Lehmann, W., Langen, P., Heldin, C.H. and Grosse, R. Identification of a polypeptide growth inhibitor from bovine mammary gland. Sequence homology to fatty acids and retinoid binding proteins. J. Biol. Chem. 262:15137–15143, 1987.

75. Jones, P.D., Carne, A., Bass, N.M. and Grigor, M.R. Isolation and characterization of fatty acid binding proteins from mammary tissue of lactating rats. Biochem. J. 251:919–925, 1988.

76. Tweedie, S. and Edwards, Y. cDNA sequence for mouse heart fatty acid binding protein, H-FABP. Nucleic Acid Res. 17:4374–4377, 1989.

77. Phelan, C.M., Larsson, C., Baird, S., Futreal, P.A., Ruttledge, M.H., Morgan, K., Tonin, P., Hung, H., Korneluk, R.G., Pollak, M.N. and Narod, S.A. The human mammary-derived growth inhibitor (MDGI) gene: genomic structure and mutation analysis in human breast tumors. Genomics 34:63–68, 1996.

78. Genuardi, M., TsI.Hira, H., Anderson, D.E. & Saunders, G.F. Distal deletion of chromosome lp in ductal carcinoma of the breast. Am. J. Hum. Genet. 45:73–82, 1989.

79. Bieche, I., Champeme, M.H. and Lidereau, R. A tumor suppressor gene on chromosome 1p32 pter controls the amplification of myc family genes in breast cancer. Cancer Res. 54:4274–4276, 1994.

80. Bieche, I., Champeme, M.H., Matifas, F., Cropp, C.S., Callahan, R. and Lidereau, R. Two distinct regions involved in 1p deletion in human primary breast cancer. Cancer Res. 53:1990–1994, 1993.

Endocrine Control of Breast Development

3.1 Introduction

The breast is a hormone-responsive organ *par excellence*. Its development is influenced by a myriad of hormones and growth factors whose stimulus selectively elicits a response consisting of cell proliferation, cell differentiation, or cell death (apoptosis) [1–11]. In either case, the response of the mammary gland to these complex influences results in developmental changes that permanently modify both the architecture and the biological characteristics of the gland [3, 4]. Among the varied hormonal influences affecting the breast, estrogens are considered to play a major role in promoting the proliferation of both the normal and the neoplastic breast epithelium [2–5, 11]. Estrogens act locally on the mammary gland stimulating DNA synthesis and promoting bud formation, an effect that has traditionally been considered to be receptor-mediated, Although this is the most widely accepted mechanism of action of this steroid hormone [10–14], at least two additional mechanisms, an autocrine/paracrine loop [15, 16] and/or a negative feedback [17] are also considered to of importance in these hormonal effects. It is generally accepted that the biological activities of estrogens are mediated by the nuclear estrogen receptor (ER) which, upon activation by cognate ligands, forms a homodimer with another ER-ligand complex and activates transcription of specific genes containing the estrogen response elements (ERE) [18]. According to this classic model, the biological responses to estrogens are mediated by the well-characterized ER, which has to be re-named estrogen receptor alpha (ERα) [19], after the cloning of a new type of

ER, the ERβ from the rat [20], mouse [21] and human [22] tissues.

From Beatson's initial report in 1896 that removal of ovaries, and concomitant reduction in circulating estrogen, could induce remission of advanced breast cancer [23], to the more sophisticated manipulation of tumors with anti-estrogenic compounds in the present day [24, 25], it is clear that a significant percentage of tumors are dependent upon estrogen for proliferation. The functions of estrogens in promoting tumor progression are partly, but not completely, understood (Fig. 3.1). In excess of 92% and 72% breast cancers express ER-α mRNA and protein, respectively [26]. The receptor is activated by binding of estrogenic ligands, translocates to the nucleus, and activates transcription of target genes associated with tumor progression. Administration of tamoxifen, a competitive antagonist of estrogen binding to ER-α, abrogates the transcriptional response, and induces tumor cell apoptosis. Mounting evidence also suggests an alternative role for estrogen in non-transcription mediated signaling pathways [19] (Fig. 3.1). Additional genetic or epigenetic factors modulate estrogen response and/or cell survival. A variety of studies have identified modulating factors including oncoproteins, growth factors, and signaling molecules such as Ha-Ras, Rafl, FGF-1 and -4, TGF-beta, HER2/NEU and Cyclin D1 [24, 25], and it is likely that more exist. Whether the action of these factors is intrinsically linked to the core estrogenic signaling pathway, or proceeds through alternative signaling pathways to result in similar biological endpoints (i.e., resistance to apoptosis; enhanced metastasis; others) need to be clarified. In vivo estrogen elicits phosphorylation of cAMP response element-binding

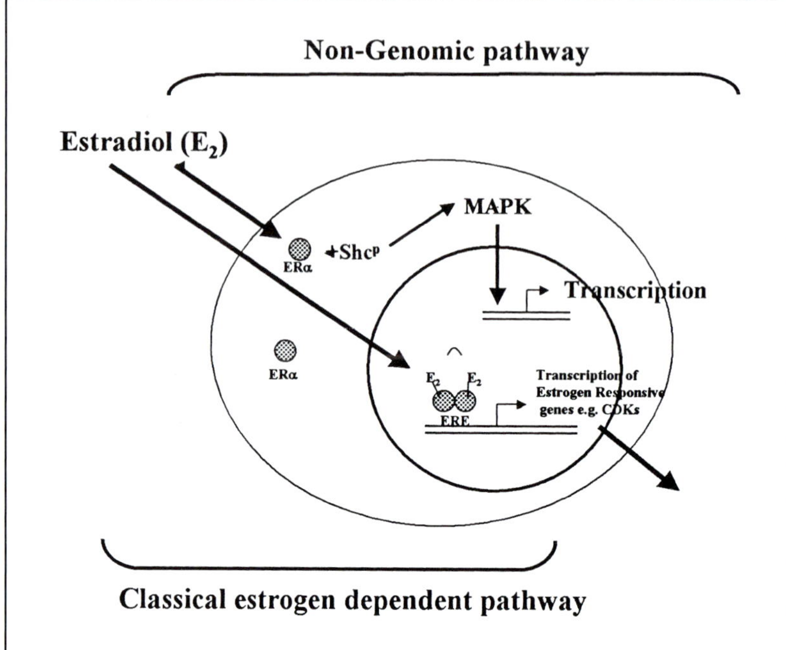

Figure 3.1

The functions of estrogens in promoting tumor progression. In the classical estrogen-dependent pathway, estradiol (*E2*) binds estrogen receptor α (*ERα*) and the resulting complex binds to estrogen-response-elements (*ERE*) resulting in the transcription of genes that promote cellular proliferation, for example cyclin-dependent kinases (*CDKs*). Recently, non-genomic (that is, not involving ERα-induced transcription) pathways of estrogenic action have been elucidated. In the indicated pathway used as an example, estradiol stimulates phosphorylation of the adapter protein Shc and interaction with ERα. Subsequently, there is activation of MAPK and downstream gene transcription

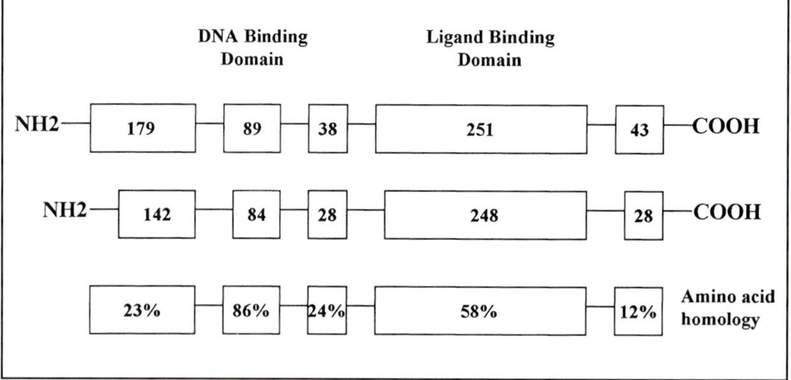

Figure 3.2

Numbers in boxes indicate number of amino acids

protein (CREB) [27, 28]. Erα is capable of activating the MAPK pathway and downstream gene transcription through estrogen-mediated stimulation of phosphorylation of the adaptor protein Shc (Fig. 3.1).

The presence of ERα in target tissue or cells is essential to their responsiveness to estrogen action. In fact, the expression levels of ERα in a particular tissue have been used as an index of the degree of estrogen responsiveness. A vast majority of human breast carcinomas are initially positive for ERα, and their growth can be stimulated by estrogens and inhibited by anti-estrogens [29–32]. ERβ and ERα share high sequence homology, especially in the regions or domains responsible for specific binding to DNA and the ligands (Fig. 3.2) [20–22, 33]. ERβ can be activated by estrogen stimulation, and blocked with anti-estrogens [20, 22, 33]. Upon activation, ERβ can form homodimers as well as heterodimers with ERα

[33–37]. The existence of two ER subtypes and their ability to form DNA-binding heterodimers suggests three potential pathways of estrogen signaling: via the ERα or ERβ subtype in tissues exclusively expressing each subtype and via the formation of heterodimers in tissues expressing both ERα and ERβ [35]. In addition, estrogens and anti-estrogens can induce differential activation of ERα and ERβ to control transcription of genes that are under the control of an AP1 element [38].

Progesterone is another major, though controversial, player in mammary gland biology. This ovarian steroidal hormone also acts, in conjunction with estrogen, through its specific receptor PgR in the normal epithelium for regulating breast development. The role of these hormones on the proliferative activity of the breast, which is indispensable for its normal growth and development, has been for a long time, and still is, the subject of heated controversies. Although estrogen is known to stimulate cell proliferation, the breast epithelium of sexually mature and normally cycling women does not exhibit maximal proliferation during the follicular phase of the menstrual cycle [8, 9, 39–44], when estrogens reach peak levels of 200–300 pg/ml while progesterone is less than 1 ng/ml [45]. Instead, the breast epithelium exhibits its maximal proliferative activity during the luteal phase, when progesterone levels reach 10–20 ng/ml and estrogen levels are 2- to 3-fold lower than those observed during the follicular phase. These observations are puzzling when analyzed in light of in vitro and experimental data, since estrogen stimulates the proliferation of cultured breast cells and breast tissues implanted in athymic nude mice. Progesterone, on the other hand, has no effect or even inhibits cell growth in the same models [43, 44].

In addition to its response to circulating hormones, the proliferative activity of the mammary epithelium in both rodents and humans varies with the degree of differentiation of the mammary parenchyma [2–5, 46–48]. In women, the highest level of cell proliferation is observed in the undifferentiated Lob 1 present in the breast of young nulliparous females [2–5]. The progressive differentiation of Lob 1 into Lob 2 and Lob 3, occurring under the hormonal influences of the menstrual cycle, and the full differentiation into lobules type 4 (Lob. 4) as the result of pregnancy leads to a concomitant reduction in the proliferative activity of the mammary epithelium [2–5, 46–48] (see Chapter 2).

3.2 Steroid Receptors, Cell Proliferation, and Breast Differentiation

The relationship of lobular differentiation, cell proliferation and hormone responsiveness of the mammary epithelium is just beginning to be unraveled. Of interest is the fact that the content of ERα and PgR in the lobular structures of the breast is directly proportional to the rate of cell proliferation. These three parameters are maximal in the undifferentiated Lob 1, decreasing progressively in Lob 2, Lob 3, and Lob 4 (Fig. 3.3, Table 3.1). The determination of the rate of

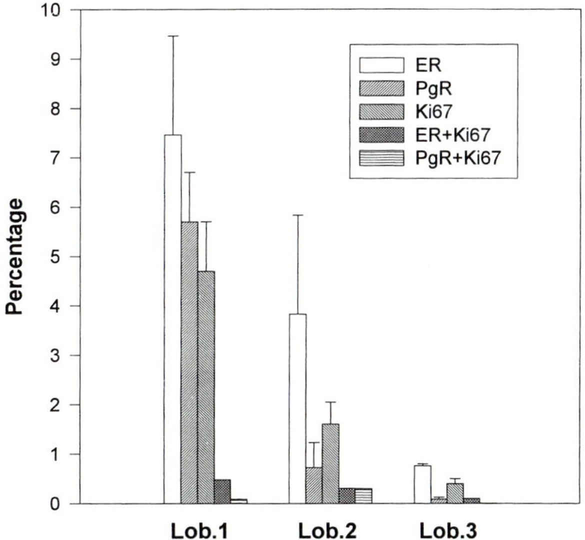

Figure 3.3

Percentage of cells positive for estrogen receptor (*ER*), progesterone receptor (*PgR*), proliferating cells (*Ki67*), and of cells positive for both ER and Ki67 (*ER+Ki67*), or PgR and Ki67 (*PgR+Ki67*) (ordinate). Cells were quantitated in Lob 1, Lob 2, and Lob 3 of the breast (abscissa) (reproduced with permission from: Russo, J., et al. Breast Cancer Research and Treatment 53:217–227, 1999)

Table 3.1. Distribution of Ki67-, ER-, and PgR-positive cells in the lobular structures of the human breast

Lobule type	Number of cells	Ki67	ER	PgR	Ki67+E	Ki67+PgR
Lob 1	19,339[a]	4.72±l.00[d,e]	7.46±2.88[h]	5.70±1.36[k]	0.48±t:0.28[h]	0.09±0.01[o]
Lob 2	8,490[b]	1.58±0.45[f]	3.83±2.44[i]	0.73±0.57[l]	0.31±0.21	0.28±0.27
Lob 3	17,750[c]	0.40±0.18[g]	0.76±0.04[j]	0.09±0.04[m]	0.01±0.01	0.01±0.01

[a] Total number of cells counted in Lob1 in breast tissue samples of 12 donors

[b] Total number of cells counted in Lob2 in breast tissue samples of five donors

[c] Total number of cells counted in Lob3 in breast tissue samples of three donors

[d] Proliferative activity determined by the percentage cells Ki67-positive, expressed as the mean ± standard deviation (SD) Differences were significant in [e] Lob 1 vs. [f] lob 2 ($t=1.98; p<0.05$), [f] Lob 2 vs. [g] Lob3 ($t=2.27; p<0.04$), and [e] Lob 1 vs. [g] Lob 3 ($t=2.56; p<0.01$)

ER-positive cells were significantly different in [h] Lob 1 vs. [i] Lob 2 and [j] Lob 3 ($t=2.04; p<0.05$). PgR-positive cells were significantly different in [k] Lob 1 vs. [l] Lob 2 ($t=2.27; p<0.05$), and [k] Lob 1 vs. [m] Lob 3 ($t=2.60; p<0.03$)

[n] Percentage of cells positive for both Ki67 and ER, expressed as the mean ± SD

[o] Percentage of cells positive for both, Ki67 and PgR, expressed as the mean ± SD

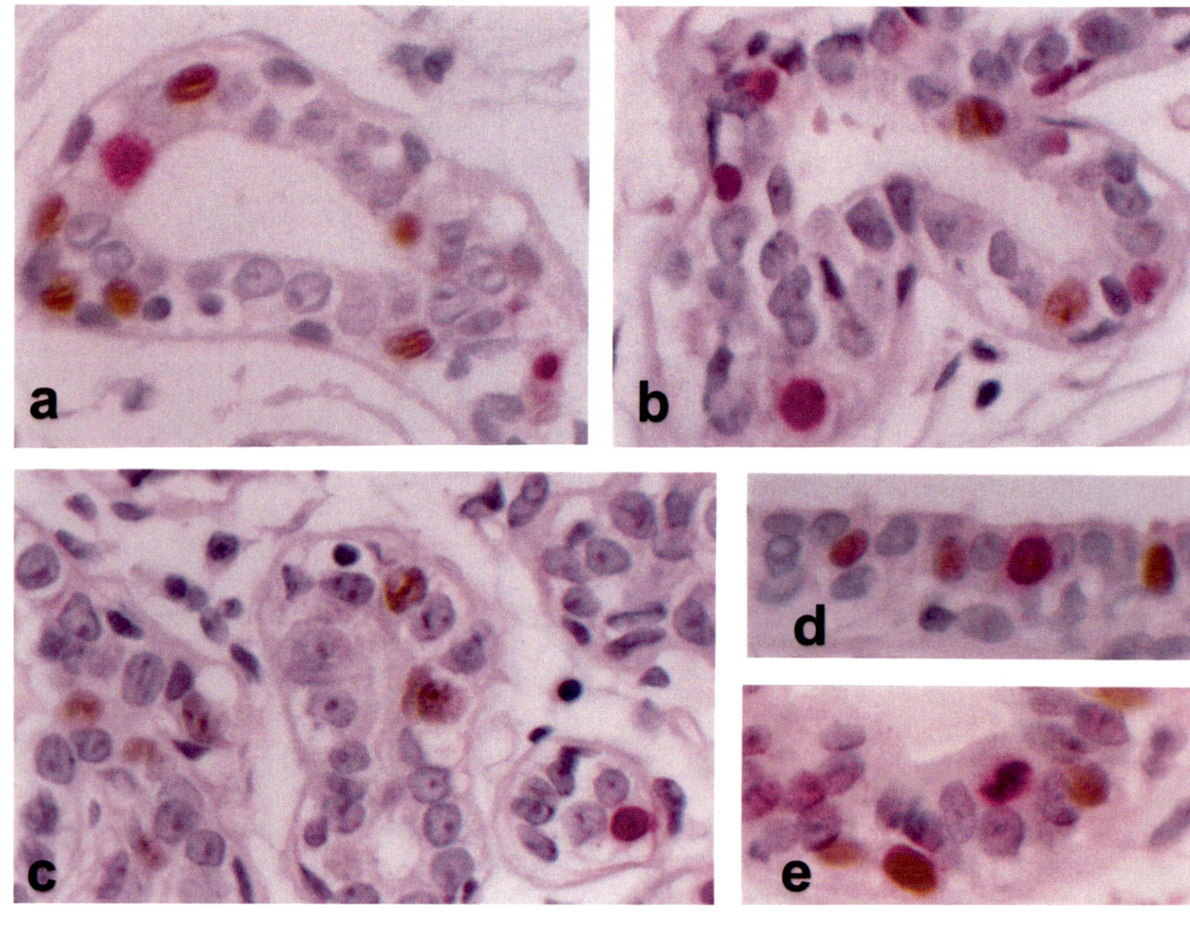

cell proliferation, expressed as the percentage of cells that stain positively with Ki67 antibody, has revealed that proliferating cells are predominantly found in the epithelium lining ducts and lobules, and less frequently in the myoepithelium and in the intralobular and interlobular stroma. Ki67-positive cells are most frequently found in Lob 1 (Fig. 3.4, Table 3.1). The percentage of positive cells is reduced by three-fold in Lob 2 and by more than ten-fold in Lob 3 (Fig. 3.3) [4, 49]. ERα- and PgR-positive cells are found exclusively in the epithelium; the myoepithelium and the stroma are totally devoid of steroid receptor containing cells. The highest number of cells positive for both receptors is found in Lob 1, decreasing progressively in Lob 2 and Lob 3 [49].

3.2.1 Relationship of Proliferating and ERα-Positive Cells in the Human Breast

We utilized a double staining procedure in order to clarify the relationship between steroid receptor positive cells and proliferating cells. A single tissue section was incubated with antibodies against Ki67 and ERα, Ki67 and PgR, or ERα and PgR. Each antibody was identified by its color reaction, brown with 3,3'-diaminobenzidine-HCl (DAB), or red with the alkaline phosphatase-vector red [49]. This procedure allowed us to quantitatively determine the spatial relationship between those cells that are proliferating and those that react with either ERα or PgR antibod-

ies. It was found that a higher percentage of cells reacted simultaneously with both ERα and PgR, appearing purple red in color (Fig. 3.4), whereas the number of cells positive for both ERα and Ki67 or PgR and Ki67 was very low (Table 3.1). The highest percentage of ERα-, PgR-, and Ki67-positive cells was observed in Lob 1. In Lob 2 the percentages of Ki67-, ERα-, and PgR-positive cells was reduced to 1.6, 3.8, and 0.7%, respectively. In Lob 3 the percentage of cells positive for these markers became negligible (Table 3.1). Of interest was the observation that even though there were similarities in the relative percentages of Ki67-, ERα- and PgR-positive cells, and in the progressive reduction in the percentage of positive cells as the lobular differentiation progressed, those cells positive for Ki67 were not the same that reacted positively for ERα or PgR (Fig. 3.4) [49]. Very few cells, less than 0.5% in Lob 1, and even fewer in Lob 2 and Lob 3, were simultaneously positive for both Ki67 and ERα (Ki67+ER) or Ki67 and PgR (Ki67+PgR) (Table 3.1). Despite their low percentage, still double labeled (Ki67+ER) cells were more numerous in Lob 1, decreasing gradually in Lob 2 and Lob 3. The percentage of cells exhibiting double labeling with Ki67 and PgR, on the other hand, were more numerous in Lob 2 than in Lob 1, but decreased to the same levels observed for ERα in Lob 3 (Table 3.1).

3.2.2 Cell Proliferation, ERα, and PgR Content in the Rat Mammary Gland

The mammary gland of young cycling virgin rats is composed of a ductal system ending in club-shaped terminal end buds (TEB) or primitive ductular, alveolar buds (AB) and lobular structures. The epithelium lining the TEB is multilayered, exhibiting active cell proliferation, as indicated by the presence of mitotic figures and active incorporation of ^{3}H-thymidine (thymidine or DNA-labeling index [DNA-LI]). Administration of ^{3}H-thymidine to 45-day-old virgin rats one hour before they were killed revealed ^{3}H-thymidine incorporation in more than 20% of the cells (Figs. 3.5, 3.6). The DNA-LI became markedly reduced in AB and lobules (Fig. 3.5, Table 3.2). Proliferating cells were also detected in the stroma, but they

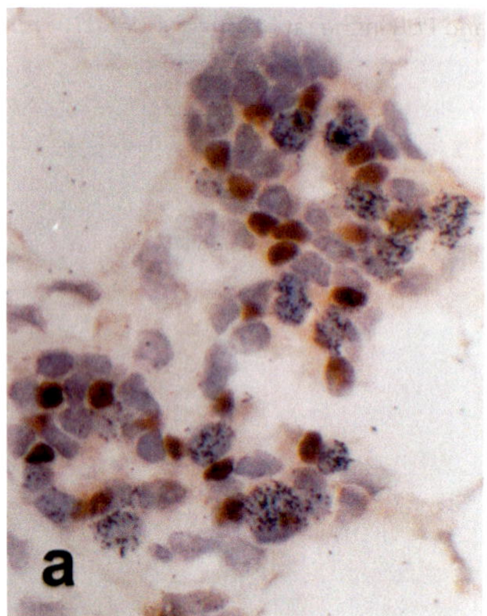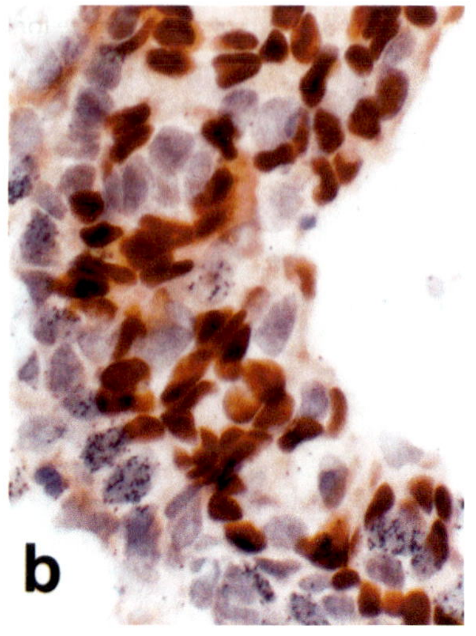

Figure 3.5 a, b

Rat mammary gland autoradiography, immunoreacted with **a** ER and **b** PgR antibodies. **a** Lob 1 ductules. The *black stippling* of *silver* grains indicates ³H-thymidine incorporation (S phase), the *brown* nuclear reaction ER-positive cells. **b** Multilayered epithelium of a terminal end bud (TEB) containing cells in the S phase of the cycle (*stippled nuclei*) and the brown reaction of PgR-positive cells (DAB-hematoxylin, ×40)

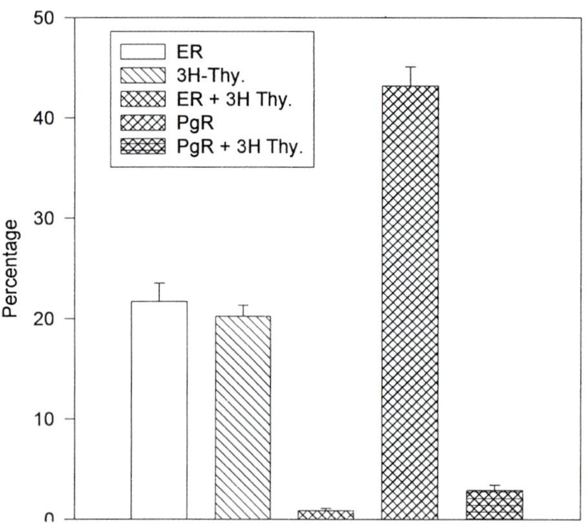

Figure 3.6

Histogram showing the percentage of cells positive for ER, ³H-thymidine incorporation during DNA synthesis (³H-thy). Double-labeled (ER + ³H-thy). PgR, and double labeled (PgR + ³H-thy) (ordinate). Cells were counted in TEB and AB + lobules (abscissa)

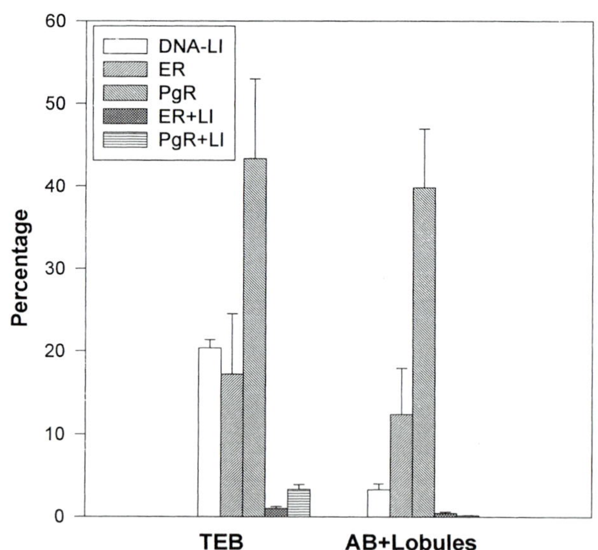

Figure 3.7

Fig. 3.7. Histogram showing the percentage of cells positive for ER, PgR and labeled in terminal end buds (*TEB*), and alveolar buds (*AB*) and lobules

Table 3.2. Distribution of cells synthesizing DNA (*DNA-LI*) and of cells positive for ER and PgR in the rat mammary gland

Type of structure	Number of cells	DNA-LI	ER	PgR	DNA-LI + ER	DNA-LI + Pg
TEB	7,092[a]	20.31±1.02[c,d]	17.21±7.35[f]	43.35±9.61[h]	1.01±0.23[j]	3.31±0.55[l]
AB + lobules	5,861[b]	3.26±0.68[e]	12.40±5.52[g]	39.81±7.15[i]	0.43±0.13[k]	0.14±0.05[m]

[a] Total number of cells counted in TEB in the mammary gland of six virgin rats
[b] Total number of cells counted in AB and lobules in the mammary gland of six virgin rats
[c] Proliferative activity, expressed as the percentage cells incorporating 3H-thymidine, or DNA labeling index (DNA-LI) expressed as the mean = SD
The DNA-LI was significantly higher in [d] TEB vs. [e] AB + lobules ($t=13.64, p<0.000001$)
The percentage of ER-positive cells was significantly lower than the percentage of PCR -positive cells in TEBs ([f] vs. [h]) ($t=11.77, p<0.00000$, and in AB + lobules ([g] vs. [i]), ($t=13.27, p<0.000000$)
ER-positive cells were significantly higher in TEB than in AB + lobules ([f] vs. [g]) ($t-2.26, p<0.02$). The percentage of PgR-positive cells in TEB ([h]) was not significantly different from that in AB + lobules ([i])
The percentage of cells doubly positive for 3H-thymidine incorporation and ER did not differ significantly in TEB ([j]) and AB + lobules ([k]). The percentage of cells doubly positive for 3H-thymidine incorporation and PgR was significantly higher in TEB than in AB + lobules ([l] vs. [m]) ($t=5.07, p<0.00000$)

were fewer in number, and they were not included in this analysis. ERα and PgR positive cells were detected only in the epithelium lining TEB, AB, ducts or lobules, but no positive cells were found in the stroma. The detection of ERα and PgR in the epithelium of TEB, AB, and lobules revealed that the number of cells positive for both receptors varied with the type of structure considered. TEB contained the highest percentage of both ERα and PgR positive cells, and both values were reduced in AB and lobules (Fig. 3.7). In contrast to what was observed in the human breast, however, the number of PgR positive cells was significantly higher than the number of ERα positive cells in the corresponding structures (Fig. 3.7, Table 3.2). It was clear that the immunocytochemical reaction with each one of the hormone receptor antibodies was positive in cells that lacked the stippling of the silver grains, whereas those cells that had incorporated 3H-thymidine had a sharp black stippling over the pale blue counterstain of hematoxylin, but were negative for both ERα and PgR (Fig. 3.6). In TEB the ratio of ERα-positive and 3H-thymidine labeled cells was roughly 1:1, while in AB and lobules it was 4:1. In all types of structures, however, the labeled cells were juxtaposed to the ERα-positive cells (Fig. 3.6a). The ratio of PgR positive and 3H-thymidine labeled cells

was 2:1 and 10:1 in TEB and AB + lobules, respectively (Fig. 3.6b, Table 3.2). PgR positive cells formed clusters surrounding isolated 3H-thymidine labeled cells (Fig. 3.6b).

3.2.3 Biological Significance

The content of ERα and PgR in the normal breast tissue varies with the degree of lobular development, in a linear relationship with the rate of cell proliferation of the same structures. The utilization of a double labeling immunocytochemical technique for staining in the same tissue section those cells containing steroid hormone receptors and those that are proliferating, i.e., Ki67-positive, allowed us to determine that the expression of the receptors occurs in cells other than the proliferating cells, confirming results reported by other authors [44]. Immunocytochemical stains for ERα, PgR, and Ki67 in human breast tissues were compared vis-a-vis with the in vivo incorporation of 3H-thymidine into cells that were synthesizing DNA in the mammary glands of young virgin Sprague-Dawley rats. The analysis of the rat mammary gland confirmed that maximal proliferative activity occurs in TEBs, as previously reported [47]. It also re-

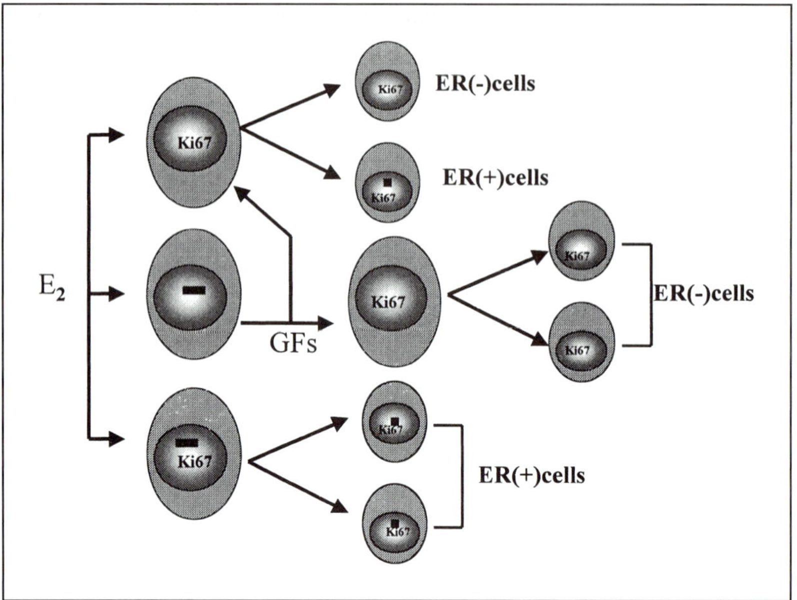

Figure 3.8

Schematic representation of the postulated pathways of estrogen actions on breast epithelial cells. Three different types of cells can be considered to be present in the mammary epithelium: Estrogen receptor-negative (*ER–*) proliferating cells (Ki67-positive), ER-positive (*ER+*) cells that do not proliferate (Ki67 negative), and a small proportion of ER+ and Ki67+ cells. Estrogen might stimulate ER+ cells to produce a growth factor that in turn stimulates neighboring ER– cells capable of proliferating. ER+Ki67+ cells can proliferate and could be stimulated by estrogen to originate ER+ daughter cells or probably tumors. ER– cells may convert to ER+ cells during neoplastic transformation (modified from: Russo, J. et al. Breast Cancer Research and Treatment 53:217–227, 1999)

vealed that the TEBs, ABs, and lobules of the virgin rat mammary gland contain receptors for both estrogen and progesterone, and that the number of cells positive for both receptors was higher in the epithelium of TEB, progressively declining in the more differentiated AB and lobules. The higher concentration of ERα and PgR in the immature mammary gland of rodents and other species has been reported by other authors [50]. Similar to what has been observed in humans, the rat mammary gland contains steroid hormone receptor positive cells only in the ductal and lobular epithelium, but no positive cells were found in the stroma. These findings contrast with results obtained by cytosolic determination that reported that a high percentage of receptors were located in the mammary stroma [50]. The findings that proliferating cells are different from those that are ERα- and PgR-positive support data that indicate that estrogen controls cell proliferation by an indirect mechanism. This phenomenon has been demonstrated using supernatants of estrogen-treated ERα-positive cells that stimulate the growth of ER-negative cell lines in culture. The same phenomenon has been shown in vivo in nude mice bearing ER-negative breast tumor xenografts [51, 52]. ER-positive cells treated with antiestrogens secrete TGF-β to inhibit the proliferation of ER-negative cells [53]. Our studies have shown that the proliferative activity and the percentage of ERα- and PgR-positive cells are highest in Lob l in comparison with the various lobular structures composing the normal breast. These findings provide a mechanistic explanation for the higher susceptibility of these structures to be transformed by chemical carcinogens in vitro [54, 55], supporting as well the observations that Lob l are the site of origin of ductal carcinomas [56]. However, the relationship between ER-positive and ER-negative breast cancers is not clear [57, 58]. It has been suggested that ER-negative breast cancers result from either the loss of the ability of the cells to synthesize ER during clinical evolution of ER-positive cancers, or that ER-positive and ER negative cancers are different entities [57, 59]. Our data allowed us to postulate that Lob l contains at least three cell types, ERα-positive cells that do not proliferate, ERα-negative cells that are capable of proliferating, and a small proportion of ERα-positive cells that can also proliferate (Fig. 3.8). Therefore, estrogen might stimulate ERα-positive cells to produce a growth factor that in turn stimulates neighboring ERα-negative cells capable of proliferating (Fig. 3.8). In the same fashion, the small proportion of cells that are ERα-positive and can proliferate could be the source of ERα-positive tumors. The possibility exists, as well, that the ERα-negative cells convert to ERα-positive cells. The conversion of ERα-negative to ERα-positive cells has been reported [60]. The newly discovered ERβ opens the possibility that those cells traditionally considered to be ERα negative might be ERβ-positive [20, 61, 62]. We have recently found that ERβ became positive during the transformation of an ERα-negative human breast epithelial cell line [63], supporting this hypothesis. The findings that proliferating cells in the human breast are different from those that contain steroid hormone receptors explain much of the in vitro data [64–67]. Of interest are the observations that while the ERα-positive MCF-7 cells respond to estrogen treatment with increased cell proliferation, and that the enhanced expression of the receptor by transfection also increases the proliferative response to estrogen [64, 68], ERα-negative cells, such as MDA-MB-468 and others, when transfected with ERα, exhibit inhibition of cell growth under the same type of treatment [65–69]. Although the negative effect of estrogen on those ERα negative cells transfected with the receptor has been interpreted as an interference with the transcription factor used to maintain estrogen independent growth [69], there is no definitive explanation for their lack of sur-

vival. These data can be explained in light of the present work, in which proliferating and ERα-positive cells are two separate populations. Furthermore, we have observed that when Lob l of normal breast tissue are placed in culture they lose the ERα-positive cells, indicating that only proliferating cells, that are also ERα-negative, can survive, and become stem cells. These observations are supported by the fact that MCF-10F, a spontaneously immortalized human breast epithelial cell line derived from breast tissues containing Lob l and Lob 2, is ERα-negative [69, 70].

Until recently, it was believed that estrogens acted through a single nuclear estrogen receptor that transcriptionally activated specific target genes, but there is mounting evidence that a membrane receptor coupled to alternative second messenger signaling mechanisms [71, 72] is also operational, and may stimulate the cascade of events leading to cell proliferation. This knowledge suggests that ERα-negative cells found in the human breast may respond to estrogens through this other pathways. Although more studies need to be done in this direction, it is clear that the findings that in the normal breast the proliferating and steroid hormone receptor positive cells are different open new possibilities for clarifying the mechanisms through which estrogens might act on the proliferating cells to initiate the cascade of events leading to cancer (see Chapter 4).

3.3 Human Chorionic Gonadotropin as a Differentiating Agent in the Human Breast and in the Rodent Mammary Gland

3.3.1 Evidence for a Receptor for Human Chorionic Gonadotropin in Human Breast Epithelial Cells

Human chorionic gonadotropin (hCG) is first synthesized by the syncytiotrophoblast of the developing embryo; it binds the granulosa cells of the ovary, inducing their luteinization and maintaining the corpus luteum of pregnancy [73, 74]. This hormone binds to a common LH/hCG transmembrane glycoprotein receptor, which is a member of the G protein-coupled receptor family. The LH/hCG receptor gene

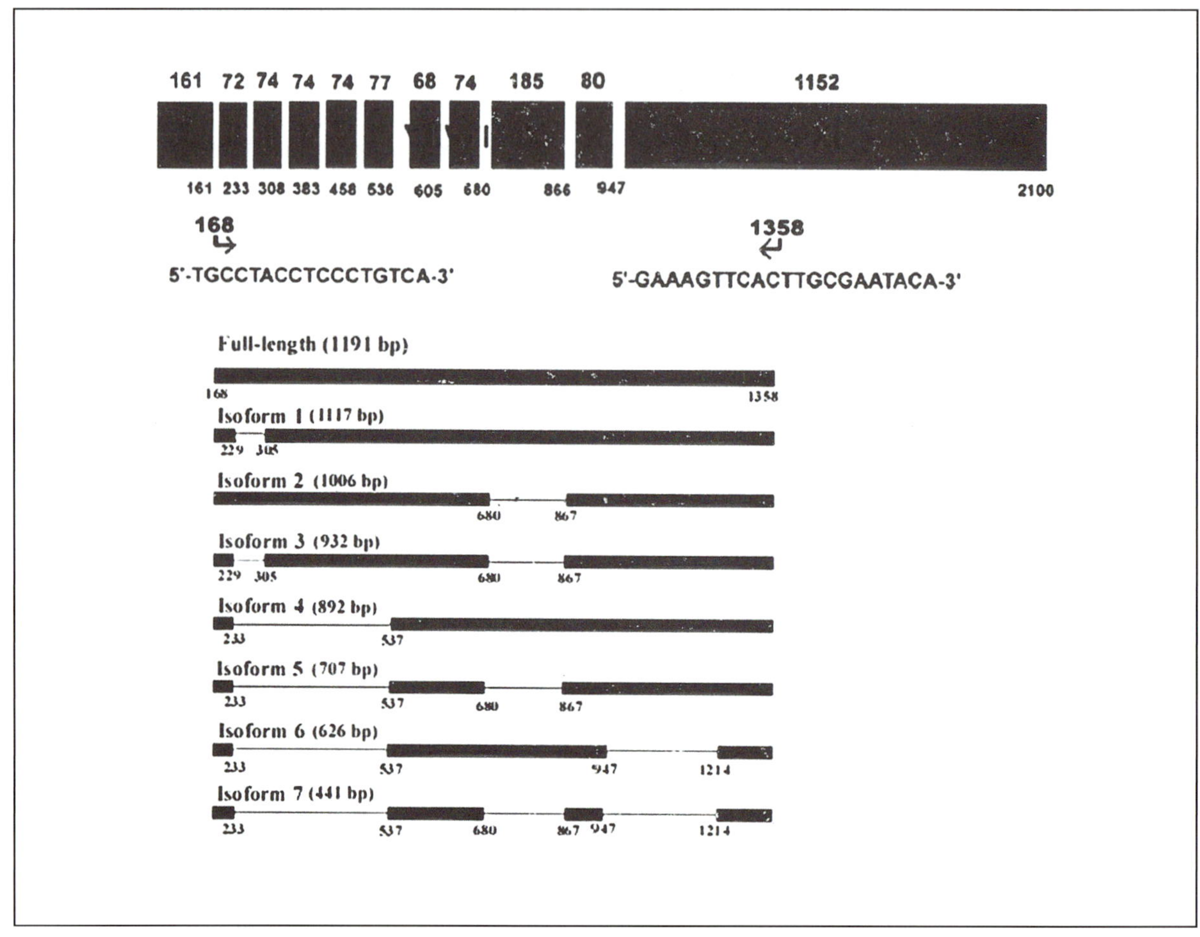

Figure 3.9

Exon organization of the LH/hCG (human chorionic gonadotropin) receptor gene and the gene specific primers for the RT-PCR

is composed of 11 exons and 10 introns and its coding region is over 60 kilobases long [75]. Aside from the full-length mRNA, various truncated forms have also been reported [76–79]. These multiple species of LH/hCG receptor mRNA are presumably derived from alternative splicing in the degree of polyadenylation of the primary transcript, which is regulated in a tissue-specific manner [75, 77–79]. Administration of hCG obtained from the urine of pregnant women (u-hCG) and of recombinant hCG (r-hCG) exerts similar effects in women and in virgin rats, stimulating the formation of corpora lutea in the ovary and inducing differentiation of the mammary gland. This phenomenon is accompanied by the synthesis of inhibin and activation of programmed cell death genes [80–84]. The same response is obtained in primary breast cancer in postmenopausal women treated with this hormone [85]. Human breast cell lines contain functional LH/hCG receptors [86] supporting the data that hCG is able to protect against DMBA-induced mammary carcinogenesis [73–77], inhibit cell proliferation of human breast epithelial cells in vitro [84] and in primary tumor of postmenopausal women treated with this hormone [87]. The human breast

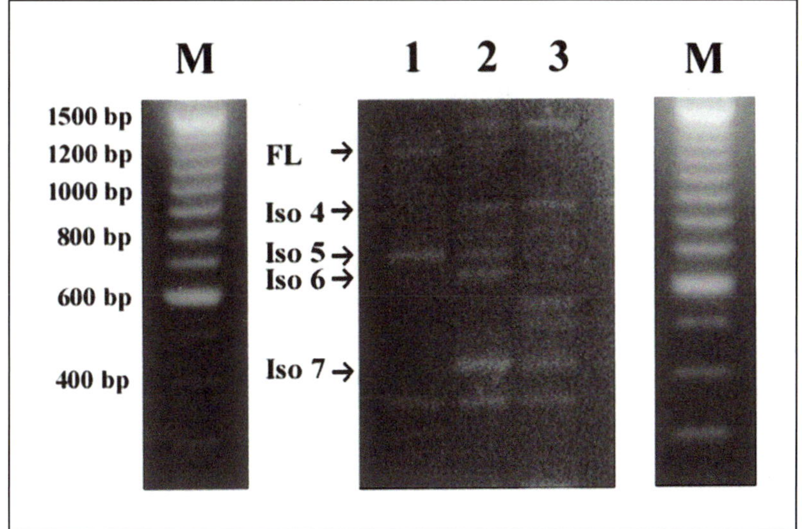

Table 3.3. Divergent expression of LH/hCG receptor isoforms in human breast epithelial cell lines. – no expression, ± very low expression, + expressed, ++ high level expression

	MCF-10-F cells	MCF-7 cells	MDA-MB-231 cells
Full length	+	±	–
Isoform 1	–	±	±
Isoform 2	–	–	–
Isoform 3	–	+	+
Isoform 4	–	+	+
Isoform 5	++	+	+
Isoform 6	–	+	±
Isoform 7	–	+	+

epithelial cells MCF-10F cells [88, 89] expressed the full-length (1191 bp) of the LH/hCG receptor (Figs. 3.9, 3.10; Table 3.3), whereas the carcinoma cell lines MCF-7 and MDA-MB-231 expressed it weakly or not at all. Isoform 1 (1117 bp) was silent in MCF-10F cells and was weakly expressed in the cancer cell lines. The isoforms 2 (1006 bp) and 3 (932 bp) of LH/hCG gene where silent in all the cell lines, whereas isoforms 4 (892 bp), 6 (626 bp) and 7 (441 bp) were silent in MCF-10F cells, but were expressed in the cancer cell lines. Instead, isoform 5 (707 bp) was expressed in the three cell lines, with stronger level of expression in MCF-10F cells (Fig. 3.10, Table 3.3) [90].

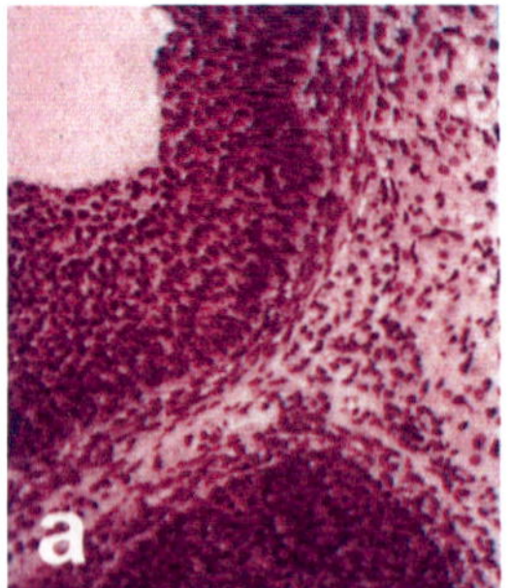

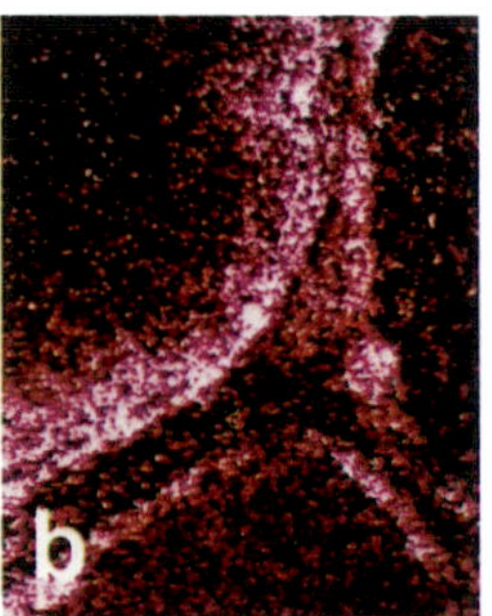

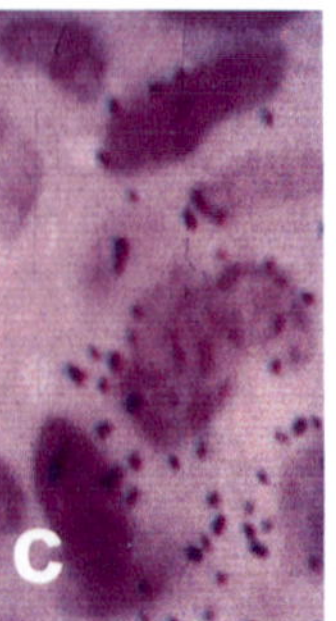

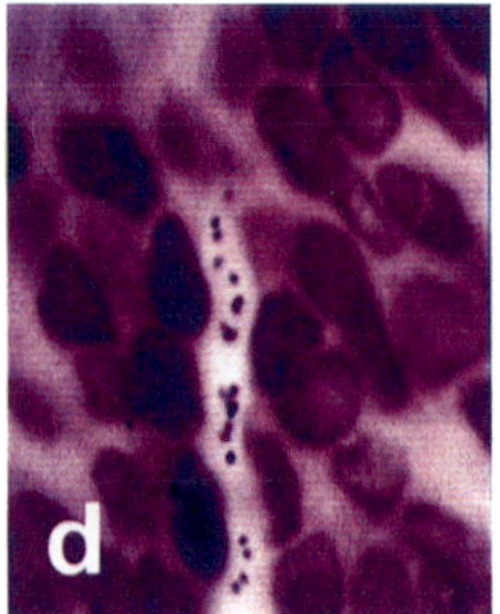

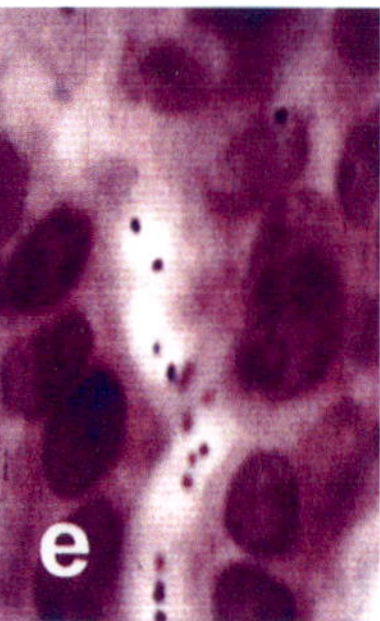

Figure 3.11 a–e

Autoradiographic detection of [^{125}I]-hCG bound to the granulose cells of a mature follicle in the ovary of a 45-day-old virgin rat in proestrus. Tissue section coated with NTB2 nuclear track emulsion, developed and counterstained with hematoxylin and eosin (H&E). **a** Bright-field ($\times$4), **b** dark-field ($\times$4), **c** view of silver grains indicating sites of [^{125}I]-hCG binding to the surface of granulose cells (H&E, $\times$40). **d, e** Silver grains showing the binding of [^{125}I]-hCG to the luminal surface of mammary epithelial cells (H&E, $\times$40)

3.3.2 Human Chorionic Gonadotropin Receptor in the Rat Mammary Gland

For detecting the location of the hCG receptor in the unprimed virgin rat we injected intraperitoneally [^{125}I]-hCG at the dose of 0.1 µCi/gram body weight (^{125}I-specific activity 86.9 µCi/µg, 79.4 µCi/µl) to 45-day-old Sprague-Dawley rats. The animals were sacrificed at 30 min, 1, 2, 4, and 6 h after hormone injection. Tissues were fixed in formalin, paraffin embedded, and sectioned at a thickness of 5 µm. Tissue sections were incubated with NTB-2, Nuclear track emulsion (Kodak, Rochester, NY) at 4°C in dark boxes for 4 weeks. The ovary was considered as the positive control (Fig. 3.11). Binding of [^{125}I]-hCG to the granulosa cells of the ovarian follicles was observed by 30 min after injection, and it remained bound up to 6 h. The silver grains were observed overlying the granulosa cells; the binding was considered positive when a cell contained four or more silver grains on its surface (Fig. 3.11a–c). In the mammary gland [^{125}I]-hCG was observed to bind to the luminal border of

epithelial cells lining lobules and terminal ducts (Fig. 3.11d, e). These observations confirmed the presence of the LH/hCG-R in the rat mammary gland.

3.3.3 Biological Significance of the LH/hCG Receptor

The alternate splicing of LH/hCG-R mRNA among the MCF-10F, MCF-7 and MDA-MB-231 cells may play a role in the different response of these cell lines to r-hCG. The LH/hCG-R, a G protein-coupled receptor, consists of two halves, the N-terminal extracellular hormone binding domain (exodomain) and the C-terminal membrane-associated, signal-generating domain (endodomain) [91, 92]. The exodomain has seven to nine Leu-rich repeats, which are generally thought to form a 1/3 donut-like structure, which upon interaction with hCG forms an hCG-exodomain complex that adjusts the structure and in its association with the endodomain results in signal generation in the endodomain. It is unclear whether the rigid 1/3 donut structure could provide the agility and versatility of this dynamic action. In addition, there is no clue as to where in the exodomain is located the endodomain contact point (the signal modulator) [93, 94]. Gonadotropin receptors are present in Leydig cells, granulosa cells of the ovary [93], in endothelial cells of target organ vessels and are involved in hormone transcytosis [94]. In human skin the receptor has been observed only in the epidermis and derived structures but not in the dermis [95]. The role of LH and hCG in skin modifications occurring during pregnancy and after the menopause is unknown. These hormones may possibly act by regulating steroidogenic enzymes or by modulating cell growth and differentiation [95]. The LH/hCG-R plays a critical role in reproductive physiology in both males and females. Naturally occurring mutations in this receptor can cause genetically transmitted disorders by producing either gain or loss of receptor function [96–100].

3.4 Effect of Human Chorionic Gonadotropin on Human Breast Epithelial Cells

Traditionally, hCG has been considered to act through its luteinizing effect on the ovary. The fact that it inhibits proliferation of HBEC in vitro required further studies for understanding the mechanism(s) of action of hCG on the mammary epithelium. For this purpose, the immortalized HBEC line MCF-10F [88, 89] was treated in vitro with hCG; the effect of hCG treatment was studied at the level of overall protein synthesis by 2-D-PAGE (Fig. 3.12), in vitro translation product of mRNA (Fig. 3.13) and synthesis of individual proteins (Fig. 3.14).

3.4.1 Effect on Protein Synthesis and In Vitro Translational Products of mRNA

The effect of hCG treatment on MCF-10F cells' protein synthesis was monitored by labeling both control and treated cells with [S^{35}]-methionine and separation by 2-D PAGE (Fig. 3.12). In MCF-10F control cells, NEPHGE resolved more than 900 polypeptides, which ranged in molecular mass from 14 to 80 kDa (Fig. 3.12a). The 2-D PAGE polypeptide profiles of hCG-treated and control cells revealed quantitative differences in both the overall spot pattern and the number of polypeptides detected in treated and control cells. The profile of hCG-treated cells revealed that at least 11 proteins were preferentially synthesized and five specific polypeptides were decreased in comparison with controls (Fig. 3.12, Table 3.4).

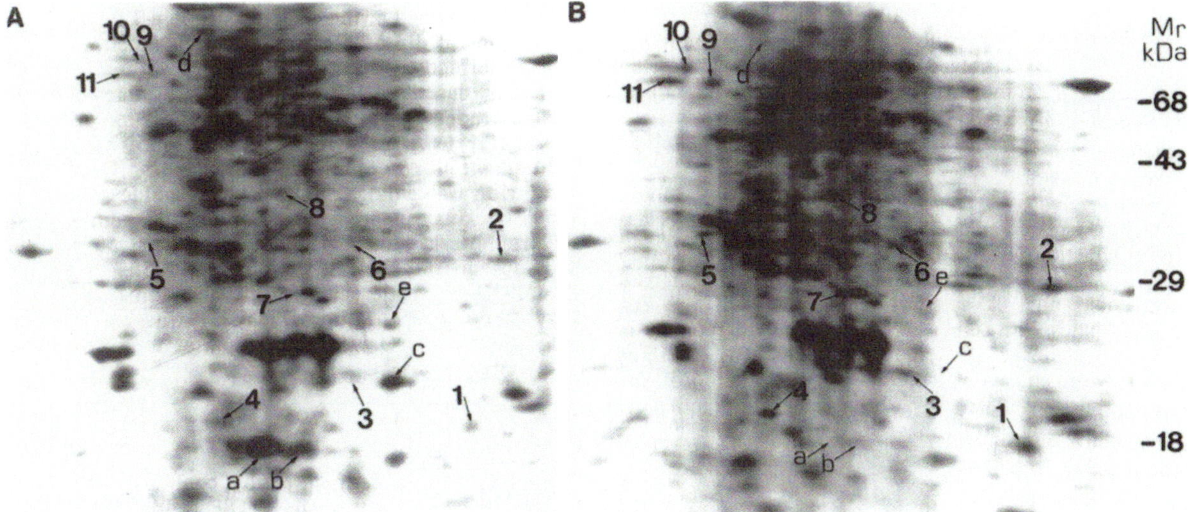

Figure 3.12 a, b

Polypeptide pattern of MC-10F cells analyzed by 2-D PAGE and fluorography. **a** Control MCF-10F cells; **b** hCG-treated cells. *Arrows (1–11)* indicate polypeptides that are more intensely labeled in hCG-treated cells; *arrows (a–e)* indicate polypeptides more intensely labeled in control than in treated cells (reprinted with permission from: from: Ho, T-Y., Russo, J., and Russo, I.H. Electrophoresis 15:746–750, 1994)

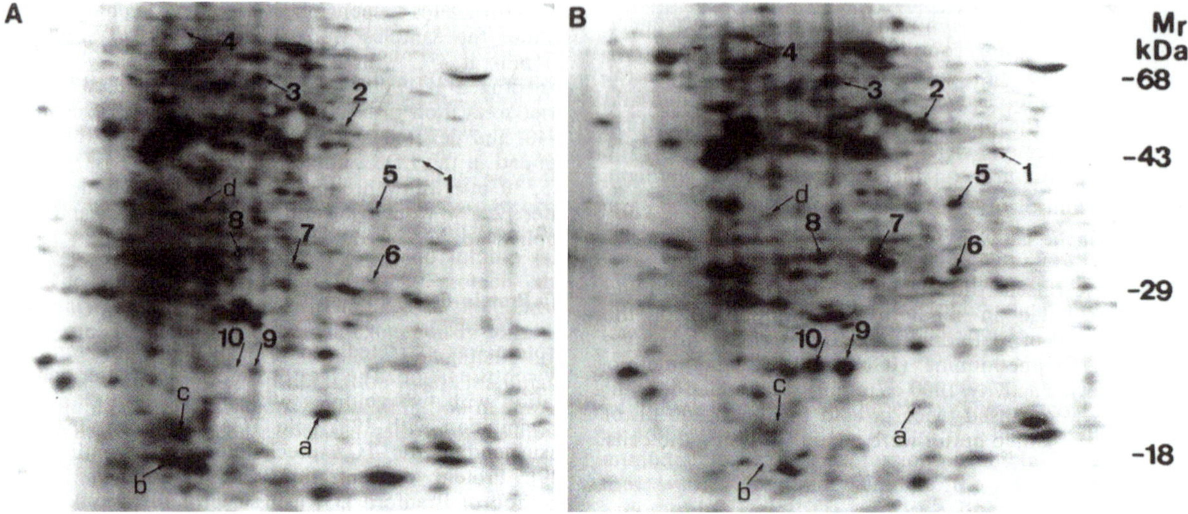

Figure 3.13 a, b

In vitro translation products of mRNA resolved by 2-D PAGE and detected by fluorography. The polypeptides shown were synthesized in vitro by rabbit reticulocyte lysates incubated with mRNA isolated from **a** control MCF-10F cells, **b** hCG treated cells. Polypeptides *1–10* were more intensely expressed by hCG-treated cells; polypeptides *a–d* indicate those exhibiting lower levels in treated than in control cells (**a**) (reprinted with permission from: Ho, T-Y., Russo, J., and Russo, I.H. Electrophoresis 15:746–750, 1994)

Figure 3.14

Effect of hCG treatment on the synthesis of inhibin by MCF-10F cells. MCF-10F control and hCG-treated cells were labeled with [S35] methionine and lysed. Aliquots containing equal number of counts were immunoprecipitated with anti-inhibin α and β antisera. *Lane 1* Total nonprecipitated samples from hCG-treated cells; *lane 2* Control cells; *lane 3* Immunoprecipitation of inhibin α from hCG-treated cells shows twofold enhanced 18 kDa band immunoprecipitation with inhibin βb antibody in comparison with control cells; (*lane 4*). Immunoprecipitation with inhibin βb antibody of hCG-treated cells showed an enhanced 14 kDa band; (*lane 5*) in comparison with control cells (*lane 6*). (Reprinted with permission from: Ho, T-Y., Russo, J., and Russo, I.H. Electrophoresis 15:746–750, 1994)

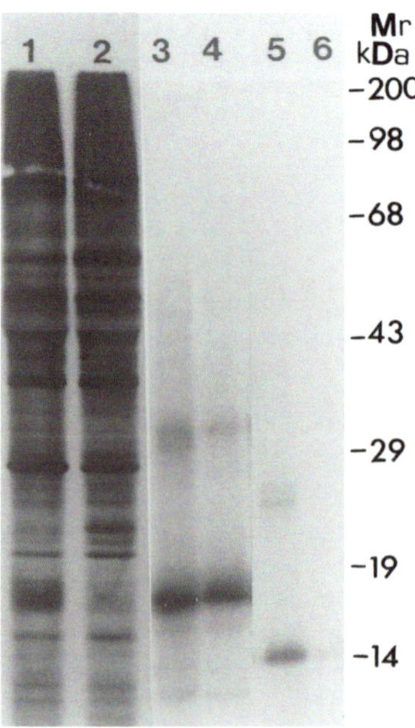

Table 3.4. Effect of hCG treatment of MCF-10F cells on protein synthesis

Polypeptide number	Molecular mass KDa	Change of abundance after hCG treatment
1	18	+
2	29	+
3	22	+
4	19.5	+
5	32.5	+
6	31	+
7	28	+
8	39	+
9	70	+
10	72	+
11	70	+
a	18	–
b	18	–
c	22	–
d	75	–
e	26	–

Under hCG treatment the regulation of gene expression at translational level appeared to be somewhat different from that of mRNA at transcriptional level. To determine whether the observed differences in polypeptide composition after hCG treatment was a reflection of changes at the RNA level, we examined in vitro translation products of mRNA isolated after treatment of MCF-10F cells with this hormone. The translation activities of total RNA preparations from hCG-treated and control cells were compared in a reticulocyte cell-free system. RNA preparations of both control and treated cells stimulated incorporation of [S^{35}]methionine into trichloroacetic acid-insoluble proteins by tenfold above the background activity of reticulocyte lysate (data not shown). Separation of the in vitro translation products on 2-D gels showed protein patterns similar to those of complete cells (Fig. 3.13). Treatment with hCG induced at least four new mRNAs (#2, 4, 7, and 10) (Fig. 3.13). The proteins encoded by the newly induced mRNAs ranged in molecular mass from 24 to 72 kDa. The hormonal treatment increased the expression of at least six mRNAs (labeled 1, 3, 5, 6, 8, and 9) and reduced the expression of at least four mRNAs (Fig. 3.13, labels a–d). Because protein synthesis in vivo might be subjected to post-translational modifications that do not occur in the in vitro translation system employed, direct correspondence of in vivo and in vitro products is not yet feasible. Nevertheless, our data suggest that transcriptional and post-transcriptional mechanisms play major roles in the control of gene expression during hCG treatment.

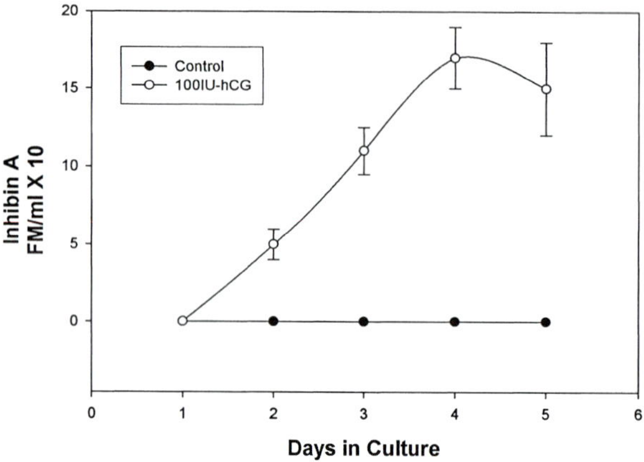

Figure 3.15

Secretion of inhibin A detected by radioimmunoassay in the culture media of MCF-10F cells treated with 100 IU of hCG at different times

3.4.2 Effect of Human Chorionic Gonadotropin Treatment on Inhibin Synthesis

Treatment of MCF-10F cells with hCG actively stimulated the synthesis of a 33 kDa polypeptide, which was not present in the autoradiographic pattern of normal MCF-10F cells. This polypeptide, which was one of the prevalent proteins in hCG-treated cells, was undetectable in the protein profile of control cells, even when the silver staining method was used (data not shown). In order to determine whether the hCG-inducible 33 kDa protein was inhibin [101, 102], two rabbit antisera directed against rat inhibin subunit α and β were utilized for immunoprecipitating [S^{35}]methionine-labeled proteins in the crude cell lysates of control and hCG-treated cells. As shown in Fig. 3.14, one-dimensional separation of immunoprecipitates with anti-α-inhibin antibody precipitated an 18kDa band, which was increased twofold by hCG treatment (lanes 3 and 4). Precipitation with anti-β-inhibin antibody revealed a 14 kDa protein band whose synthesis was stimulated six-fold by hCG (lanes 5 and 6). MCF-10F cells treated with 100 IU of hCG release Inhibin A in the culture medium (Fig. 3.15). This observation suggested that the polypeptide is released from the cells and may exert au-

Figure 3.16a–f ▶

Dose-effect of hCG treatment on the growth of: **a** MCF-10F cells; **b** MCF-7 cells; and **c** T-24 cell. Cells were treated with 1, 10, or 100 IU hCG and growth was evaluated at 24, 48, 72, 96, and 120 h of treatment. For cell growth evaluation control and treated cells were trypsinized and counted with a hemocytometer or with an EL-312 microplate reader using a modified MTT [3,(4,5 di-methythiazol-2-yl) 2,5-diphenyl-tetrazolium bromide] method. The correlation coefficient between cell counts obtained with the hemocytometer and optical densities obtained with the microplate reader was $r^2 = 0.99$. Statistical analysis was performed by unpaired t-test or analysis of variance, where appropriate. Each point represents the mean ($\pm$ SD) number of cells in four wells. $p < 0.01$ vs. control by Student's t-test. **d** Percentage of cell growth after hCG treatment vs. the control in MCF-10F, MCF-7 and T-24 cells at different concentrations of hCG; **e, f** Effect of inhibin and transforming growth factor beta (TGF-β) on MCF-10F cell proliferation. MCF-10F cells were treated with inhibin A at the doses of 0.1, 1.0, 10.0 and 20.0 ng/ml or with TGF-β at the doses of 0.1, 1.0, and 10.0 ng/ml. Cells were collected at 24, 48, 72, 96, and 120 h of treatment. Inhibin treatment depressed cell proliferation as early as at 24 h of treatment. The rate of cell growth progressively recovered from 48 to 120 h, when the cells reached the same level of growth of control cells. TGF-β treatment depressed cell proliferation in a progressive and dose dependent manner with time of treatment, reaching a maximal inhibitory effect at 96 h of treatment, with recovery of cell growth thereafter to control levels in the 0.1 ng treated group, but negligible change in the 10.0 ng treated group

tocrine and/or paracrine effects. Although in the results reported here only inhibin A has been identified to be secreted into the medium under hCG stimulus, other polypeptides were observed to be either stimulated or depressed by hCG treatment; they, in turn, might play a role in the control of cell proliferation.

Inhibins are growth factors with structural homology to the transforming growth factor (TGF) βs, and Mullerian inhibiting substance (MIS), among others [101, 102]. These non-steroidal glycoprotein hormones are produced by the gonads and the placenta [103–106]. They feed back to the anterior pituitary gland to inhibit specifically the production and/or secretion of follicle stimulating hormone

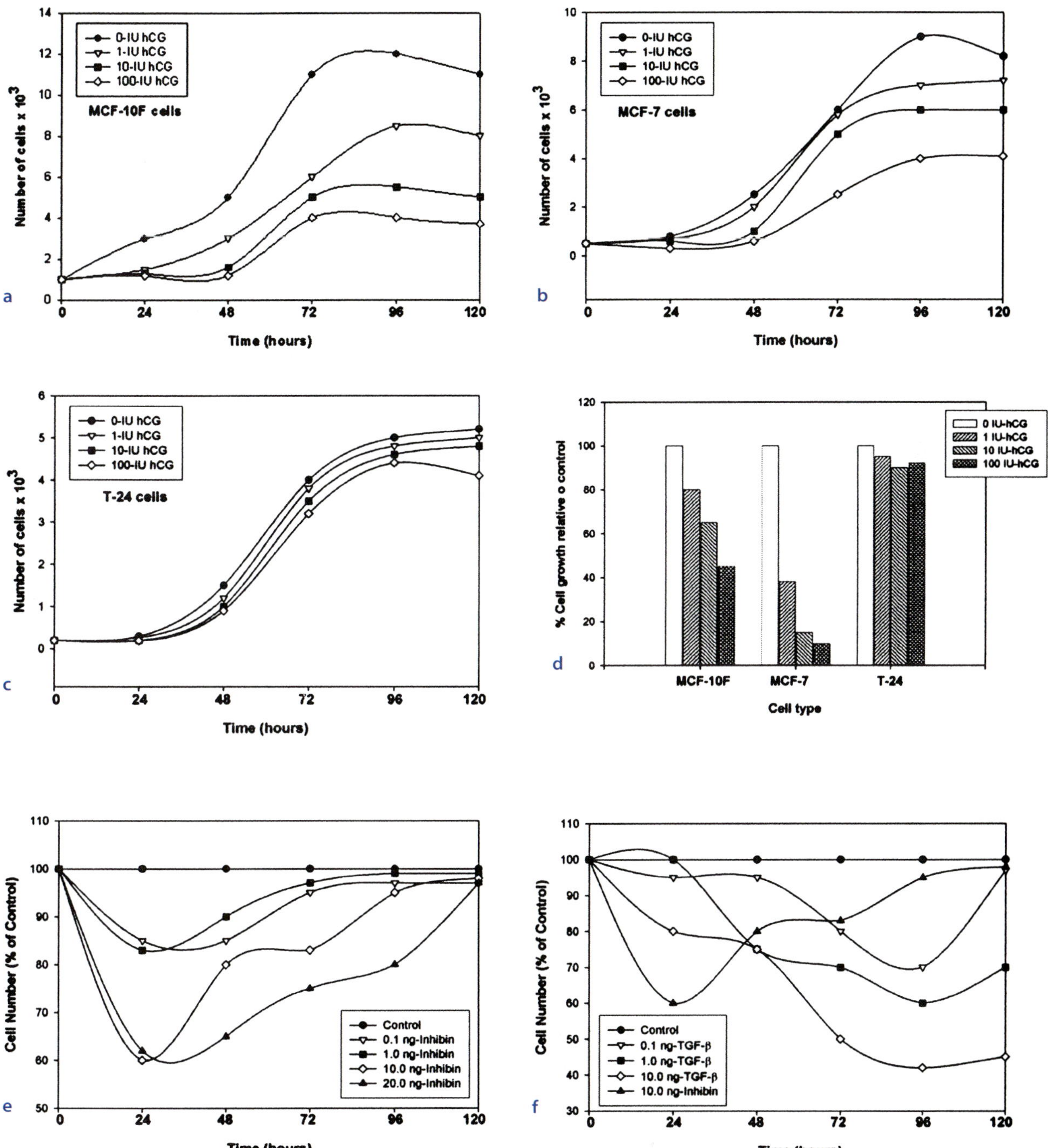
MCF-10F cells
0-IU hCG
1-IU hCG
10-IU hCG
100-IU hCG
Number of cells x 10³
Time (hours)
a

MCF-7 cells
0-IU hCG
1-IU hCG
10-IU hCG
100-IU hCG
Number of cells x 10³
Time (hours)
b

T-24 cells
0-IU hCG
1-IU hCG
10-IU hCG
100-IU hCG
Number of cells x 10³
Time (hours)
c

% Cell growth relative o control
0 IU-hCG
1 IU-hCG
10 IU-hCG
100 IU-hCG
MCF-10F
MCF-7
T-24
Cell type
d

Cell Number (% of Control)
Control
0.1 ng-Inhibin
1.0 ng-Inhibin
10.0 ng-Inhibin
20.0 ng-Inhibin
Time (hours)
e

Cell Number (% of Control)
Control
0.1 ng-TGF-β
1.0 ng-TGF-β
10.0 ng-TGF-β
10.0 ng-Inhibin
Time (hours)
f

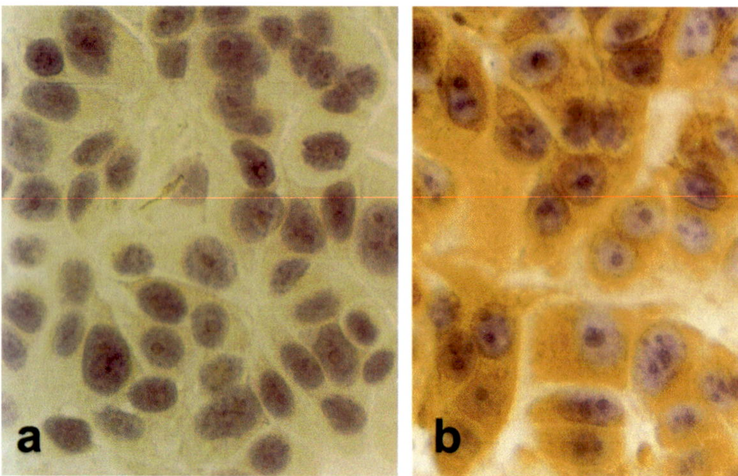

Figure 3.17 a, b

Inhibin α-immunostain of **a** control and **b** hCG treated MCF-10F cells, Magnification ×600. Antibodies to inhibin were raised in rabbit against polypeptides synthesized at our facilities

(FSH) [107] and in the placenta they regulate the synthesis of hCG [105]. The granulosa cells of the ovary in the female have been identified as the site of inhibin synthesis [108]. The major form of this protein is a disulfide-linked heterodimer, consisting of an α-chain and one of two highly homologous β chains, designated A and B [101, 102]. The A chain is an 18-Kd peptide and the B chain is 14-Kd peptides, which lead to the formation of a 32-Kd a-13 dimer in most species. Depending on the β chain (A or B), inhibin is termed Inhibin A or Inhibin B [101, 102].

Treatment of MCF-7, a breast adenocarcinoma cell line, with 100 IU hCG/ml for 24 h induced the expression of α and β chain immunoreactive inhibin in a pattern similar to that induced in the immortalized HBEC MCF-10F. However, it did not induce inhibin expression in the human bladder carcinoma cell line T24. There was a direct correlation between the intensity of expression of inhibin by treated cells and the inhibitory effect of hCG treatment on cell proliferation (Fig. 3.16). Control cells did not exhibit any significant immunocytochemical positivity when reacted with anti-inhibin antibodies, whereas hCG treated MCF-10F and MCF-7 cells showed a strong (2+ to 3+) positive immunoreactivity in nearly 100% of the cells. The reaction was stronger in MCF-10F cells, in which it appeared as a homogeneous brown staining throughout the cytoplasm (Fig. 3.17). Neither control nor hCG treated T-24 bladder carcinoma cells, on the other hand, showed any immunoreactivity with the antibodies tested [81]. In order to verify whether the expression of inhibin detected by immunocytochemistry was the result of increased synthesis, RNA of control and hCG-treated MCF-1OF cells was collected for Northern blot analysis. The hormonal treatment induced a 10-fold amplification of inhibin α and β mRNA, while TGF-α and TGF-β mRNAs were not amplified (Fig. 3.18). An additional experiment was performed to determine whether the synthesis of inhibin induced by hCG was dose dependent, similarly to what was observed on cell growth. MCF-10F cells were treated with 1, 10 or 100 IU hCG/ml for 24 h, and then RNA was extracted. Inhibin mRNA was amplified in MCF-1OF cells in a dose

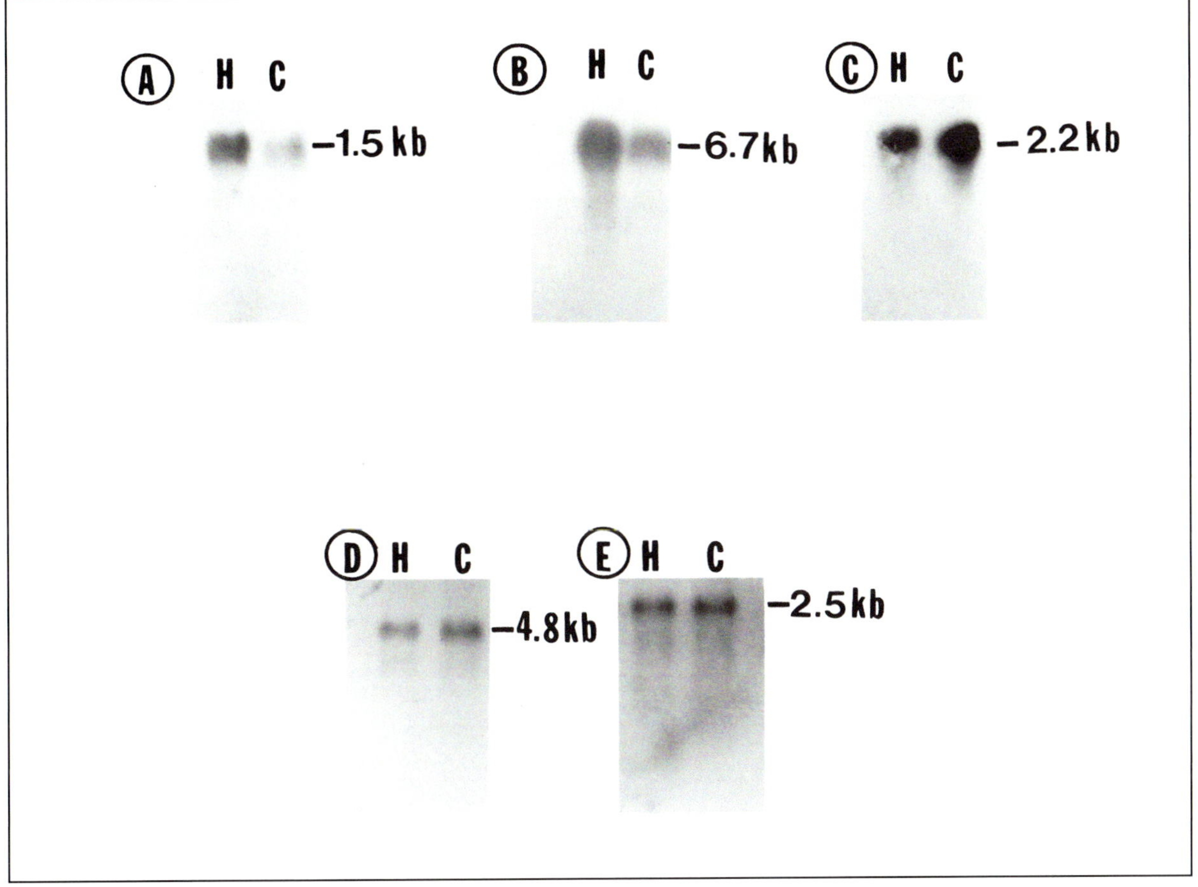

Figure 3.18 a–e

Northern blot analysis showing MCF-10F cells treated with 100 IU hCG (*H*) compared with treated with solvent (*C*). **a** Inhibin βA-subunit; **b** inhibin α-subunit; **c** β-actin; **d** TGF-α; **e** TGF-β

dependent manner, with maximal response being elicited by 100 IU.

It is well known that hCG acts on ovarian and testicular cells by binding to the LH/hCG-R, thus activating a G protein which in turn stimulates adenyl cyclase, resulting in elevations in circulating levels of estradiol and inhibin [109]. Thus, inhibin secretion and circulating serum levels are a good marker of ovarian responsiveness to hCG stimulation. The main known functions of inhibin are the suppression of follicle stimulating hormone (FSH) secretion by the pituitary gland and regulation of hCG production by the placenta. Although no specific effects of inhibin on the mammary epithelium have been previously described, our findings that hCG induces the synthesis of inhibin both in vivo and in vitro [81, 83], suggest that a direct mechanism similar to that described in the ovary might be operating in our experimental systems. Our data acquire significance in light of the knowledge that inhibin has been shown to be a critical negative regulator of gonadal stromal cell proliferation and the first secreted protein identified as having tumor suppressor activity [110].

The isolation and characterization of hCG-induced genes would eventually aid in elucidation of the molecular bases of the effect of this hormone on mammary gland differentiation and carcinogenesis. Our results allowed to postulate that one of the pathways through which hCG inhibits cell proliferation is through the increased expression of the inhibin gene.

3.4.3 Effect of Hormones on the Proliferative Activity of Cultured Normal and Neoplastic Human Breast Epithelial Cells

Treatment of MCF-10F cells with hCG at the doses of 1, 10, or 100 IU inhibited the growth of the cells in a dose dependent manner (Fig. 3.16a). The same doses of hCG inhibited MCF-7 cell growth also in a dose-dependent manner, although a greater inhibition of growth occurred at lower hCG doses than in MCF-10F cells (Fig. 3.16b). The growth of the urothelial cell line T24 was not affected by hCG treatment (Fig. 3.16c,d) [81]. Treatment of MCF-10F cells with inhibin A at the doses of 0.1, 1.0, 10.0 and 20.0 ng/ml resulted in a depression in cell proliferation which became evident during the first 24 h of treatment. The rate of cell growth progressively recovered from 48 to 120 h, when the cells reached the same level of growth of control cells (Fig. 3.16e). Treatment of MCF-10F cells with transforming growth factor beta (TGF-β) at the doses of 0.1, 1.0, and 10.0 ng/ml depressed cell proliferation in a progressive and dose dependent manner with time of treatment, reaching a maximal inhibitory effect at 96 hours of treatment, Cell growth recovered thereafter to control levels in the 0.1 ng treated group, but the change was negligible in the 10.0 ng treated group (Fig. 3.16f).

For detecting the effect of hCG on cell cycle parameters MCF-7 cells were plated at a density of 3×10^4 cells in Earle's Minimal Essential Medium with 5% dextran-charcoal-stripped serum and 100 IU/

Table 3.5. Effect of hCG on MCF-7 cell kinetic parameters

Group	DNA labeling index[a] Mean ± SD	Mitotic index[b] Mean ± SD
Control	25.4±6.2	2.2±1.6
HCG (100 IU/ml)	12.7±4.7	1.2±0.9

[a] DNA-labeling index was determined by counting the number of cells incorporating ^{3}H-thymidine; it is expressed as number of labeled cells per 100 cells
[b] Mitotic index was determined by counting the number of cells in mitosis per 100 cells. Mean of four dishes per group

Table 3.6. Effect of hCG on MCF-7 cell cycle parameters. *CV* coefficient of variation

Group	Length of treatment	Phases of the cell cycle				
		G^1 (%)	CV	S (%)	G2 (%)	CV
Control	–	28.7	2.58	51.2	20.1	3.17
hCG	1 h	37.1	2.83	46.2	16.7	2.37
	3 h	32.0	2.22	39.4	28.6	2.18
	6 h	32.8	2.07	30.09	36.3	1.08
	48 h	61.6	3.99	20.0	18.3	2.70

HCG/ml were added at the time of plating. Cell growth, mitotic index and DNA-labeling index (DNA-LI), measured by ^{3}H-thymidine incorporation autoradiography, were evaluated at 24 h of treatment. hCG treatment significantly inhibited cell proliferation and DNA synthesis measured as mitotic activity (Table 3.5). For flow cytometric analysis of the cell cycle, the cells treated with 100 IU were evaluated at 1, 3, 6 and 48 h of treatment (Table 3.6). Flow cytometric analysis showed that hCG produced an accumulation of cells in G1 phase and reduction of cells in S phase (Table 3.6). These data are similar to the response effect of tamoxifen on asynchronous and synchronized cultures of MCF-7 cells in which growth inhibition was associated with the accumulation of cells in the G0-G1 phase of the cell cycle [111, 112]. The number of cells in S phase decreased with time of treatment, with maximal reduction in the percentage of cells in S phase at 48 h, value that inversely correlated with the accumulation of cells in G1.

3.4.4 Biological Significance of the hCG-Inhibin Pathway

Human chorionic gonadotropin stimulates the synthesis of inhibin in mammary epithelial cells, both in vivo and in vitro [81]. Inhibin might serve as a local mediator of the action of hCG, acting as an inhibitor growth regulating factor. We observed that hCG treatment increases inhibin immunoreactivity in the mammary epithelial cells of virgin female rats [73], and has an effect on rat and human breast epithelial cells in vitro [81]. This hypothesis was tested by treating the immortalized non-neoplastic human breast epithelial cell line, MCF-10F, the breast cancer cell line MCF-7 and a urothelial cancer cell line T-24 in vitro with hCG at various concentrations, in order to evaluate the influence of this treatment on cell growth and on the expression of inhibin. hCG significantly inhibited the growth of both MCF-10F and MCF-7 cells in a dose dependent manner. The antiproliferative effect observed was accompanied by increased expression of inhibin immunoreactivity in the cytoplasm of treated cells. The malignant bladder carcinoma cell line T-24, on the other hand, was not affected in its cell growth nor in its expression of inhibin immunoreactivity by this hormonal treatment. These results suggest that hCG might have a specificity in its action towards hormone dependent cells. Furthermore, it is possible to postulate that inhibin might act as a mediator of the action of hCG on mammary epithelial cells [15, 81, 85]. A specific receptors for hCG have been shown in the mammary epithelium, supported by its direct hormonal effect of hCG in vitro. This receptor, which was thought to be expressed solely in gonadal cells, has also been isolated from uterus [113] and from a human thyroid library [114], supporting the existence of extragonadal locations for this receptor. On binding hCG, the LH-CG-R resulting increase in cAMP stimulates cAMP-dependent protein-kinase, increasing in turn the synthesis and secretion of steroids [109]. Interestingly, the production of inhibin is also regulated via a cAMP-mediated pathway, suggesting that a similar mechanism might be operational in the hCG-mediated stimulation of inhibin synthesis by human breast epithelial cells. Specific growth factors have been shown to regulate the growth and differentiation of normal tissue, while their inappropriate expression has been implicated in the uncontrolled proliferation observed in neoplastically transformed cells [115–117]. Rapid proliferation of tumor cells in culture under conditions where normal cells would be quiescent may be a consequence of the secretion of autocrine acting growth factors, expression of their cell surface receptors, and in some cases activation of specific intracellular proliferative signals [118]. The precise mechanism involved in the secretion of growth factors by epithelial cells in vivo is largely unknown. It is conceivable that tumor cell-derived mitogens may also affect growth and gene expression of normal cells surrounding the tumor. Thus, growth factors secreted by tumor cells may act in vivo as paracrine and/or autocrine regulators of tumor growth. Although the actions of growth promoting factors such as epidermal growth factor (EGF), TGF-α, or IGF-I are well documented [119–121], considerably less is known about the influence of growth factors on the inhibition of epithelial tumor cell growth. A wide range of extracellular regulatory signaling molecules, including steroid hormones, interferons, and TGF-β, can inhibit the proliferation of certain tumor cell lines. For example, glucocorticoids have been shown to inhibit somatic growth, the growth of several tumors in vivo [122–124] and to suppress the proliferation of cell cultures in vitro [125–127]. These effects have been attributed to either an increase in the synthesis of tumor cell growth inhibitors, to the inhibition of synthesis of growth stimulatory genes and of their receptors or to a combination of both mechanisms.

Induction of tumor differentiation is another mechanism of inhibition of cell growth. Tumor cell differentiation has been obtained with specific agents, such as retinoic acid (RA), which induces terminal differentiation, and ultimately complete remission of acute promyelocytic leukemia [128]. RA also induces a mouse teratocarcinoma cell line to irreversibly differentiate into endoderm-like cells, increasing, among others, the levels of *c-jun* mRNA, a differentiation associated gene [129]. Leukemic cells and teratocarcinomas are the models most widely utilized for testing differentiation-inducing agents. The transfer of cells to mouse blastocyst or the induction of differentiation of breast cancer by embryonic tissue are other methods utilized for the control of tumor growth by induction of differentiation [130–133].

Most studies examining the hormonal regulation of epithelial cell growth have focused on the well characterized polypeptide epithelial cell growth inhibitor TGF-β [10]. In contrast, although hCG has been shown to inhibit both in vivo and in vitro growth of HBEC, and inhibin has been reported to be expressed under hCG stimulation, relatively little is known about the mechanism of these actions. The observed preventive and tumoristatic effect of hCG on mammary tumors strongly support a role for this hormone in the control of tumor growth through either inhibition of cell proliferation, induction of programmed cell death or induction of differentiation; this latter one is defined as decreased cell proliferation, leading to an arrest of cell division, modifications of cell morphology and expression of specific gene products such as inhibin [134]. In eukaryotic cells, protooncogenes are involved in virtually every step in the signal transduction pathway that controls cell proliferation [135]. Expression of several genes, including c-fos, c-jun and c-myc, is required for cells to transit the G1 phase and to initiate DNA synthesis [136, 137]. Although initial studies on the regulation of c-fos and c-jun expression were concerned primarily with mitogenic stimuli, it has become clear that these genes function as components of a relatively common signal transduction cascade that operates in several different cell types. Both c-fos and c-jun are members of the set of genes known as cellular immediate-early genes [138, 139]. This set of genes has been defined operationally by the fact that their expression is induced rapidly by extracellular stimuli even in the presence of protein synthesis inhibitors. This feature is shared with the immediate-early genes of several viruses. Furthermore, like many of the viral immediate-early genes, both c-fos and c-jun encode proteins (Fos and Jun, respectively) that function in transcriptional regulation. These proteins are thought to regulate expression of cell type-specific target genes whose products contribute to long-term cellular responses to stimulation. Fos and Jun form a heterodimeric complex that interacts with the regulatory element known as the transcription factor AP-1 (Activator Protein-1) binding site [140]. Thus, two independently isolated oncogenes encode proteins that function cooperatively as a bimolecular complex to regulate target gene expression in response to cell stimulation. In fact, Jun was first identified as a Fos-binding protein. We hypothesize that hCG mediates its effect on inhibiting cell proliferation by inducing inhibin, through activation of the early response gene pathway, a postulate supported by the observation that hCG induces the expression of c-fos and c-myc mRNA in testicular tumor cells [141]. On the other hand, since the deregulated expression of c-myc is associated with increased incidence of programmed cell death/apoptosis, which also accompanies the elevated expression of c-myc in physiological conditions, such as the involution of breast and prostate, it is possible to postulate that the inhibitory effect of hCG on cell proliferation might be due to the arrest of the cells in the G1 or G0 compartments by a process of terminal differentiation, or as a result of cell death by apoptosis [142–144]. There is evidence that apoptosis appears to be related to the cell cycle, and many apoptotic agents cause also a block in the G1, S or G2 phases of the cell cycle [145–147]. Induction of apoptosis in mammalian cells has been also associated with the increased expression of the TRPM-2 gene [148]. This gene displays homology to the sulfated glycoprotein-2 gene, which is constitutively expressed in rodent Sertoli and epididymal epithelial cells. Expression of the wild-type p53 protein in both human and mouse tumor cell lines has been demonstrated to induce apoptosis [139–151]. Expression of bc1-2 has been shown to inhibit glucocorticoid induced apoptosis in thymocytes and B-lymphocytes and to abrogate c-myc induced apoptosis without affecting the c-myc mitogenic function [151,152]. Since inhibin has been shown to be a critical negative regulator of gonadal stromal cell proliferation and the first secreted protein identified to have tumor suppressor activity [110], it is possible to expect that inhibin will inhibit the growth of HBEC in culture by either arrest of the cells in a specific phase of the cell cycle or by apoptosis.

3.5 Homeobox Genes' Expression and Their Modulation by Human Chorionic Gonadotropin in Human Breast Epithelial Cells

Human chorionic gonadotropin is a glycoprotein hormone containing a cystine-knot folding motif that is found in peptide growth factors known to activate the expression of homeogenes [153]. Homeobox genes (HOX) are a family of regulatory genes encoding a closely related subset of homeobox containing transcription factors that primarily play a crucial role in embryogenesis [154–163]. The homeobox of these factors encodes a 61 amino acid homeodomain that binds specifically to DNA. After embryogenesis, HOX genes may continue to be transcribed according to a tissue-specific pattern of expression. To date, 39 class I homeobox genes have been identified in humans. They are organized in four clusters (HOX A, B, C and D), which are located on chromosomes 7, 17, 12 and 2, respectively [155, 156]. Several homeobox-containing genes have been observed to display an altered pattern of expression in some malignancies when compared with the corresponding normal tissues [157, 158]. Moreover, misregulation of certain homeobox genes can lead to cellular transformation in culture, as well as tumor formation in vivo [159–162]. There is evidence that some of the HOX genes are involved in the development of various solid tumors including human breast cancer [162, 163]. These observations suggest that in addition to their role in embryogenesis, homeobox-containing genes may play an important role both in controlling cell differentiation and in the multistep process of tumorigenesis. However, few data are presently available on HOX gene regulation in normal or malignant human breast epithelial cells. It is known that some peptide growth factors activate the expression of homeobox genes trough a cystine-knot-folding motif. Human chorionic gonadotropin (hCG) is a glycoprotein hormone containing a cystine-knot folding motif that suggests that it also could interact with a homeodomain. HCG is the first hormone secreted by embryonal tissues and therefore it is possible to postulate that it could be an important developmental factor. In previous studies, hCG has been proven to be an efficacious physiological protector in rats against the initiation and progression of mammary tumors induced by carcinogen 7, 12-dimethylbenz(a)anthracene (DMBA), accompanied by the induction of cellular differentiation [164, 165], depression of the proliferation of breast tumor cells in vitro and activation of programmed cell death [166, 167]. In addition, it has been reported that hCG suppresses the activation of nuclear transcription factor-kappa B and activator protein-1 (AP-1) induced by tumor necrosis factor (TNF) [168]. Altogether, these data suggested that hCG effect on mammary epithelial cells could be mediated by HOX gene expression, probably through inhibiting AP-1 transcription activities. Class I homeobox genes are expressed in human breast epithelial cell lines. We have observed that the expression of these genes and the divergent expression of HOXA1 in human breast epithelial cells is modulated by recombinant (r-)hCG. R-hCG also modulates the expression of HOX2, a gene that is silent in MCF-10F cells, showing its potential role in inhibiting the expression of AP-1 transcription factor. Treatment of MCF-10F cells with hCG down-regulated all the three transcripts of HOXA1 at an early stage of treatment, whereas HOXA1-S1, the largest transcript, and

HOXA1-S3, the smallest transcript, were up-regulated in the cancer cell lines MDA-MB-231 and MCF-7, respectively [154].

3.5.1 Class I Homeobox Gene Expression in Human Breast Epithelial Cell Lines

Despite extensive literature on the role in embryonic and fetal development, HOX gene expression in adult cells has been reported only recently in a few tissues, including kidney, intestine, testis, colon, and the mouse mammary gland [169–174]. Because RT-PCR amplification of HOX gene transcripts with primers that recognize specific HOX genes has been widely used for analyzing the expression level of HOX genes in various human cancer or normal cells [169, 170], we utilized this methodology for analyzing the expression of class I homeobox genes in MCF-10F, MDA-MB-231, and MCF-7 cells. From 39 class I homeobox genes tested, 33 were expressed in MCF-10F cells, 35 in MCF-7, and 36 in MDA-MB-231 cells. Only four, HOXA2, B1, C4, and C9 were silent or not detected in any of the three cell lines tested by RT-PCR method. HOXB7 was silent in MCF-10F cells and C10 in MDA-MB-231 cells; B13 was expressed only in MCF-7 cells (Fig. 3.19); gene expression pattern is schematically summarized in Fig. 3.20. HOXA1 gene amplification and sequence analysis confirmed that there were three fragments that corresponded to three alternatively spliced transcripts of HOXA1 described by Chariot [171]; the 1,121 bp was expressed in MDA-MB-231 cells, but was absent in MCF-10F and MCF-7 cells; the 655 bp and 452 bp fragments, on the other hand, were strongly expressed in MCF-10F cells, more weakly in MCF-7 cells, and were absent in MDA-MB-231 cells (Fig. 3.21).

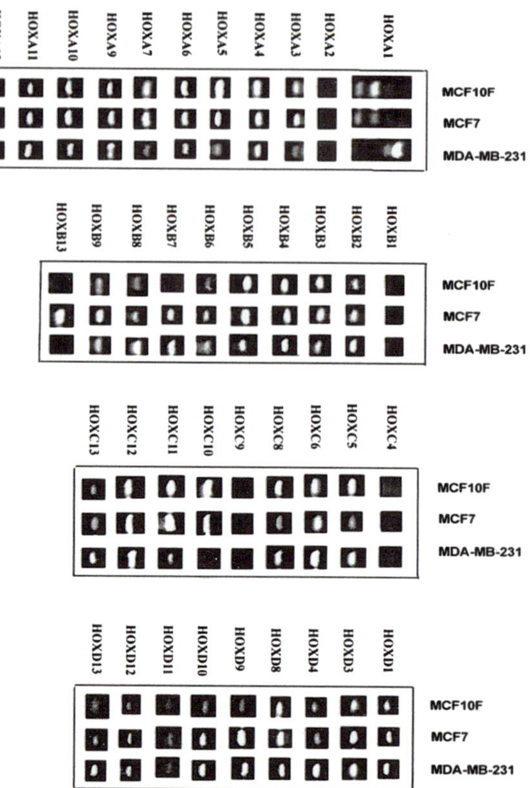

Figure 3.19

RT-PCR analysis of the HOXA, B, C and D gene expression in MCF10F, MCF7 and MDA-MB-231 cell lines. Cellular total RNA was isolated from cultured cells. After 40 cycles of amplification with the specific primers, RT-PCR products were electrophoresed on 2% agarose gels. All the amplified products exhibit the expected size

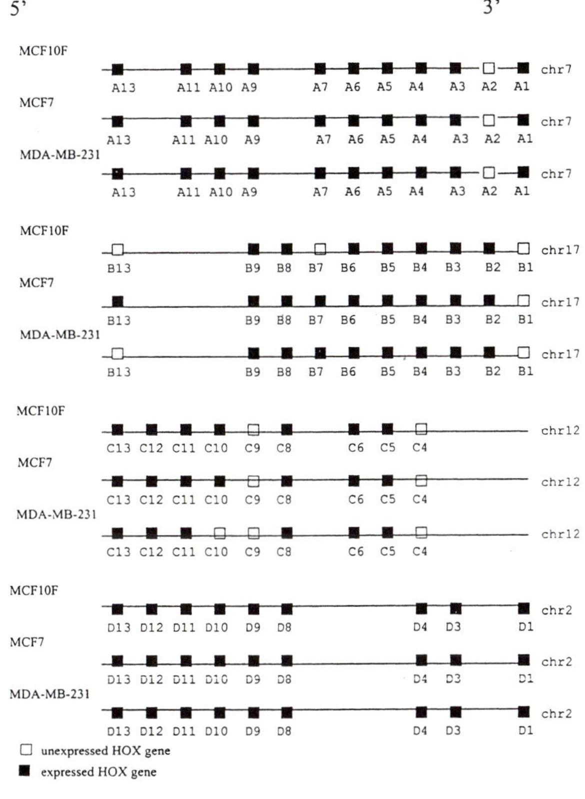

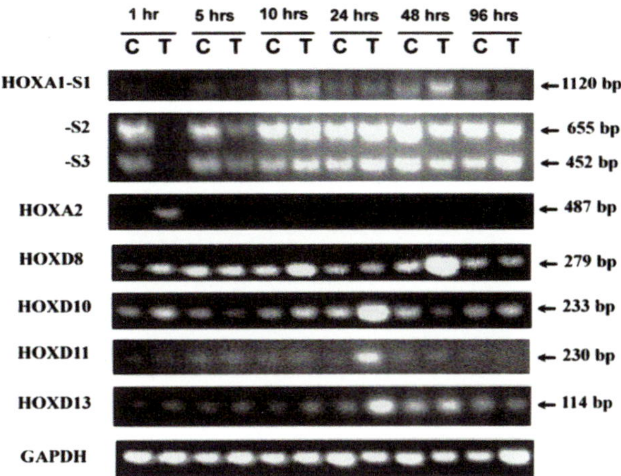

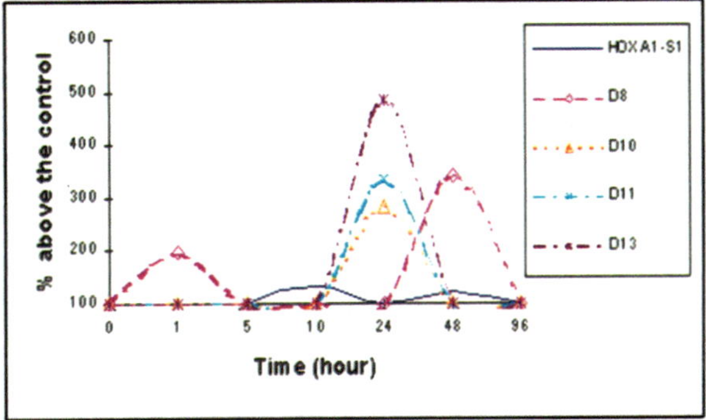

Figure 3.20

Diagram of HOX gene expression in MCF10F, MCF7 and MDA-MB-231 cells. Homeobox clusters are shown according to their physical position on the chromosomes

Figure 3.21

Expression and structures of HOXA1 mRNA isoforms in human breast epithelial cells. *Straight lines* indicate introns and the *black boxes* correspond to the detection portions (1121 bp, 655 bp and 452 bp) of alternatively spliced HOXA1 gene (S1–S3) by RT-PCR

3.5.2 Human Chorionic Gonadotropin Modulates Expression of Homeobox Genes

Treatment of the human breast epithelial cells MCF-10F, MCF-7, and MDA-MB-231 with 5 µg r-hCG per ml culture medium for 1, 5, 10, 24, 48, and 96 h induced the following effects on gene expression: In MCF-10F cells, r-hCG rapidly down-regulated all the three transcripts of HOXA1(HOXA1-S1, -S2 and -S3) at 1- and 5-h points, and a 24-h treatment resulted in up-regulation of HOXD10 (3.8-fold), D11 (4.2-fold) and D13 (5.8-fold), whereas at 48 h of treatment only

D8 was up-regulated by 4.2-fold (Fig. 3.22); In MCF-7 cells, r-hCG treatments of 5 and 10 h resulted in up-regulation of HOXA1-S3 (3.1-fold), B3 (4.2-fold), B8 (4.1-fold) and D11 (3.6-fold) (Fig. 3.23), and in MDA-MB-231 cells the 5- and 10-h treatments up-regulated HOXA1-S1(3.6-fold), C8 (2.0-fold), D8 (2.4-fold) and D11 (3.8-fold) (Fig. 3.24). Minimal or no effects were seen on the expression of other HOX genes. A significant finding of this study was that hCG rapidly induced the transient expression of HOXA2, the silent gene in MCF-10F (Fig. 3.22).

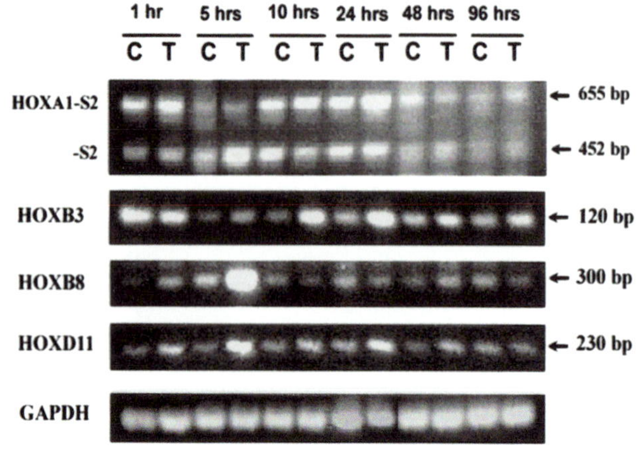

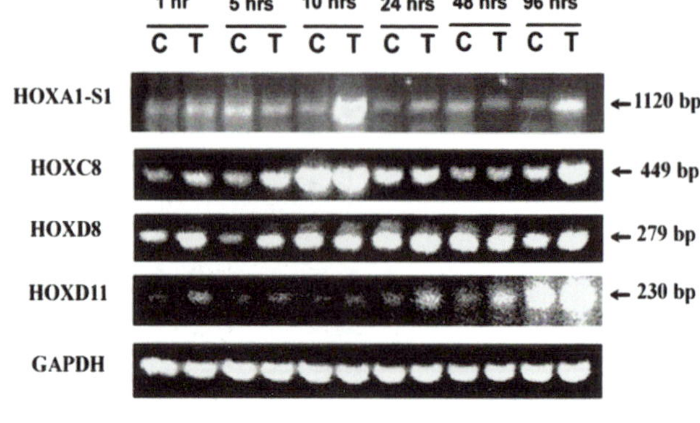

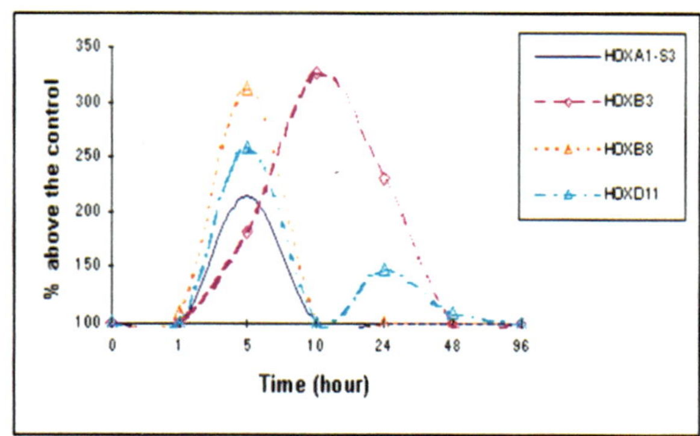

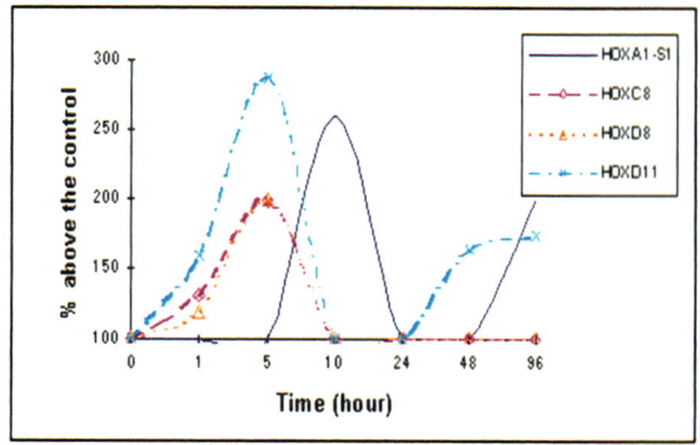

Figure 3.22

Results of the semi-quantitative RT-PCR analyses with total RNAs from MCF-10F cells treated with r-hCG for 1, 5, 10, 24, 48 and 96 h, compared to untreated cells and normalized by glyceraldeyele-3-phosphate dehydrogenase (*GAPDH*) gene. *C* control cells, *T* hCG-treated cells, *S1~S3* alternatively spliced HOXA1 gene

Figure 3.23

Results of the semi-quantitative RT-PCR analyses with total RNAs from MCF-7 cells treated with r-hCG for 1, 5, 10, 24, 48 and 96 h, compared to untreated cells and normalized by GAPDH gene. *S2, S3* alternatively spliced HOXA1 genes

3.5.3 Human Chorionic Gonadotropin and HOXA2 Inhibit AP-1

Treatment of MCF-10F cells with hCG alters the expression of AP-1 (Table 3.7), as demonstrated by electrophoretic mobility shift assay (EMSA) (Fig. 3.25). This test was performed using cell extracts of MCF-10F cells treated with 5 μg r-hCG for 1, 12 and 24-h. Protein binding remained unchanged from control levels after 1 and 12 h of r-hCG treatment. There was significant reduction in AP-1 protein binding expression in cells treated for 24 h (Fig. 3.25 a, lane 6), which reverted to control levels by 24 h post-treatment (Fig. 3.25 a, lanes 7–9).

Because the expression of HOXA2, which is silent in MCF-10F cells, was induced by hCG treatment in vitro, we postulated that HOXA2 could be involved in the activation of the AP-1 pathway. Using EMSA we

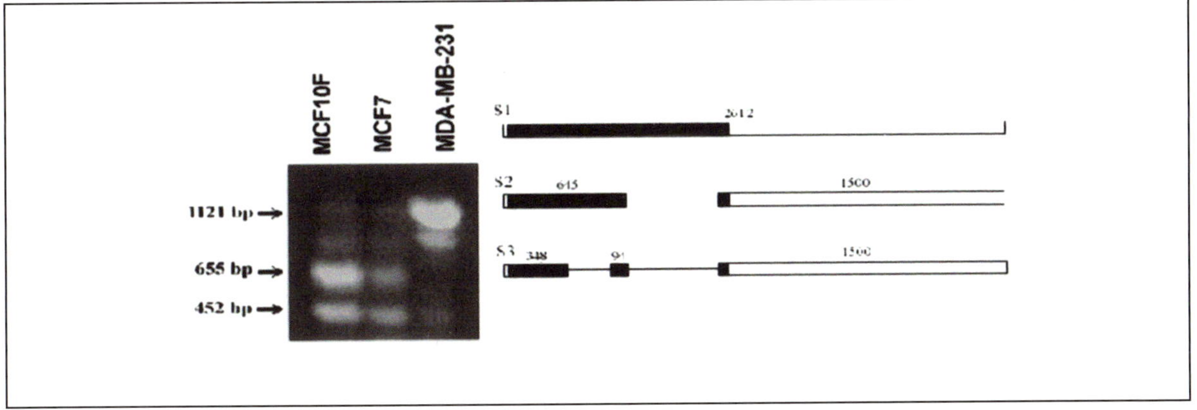

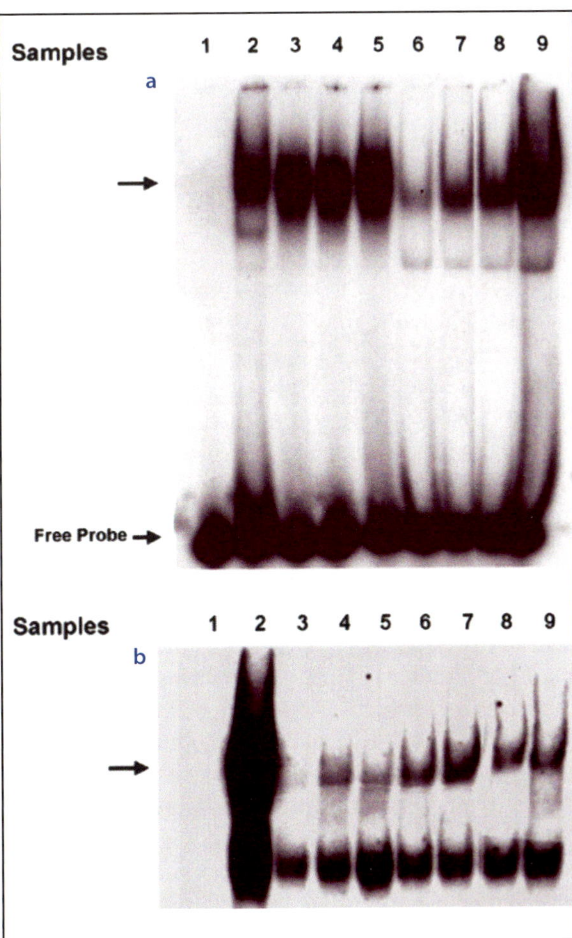

Figure 3.24

Results of the semi-quantitative RT-PCR analyses with total RNAs from MDA-MB-231 cells treated with r-hCG for 1, 5, 10, 24, 48 and 96 h, compared to untreated cells and normalized by GAPDH gene. *S1* alternatively spliced HOXA1 gene

Figure 3.25 a, b ▶

Electrophoretic mobility shift assay (EMSA) was performed using 3 µg of nuclear extracts from MCF-10F cells treated with 5 µg of r-hCG. *Lane 1*, no extract (negative control); *lane 2*, HeLa extract (positive control); *lane 3*, MCF-10F control cells; *lane 4*, MCF-10F cells with 1-h-treatment of r-hCG; *lane 5*, MCF-10F cells with 12-h-treatment of r-hCG; *lane 6*, MCF-10F 24-h treatment with r-hCG. **b** EMSA were performed using 3 µg of nuclear extracts from MCF-10F cells transfected with or without pCMV-HOXA2 plasmid. *Lane 1*, no extract (negative control); *lane 2*, HeLa extract (positive control); *lane 3*, MCF-10F control cells; *lane 4*, MCF-10F cells with 1-h-treatment of RANK ligand; *lane 5*, MCF-10F cells with 12-h-treatment of RANK ligand; *lane 6*, MCF-10F cells transfection with pCMV-HOXA2 plasmid (MCF-10F-A2+); *lane 7*, MCF-10F-A2+ cells with 1-h-treatment of RANK ligand; *lane 8*, MCF-10F-A2+ cells with 12-h-treatment of RANK ligand; *lane 9*, MCF-10F-A2+ cells with 24-h-treatment of RANK ligand. **a** AP-1 EMSA; **b** NF-κB EMSA

Table 3.7. hCG-modulated genes that encode transcription factors/DNA binding protein

Gene/protein name	Accession number	Fold	Classification/function
c-myc	P01106	1.5	Oncogene and tumor suppressor, other transcription protein
Puf	P22392	2.02	Transactivating factor; interaction with an element located upstream from the c-myc gene
RhoE	P52199	2.00	Oncogene and tumor suppressor; Rho-related GTP-binding protein
EIF-I	P32519	3.12	Transcription activators and repressor; regulating differential gene expression
GSPTI (GSTI-HS)	P15170	−5.0	A GTP-binding protein essential for the G1- to S-phase transition of the cell cycle
AP-1	P05412	−6.0	Transcription activator and repressor
DNA binding protein CPBP	Q99612	−3.0	DNA binding protein involved in the regulation of TATA box-less gene
G rich sequence factor I (GRSFI)	Q12849	−3.10	mRNA binding protein involved in mRNA processing

observed a higher level of AP-1 activation by TNF in MCF-10F cells (Fig. 3.25b). However, after transient transfection with HOXA2 cDNA expression construct, the AP-1 binding activity was significantly decreased, producing the same effect that r-hCG alone (Fig. 3.25b), suggesting that the effect of this hormone on AP-1 expression is modulated by HOXA2.

Our data have demonstrated for the first time that most of the 39 cluster I homeobox known genes are expressed in both normal and neoplastic human breast epithelial cells. Our observations allowed us to conclude that homeobox gene expression is independent of the estrogen receptor status of the cells, since a similar number of genes were expressed in the ER-negative immortalized MCF-10F and malignant cell lines MDA-MB-231, as well as in the ER-positive cells MCF-7. A similar number of genes has been also detected in other human adult tissues and cells, such as colon (29/38), kidney (30/38) and cervix keratinocytes (34/39) [157, 158, 170]. The fact that HOXB7 was absent in MCF-10F cells, but was expressed in the neoplastic cell lines, suggested that its expression might be associated with oncogenic transformation in the human breast epithelium. However, in mouse mammary gland HOXB7 may play a role in remodeling and in reestablishing ductal branching [173]. The transduction of HOXB7 has been shown to induce βFGF expression and alter growth characteristic of human breast cancer cells. Altogether these data suggest that the expression of most class I HOX genes in human breast epithelial cells may play some role in the control of differentiation and neoplastic transformation of these cells.

The types of genes activated vary with the biological characteristics of the cells, suggesting that the expression and regulation of HOX genes are cell type-specific. The exact mechanism of their actions, however, is still poorly understood. Some homeobox genes may be targets for TGF-β superfamily members, such as activin, a homodimer composed of two inhibin β chains [176]. Our previous studies have found that the effect of hCG in inhibition of rat mammary tumorigenesis was associated with increased expression of inhibin [177]. HOX gene expression, in general, affects cell growth, differentiation, and fate [178]. We identified three fragments of the HOXA1 gene that were amplified in human breast epithelial cells: 1,121 bp, 655 bp and 452 bp. Sequence analysis confirmed that they belong to three alternatively spliced transcripts of HOXA1 described by Chariot [175]. In addition to its role in development, HOXA1 is involved in murine cellular transformation and/or mammary gland tumorigenesis [161, 174]. Data presented here indicate that r-hCG down-regulates the three transcripts of HOXA1 at very early stage in the immortalized human breast epithelial cells MCF-10F, whereas HOXA1-S1, the largest transcript, as well as HOXA1-S3, the smallest transcript, were up-regulated in the cancer cell lines MDA-MB-231 and MCF-7, respectively. The relationship between HOXA1 expression and breast cancer has been reported [163]. It has been reported that HOXA1 transcripts are induced by retinoic acid in MCF-7 cells [175]. Our results, combined with these data, suggest that HOXA1 may play a role in breast epithelial differentiation and neoplastic transformation depending upon the stimulus received by the cell.

A significant finding of this study is that hCG rapidly induces the transient expression of HOXA2, the silent gene in MCF-10F. So far, there are insufficient data available for understanding the biological function of HOXA2 in adult tissues, and the mechanisms that regulate its expression are still totally unclear. To explore if hCG effect is mediated by some of the HOX genes, we performed the electrophoretic mobility shift assay (EMSA) for AP-1 transcription factor using cell extracts of MCF-10F cells treated with r-hCG. We observed a significant reduction in protein binding expression. We further demonstrated that HOXA2 is involved in the modulation of AP-1, a higher level of AP-1 activation by TNF was observed in MCF-10F cells. However, after transient transfection with HOXA2 cDNA expression construct, the AP-1 biding activity was significantly decreased. Suggesting that HOX A2 modulates the effect of r-hCG on AP1 expression. Whereas other transcription factors/DNA binding proteins are also of great interest [179–193] for our understanding the action of hCG we have concentrated in this work in the AP-1. The activation of AP-1 is mediated through the activation of a stress-activated protein kinase called c-jun N-terminal kinase (JNK) [194]. E6/E7 immortalized human keratinocytes transfected with dominant negative c-jun TAM67 showed a reduction in the elevated

AP-1 activities seen with progression and suppression of tumor phenotype [195]. In addition, cotransfection of MCF-7 cells with a c-jun expression vector and the EGFR promoter reporter resulted in a 7-fold increase in promoter activity [196], and an elevated level of c-jun activation related to poorer quality and shortened duration of endocrine response in estrogen-receptor-positive breast cancer patients [197]. Transfection of JB6 cells with pdcd4, a novel transformation suppressor gene, resulted in inhibition of AP-1 transactivation [198]. Our data indicate that the over-expression of HOXA2 protein alone was not sufficient to block the TNF-induced AP-1 activation, however, hCG that has been reported to be a suppressor on TNF-induced AP-1 activation [168], could be due through the activation of HOXA2.

Altogether, our data have shown that the majority of HOX genes are active in human breast epithelial cells and they have a divergent expression pattern that is modulated by exogenous hCG. These observations not only imply that HOX genes play a role in the process of differentiation and transformation of human breast epithelial cells, but also identifies hCG as a novel regulator in the complicated HOX network. The finding that human breast epithelial cells present different splicing forms of hCG receptor may explain why hCG does not exert the same effect in MCF-10F, MCF-7 and MDA-MB-231 cells in the activation of the HOXA1 gene. In addition to its role in development, Hox-a1 is involved in murine cellular transformation and/or mammary gland tumorigenesis [161, 199]. Data presented here indicate that r-hCG down-regulated all the three transcripts of HOXA1 at very early stage in the immortalized human breast epithelial cells MCF-10F, probably due to the presence of the full length LH/hCG receptor. HOXA1-S1, the largest transcript, as well as HOXA1-S3, the smallest transcript, were up regulated in the cancer cell lines MDA-MB-231 and MCF-7, respectively. These two cell lines did express weakly or not express the full-length LH/hCG receptor. Our present level of knowledge does not allow us to completely rule out the possibility that other mechanisms may be implicated or that other splicing forms of the LH/hCG receptor may be responsible for the effect of r-hCG in the cancer cell lines. HOXA1 gene is the most near to the 3' position in the HOXA chromosomal cluster on chromosome 7. In the developing embryo, murine homologue HOXA1 protein may regulate the expression of other HOX genes in its rostral domain of expression, suggesting that this gene probably plays a key role in modulating the expression of other HOX genes. In studies performed in human tissues and cell lines HOXA1 could be an important gene that plays a crucial role in the establishment of the phenotype of the human breast cancer cell and could be one of the orchestrators that regulate breast epithelial cell differentiation [175, 200]. Our results suggest that the differential effect of h-hCG on HOXA1 could be due to differences in LH/hCG receptor expression and demonstrate that it plays a role in breast epithelial differentiation and neoplastic transformation.

3.6 Human Chorionic Gonadotropin and Histone Acetylation

Human chorionic gonadotropin or hCG-induced differentiation of the mammary gland is associated with the synthesis of inhibin, a heterodimeric protein that is structurally related to the transforming growth factor-β (TGF-β) family [81, 201]. The expression of both inhibin A, and B is increased by hCG treatment both in vitro and in vivo [81, 201]. The effect of hCG was accompanied by a significant activation of c-myc and c-jun, while c-fos was not modified by the treatment. These early genes remained activated, even after the cessation of hCG treatment, an indication that their expression was regulated by the hCG treatment in a fashion similar to that described for inhibin. Even though inhibin belongs to the TGF-β family, hCG treatment did not affect the level of expression of TGF-β, or of other members of this family. The data support the concept that hCG acts as an inducer of inhibin, and immediate early-gene. hCG increases the expression of testosterone repressed prostate message 2 (TRPM2) and interleukin-l-converting enzyme (ICE) transcripts as early as 5 days after initiation of treatment and their values remained elevated up to 20 days post-treatment [201]. The product of the proto-oncogene, bc12 and one of its family members, bcl-XL, are known to play a role in promoting cell survival and inhibiting apoptosis, and expression of bcl-XS is associated with the induction of apoptosis. hCG treatment had no effect on the expression of bc12 and bcl-XL at any of the time periods tested, instead, it induced the expression of bcl-XS [165, 201–203]. Gene transcription has been shown to be regulated by acetylation and deacetylation of histones [204]. Eukaryotic transcription is a highly regulated process, and the acetylation is now known to play a major role in this regulation. DNA typically exists in vivo as a repeating array of nucleosomes, in which 146 bp of DNA are around a histone octamer that consisting of two each of histone protein H2A, H2B, H3, and H4. This chromatin structure could be affected by histone acetylation. Histone acetylation eliminates the positive charge of E-amino group on lysine residue, which could lead to destabilization and consequent dissociation of nucleosomes, thus allowing access of transcription factors and RNA polymerase to the DNA. In addition, histone acetylation inhibits the stacking of nucleosomes into the solenoid structure and thus the formation of higher-order structure [205]. hCG and inhibin induce acetylated histone accumulation in MCF-1OF cells. Figure 3.26 shows the levels of acetylated histone H3 and H4 in MCF10 F cells treated with different concentration of hCG as well as inhibin β-subunit at various time points. In the Western blot analysis, both acetylated histone H3 and H4 were significantly increased by hCG treatment over 12 h in MCF-1OF cells at all the doses tested. Inhibin induced the accumulation of acetylated histone H3 after 4-h treatment at the concentration of 1 ng/ml or at all the time points with higher concentration (10–1,000 ng/ml). However, only slight induction of acetylated histone H4 was detected in the cells treated with higher concentration of inhibin (100 ng/ml) over 12 h (Fig. 3.27). Both hCG and inhibin increase acetylation levels of histone H3 and H4 in MCF-l0F cells, however inhibin is able to produce its effect at 4 h instead of 12 h with the lower doses of hCG. At higher doses both hCG and inhibin has a faster action of the H3-acetylation. For H4 acetylation it was a late effect with not a clear dose depended effect. These data are the first to demonstrate that these hormones are histone acetylators. These data acquire relevance to the light that chro-

Figure 3.26

Western blot analysis. hCG increases the accumulation of acetylated histone H3 and H4 in MCF-10F cells

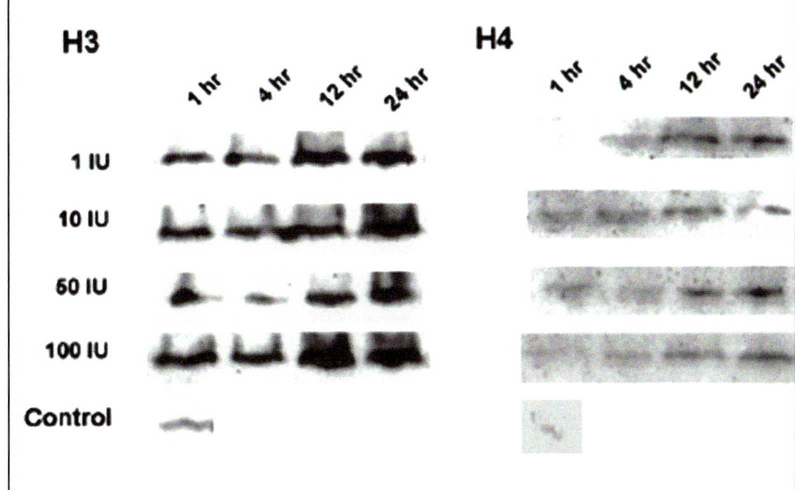

Figure 3.27

Western blot analysis of the accumulation of acetylated histone H3 and H4 in MCF-10F cells. Cells were treated with inhibin at 1, 10, 100, or 1,000 ng/ml for 1, 4, 12, or 24 h, respectively

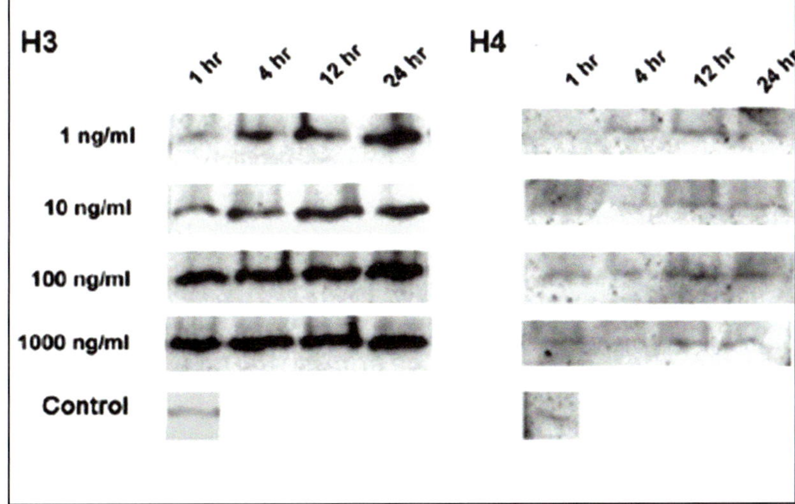

matin fractions enriched in actively transcribed genes are also enriched in highly acetylated core histones [206], whereas silent genes are associated with nucleosomes with a low level of acetylation. Allfrey [207] first suggested that histone acetylation was involved in the regulation of transcription. During the past decade, considerable evidence has accumulated to establish the role of acetylation and deacetylation of histones in the regulation of transcription [206–209]. Acetylation neutralizes the charge of the histones and generates a more open DNA conformation. Transcription factors and the transcription apparatus then have access to the DNA, and expression of the corresponding genes is promoted. In the breast epithelial cells H3 acetylation seems to play a more important role than H4, instead in amphibian metamorphosis thyroid hormone treatment induces gene activation and histone H4 acetylation regulating the expression [210]. This type of organ specific effect is also observed in the gene encoding hepatic nuclear factor 1-alpha (HNF1-alpha). HNF1-alpha is essential for the expression of glut2 glucose transporter and L-type pyruvate kinase (pklr) genes in pancreatic insulin-producing cells, whereas in liver, kidney, or duodenum tissue, glut2 and pklr expression is maintained in the absence of HNF1-alpha. However, it is indispensable for hyperacetylation of histones in glut2 and pklr promoter nucleosomes in pancreatic islets but not in liver cells, where glut2 and pklr chromatin remains hyperacetylated in the absence of HNF1-alpha [211]. Whereas it is not clear how the histone 3 acetylation is involved in the activation of early genes like c-myc and c jun or those controlling programmed cell death in the mammary epithelial cells by the hCG and inhibin, there are evidence histone acetylase plays a role in regulation of transcription, cell cycle progression, differentiation and DNA repair [212–222]. In addition, nuclear estrogen receptors have been postulated to regulate gene expression via their association with histone acetylase (HAT) or deacetylase complexes [223]. Altogether, our data provide in vivo evidence that hCG and inhibin effect on mammary epithelial cells could be mediated by histone acetylation and indicate that acetylation could act as a regulator in the mechanism of action of these hormones.

3.7 Conclusions

The breast epithelium not only responds to estrogen but also to other myriad of hormones and growth factors. We have made special emphasis in the novel effect of hCG due to is importance in breast cancer prevention. Figure 3.28 summarizes the findings described in this chapter. The hormone binds to a spe-

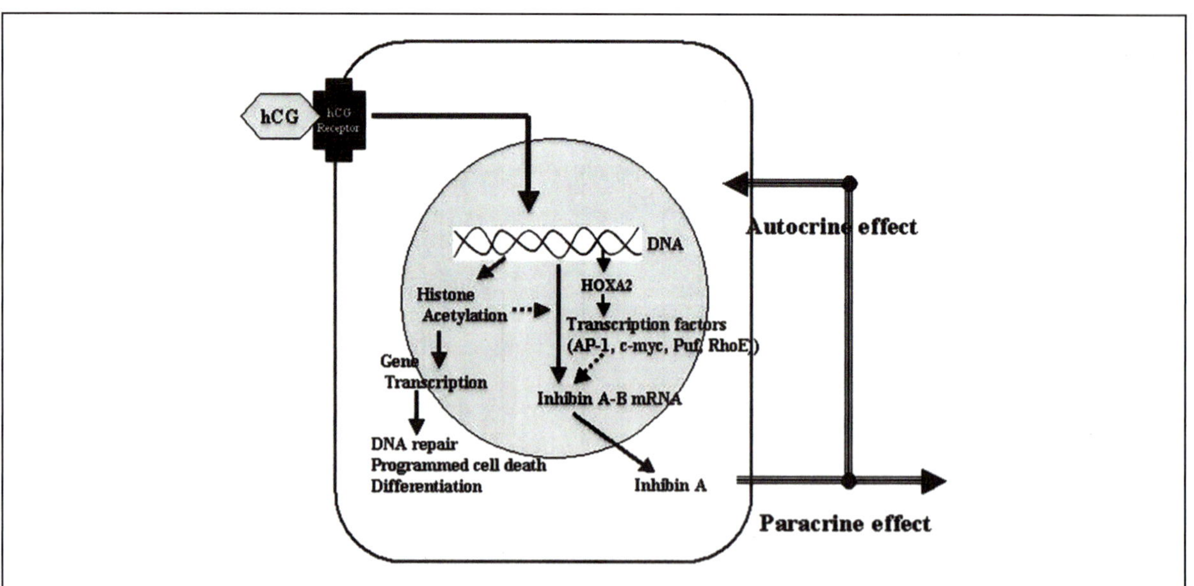

Figure 3.28

The hormone binds to a specific membrane receptor, activating several homeobox genes, among them HOXA2, a silent gene that is significantly up regulated by the hormone resulting in activation of several transcription factors, either by down-regulation or by up-regulation. Among them is the down-regulation of AP-1 that could be related to the synthesis of inhibin. Inhibin is secreted and may act as a paracrine and/or autocrine factor regulating cell proliferation and sustain the effect on HOXA2 and AP-1. The acetylation of H4 by both inhibin and hCG indicates that through this pathway they regulate gene transcription controlling DNA repair, programmed cell death, and differentiation cific membrane receptor, activating several homeobox genes, among them HOXA2, a silent gene that is significantly up regulated by the hormone resulting in activation of several transcription factors (Table 3.7), either by down-regulation or by up-regulation. Among them is the down-regulation of AP-1 that could be related to the synthesis of inhibin. The non-steroidal glycoprotein inhibin is secreted and may act as a paracrine and/or autocrine factor regulating cell proliferation and sustain the effect on HOXA2 and AP-1. The acetylation of H4 by both inhibin and hCG could indicate that through this pathway gene transcription of cell cycle related genes such as p53 and ICE that may lead to apoptosis or through p21 to cell growth arrest, programmed cell death and DNA repair.

References

1. Russo, I.H., Russo, J. Mammary gland neoplasia in long-term rodent studies. Env. Health Perspectives. 104:938–967, 1996.
2. Russo, J., Russo, I.H. Role of hormones in human breast development- the menopausal breast. In: Progress in the Management of Menopause. London: Parthenon Publishing; 1997. P. 1–10.
3. Russo, I.H., Russo, J. Role of hormones in cancer initiation and progression. J. Mam. Gland. Biol. Neoplasia 3:49–61, 1998.
4. Russo, J., Russo, I.H. Role of differentiation in the pathogenesis and prevention of breast cancer. Endocr. Related Cancer 4:7–21, 1997.
5. Calaf, G., Alvarado, M.E., Bonney, G.E., Amfoh, K.K., Russo, J. Influence of lobular development on breast epithelial cell proliferation and steroid hormone receptor content. Int. J. Oncol. 7:1285–1288, 1995.
6. Lippman, M.E., Dickinson, R.B., Gelmann, E.P., Rosen N, Knabbe, C, Bates S, et al. Growth regulation of human breast carcinoma occurs through regulated growth factor secretion. J. Cell Biochem. 35:1–16, 1987.
7. Meyer, J.S. Cell proliferation in normal human breast ducts fibroadenomas and other duct hyperplasias measured by nuclear labeling with tritiated thymidine. Hum. Path. 8:67–81, 1977.
8. Masters, J.R.W., Drife, J.O., Scarisbrick, J.J. Cyclic variations of DNA synthesis in human breast epithelium. J. Natl. Cancer Inst. 58:1263–65, 1977.
9. Ferguson, D.J.P., Anderson, T.J. Morphologic evaluation of cell turnover in relation to the menstrual cycle in the "resting" human breast. Br. J. Cancer 44:177–181, 1981.
10. Anderson, T.J., Ferguson, D.J.P., Raab, GM. Cell turnover in the "resting" human breast: influence of parity, contraceptive pill, age and laterality. Br. J. Cancer 46:376–82, 1982.
11. Russo, J., Russo, I.H. Estrogens and Cell Proliferation in the Human Breast. J. Cardiovascular. Pharmacol. 28:19–23, 1996.
12. Kumar, V., Stack, G.S., Berry, M., Jin, J.R., Chambon, P. Functional domains of the human estrogen receptor. Cell 51:941–951, 1987.
13. King, R.J.B. Effects of steroid hormones and related compounds on gene transcription. Clin. Endocrinol. 36:1–14, 1992.
14. Huseby, R.A., Maloney T.M., McGrath, C.M. Evidence for a direct growth-stimulating effect of estradiol on human MCF-7 cells in vitro. Cancer Res. 144:2654–2659, 1987.
15. Huff, K.K., Knabbe, C, Lindsey, R., Kaufman, D., Bronzert, D., Lippman, M.E., Dickson, R.B. Multihormonal regulation of insulin-like growth factor 1-related protein in MCF-7 human breast cancer cells. Mol. Endocrinol. 2:200–208, 1988.
16. Dickson, R.B., Huff, K.K., Spencer, E.M., Lippman, M.E. Induction of epidermal growth factor related polypeptides by 17β-estradiol in MCF-7 human breast cancer cells. Endocrinology 118:138–142, 1986.
17. Soto, A.M., Sonnenschein, C. Cell proliferation of estrogen-sensitive cells: the case for negative control. Endocr. Rev. 48:52–58, 1987.
18. Tsai, M.J., O'Malley, B.W. Molecular mechanisms of steroid/thyroid receptor super-family members. Annu. Rev. Biochem. 63:451–486, 1994.
19. Song, X-D., McPherson, R.A., Adam, L., Bao, Y., Shupnik, M., Kumar, R., and Santen, R.J. Linkage of rapid estrogen action to MAPK activation by ER-alpha-SHC association and SHC pathway activation. Mol Endo. 16:116–127, 2002.
20. Kuiper, G.G.J.M., Enmark, E, Pelto-Huikko, M, Nilsson S, Gustaffson, JA. Cloning of a novel estrogen receptor expressed in rat prostate and ovary. Proc. Natl. Acad. Sci. USA 93:5925–5930, 1996.
21. Tremblay, G.B., Tremblay, A., Copeland, N.G., Gilbert, D.J., Jenkins. N.A., Labrie, F., Giguere, V. Cloning, chromosomal localization, functional analysis of the murine estrogen receptor β. Mol. Endocrinol. 11:353–65, 1997.
22. Mosselman, S., Polma, J., Dijkema, R. ER β: identification and characterization of a novel human estrogen receptor. FEBS Lett. 392:49–53, 1996.
23. Leake, R. 100 years of the endocrine battle against breast cancer. Lancet, 347:1780–1781,1996.
24. Clarke, R., Skaar, T.C., Bouker, K.B., Davis, N., Lee, Y.R., Welch, J.N., and Leonessa, F., Molecular and pharmacological aspects of anti-estrogen resistance. J. Steroid Biochem. Mol. Biol. 76:71–84, 2001.
25. Dorssers, L.C., vanderFlier, S., Brickman, A., van Agthover, T., Veldscholte, J., Berns, E.M., Klijn, J.G., Beex, L.V. and Foekens, J.A. Tamoxifen resistance in breast cancer: elucidating mechanisms. Drugs 61:1721–1733, 2001.

26. Shaw, J.A., Udokang, K., Mosquera, J.-M., Chauhan, H., Jones, J.L., Walker, R.A. Oestrogen receptors alpha and beta differ in normal human breast and breast carcinomas. J. Pathol. 198:450–457, 2002.

27. Wade, C.B., Dorsa, D.M. Estrogen activation of cyclic adenosine 5'-monophosphate response element-mediated transcription requires the extracellularly regulated kinase/mitogen-activated protein kinase pathway. Endocrinol. 144:832–838, 2003.

28. Coleman, K.M., Dutertre, M., El-Gharbawy, A., Rowan, B.G., Weigel, N.L., Smith, C.L. Mechanistic differences in the activation of estrogen receptor alpha (ERalpha)- and ERbeta-dependent gene expression by cAMP signaling pathway (s). J. Biol. Chem. 278:12834-12845, 2003.

29. Katzenellenbogen, B.S. Dynamics of steroid hormone receptor action. Annu. Rev. Physiol. 42:17–35, 1980.

30. Topper, J., Freedman, C. Multiple hormone interactions in the developmental biology of the mammary gland. Physiol. Rev. 60:1049–1060, 1980.

31. Dickson, R.B., Lippman, M.E. Cellular and molecular biology. In: Lippman, M.E, Dickson, R.B., editors. Breast cancer. Boston: Kluwer Academic Publishers, pp119–165, 1988.

32. Jordan, C. Tamoxifen: the herald of a new era of preventive therapeutics. J. Natl. Cancer Inst. 89:747–749, 1997.

33. Kuiper, G.G.J.M., Carlsson, B., Grandien, K., Enmark, E., Haggblad, J., Nilsson, S., Gustafsson, J.A. Comparison of the ligand binding specificity and transcript tissue distribution of estrogen receptors α and β. Endocrinology 138:863–870, 1997.

34. Cowley, S.M., Hoare, S., Mosselman, S., Parker, M.G. Estrogen receptors α and β form heterodimers on DNA. J. Biol. Chem. 272:19858–19862, 1997.

35. Kuiper, G.G.J.M., Gustafsson, J.A. The novel estrogen receptor-β subtype: potential role in the cell- and promotor-specific actions of estrogens and anti-estrogens. FEBS Lett. 410:87–90,1997.

36. Pace, P., Taylor, J., Suntharalingam, S., Coombes, R.C., Ali, S. Human estrogen receptor β binds DNA in a manner similar to and dimerizes with estrogen receptor α. J. Biol. Chem. 272:25832–25838, 1997.

37. Ogawa, S., Inoue, S., Watanabe, T., Hiroi, H., Orimo, A., Hosoi T., Ouchi, Y., Muramatsu, M. The complete primary structure of human estrogen receptor β (hERβ) and its hetero-dimerization with ER α in vivo and in vitro. Biochem. Biophys. Res. Commun. 243:122–126, 1998.

38. Paech, K., Webb, P., Kuiper, G.G.J.M., Nilsson, S., Gustafsson, J.A., Kushner, P.J., Scanlan, T.S. Differential ligand activation of estrogen receptors ERα and ERβ at AP1 sites. Science 277:1508–1510, 1997.

39. Longacre, T.A., Bartow, S.A. A correlative morphologic study of human breast and endometrium in the menstrual cycle. Am. J. Surg. Pathol. 10:382–393, 1986.

40. Going, J.J., Anderson, T.J., Battersby, S. Proliferative and secretory activity in human breast during natural and artificial menstrual cycles. Am. J. Pathol. 130:193–204, 1988.

41. Potten, C.S., Watson, R.J., Williams, G.T. The effect of age and menstrual cycle upon proliferative activity of the normal human breast. Br. J. Cancer 58:163–170, 1988.

42. Clark, R.B., Howell, A., Potter, C.S., Anderson, E. Dissociation between steroid receptors expression and cell proliferation in the human breast. Cancer Res. 57:4987–4991, 1997.

43. Laidlaw, I.J., Clark, R.B., Howell, A., Owen, A.W.M.C., Potten, C.S., Anderson, E. Estrogen and progesterone stimulate proliferation of normal human breast tissue implanted in athymic nude mice. Endocrinology 136:164–171, 1995.

44. Clarke, R.B., Howell, A., Anderson, E. Estrogen sensitivity of normal human breast tissue in vivo and implanted into athymic nude mice: analysis of the relationship between estrogen-induced proliferation and progesterone receptor expression. Breast Cancer Res. Treat. 45:121–183, 1997.

45. Goodman, H.M., editor. Basic medical endocrinology. New York: Raven Press, 1994: pp 288–290.

46. Russo, J., Rivera, R., Russo, I.H. Influence of age and parity on the development of the human breast. Breast Cancer Res. Treat. 23:211–218, 1992.

47. Russo, J., Russo, I.H. Influence of differentiation and cell kinetics on the susceptibility of the rat mammary gland to carcinogenesis. Cancer Res. 40:2677–2687, 1980.

48. Russo, J., Russo, I.H. Biology of disease. Biological and molecular bases of mammary carcinogenesis. Lab. Invest. 57:112–137, 1987.

49. Russo, J., Ao, X., Grill, C., and Russo, I.H. Pattern of distribution for estrogen receptor a and progesterone receptor in relation to proliferating cells in the mammary gland. Breast Cancer Res. and Treat. 53:217–227, 1999.

50. Haslam, S. Role of sex steroid hormones in normal mammary gland function. In: Neville M. C., Daniel C.W. (eds) The Mammary Gland: Development, Regulation and Function. Plenum Press, New York, 1987, pp 499–533.

51. Clarke, R., Dickson, R.B., Lipton, M.E. Hormonal aspects of breast cancer. Growth factors, drugs and stromal interactions. Crit. Rev. Oncol. Hematol. 12:1–23, 1992.

52. Knabbe, C., Lipton, M.E., Wakefield, L.M., Flanders, K.C., Kasid, A., Derynck, R., et al. Evidence that transforming growth factor β is a hormonally regulated negative growth factor in human breast cancer cells. Cell 48:417–428, 1987.

53. Dickson, R., Lipton, M. Control of human breast cancer by estrogen, growth factors and oncogenes. In: Lipman, M.E., Dickson, R.B., editors. Estrogen receptors in human breast cancer. New York: Raven Press, 1975.

54. Russo, J., Calaf, G., Russo, I.H. A critical approach to the malignant transformation of human breast epithelial cells. CRC Crit. Rev. Oncog. 4:403–417, 1993.

55. Russo, J., Reina, D., Frederick, J., Russo, I.H. Expression of phenotypical changes by human breast epithelial cells treated with carcinogens in vitro. Cancer Res. 48:2837–2857, 1988.

56. Russo, J., Gusterson, B.A., Rogers, A., Russo, I.H., Wellings, S.R., van Zwieten, M.J. Biology of the Disease. Comparative

study of human and rat mammary tumorigenesis. Lab. Invest. 62:244–278, 1990.

57. Habel, L. A., Stamford, J.L. Hormone receptors and breast cancer. Epidemiol. Rev. 15:209–219, 1993.

58. Harlan, L.C., Coates, R.J., Block, G. Estrogen receptor status and dieting intakes in breast cancer patients. Epidemiology 4:25–31, 1993.

59. Moolgavkar, S.H., Day, N.E., Stevens, R.G. Two-stage model for carcinogenesis: epidemiology of breast cancer in females. J. Natl. Cancer Inst. 65:559–569, 1980.

60. Kodama, P., Green, G.L., Salmon, S, S.E. Relation of estrogen receptor expression to clonal growth and antiestrogen effects on human breast cancer cells. Cancer Res. 45:2720–2724, 1985.

61. Kuiper, G.G.J.M., Enmark, E., Pelto-Huikko, M., Nilsson, S., Gustaffson, J-A: Cloning of a novel estrogen receptor expressed in rat prostate and ovary. Proc. Natl. Acad. Sci. USA 93:5925–5930, 1996.

62. Byers, M., Kuiper, G.G.J.M., Gustaffson, J-A., Park-Sarge, O.K. Estrogen receptor-β mRNA expression in rat ovary: down-regulation by gonadotropins. Mol. Endocrinol. 11:172-l82, 1997.

63. Vladusic, E.A., Hornby, A.E., Guerra-Vladusic, F.K., Lupu, R. Expression of estrogen receptor-β messenger RNA variant in human breast cancer. Cancer Res. 58:210–214, 1998.

64. Foster, J.S., Wimalasena, J. Estrogen regulates activity of cyclin-dependent kinases and retinoblastoma protein phosphorylation in breast cancer cells. Mol. Endocrinol. 10:488–498, 1996.

65. Wang, W., Smith, R., Burghardt, R., Safe, SH. 17β estradiol-mediated growth inhibition of MDA-MB 468 cells stably transfected with the estrogen receptor: cell cycle effects. Mol. Cell Endocrinol. 133:49–62, 1997.

66. Levenson, A.S., Jordan, V.C. Transfection of human estrogen receptor (ER) cDNA into ER negative mammalian cell lines. J. Steroid Biochem. Mol. Biol. 51:229–239, 1994.

67. Weisz, A., Bresciani, F. Estrogen regulation of proto-oncogenes coding for nuclear proteins. Crit. Rev. Oncogen. 4:361–388, 1993.

68. Zajchowski, D.A., Sager, K., Webster, L. Estrogen inhibits the growth of estrogen receptor negative, but not estrogen receptor positive, human mammary epithelial cells expressing a recombinant estrogen receptor. Cancer Res. 53:5004–5011, 1993.

69. Pilat, M.J., Christman, J.K., Brooks, S.C. Characterization of the estrogen receptor transfected MCF-10A breast cell line 139B6. Breast Cancer Res. Treat. 37:253–266, 1996.

70. Calaf, G., Tahin, Q., Alvarado, M.E., Estrada, S., Cox, T., Russo, J. Hormone receptors and cathepsin D levels in human breast epithelial cells transformed by chemical carcinogens. Breast Cancer Res. Treat. 29:169–177, 1993.

71. Aronica, S.M., Kraus, W.L., Katzenellenbogen, B.S. Estrogen action via the cAMP signaling pathway. Stimulation of adenylate cyclase and cAMP regulated gene transcription. Proc. Natl. Acad. Sci. USA 91:8517–8521, 1994.

72. Pappos, T.C., Gametahu, B., Watson, C.S. Membrane estrogen receptors identified by multiple antibody labeling and impeded-ligand binding. FASEB J. 9:404–410, 1994.

73. Alvarado, M.V., Russo, J., Russo, I.H. Immunolocalization of inhibin in the mammary gland of rats treated with hCG. J. Histochem. Cytochem. 41:29–34, 1993.

74. Russo, I.H., and Russo, J. Role of hormones in mammary cancer initiation and progression. J. Mammary Gland Biol. Neoplasia. 3:49–61, 1998.

75. Segaloff, D.L., Ascoli, M. The lutropin/choriogonadotropin receptor- 4 years later. Endocr. Rev. 4: 324–347, 1993.

76. Minegishi, T., Nakamura, K., Takakura, Y., Miyamoto, K., Hasegawa, Y., Ibuki, Y., Igarashi, M. Cloning and sequencing of human LH/hCG receptor cDNA. Biochem. Biophys. Res. Commun. 172:1049–1054, 1990.

77. Frazier, A.L., Robbins, L.S., Stork, P.J., Sprengel, R., Segaloff, D.L., Cone, R.D. Isolation of TSH and LH/CG receptor cDNAs from human thyroid: regulation by tissue specific splicing. Mol. Endocrinol. 4:1264–1276, 1990.

78. Sokka, T., Hamalainen, T., Huhtaniemi, L. Functional LH receptor appears in the neonatal rat ovary after changes in the alternative splicing pattern of the LH receptor mRNA. Endocrinology 130:1738–1740, 1992.

79. Reinholz, M.M., Zschunke, M.A., Roche, P.C. Loss of alternately spliced messenger RNA of the luteinizing hormone receptor and stability of the follicle-stimulating hormone receptor messenger RNA in granulosa cell tumors of the human ovary. Gynecol. Oncol. 79: 264–271, 2000.

80. Srivastava, P., Russo, J., Russo, I.H. Chorionic gonadotropin inhibits rat mammary carcinogenesis through activation of programmed cell death. Carcinogenesis, 18:1799–1808, 1997.

81. Russo, I.H. and Russo, J. Role of hCG and inhibin in breast cancer. Int. J. of Oncology 4:297–306, 1994.

82. Russo, I.H. and Russo, J. Hormonal approach to breast cancer prevention. J. Cell Biochem. Suppl. 34:1–6, 2000.

83. Russo, J. and Russo, I.H. Human Chorionic Gonadotropin in Breast Cancer Prevention. In: Endocrine Oncology, (S.P. Ethier, editor), Humana Press Inc., Totowa, NJ, pp121–136, 2000.

84. Russo, I.H., Koszalka, M., Russo, J. Effect of human chorionic gonadotropin on mammary gland differentiation and carcinogenesis. Carcinogenesis 11:1849–1855, 1990.

85. Alvarado, M.V., Alvarado, N.E., Russo, J., Russo, I.H. Human chorionic gonadotropin inhibits proliferation and induces expression of inhibin in human breast epithelial cells in vitro. In Vitro Cell Dev. Biol. Anim. 30:4–8, 1994.

86. Lojun, S., Bao, S., Lei, Z.M., Rao, C.V. Presence of functional luteinizing hormone/ chorionic gonadotropin (hCG) receptors in human breast cell lines: implications supporting the premise that hCG protects women against breast cancer. Biol. Reprod. 57:1202–1210, 1997.

87. Russo, J., Janssens, J.P., Russo, I.H. Recombinant human chorionic gonadotropin (r-hCG) significantly reduces primary tumor cell proliferation in patients with breast cancer. Breast Cancer Res. and Treat. 64:161a, 2000.

88. Soule, H.D., Maloney, T.M., Wolman, S.R., Peterson, N.D., Brenz, R., McGrath C.M., Russo, J., Pauley, R.J., Jones, R.F., and Brooks, S.C. Isolation and characterization of a spontaneously immortalized human breast epithelial cell line, MCF-10. Cancer Research, 50:6075–6086, 1990.

89. Tait, L.R., Soule, H.D., and Russo, J. Ultrastructural and immunocytochemical characterization of an immortalized human breast epithelial cell line, MCF-10. Cancer Research, 50:6087–6094, 1990.

90. Jian, X., Russo, I.H., Russo, J. Alternately spliced luteinizing hormone/human chorionic gonadotropin receptor mRNA in human breast epithelial cells. Int. J. Oncol. 20: 735–738, 2002.

91. Zeng, H., Phang, T., Song, Y.S., Ji, I., Ji, T.H. The role of the hinge region of the luteinizing hormone receptor in hormone interaction and signal generation. J. Biol. Chem. 276: 3451–3458, 2001.

92. Song, Y.S., Ji, I., Beauchamp, J,. Isaacs, N.W., Ji, T.H. Hormone interactions to Leu-rich repeats in the gonadotropin receptors. II. Analysis of Leu-rich repeat 4 of human luteinizing hormone/ chorionic gonadotropin receptor. J. Biol. Chem.. 276:3436–3442, 2001.

93. Kuroda, H., Mandai, M., Konishi, I., Tsuruta, Y., Kusakari, T.. Kariya, M., Fujii, S. Human ovarian surface epithelial (OSE) cells express LH/hCG receptors, and hCG inhibits apoptosis of OSE cells via up-regulation of insulin-like growth factor-1. International Journal of Cancer 91:309–315, 2001.

94. Hai, M.V., De Roux, N., Ghinea, N., Beau, I., Loosfelt, H., Vannier, B., Meduri, G., Misrahi, M., Milgrom, E. Gonadotropin receptors. Annales d Endocrinologie. 60:89–92, 1999.

95. Venencie, P.A.Y., Meduri, G., Pissard, S., Jolivet, A., Loosfelt, H., Milgrom, E., Misrahi, M. Luteinizing hormone/human chorionic Gonadotrophin receptors in various epidermal structures. British Journal of Dermatology. 141:438–446, 1999.

96. Latronico, A.C. Naturally occurring mutations of the luteinizing hormone receptor gene affecting reproduction. Seminars in Reproductive Medicine. 18:17–20, 2000.

97. Munshi, U.M., Peegel, H., Menon, K.M. Palmitoylation of the luteinizing hormone/human chorionic gonadotropin receptor regulates receptor interaction with the arrestin-mediated internalization pathway. European Journal of Biochemistry. 268:1631–1639, 2001.

98. Lei, Z.M., Mishra, S., Zou, W., Xu, B., Foltz, M., Li, X., Rao, C.V. Targeted disruption of luteinizing hormone/human chorionic gonadotropin receptor gene. Molecular Endocrinology. 15:184–200, 2001.

99. Yano, K., Kohn, L.A.D., Saji, M., Okuno, A., Cutler, G.B., Jr. Phe576 plays an important role in the secondary structure and intracellular signaling of the human luteinizing hormone/chorionic gonadotropin receptor. J. Clin. Endocrinol. Metab. 82:2586–2591, 1997.

100. Licht, P., Cao, H., Zuo, J., Lei, Z.M., Rao, V., Merz, W.E., Day, T.G. Jr. Lack of self-regulation of human chorionic gonadotropin biosynthesis in human choriocarcinoma cells. J. Clin. Endocrinol. Metab. 78:1188–1194, 1994.

101. Ying, S-Y. Inhibins, activins and follistatins. J. Steroid Biochem. 33:705–713, 1989.

102. Meunier, H., Rivier, C., Evans, R.M. and Vale, W. Gonadal and extragonadal expression of inhibin α, βA and βB subunits in various tissues predicts diverse functions. Proc. Natl. Acad. Sci. USA. 85:247–251, 1988.

103. Roberts, V., Meunier, H., Sawchenko, P.E., Vale, W. Differential production and regulation of inhibin subunits in rat testicular cell types. Endocrinology 125:2350–2359, 1989.

104. Veeramachaneni, D.N.R., Schanbacher, B.D., Amann, R.P. Immuno-localization and concentrations of inhibin A in the ovine testis and excurrent duct system. Biol. Reprod. 41:499–503, 1989.

105. Petraglia, F., Vaughan, J., Vale, W. Inhibin and activin modulate the release of gonadotropin-releasing hormone, human chorionic gonadotropin and progesterone from cultured human placental cells. Proc. Natl. Acad. Sci. USA 85:5114–5l17, 1989.

106. Roberts, V.J., Sawchenko, P.E., Vale, W. Expression of inhibin/activin subunit messenger ribonucleic acids during rat embryogenesis. Endocrinol. 128:3122–3129, 1991.

107. McLachlan, R.I., Matsumoto, A.M., Burger, H.G., DeKretser, D.M., Bremmer, W.J. Relative roles of follicle stimulating hormones in the control of inhibin secretion in normal men. J. Clin. Inv. 82:880–884, 1988.

108. Woodruff, T.K., Mayo, K.E. Regulation of inhibin synthesis in the rat ovary. Annu. Rev. Physiol. 52:807–821, 1990.

109. Hunzicker-Dunn, M., Birnbauer, L. The involvement of adenylyl cyclase and cyclic AMP-dependent protein kinases in luteinizing hormone actions. In: Luteinizing Hormone Action and Receptors. Ascoli M. (ed.) Florida, CRC Press, pp57–134, 1990.

110. Matzuk, M., Milton, J., Su, J., Hsuch, W., Bradley, A. α-inhibin is a tumor suppressor gene with gonadal specificity in mice. Nature 360:313–319, 1992.

111. Sutherland, R.L., Green, M.D., Hall, R.E., Reddell, R.R. and Taylor, I.W. Tamoxifen induces accumulation of MCF-7 human mammary carcinoma cells in the G_0/G_1 phase of the cell cycle. Eur. J. Cancer Clin. Oncol. 19:615–621, 1983.

112. Taylor, I.W., Hodson, P.J, Green, M.D. and Sutherland, R.L. Effects of tamoxifen on cell cycle progression of synchronous MCF-7 human mammary carcinoma cells. Cancer Res. 43:4007–4010, 1983.

113. Ziecick, A.J., Stanchev, P.D., Tilton, J.E. Evidence for the presence of luteinizing hormone/human chorionic gonadotropin-binding sites in the porcine uterus. Endocrinology 119:1159–1163, 1986.

114. Frazier, A.L., Robbins, L.S., Stork, P.J., Sprengel, R., Segaloff, D.L., Cone, R.D. Isolation of TSH and LH/CG receptor cDNAs from human thyroid: Regulation by tissue specific splicing. Mol. Endocrinol. 4:1264–1276, 1990.

115. Goustin, A.S., Leof, E.B., Shipley, G.D., and Moses, H.L. Growth factors and cancer. Cancer Res. 46:1015–1029, 1986.

116. Heldin, C-H., and Westermark, B. Growth factors: mechanism of action and relation to oncogenes. Cell 37:9–20, 1984.

117. Bishop, J.M. The molecular genetics of cancer. Science 235:305–311, 1977.
118. Ullrich, A. and Schlessinger, J. Signal transduction by receptors with tyrosine kinase activity. Cell 61:203–212, 1990.
119. Peres, R., Betsholtz, C., Westermark, B. and Heldin, C-H. Frequent expression of growth factors for mesenchymal cells in human mammary carcinoma cell lines. Cancer Res. 47:3425–3429, 1987.
120. Halper, J. and Moses, H.L. Purification and characterization of a novel transforming growth factor. Cancer Res. 47:4552–4559, 1987.
121. Bronzert, D.A., Pantazis, P., Antoniades, H.N., Kasid, A., Davidson, N., Dickson, R.B. and Lippman, M.E. Synthesis and secretion of platelet-derived growth factor by human breast cancer cell lines. Proc. Natl. Acad. Sci. USA. 84:5763–5767, 1987.
122. Dickson, R.B. and Lippman, M.E. Estrogenic regulation of growth and polypeptide growth factor secretion in human breast carcinoma. Endocrine Rev. 8:29–43, 1987.
123. Huang, D-P., Schwartz, C.E., Chiu, J-F., and Cook, J.R. Dexamethasone inhibition of rat hepatoma growth and α fetoprotein synthesis. Cancer Res. 44:2976–2980, 1984.
124. Mira-y-Lopez, R., Reich, E., Stolfi, R.L., Martin, D.S. and Ossowski, L. Coordinate inhibition of plasminogen activator and tumor growth by hydrocortisone in mouse mammary carcinoma. Cancer Res. 45:2270–2276, 1985.
125. Cook, P.W., Swanson, K.T., Edwards, C.P. and Firestone, G.L. Glucocorticoid receptor-dependent inhibition of cellular proliferation in dexa-methasone-resistant and hypersensitive rat hepatoma cell variants. Mol. Cell Biol. 8:1449–1459, 1988.
126. Smith, R.G., Syms, A.J., Nag, A., Lerner, S. and Noms, J.S. Mechanism of the glucocorticoid regulation of growth of the androgen-sensitive prostate-derived R3327H-G8-A1 tumor cell line. J. Biol. Chem. 260:12454–12463, 1985.
127. Syms, A.J., Norris, J.S. and Smith, R.G. Autocrine regulation of growth: I. Glucocorticoid inhibition is overcome by exogenous platelet derived growth factor. Biochem. Biophys. Res. Commun. 122:68–74, 1984.
128. Miller Jr., W.H., Dmitrovsky, E. Retinoid acid audits rearranged receptor in the treatment of acute promyelocytic leukemia. In: Important Advances in Oncology. DeVita V, Hellman S and Rosenberg SA (eds). JB Lippincott Co, Philadelphia, pp81–90,
129. Iwai, S.A., Kosaka, N.M., Nishinu, Y., Sumi, T.. Sakuda, M., Nishimune, Y. Changes in Hoxl.6, cqun and Oct-3 gene expressions are associated with teratocarcinoma F9 cell differentiation in three different ways of induction. Exptl. Cell Res. 205:39–43, 1993.
130. DeCosse, J.J., Gossens, C.L. and Kuzma, J.F. Breast cancer: induction of differentiation by embryonic tissues. Science 181:1057–1058, 1973.
131. Evan. G.L., Littlewood, T.D. The role of c-myc in cell growth. Current Opin. Genet. Develop. 3:44–49, 1993.
132. Illmensee, K. and Mintz, B. Totipotency and normal differentiation of single teratocarcinoma cells cloned by injection into blastocysts. Proc. Natl. Acad. Sci. USA. 73:549–553, 1976.
133. Ki Hong, W., Wittes, R.E., Hadju, S.T., Cvitkovic, E., Whitmore, W. and Golbey, R.B. The evaluation of mature teratoma from malignant testicular tumors. Cancer 40:2987–2992, 1977.
134. Contractor, S.F., Davies, H.. Effect of human chorionic somatomammotrophin and human chorionic gonadotropin on phytohaemagglutinin-induced lymphocyte transformation. Nature 243:284–286, 1973.
135. Heintz, N.H., Dailey, L., Held, P. and Heintz, N. Eukaryotic replication origins as promoters of bi-directional DNA synthesis. Trends in Genetics 8:376–381, 1992.
136. Draetta, G. Cell cycle control in eukaryotes. Trends Biochem. Sci. 15:378, 1990.
137. Ransone, L.J. and Verman, I.M. Nuclear proto-oncogenes *fos* and *jun*. Annu. Rev. Cell Biol. 6:539, 1990.
138. Curran, T. and Morgan, J.I. Memories of Fos. Bio Essays 7:255–258, 1987.
139. Lau, L.F. and Nathans, D. Expression of a set of growth-related immediate early genes in Balb/c 3T3 cells. Coordinate regulation with c-fos and c-myc. Proc. Natl. Acad. Sci. USA. 84:1182–1186, 1987.
140. Curran, T. and Franza, B.R. Fos and Jun: the AP-I connection. Cell 55:395–397, l988.
141. Czerwiec, F.S., Meimer, M.H., Puitt, D. Transiently elevated levels of c-fos and c-myc oncogene messenger ribonucleic acids in cultured murine Leydig tumor cells after addition of human chorionic gonadotropin. Mol. Endocrinol. 3:105–109. 1989.
142. Wyllie, A.H. Glucocorticoid-induced thymocyte apoptosis is associated with endogenous endonuclease activation. Nature 284:555–556, 1980.
143. Wyllie, A.H., Kerr, J.F.R., Currie, A.R. Cell death. The significance of apoptosis. Int. Rev. Cytol. 68:251–306, 1980.
144. Cohen, J.J. and Duke, R.C. Glucocorticoid activation of a calcium-dependent endonuclease in thymocyte nuclei leads to cell death. J. Immunol. 132:38–42, 1984.
145. O'Connor, P.M., Wassermann, K., Sarang, M., Magrath, I.,. Bohr, V.A., Kohn, K.W. Relationship between DNA crosslinks, cell cycle, and apoptosis in Burkitt's Lymphoma cell lines differing in sensitivity to nitrogen mustard. Cancer Res. 51:6550–6557, 1991.
146. Kerr, J.F.R., Harmon, B.V. Definition and incidence of apoptosis: a historical perspective. In: Apoptosis: The Molecular Basis of Cell Death. L.D. Tomei and F.O. Cope (eds.) Plainview: Cold Spring Harbor Press, pp5–29, 1991.
147. Gerschenson. L.E., Rotell, R.J. Apoptosis and cell proliferation are terms of the growth equation. In: Apoptosis: The Molecular Basis of Cell Death. L.D. Tomeik and F.O. Cope (eds.) Cold Spring Harbor Laboratory Press, ppl39–155, 1991.
148. Buttyam, R,. Olsson, C.A., Pintar, J., Chang, C. Bandyk, M., Ng, P-Y. and Sawczuk, I.S. Induction of the TRPM-2 gene in cells undergoing programmed death. Mol. Cell Biol. 9:3473–3481, 1989.

149. Yonish-Rouach, E.. Resnitzky, D., Lotem, J., Sachs, L., Kimchi, A. and Oren, M. Wild-type pS3 induces apoptosis of myeloid leukaemic cell that is inhibited by interleukin-6. Nature 353:345–347, 1991.

150. Shaw, P., Bovey, R., Tardy, S., Sahli, R., Sordat, B. and Costa, J. Induction of apoptosis by wild-type p53 in a human colon tumor-derived cell line. Proc. Natl. Acad. Sci. USA. 89:4495–4499, 1992.

151. Alneri, E.S., Femades, T.F., Haldar, S., Croce, C.M., Litwack, G. Involvement of bc1–2 in glucorticoid- induced apoptosis of human pre-B-leukemias. Cancer Res. 52:491–495, 1992.

152. Sentman, C.L., Shutter, J.R., Hockenberry, D., Kanagawa, O. and Korsmeyer, S.J. hcl-2 inhibits multiple forms of apoptosis but not negative selection in thymocytes. Cell 67:879–888, 1991.

153. Sun, P.D., and Davies, D.R. The cystine-knot growth factor super-family. Annu. Rev. Biophys. Biomol. Struct. 24:269–291, 1995.

154. Russo, J., Lareef, M.H., Russo, I.H., and Jiang, X. Modulation of Hox gene expression in human breast epithelial cells by human chorionic gonadotropin, Proc. Am. Assoc. Cancer Res. 42:2649a, 2001.

155. Acampora, D., D'Esposito, M., Faiella, A., Pannese, M., Migliaccio, E., Morelli, F., Stornaiuolo, A., Nigro, V., Simeone, A., Boncinelli, E. The human HOX gene family. Nucleic Acids Res. 17:10385–10402, 1989.

156. Apiou, F., Flagiello, D., Cillo, C., Malfoy, B., Poupon, M.F., Dutrillaux, B. Fine mapping of human HOX gene clusters. Cytogenet. Cell Genet. 73:114–115, 1996.

157. De Vita, G., Barba, P., Odartchenko, N., Givel, J.C., Freschi, G., Bucciarelli, G., Magli, M.C., Boncinelli, E., Cillo, C. Expression of homeobox-containing genes in primary and metastatic colorectal cancer. Eur. J. Cancer 29A: 887–893, 1993.

158. Cillo, C., Barba, P., Freschi, G., Bucciarelli, G., Magli, M.C., Boncinelli, E. HOX gene expression in normal and neoplastic human kidney. Int. J. Cancer 51:892–897, 1992.

159. Aberdam, D., Negreanu, V., Sachs, L., Blatt, C. The oncogenic potential of an activated Hox-2.4 homeobox gene in mouse fibroblasts. Mol. Cell Biol. 11:554–557, 1991.

160. Song, K., Wang, Y., Sassoon, D. Expression of Hox-7.1 in myoblasts inhibits terminal differentiation and induces cell transformation. Nature 360:477–481, 1992.

161. Maulbecker, CC, Gruss, P. The oncogenic potential of deregulated homeobox genes. Cell Growth Differ. 4:431–441, 1993.

162. Cillo, C., Faiella, A., Cantile, M., Boncinelli, E. Homeobox genes and cancer. Exp. Cell Res. 248:1–9, 1999.

163. Chariot, A., Castronovo, V. Detection of HOXA1 expression in human breast cancer. Biochem. Biophys. Res. Commun. 222:292–297, 1996.

164. Russo, I.H., Koszalka, M., Russo, J. Effect of human chorionic gonadotropin on mammary gland differentiation and carcinogenesis. Carcinogenesis 11:1849–1855, 1990.

165. Russo, I.H., Russo, J. Hormonal approach to breast cancer prevention. J. Cell Biochem. 34:1–6, 2000.

166. Alvarado, M.V., Alvarado, N.E., Russo, J., Russo, I.H. Human chorionic gonadotropin inhibits proliferation and induces expression of inhibin in human breast epithelial cells in vitro. In Vitro Cell Dev. Biol. Anim., 30A:4–8, 1994.

167. Srivastava, P., Russo, J., Mgbonyebi, O.P., Russo, I.H. Growth inhibition and activation of apoptotic gene expression by human chorionic gonadotropin in human breast epithelial cells. Anticancer Res, 18:4003–4010, 1998.

168. Manna, S.K., Mukhopadhyay, A., Aggarwal, B.B. Human chorionic gonadotropin suppresses activation of nuclear transcription factor-kappa B and activator protein-1 induced by tumor necrosis factor. J. Biol. Chem. 275:13307–13314, 2000.

169. Flagiello, D, Gibaud, A, Dutrillaux, B, Poupon, M.F., Malfoy, B. Distinct patterns of all-trans retinoic acid dependent expression of HOXB and HOXC homeogenes in human embryonal and small-cell lung carcinoma cell lines. FEBS Lett. 415:263–267, 1997.

170. Alami, Y, Castronovo, V, Belotti, D, Flagiello, D, Clausse, N. HOXC5 and HOXC8 expression are selectively turned on in human cervical cancer cells compared to normal keratinocytes. Biochem. Biophys. Res. Commun. 257:738–745, 1999.

171. Wolgemuth, D.J., Viviano, C.M., Gizang-Ginsberg, E., Frohman, M.A., Joyner, A.L., Martin, G.R. Differential expression of the mouse homeobox-containing gene Hox-1.4 during male germ cell differentiation and embryonic development. Proc. Natl. Acad. Sci. USA 84:5813–5817, 1987.

172. James, R., Kazenwadel, J. Homeobox gene expression in the intestinal epithelium of adult mice. J. Biol. Chem. 266:3246–3251, 1991.

173. Srebrow, A., Friedman, Y., Ravanpay, A., Daniel, C.W., Bissell M.J. Expression of Hoxa-1 and Hoxb-7 is regulated by extracellular matrix-dependent signals in mammary epithelial cells. J. Cell Biochem. 71:310–312, 1998.

174. Care, A., Silvani, A., Meccia, E., Mattia, G., Peschle, C., Colombo M.P.. Transduction of the SkBr3 breast carcinoma cell line with the HOXB7 gene induces bFGF expression, increases cell proliferation and reduces growth factor dependence. Oncogene; 16:3285–3289, 1998.

175. Chariot, A., Moreau, L., Senterre, G., Sobel, M.E., Castronovo, V. Retinoic acid induces three newly cloned HOXA1 transcripts in MCF-7 breast cancer cells. Biochem. Biophys. Res. Commun. 215:713–720, 1995.

176. Kloen, P., Visker, M.H., Olijve, W., van Zoelen, E.J., Boersma, C.J. Cell-type-specific modulation of Hox gene expression by members of the TGF-beta super-family: a comparison between human osteosarcoma and neuroblastoma cell lines. Biochem. Biophys. Res. Commun. 233:365–369, 1997

177. Srivastava, P., Russo, J., and Russo, I.H. Inhibition of rat mammary tumorigenesis by human chorionic gonadotropin is associated with increased expression of inhibin. Molecular Carcinogenesis, 26:1–10, 1999.

178. Chariot, A., Gielen, J., Merville, M.P., Bours, V. The homeo-domain-containing proteins: an update on their interacting partners. Biochem. Pharmacol. 58:1851–1857, 1999.

179. Gupta, S., Seth, A., Davis, R.J. Transactivation of gene expression by Myc is inhibited by mutation at the phosphorylation sites Thr-58 and Ser-62. Proc. Natl.. Acad. Sci. USA 90:3216–3220, 1993.

180. Gilles, A.M., Presecan, E., Vonica, A., Lascu, I. Nucleoside diphosphate kinase from human erythrocytes. Structural characterization of the two polypeptide chains responsible for heterogeneity of the hexameric enzyme. J. Biol. Chem. 266:8784–8789, 1991.

181. Postel, E.I.I., Ilerberich, S.J., Flint, S.J., Ferrone, C.A. Human c-myc transcription factor PuF identified as nm23-H2 nucleoside diphosphilate kinase, a candidate suppressor of tumor metastasis. Science 261:478–480, 1993.

182. Nobes, C.D., Lauritzen, I., Mattei, M.G., Paris, S., Hall, A., Chardin, P. A new member of the Rho family, Rndl, promotes disassembly of actin filament structures. and loss of cell adhesion. J. Cell Biol. 141:187–197, 1998.

183. Foster, R., Hu, K.Q., Lu, Y., Nolan, K.M., Thissen, J., Settleman, J. Identification of a novel human Rho protein with unusual properties: GTPasc deficiency and in vivo farnesylation. Mol. Cell Biol. 16:2689–2699, 1996.

184. Wang, C.Y., Petryniak, B., Thompson, C.B., Kaelin, W.G., Leiden, J.M. Regulation of the Ets-related transcription factor Elf-1 by binding to the retinoblastoma protein. Science 260:1330–1335, 1993.

185. Thompson, C.B., Wang, C.Y., Ho, I.C., Bohjanen, P.R., Petryniak, B., June, C.H., Miesfeldt, S., Zhang, L., Nabel, G.J., Karpinski, B., et al. cis-acting sequences required for inducible interleukin-2 enhancer function bind a novel Ets-related protein, Elf-1. Mol. Cell Biol. 12:1043–1053, 1992.

186. Hoshino, S., Miyazawa, H., Enomoto, T., Hanaoka, F., Kikuchi, Y., Kikuchhhhi, A., Ui, M. 1989 A human homologue of the yeast GST1 gene codes for a GTP-binding protein and is expressed in a proliferation-dependent manner in mammalian cells. EMBO J. 8:3807–3814, 1989.

187. Glover, J.N., Harrison, S.C. Crystal structure of the heterodimeric bZIP transcription factor c-Fos-c-Jun bound to DNA. Nature 373:257–261, 1995.

188. Junius, F.K., O'Donoghue, S.I., Nilges, M., Weiss, A.S., King, G.F. High resolution NMR solution structure of the leucine zipper domain of the c-Jun homodimer. Biol. Chem. 271:13663–13667, 1996.

189. Hattori, K., Angel, P., Le Beau, M.M., Karin, M. Structure and chromosomal localization of the functional intronless human JUN proto-oncogene. Proc. Natl. Acad. Sci. USA 85:9148–9152, 1988.

190. Bohmann, D., Bos, T.J., Admon, A., Nishimura, T., Vogt, P.K., Tjian, R. Human proto-oncogene c-jun encodes a DNA binding protein with structural and functional properties of transcription factor AP-1. Science 238:1386–1392, 1987.

191. Slavin, D., Sapin, V., Lopez-Diaz, F., Jacquemin, P., Koritschoner, N., Dastugue, B., Davidson, I., Chatton, B., Bocco, J. The Kruppel-like core promoter binding protein gene is primarily expressed in placenta during mouse development. Biol. Reprod. 61:1586–1591, 1999.

192. Koritschoner, N.P., Pocco, J.L., Panzetta-Dutari, G.M., Dumur, C.I., Flury, A, Patrito, L.C. A novel human zinc finger protein that interacts with the core promoter element of a TATA box-less gene. J. Biol. Chem. 272:9573–9580, 1997.

193. Qian, Z, Wilusz, J. GRSF-1: a poly(A)+ mRNA binding protein which interacts with a conserved G-rich element. Nucleic Acids Res. 22:2334–2343, 1994.

194. Karin, M., Delhase, M. JNK or IKK, AP-1 or NF-kappaB, which are the targets for MEK kinase 1 action? Proc. Natl. Acad. Sci. USA, 95:9067–9069, 1998.

195. Lie, J.J., Rhim, J.S., Schlegel, R., Vousden, K.H., Colburn, N.H. Expression of dominant negative Jun inhibits elevated AP-1 and NF-kappaβ transactivation and suppresses anchorage independent growth of HPV immortalized human keratinocytes. Oncogene 16:2711–2721, 1998.

196. Johnson, A.C., Murphy, B.A., Matelis, C.M., Rubinstein., Y., Piebenga, E.C., Akers, L.M., Neta, G., Vinson, C., Birrer, M. Activator protein-1 mediates induced but not basal epidermal growth factor receptor gene expression. Mol. Med. 6:17–27, 2000.

197. Gee, J.M., Barroso, A.F., Ellis, I.O., Robertson J.F., Nicholson, R.I. Biological and clinical associations of c-jun activation in human breast cancer. Int. J. Cancer. 89:177–186, 2000.

198. Yang, H.S., Jansen, A.P,. Nair, R., Shibahara, K., Verma, A.K., Cmarik, J.L., Colburn, N.H. A novel transformation suppressor, Pdcd4, inhibits AP-1 transactivation but not NF-kappaβ or ODC transactivation. Oncogene 20:669–676, 2001.

199. Friedmann, Y., Daniel, C.A., Strickland, P., Daniel, C.W. Hox genes in normal and neoplastic mouse mammary gland. Cancer Res. 54:5981–5985, 1994.

200. Chariot, A., Castronovo, V. Detection of HOXA1 expression in human breast cancer. Biochem. Biophys. Res. Commun. 222:292–297, 1996.

201. Russo, J. and Russo, I.H. Human Chorionic Gonadotropin in Breast Cancer Prevention In: Endocrine Oncology. Ethier SP, (ed.) Humana Press Inc., Totowa, NJ., pp 121–136, 2000.

202. Russo, I.H., Srivastava, P., Mgbonyebi, O.P. and Russo, J. Activation of programmed cell death by human-chorionic gonadotropin in breast cancer therapy. Acta Haematol. 98:16, 1997.

203. Srivastava, P., Russo, J. and Russo, I.H. Chorionic gonadotropin inhibits rat mammary carcinogenesis through activation of programmed cell death. Carcinogenesis 18:1799–1808, 1998.

204. Grunstein, M. Histone acetylation and chromatin structure and transcription. Nature 389:349–352, 1997.

205. Kornberg, R.D. and Lorch, Y. Twenty-five years of the nucleosome particle of the eukaryote chromosome. Cell 98:285–294, 1999.

206. Kouzarides, T. Histone acetylases and deacetylases in cell proliferation. Curr. Opin. Genet Dev. 9:40–48, 1999.

207. Allfrey, V.G. Post synthetic modifications of histone: a mechanism for the control of chromosome structure by the modulation of histones – DNA interactions. In: Chromatin and Chromosome structure. Li, T., Eckhardt, R.C.A. (eds.) Academic Press, New York, pp167–191, 1977.

208. Luger, K., Mader, A.W., Richmond, R.K., Sargent, D.F., Richmond, T.J. Crystal structure of the nucleosome core particle at 2.8A resolution. Nature 389:251–260, 1997.

209. Davie, J.R. Covalent modifications of histones: expression from chromatin templates. Curr. Opin. Genet. Dev. 8:173–178, 1997.

210. Sachs, L.M. and Shi, Y.B. Targeted chromatin binding and histone acetylation in vivo by thyroid hormone receptor during amphibian development. Proceedings of the National Academy of Sciences of the United States of America 97:13138–13143, 2000.

211. Parrizas, M., Maestro, M., Boj, S., Paniagua, A., Casamitjana, R., Gomis, R., Rivera, F. and Ferrer, J. Hepatic nuclear factor 1-alpha directs nucleosomal hyperacetylation to its tissue-specific Molecular & Cellular Biology 21:3234–3243, 2001.

212. Ogryzko, V.V., Kotani, T., Zhang, X., Schiltz, R.L., Howard, T., Yang, X.J., Howard, B.H., Qin, J. and Nakatani, Y, Histone-like TAFs within the PCAF histone acetylase complex. Comment in: Cell 94(1):1–4, 1998 Cell 94:35–44, 1998.

213. Deckert, J. and Struhl, K. Histone acetylation at promoters is differentially affected by specific activators and repressors. Molecular & Cellular Biology 21:2726–2735, 2001.

214. Bhadra, U., Pal-Bhadra, M. and Birchler., J.A. Histone acetylation and gene expression analysis of sex lethal mutants in Drosophila. Genetics 155:753–763, 2000.

215. Ikura, T., Ogryzko, V.V., Grigoriev, M., Groisman, R., Wang, J., Horikoshi, M., Scully, R., Qin, J. and Nakatani, Y. Involvement of the TIP60 histone acetylase complex in DNA repair and apoptosis. Cell 102:463–473, 2000.

216. Zhang, Q., Vo, N. and Goodman, R.H. Histone binding protein RbAp48 interacts with a complex of CREB binding protein and phosphorylated CREB. Molecular & Cellular Biology 20:4970–4978, 2000.

217. Herrera, J.E., Schiltz, R.L., and Bustin, M. The accessibility of histone H3 tails in chromatin modulates their acetylation by P300/CBP-associated factor. Journal of Biological Chemistry 275:12994–12999, 2000.

218. Garrison, P.M., Rogers, J.M., Brackney, W.R. and Denison, M.S. Effects of histone deacetylase inhibitors on the Ah receptor gene promoter. Archives of Biochemistry & Biophysics. 374:161–171, 2000.

219. McMahon, S.B., Wood, M.A. and Cole, M.D. The essential cofactor TRRAP recruits the histone acetyltransferase hGCN5 to c-Myc. Molec. & Cellular Biolog. 20:556–562, 2000.

220. Masumi, A., Wang, I.M., Lefebvre, B., Yang, X.J., Nakatani, Y. and Ozato, K. The histone acetylase PCAF is a phorbol-ester-inducible coactivator of the IRF family that confers enhanced interferon responsiveness. Molecular & Cellular Biology 19:1810–1820, 1999.

221. Vassilev, A., Yamauchi, J., Kotani, T., Prives, C., Avantaggiati, M.L., Qin, J. and Nakatani, Y. The 400 kDa subunit of the PCAF histone acetylase complex belongs to the ATM superfamily. Molecular Cell 2:869–875, 1998.

222. Randhawa, G.S., Bell, D.W., Testa, J.R., Feinberg, A.P. Identification and mapping of human histone acetylation modifier gene homologues. Genomics 51:262–269, 1998.

223. Chen, H., Lin, R.J., Xie, W., Wilpitz, D. and Evans, R.M. Regulation of hormone-induced histone hyperacetylation and gene activation via acetylation of an acetylase. Cell 98:675–686, 1999.

The Role of Estrogen in Breast Cancer

4.1 Introduction

Intensive epidemiological studies have identified a number of genetic risk factors associated with breast cancer, including evidence of *BRCA1* and *BRCA2* susceptibility genes, familiar history of cancer in the breast, ovary or endometrium and individual history of breast diseases [1]. An increased risk has also been associated with early onset of menstruation, nulliparity or delayed first childbirth, short duration of breast feeding, late menopause, use of hormone replacement therapy and increased bone density [2–4]. A principal culprit common for all these endocrine-related risk factors is the prolonged exposure to female sex hormones [5–8]. The hormonal influences have been mainly attributed to unopposed exposure to elevated levels of estrogens [5], as has been indicated for a variety of female cancers, namely, vaginal, hepatic and cervical carcinomas [9–11]. Exposure to estrogens, particularly during the critical developmental periods (e.g., in utero, puberty, pregnancy, menopause), also affects affective behaviors (e.g., depression, aggression, alcohol intake) and increases breast cancer risk [12]. In addition, both environmental and genetic factors are believed to exert their influence by a hormonal mechanism [13–18].

It is generally accepted that the biological activities of estrogens are mediated by nuclear estrogen receptors (ER) which, upon activation by cognate ligands, form homodimers with another ER-ligand complex and activate transcription of specific genes containing the estrogen response elements (ERE) (Fig. 4.1) [19]. According to this classical model, the biological responses to estrogens are mediated by the ER universally identified until recently, which has

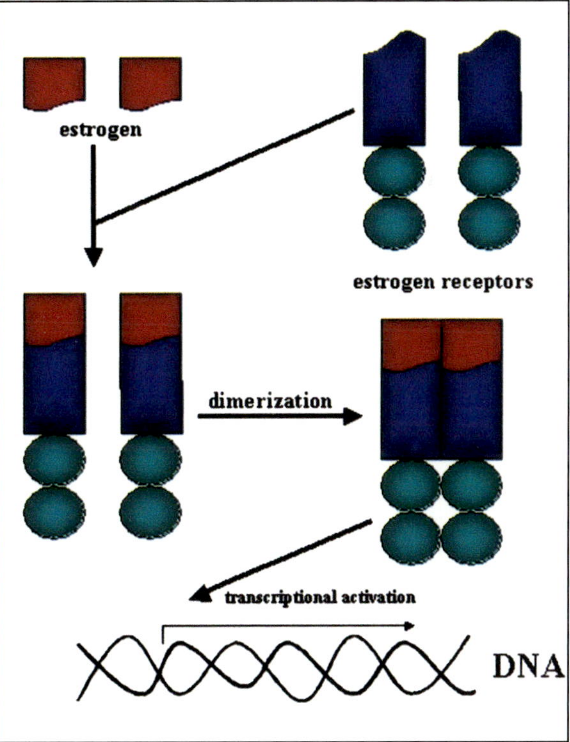

Figure 4.1

Classical model of receptor-mediated estrogen action

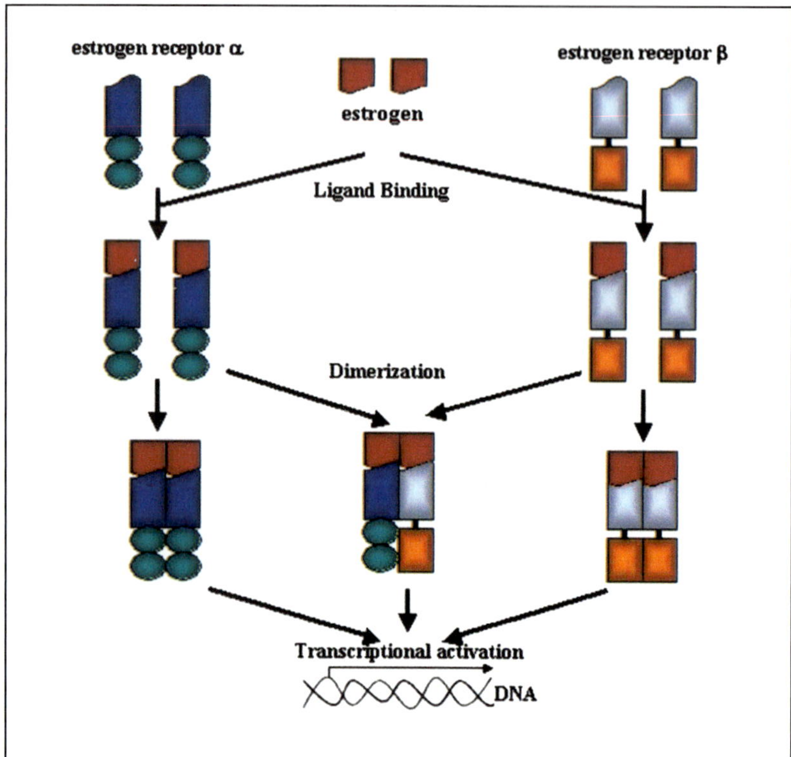

Figure 4.2

Proposed interactions of ERα and ERβ-mediated signal transduction pathways

been termed as ERα after the discovery of a second type of ER (ERβ). The presence of ERα in target tissues or cells is essential to their responsiveness to estrogen action. In fact, the expression levels of ERα in a particular tissue have been used as an index of the degree of estrogen responsiveness [20]. A vast majority of human breast carcinomas are initially positive for ERα, and their growth can be stimulated by estrogens and inhibited by anti-estrogens [19, 20]. The ERβ has been cloned from the rat, mouse, and human [21, 22]. ERβ and ERα share high sequence homology, especially in the regions or domains responsible for specific binding to DNA and the ligands (see Chapter 3). ERβ can be activated by estrogen stimulation, and blocked with anti-estrogens [21, 22]. Upon activation, ERβ can form homodimers as well as heterodimers with ERα [22, 23]. The existence of two ER subtypes and their ability to form DNA-binding heterodimers suggests three potential pathways of estrogen signaling: via the ERα or ERβ subtype in tissues exclusively expressing each subtype and via the formation of heterodimers in tissues expressing both ERα and ERβ (Fig. 4.2) (see Chapter 3). The pathways of the ER-mediated signal transduction have become even more complicated by the recent discovery of other types of ER [24, 25]. In addition, estrogens and anti-estrogens can induce differential activation of ERα and ERβ to control transcription of genes that are under the control of an AP1 element [23].

4.2 Sources of Estrogens in Human Breast Tissue

The most biologically active estrogen in breast tissue is 17β-estradiol. Circulating estrogens are mainly originated from ovarian steroidogenesis in premenopausal women and peripheral aromatization of ovarian and adrenal androgens in postmenopausal women [26]. The importance of ovarian steroidogen-

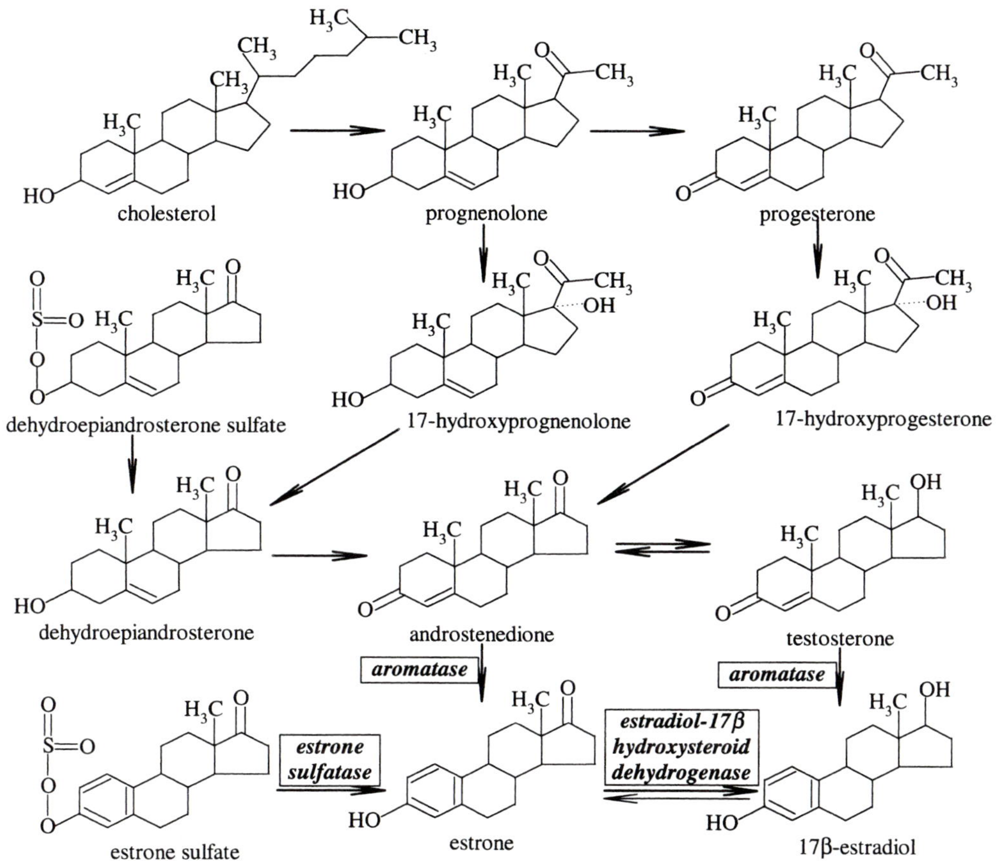

Figure 4.3

Steroidogenic pathways leading to the biosynthesis of estrogens

esis in the genesis of breast cancer is highlighted by the fact that occurring naturally or induced early menopause prior to age 40 significantly reduces the risk of developing breast cancer [26]. However, the uptake of 17β-estradiol from the circulation does not appear to contribute significantly to the total content of estrogen in breast tumors, since the majority of estrogen present in the tumor tissues is derived from de novo biosynthesis [26]. In fact, the concentrations of 17β-estradiol in breast cancer tissues do not differ between premenopausal and postmenopausal women, even though plasma levels of 17β-estradiol decrease by 90% following menopause [27]. This phenomenon might be explained by the observation that enzymatic transformations of circulating precursors in peripheral tissues contribute 75% of estrogens in premenopausal women and almost 100% in postmenopausal women [28, 29], the data that highlight the importance of in situ metabolism of estrogens. Three main enzyme complexes that are involved in the synthesis of biologically active estrogen (i. e., 17β-estradiol) in the breast are:

1. Aromatase that converts androstenedione to estrone
2. Estrone sulfatase that hydrolyses the estrogen sulfate to estrone
3. 17β-estradiol hydroxysteroid dehydrogenase that preferentially reduces estrone to 17β-estradiol in tumor tissues (Fig. 4.3) [30, 31]

Aromatase (estrogen synthetase) is the enzyme complex responsible for the final step in estrogen synthesis, the conversion of androstenedione and testosterone to estrone and 17β-estradiol, respectively (Fig. 4.3). Circulating free and conjugated dehydroepiandrosterone (DHEA) is the major androgen precursor for estrogen synthesis in the peripheral tissues, especially in postmenopausal women. The circulating DHEA is extensively converted to androstenedione and estrone in human breast cancer stromal cells, resulting in a tissue plasma concentration gradient of up to an eight-fold higher accumulation of androstenedione in breast cancer tissues [26]. Higher aromatase activities have been observed in areas of the breast bearing cancer than in non-involved quadrants [26]. It has also been shown that local synthesis of estrogen via the aromatase enzyme present predominantly in tumor stromal tissue [32] can increase tumor estrogen levels and growth rate [33–35]. In fact, the aromatase-positive macrophages, the predominant population of leukocytes in some breast carcinomas [26], have been identified as the major source of local estrogen production in breast tissues and breast cancer [36]. In addition, an increase in breast cancer susceptibility has been associated with aberrant aromatase activities [37] as well as genetic polymorphisms in the aromatase gene [38]. It has been suggested that an increase in aromatase expression or activity is related to the malignant phenotype, but not necessarily the biological behavior or clinical course, of breast cancer [39]. In contrast, an increase in aromatase in the stromal cells of breast adipose tissue may be correlated with the development of, or predisposition to, breast cancer [39]. Ironically, the plasma concentration of DHEA sulfate

peaks in the second decade of life and declines markedly during adulthood [40], supporting the notion that concentrations of circulating DHEA are inversely correlated with the risk of breast cancer [26]. Nevertheless, aromatization of the androgenic C19 steroids by aromatase activity is one of the most important pathways for the biosynthesis of the estrogenic C18 steroids.

Even though the major pathway of estrone synthesis is via aromatization of the precursor androgens in the ovary or peripheral tissue, much of the estrone synthesized is converted by estrone sulfotransferase to estrone sulfate, which can be converted back to estrone by estrone sulfatase-mediated hydrolysis. Sulfation is an important process in the metabolism and inactivation of steroids, including estrogens, because the addition of the charged sulfonate group protects the hormones from binding to their receptors and serves as reserve material for the biosynthesis of active hormones through the action of endogenous sulfatases [41]. Breast cancer cells lack estrogen sulfotransferase to inactivate estrogens and faced expression of the enzyme in breast carcinoma cells decreases their responsiveness to estrogen-induced growth stimulation [41]. In contrast, breast cancer tissues contain 10–100 times higher sulfatase activity than the aromatase activity and produce estrone mainly through the hydrolysis of estrone sulfate [30, 42]. In fact, it has been proposed that estrone production by sulfatase activity is ten-fold more than that by aromatase activity [43]. A large amount of estrone sulfate and estrone sulfatase activity have been observed in breast tumor tissues, especially in those from postmenopausal women [30]. Thus, estrone sulfate is quantitatively the most important circulating estrogen in women and acts as a large reservoir for the formation of estrone [26].

17β-hydroxysteroid dehydrogenases (17β-HSD) belong to a family of HSD enzymes that are involved in the interconversion of the oxidized form and the reduced form of steroid hormones. Members of HSD family include 3β-HSD that catalyze the conversion of 5-ene-3β-hydroxysteroids (e. g., pregnenolone) to corresponding 4-ene-3-keto-steroids (e. g., progesterone), 11β-HSD that catalyze the conversion of glucocorticoids and their inactive metabolites and 17β-

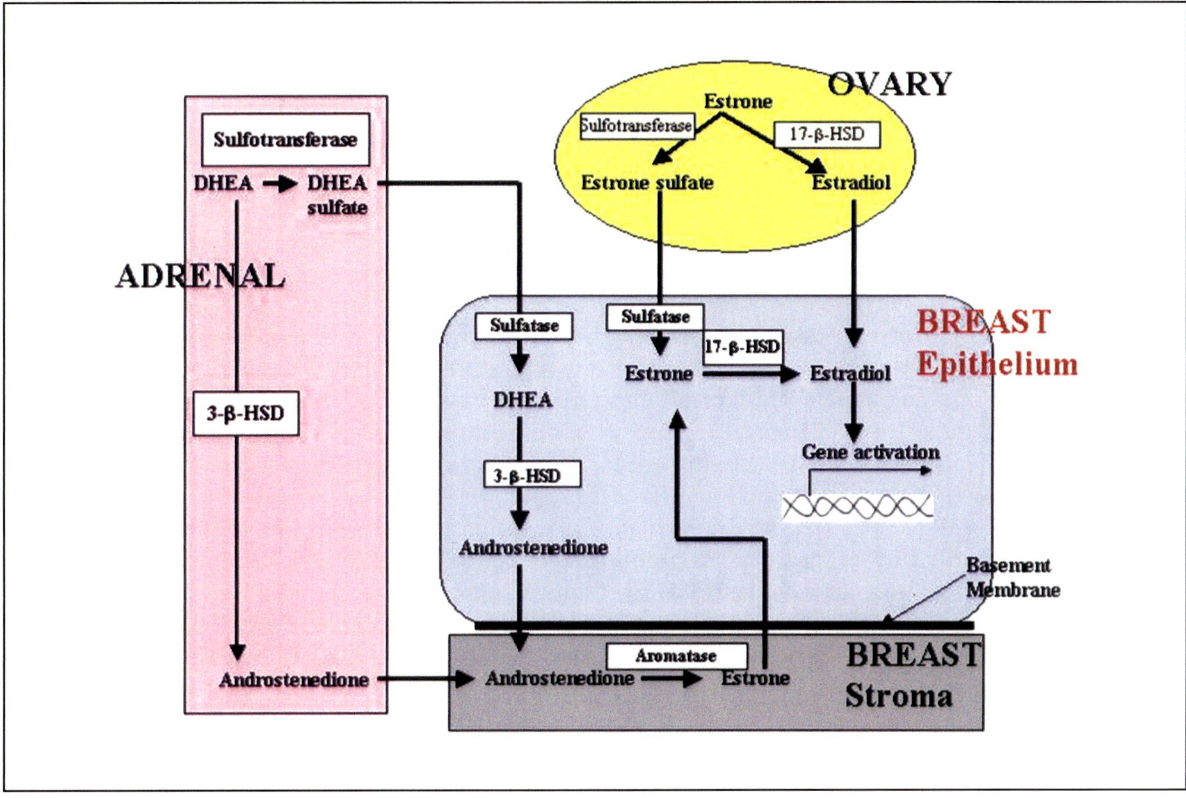

Figure 4.4

Tissue interactions in the biosynthesis and action of estrogens in human breast tissues

HSD that catalyze the oxido-reduction at carbon 17 of C-18 and C-19 steroids [26]. There are seven types of 17β-HSD that have been characterized so far (see review 26). Type I 17β-HSD, which is expressed mainly in the placenta, ovary and breast, catalyzes the reduction of estrone to 17β-estradiol, the most potent estrogen [43, 44]. Expression of type I 17β-HSD has also been reported in human breast carcinoma, but its level is variable and not necessarily higher than in non-neoplastic breast tissue. In addition, type I 17β-HSD is expressed in both stromal and epithelial components of the breast. However, the level of type I 17β-HSD expression is higher in normal, but not can-

cerous, breast epithelial cells as compared to their respective stromal counterparts [26]. More importantly, the activity of type I 17β-HSD favors reduction of estrone to 17β-estradiol in primary epithelial and stromal cells derived from cancerous breast, while the oxidative activity of type I 17β-HSD predominates in primary cultures of normal breast epithelial and stromal cells. Similarly, the reductive pathway of type I 17β-HSD is more active in breast tumors [26]. Both the expression and the reductive activity of type I 17β-HSD can be up regulated by cytokines and growth factors rich in breast tumors. These data suggest an important role of type I 17β-HSD in the local production of biologically active estrogen in human breast [26].

It should be noted, however, that de novo biosynthesis of active estrogen is also influenced by activity of other enzymes along the steroidogenesis pathways (Fig. 4.3). For instance, 3β-HSD activity is essential to the formation of androgenic steroids that serve as the substrates for aromatase activity in the breast [45]. It should also be noted that local synthesis of active estrogen could confer growth advantage only if type I 17β-HSD, aromatase and estrogen receptors are coordinately expressed [39]. In this regard, a significant correlation between the expression of type I 17β-HSD and aromatase has been observed in invasive lobular carcinoma, but not in ductal carcinoma [46]. In addition, no consistent correlation has been found between the expression of estrogen receptors and aromatase activity [47, 48]. Since local synthesis of estrogen in the stromal component can increase the estrogen levels and growth rate of breast carcinoma [33–35], a paracrine mechanism has been proposed to account for stromal-epithelial interactions in the biosynthesis and action of estrogens in human breasts (Fig. 4.4). Clearly, further studies are warranted to investigate the regulatory mechanisms that are involved in the control of expression of aromatase, type I 17β-HSD and estrogen receptors in the epithelial and stromal components of the breasts.

4.3 Role of Estrogens in Human Breast Proliferation

Even though the breast is influenced by a myriad of hormones and growth factors [49–52], estrogens are considered to play a major role in promoting the proliferation of both the normal and the neoplastic breast epithelium [49, 50]. Estradiol acts locally in the mammary gland, stimulating DNA synthesis and promoting bud formation, probably through an ER-mediated mechanism [49]. It is also known that the prevailing metabolic condition of an individual animal or human may significantly influence mammary gland responses to hormones. In addition, the mammary gland responds selectively to given hormonal stimuli for either cell proliferation or differentiation, depending upon specific topographic differences in gland development. In either case, the response of the mammary gland to these complex hormonal and metabolic interactions results in developmental changes that permanently modify both the architec-

ture and the biological characteristics of the gland [49, 51].

The fact that the normal epithelium contains receptors for both estrogen and progesterone lends support to the receptor-mediated mechanism as a major player in the hormonal regulation of breast development. The role of these hormones on the proliferative activity of the breast, which is indispensable for its normal growth and development, has been for a long time, and still is, the subject of heated controversies [26]. There is little doubt, however, that the proliferative activity of the mammary epithelium in both rodents and humans varies with the degree of differentiation of the mammary parenchyma [49–55]. In humans, the highest level of cell proliferation is observed in the undifferentiated lobules type (Lob 1) present in the breast of young nulliparous females [49–52]. The progressive differentiation of Lob 1 into lobules types 2 (Lob 2) and 3 (Lob 3), occurring under the hormonal influences of the menstrual cycle, and the full differentiation into lobules type 4 (Lob 4), as a result of pregnancy, leads to a concomitant reduction in the proliferative activity of the mammary epithelium [49–55]. The content of ERα and progesterone receptor (PgR) in the lobular structures of the breast is directly proportional to the rate of cell proliferation, being also maximal in the undifferentiated Lob1, and decreasing progressively in Lob 2, Lob 3, and Lob 4 [51, 56] (see Chapter 2). In all cases, the proliferating cells are almost exclusively found in the epithelium lining ducts and lobules. Only occasionally are positive cells found in the myoepithelium, or in the intralobular and interlobular stroma. The same pattern of reactivity is also observed in tissue sections incubated with the ERα and PgR antibodies. Positive cells are found exclusively in the epithelium. The number of cells positive for ERα or PgR is highest in the Lob 1, decreases progressively in Lob 2 and Lob 3 [56]. It should be noted, however, that it remains unclear from the above studies whether the cells that are positive for steroid receptors are those that are proliferating. The use of the double staining procedure for Ki67 and ERα or PgR has allowed to quantitatively determine in the same tissue sections the spatial relationship between those cells that are proliferating and those that react with the ERα or

PgR antibody (see Chapter 2). The utilization of a double labeling immunocytochemical technique to stain the same tissue section for steroid hormone receptors and Ki67 proliferating antigen has allowed to conclude that the expression of the receptors occurs in cells other than the proliferating cells, confirming results reported by others [57]. The findings that proliferating cells are different from those that are ERα- and PgR-positive support data that indicate that estrogen controls cell proliferation by an indirect mechanism. This phenomenon has been demonstrated using supernatant of estrogen-treated ERα-positive cells that stimulates the growth of ERα-negative cell lines in culture. The same phenomenon has been shown in vivo in nude mice bearing ER-negative breast tumor xenografts [57]. ERα-positive cells treated with antiestrogens secrete transforming growth factor-β that inhibits the proliferation of ERα-negative cells [58]. The findings that proliferating cells in the human breast are different from those that contain steroid hormone receptors explain many of the in vitro data [59, 60]. Of interest are the observations that while the ERα-positive MCF-7 cells respond to estrogen treatment with increased cell proliferation, and that the enhanced expression of the ERα by transfection also increases the proliferative response to estrogen [59–61], ERα-negative cells, such as MDA-MB 468 and others, when transfected with ERα, exhibit inhibition of cell growth under the same type of treatment [60]. Although the negative effect of estrogen on those ERα-negative cells transfected with the ERα has been interpreted as an interference of the transcription factor used to maintain estrogen independent growth [61], there is no definitive explanation for their lack of survival. However, it can be explained by the finding that proliferating and ERα-positive cells are two separate populations. Further support is the finding that when Lob 1 of normal breast tissue are placed in culture, they lose the ERα-positive cells, indicating that only proliferating cells that are also ERα-negative can survive and constitute the stem cells [62, 63] (see Chapter 2).

4.4 Estrogens in Human Breast Carcinogenesis

Although 67 % of breast cancers are manifested during the postmenopausal period, a vast majority, 95 %, is initially hormone-dependent [26]. This indicates that estrogens play a crucial role in their development and evolution. It has been established that in situ metabolism of estrogens through aromatase-mediated pathway is correlated with the risk of developing breast cancer [37, 38]. A recent finding that expression of estrone sulfatase is inversely correlated with relapse-free survival of human breast cancer patients [42] reiterates the importance of estrone sulfatase-mediated local production of estrogen in the development and progression of human breast cancer. However, it is still unclear whether estrogens are carcinogenic to the human breast. Most of the current understanding of carcinogenicity of estrogens is based on studies in experimental animal systems and clinical observations of a greater risk of endometrial hyperplasia and neoplasia associated with estrogen

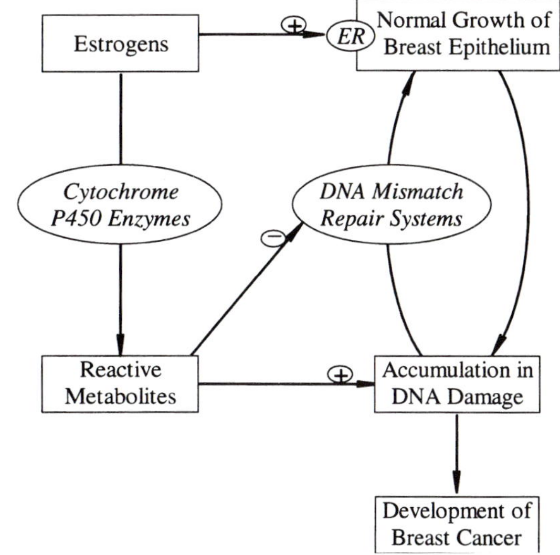

Figure 4.5

Potential mechanisms of estrogen-induced carcinogenesis in human breast tissues supplementation or polycystic ovarian syndrome [26].

There are three mechanisms that have been considered to be responsible for the carcinogenicity of estrogens: receptor-mediated hormonal activity, which has generally been related to stimulation of cellular proliferation, resulting in more opportunities for accumulation of genetic damages leading to carcinogenesis [63], a cytochrome P450-mediated metabolic activation, which elicits direct genotoxic effects by increasing mutation rates (Fig. 4.5) [64], and the induction of aneuploidy by estrogen [65–73]. There is also evidence that estrogen compromises the DNA repair system and allows accumulation of lesions in the genome essential to estrogen-induced tumorigenesis [74].

4.4.1 Receptor-Mediated Pathway

The receptor-mediated activity of estrogen is generally related to induction of expression of the genes involved in the control of cell cycle progression and growth of human breast epithelium. The biological response to estrogen depends upon the local concentrations of the active hormone and its receptors. The level of ER expression is higher in breast cancer patients than in control subjects and is related to breast cancer risk in postmenopausal women. It has been suggested that overexpression of ER in normal human breast epithelium may augment estrogen responsiveness and hence the risk of breast cancer. The proliferative activity and the percentage of ERα-positive cells are highest in Lob 1 in comparison with the various lobular structures composing the normal breast. These findings provide a mechanistic explanation for the higher susceptibility of these structures to be transformed by chemical carcinogens in vitro [75–77], supporting as well the observations that Lob 1 are the site of origin of ductal carcinomas [77].

The presence of ERα-positive and ERα-negative cells with different proliferative activity in the normal human breast may help to elucidate the genesis of ERα-positive and ERα-negative breast cancers [78–80]. It has been suggested that either ERα-nega-tive breast cancers result from the loss of the ability of the cells to synthesize ERα during clinical evolution of ERα-positive cancers, or that ERα-positive and ERα-negative cancers are different entities [80]. Based on these observations, it is postulated that Lob 1 contain at least three cell types, ERα-positive cells that do not proliferate, ERα-negative cells that are capable of proliferating, and a small proportion of ERα-positive cells that can proliferate as well (Fig. 4.6) [56]. Therefore, estrogen might stimulate ERα-positive cells to produce a growth factor that in turn stimulates neighboring ERα-negative cells capable of proliferating (Fig. 4.6) [56]. In the same fashion, the small proportion of cells that are ERα-positive and can proliferate could be the stem cell of ERα-positive tumors. The possibility exists, as well, that the ERα-negative cells convert to ERα-positive cells [56] or that they express ER-β.

The newly discovered ERβ opens another possibility that those cells traditionally considered negative for ERα might be positive for ERβ [21–23]. It has recently been found that ERβ is expressed during the immortalization and transformation of ER-negative human breast epithelial cells [81], supporting the hypothesis of conversion from a negative to a positive receptor cell. The functional role of ERβ-mediated estrogen signaling pathways in the pathogenesis of malignant diseases is essentially unknown. In the rats, ERβ-mediated mechanisms have been implicated in the upregulation of PgR expression in the dysplastic acini of the dorsolateral prostate in response to treatment of testosterone and 17β-estradiol [82]. In the human, ERβ has been detected in both normal and cancerous breast tissues or cell lines, and is the predominant ER type in normal breast tissue. Expression of ERβ in breast tumors is inversely correlated with the PgR status and variant transcripts of ERβ have been observed in some breast tumors [26]. ERβ and ERα are co-expressed in some breast tumors and a few breast cell lines, suggesting an interesting possibility that ERα and ERβ proteins may interact with each other and discriminate between target sequences leading to differential responsiveness to estrogens (Fig. 4.2). In addition, estrogen responses mediated by ERα and ERβ may vary with different composition of their co-activators that transmit the

Figure 4.6

Schematic representation of the postulated pathways of estrogen actions on breast epithelial cells

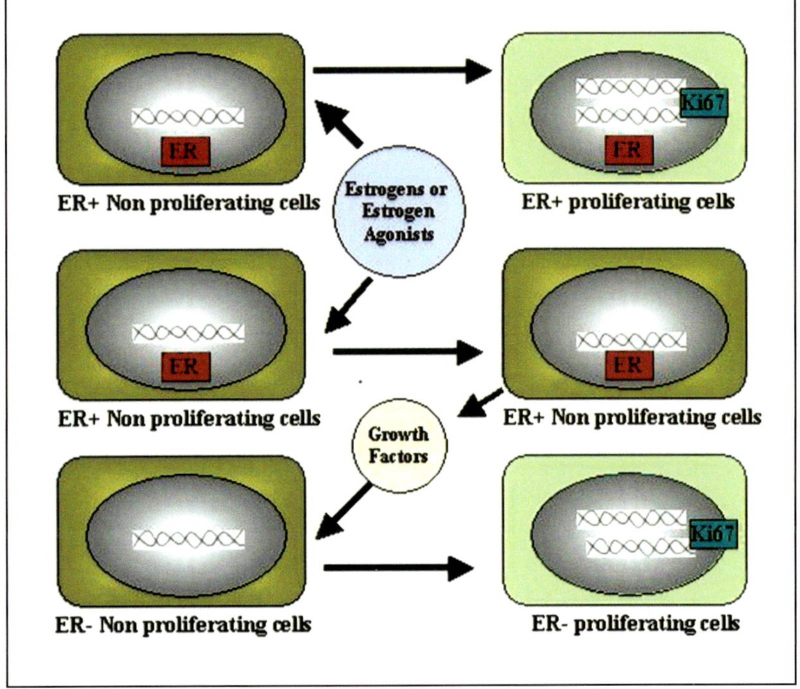

effect of ER-ligand complex to the transcription complex at the promoter of target genes. Recently, it has been shown that an increase in the expression of ERα with a concomitant reduction in ERβ expression occurs during tumorigenesis of the breast and ovary [83], but breast tumors expressing both ERα and ERβ are lymph node-positive and tend to be of higher histopathological grade. These data suggest a change in the interplay of ERα- and ERβ-mediated signal transduction pathways during breast tumorigenesis.

Even though it is now generally believed that alterations in the ER-mediated signal transduction pathways contribute to breast cancer progression toward hormonal independence and more aggressive phenotypes, there is also mounting evidence that a membrane receptor coupled to alternative second messenger signaling mechanisms (see Chapter 3, and [84, 85]) are operational, and may stimulate the cascade of events leading to cell proliferation. This knowledge suggests that ERα-negative cells found in the human breast may respond to estrogens through this or other pathways. The biological responses elicited by estrogens are mediated, at least in part, by the production of autocrine and paracrine growth factors from the epithelium and the stroma in the breast [86]. In addition, evidence has accumulated over the last decade supporting the existence of ER variants, mainly a truncated ER and an exon deleted ER. It has been suggested that expression of ER variants may contribute to breast cancer progression toward hormone independence. Although more studies need to be done in this direction, it is clear that the findings that in the normal breast the proliferating and steroid hormone receptor positive cells are different open new possibilities for clarifying the mechanisms through which estrogens might act on the proliferating cells to initiate the cascade of events leading to cancer.

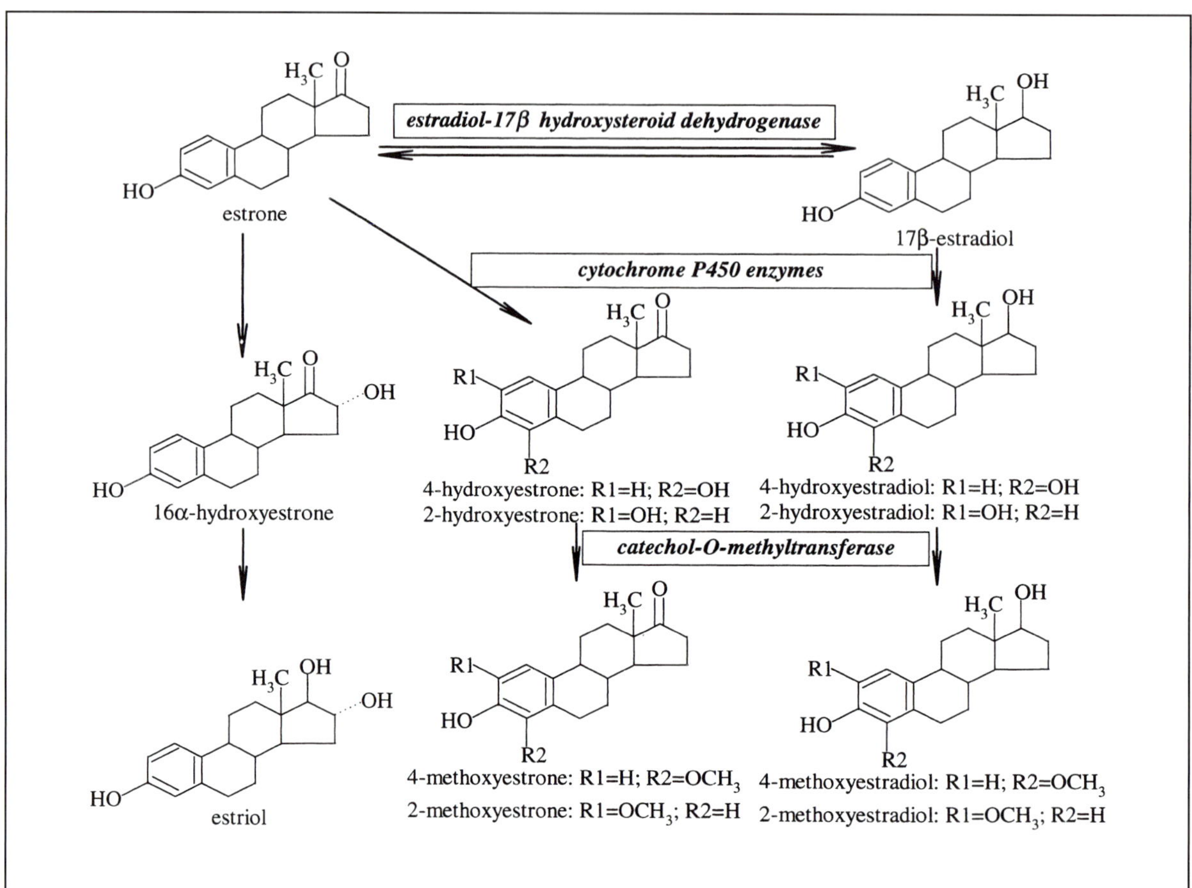

4.4.2 Oxidative Metabolism of Estrogen

There is evidence that oxidative catabolism of estrogens mediated by various cytochrome P450 (CYP) complexes constitutes a pathway of their metabolic activation and generates reactive free radicals and intermediate metabolites reactive intermediates that can cause oxidative stress and genomic damage directly [64, 65]. 17β-estradiol and estrone, which are continuously interconverted by 17β-estradiol hydroxysteroid dehydrogenase (or 17β-oxidoreductase), are the two major endogenous estrogens (Fig. 4.7). They are generally metabolized via two major pathways: hydroxylation at C-16α position and at the C-2 or C-4 positions (Fig. 4.7) [87–89]. The carbon position of the estrogen molecules to be hydroxylated dif-

Figure 4.7

Biosynthesis and steady-state control of catechol estrogens in human breast tissues

fers among various tissues and each reaction is probably catalyzed by various CYP isoforms. For example, in MCF-7 human breast cancer cells, which produce catechol estrogens in culture, CYP 1A1 catalyzes hydroxylation of 17β-estradiol at C-2, C-15α and C-16α, CYP 1A2 predominantly at C-2 [26, 90], and a member of the CYP 1B subfamily is responsible for the C-4 hydroxylation of 17β-estradiol. CYP3A4 and CYP3A5 have also been shown to play a role in the 16α-hydroxylation of estrogens in human [26].

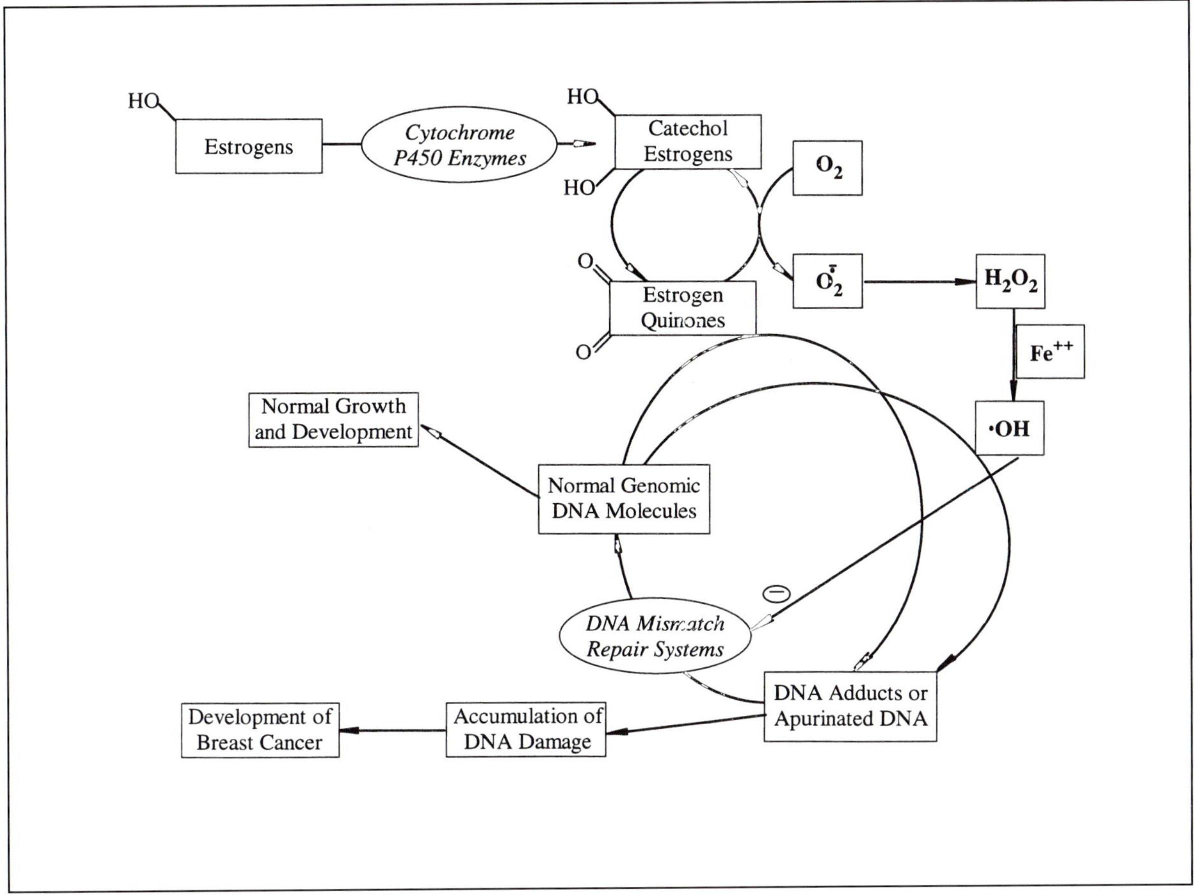

Figure 4.8

Carcinogenic effects associated with the metabolisms of catechol estrogens in human breast tissues

The hydroxylated estrogens are catechol estrogens that will easily be auto-oxidized to semiquinones and subsequently quinones, both of which are electrophiles capable of covalently binding to nucleophilic groups on DNA via a Michael addition and, thus, serve as the ultimate carcinogenic reactive intermediates in the peroxidatic activation of catechol estrogens (Fig. 4.8). In addition, a redox cycle consisting of the reversible formation of the semiquinones and quinones of catechol estrogens catalyzed by microso-mal P450 and cytochrome P450-reductase can locally generate superoxide and hydroxyl radicals to produce additional DNA damage (Fig. 4.8). Furthermore, catechol estrogens have been shown to interact synergistically with nitric oxide present in human breast generating a potent oxidant that induces DNA strand breakage [26].

Steady state concentrations of catechol estrogens are determined by the cytochrome P450-mediated hydroxylations of estrogens and monomethylation of catechols catalyzed by blood-borne catechol *o*-methyltransferase (Fig. 4.7) [91]. Increased formation of catechol estrogens as a result of elevated hydroxylations of 17β-estradiol at C-4 and C-16α [26, 92] positions occurs in human breast cancer patients and in women at a higher risk of developing this disease.

There is also evidence that lactoperoxidase, present in milk, saliva, tears and mammary glands, catalyzes the metabolism of 17β-estradiol to its phenoxyl radical intermediates, with subsequent formation of superoxide and hydrogen peroxide that might be involved in estrogen-mediated oxidative stress [93]. A substantial increase in base lesions observed in the DNA of invasive ductal carcinoma of the breast [94] has been postulated to result from the oxidative stress associated with metabolism of 17β-estradiol [93].

4.4.2.1 Estrogen as Mutagenic Agents

The detection of various types of DNA damage induced by estrogen metabolites in cell-free systems or in cells in culture and by parent hormones in vivo [95–99] has led to the hypothesis of an additional role of estrogen as mutagen and tumor initiator [100, 101]. The induction of mutations by estrogens or their metabolites has been demonstrated [102, 103] supporting the hypothesis that estrogens are mutagenic and that metabolic conversion of E_2 to catechol estrogen is required for the induction of such mutations. In addition to mutations, E_2 also induces microsatellite instability. Changes in DNA fragments containing microsatellite repeat sequences have been detected in E_2-induced hamster kidney tumors, in surrounding kidney tissue [104] and in MCF-10F HBEC transformed by E_2 [105]. Microsatellite instability is a relatively common genetic modification [106–108], induced by the natural hormone E_2 in cells in culture [105], in Syrian hamster kidney tumors, and in surrounding tissues [104]. It has also been detected with high frequency in human vaginal tumors in daughters of women treated with diethylstilbestrol (DES) [109]. Microsatellite instability has also been detected in human breast tumors [110–117].

4.4.2.2 The Mechanism by Which Estrogens Induce Mutations

Chemical carcinogens covalently bind to DNA to form two types of adducts: stable ones that remain in DNA unless removed by repair and depurinating ones that are lost from DNA by destabilization of the glycosyl bond [118, 119]. Evidence that depurinating polycyclic aromatic hydrocarbon-DNA adducts play a major role in tumor initiation [118–120] and that estrogen metabolites form depurinating DNA adducts strongly indicates that estrogen is an endogenous initiators of cancer [95]. Catechol estrogens (CE) are among the major metabolites of estrone (E_1) and estradiol (E_2). If these metabolites are oxidized to the electrophilic CE quinones (CE-Q), they may react with DNA. Specifically, the carcinogenic 4-CE [96, 121] are oxidized to CE-3,4-Q, which react with DNA to form depurinating adducts [95, 122]. These adducts generate apurinic sites that may lead to oncogenic mutations [74, 120, 122, 123], thereby initiating cancer.

4.4.2.3 Additional Factors Contributing to the Carcinogenic Effect of Estrogen

The breast is an endocrine organ and can synthesize E_2 in situ from precursor androgens via the enzyme aromatase [26]. Breast tissue contains aromatase and produces amounts of E_2 that exert biologic effects on proliferation. The effects of local production exceed those exerted in a classical endocrine fashion by uptake of E_2 from plasma. One critical factor is excessive synthesis of E_2 by overexpression of CYP19 in target tissues [124–128] and/or the presence of excess sulfatase that converts stored E_1 sulfate to E_1 [129]. The observation that breast tissue can synthesize E_2 in situ suggests that much more E_2 is present in some locations of target tissues than would be predicted from plasma concentration [128]. A second critical factor might be high levels of 4-CE due to overexpression of CYP1B1, which converts E_2 predominantly to 4-OHE$_2$ [130–132]. This could result in relatively large amounts of 4-CE and, subsequently, more extensive oxidation to their CE-3, 4-Q. A third factor could be a lack or low level of COMT activity. If this enzyme is insufficient, either through a low level of expression or its low activity allele, 4-CE will not be effectively methylated, but will be oxidized to the ultimate carcinogenic metabolite, CE-3, 4-Q. Fourth, a low level of GSH and/or low levels of quinone reductase and/or CYP reductase can leave available a higher level of CE-Q that may react with DNA.

The effects of some of these factors have already been observed in analyses of breast tissue samples from women with and without breast cancer [133]. The levels of E_1 (E_2) in women with carcinoma were higher. In women without breast cancer, a larger amount of 2-CE than 4-CE was observed. In women with breast carcinoma, the 4-CE were 3.5 times more abundant than the 2-CE and were 4 times higher than in the women without breast cancer. Furthermore, a statistically lower level of methylation was observed for 2-CE and 4-CE in cancer cases vs. controls. Finally, the level of CE-Q conjugates in women with cancer was three times that in the controls, suggesting a larger probability for the CE-Q to react with DNA in the breast tissue of women with carcinoma. The levels of E_1(E_2) ($p<0.02$) and quinone conjugates ($p<0.01$) are highly significant predictors of breast cancer, and the levels of methylated CE ($p<0.02$) are significant predictors of protection against breast cancer. Altogether, these data are supporting the concept that estrogen and its metabolites can be found at high concentration in the breast tissue indicating a direct carcinogenic effect in the breast epithelial cells [133].

4.4.3 Estrogens as Inducers of Aneuploidy

Breast cancer is considered the result of sequential changes that accumulate over time. DNA content changes, i.e., loss of heterozygosity (LOH) and aneuploidy, can be detected at early stages of morphological atypia, supporting the hypothesis that aneuploidy is a critical event driving neoplastic development and progression [134, 135]. Aneuploidy is defined as the gain or loss of chromosomes; it is a dynamic, progressive, and accumulative event that is almost universal in solid tumors [136, 137]. The extensive array of altered gene expression observed in tumors and the numerous altered chromosomes de-

tected by CGH [72, 138] provide striking evidence that aneuploidy can totally disrupt cell homeostatic control. The main question is whether aneuploidy is a consequence of neoplastic development or a cause of neoplastic development [72, 73, 138]. One of the several mechanisms proposed for the development of aneuploidy is the failure to appropriately segregate chromosomes [73, 74, 139], for example, interference with mitotic spindle dynamics, abnormal centrosome duplication, altered chromosome condensation and cohesion, defective centromeres, and loss of mitotic checkpoints [139]. Functional consequences of centrosome defects may play a role during neoplastic transformation and tumor progression, increasing the incidence of multipolar mitoses that lead to chromosomal segregation abnormalities and aneuploidy. In considering estrogens as carcinogenic agents there is evidence that they affect microtubules [140] and a recently report indicates that progesterone may facilitate aneuploidy [141]. The importance of these findings is magnified with the recent publications that demonstrate women on hormone replacement treatments that include progesterone have increased mammographic breast density and increased breast cancer risk than women taking only estrogen [142–144].

In the center stage of the research endeavor on aneuploidy are the centrosomes that are organelles that nucleate microtubule growth and organize the mitotic spindle for segregating chromosomes into daughter cells, establishing cell shape and cell polarity, processes essential for epithelial gland organization [72, 139]. Centrosomes also coordinate numerous intracellular activities, in part by providing a site enriched for regulatory molecules, including those that control cell cycle progression, centrosome and spindle function, and cell cycle checkpoints [73, 145–148]. Although the underlying mechanisms for the formation of abnormal centrosomes are not clear, several possibilities have been proposed and implicated in the development of cancer such as alterations of checkpoint controls initiating multiple rounds of centrosome replication within a single cell cycle and failure of cytokinesis, cell fusion, and cell cycle arrest in S-phase uncoupling DNA replication from centrosome duplication [146].

4.5 Biological Demonstration That Estrogens Are Carcinogenic in the Human Breast

4.5.1 The Proof of Principle

To fully demonstrate that estrogens are carcinogenic in the human breast through one or more of the mechanisms explained above it will require an experimental system in which, estrogens by themselves or one of their metabolites would induce transformation phenotypes indicative of neoplasia in HBEC in vitro and also induce genomic alterations similar to those observed in spontaneous malignancies, such as DNA amplification and loss of genetic material that may represent tumor suppressor genes [149–164].

4.5.2 The In Vitro Model of Cell Transformation

The transforming potential of estrogens on human breast epithelial cells (HBEC) in vitro, have being evaluated by utilizing the spontaneously immortalized HBEC MCF-10F [165, 166]. In order to mimic the intermittent exposure of HBEC to endogenous estrogens, all cells were first treated with 0, 0.007 nM, 70 nM and 1 µM of E_2, DES, BP, Progesterone, 2-OH-E_2, 4-OH-E_2 and 16-α-OH E_2 at 72 h and 120 h post plating. Treatments were repeated during the second week, and cells were collected at the 14th day for phenotypic and genotypic analysis (Fig. 4.9). At the end of each treatment period, the culture medium was replaced with fresh medium. At the end of the second week of treatment, the cells were assayed for determination of, survival efficiency (SE), colony efficiency (CE), colony size (CS), ductulogenic capacity and invasiveness in a reconstituted basement membrane. All phenotypes indicative of cell transformation [167, 168].

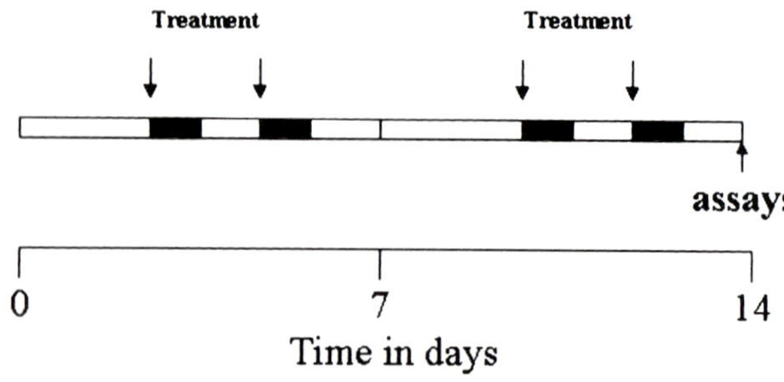

Figure 4.9

MCF-10-F cells were treated with E_2, DES, BP, 2-OH-E_2, 4-OH-E_2, 16-α-OH-E_2, progesterone or cholesterol, at 72 h and 120 h post plating. Treatments were repeated during the second week, and cells were collected at the 14th day for phenotypic and genotypic analysis

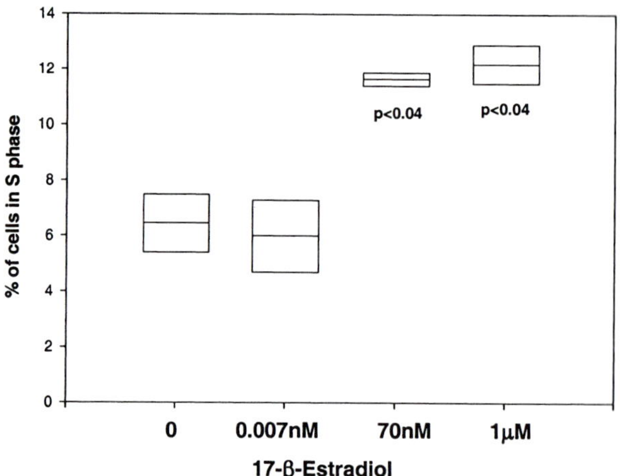

Figure 4.10

Flow cytometric data of MCF-10F transformed with 17β-estradiol at different concentrations as indicated in Fig. 4.9. The cells obtained from these treatments were used for measuring the S-phase of the cell cycle

4.5.2.1 Transformation Effect of Estrogen in MCF-10F Cells

We have determined the optimal doses for the expression of the cell transformation phenotype by treating the immortalized human breast epithelial

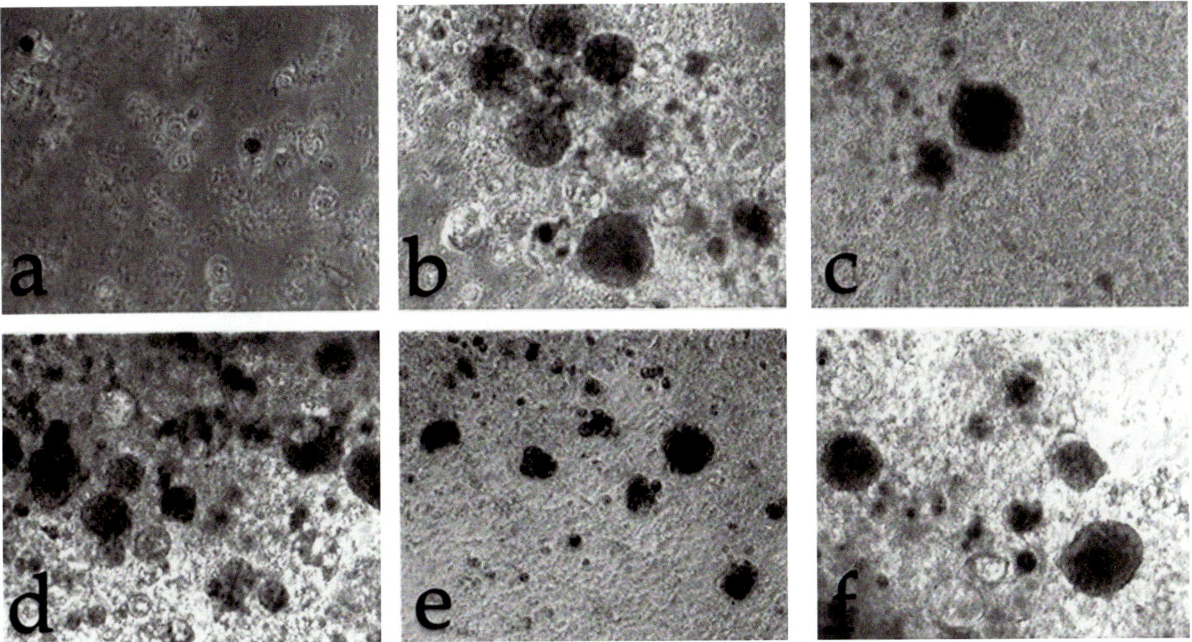

Figure 4.11 a–f

MCF-10F cells plated in agar-methocel for colony assay. Control cells do not form colonies. **a** Only isolated cells are present; **b–d** colonies formed by E_2, DES, and BP-treated MCF-10F cells respectively; **e** colonies of MCF-10F cells transformed with 70 nM of 2-OH-E_2; **f** colonies of MCF-10F cells transformed with 0.007 nM of 4-OH-E_2. All the photographs were taken at ×4 in a phase contrast microscope

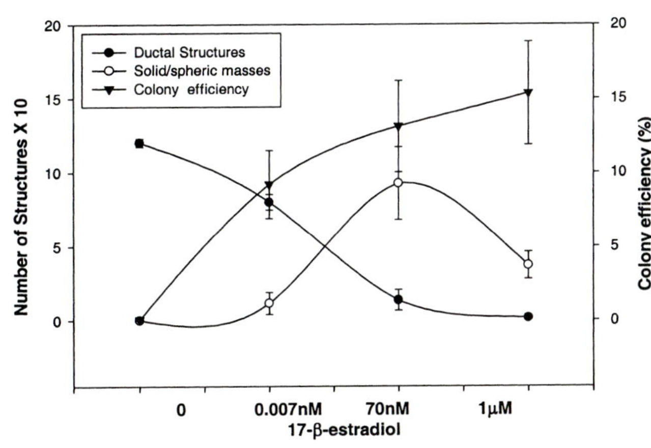

Figure 4.12

Curves showing the dose response effect of MCF-10F cells to the transforming effect of 17β-estradiol. The left ordinate expresses the number of structures (ductules and solid masses) detected by 10,000 cells plated in collagen matrix. The right ordinate depicts the percentage of colonies or colony efficiency (CE) of MCF-10F cells. The CE was determined by a count of the number of colonies greater than 100 µm in diameter, and expressed as percentage of the original number of cells plated per well

cells (HBEC) MCF-10F with 17β-estradiol (E_2) with 0.0, 0.07 nM, 70 nM, or 1 µM of E_2 twice a week for 2 weeks (Fig. 4.9). The survival efficiency (SE) was increased with 0.007 nM and 70 nM of 17β-estradiol and decrease with 1 µM and the proliferative activity of these E_2 transformed cells, measured by the percentage of cells in the S phase of the cell cycle, was also increased in a dose dependent fashion (Fig. 4.10). The cells treated with either doses of E_2 formed colonies in agar methocel (Fig. 4.11) and the size was not

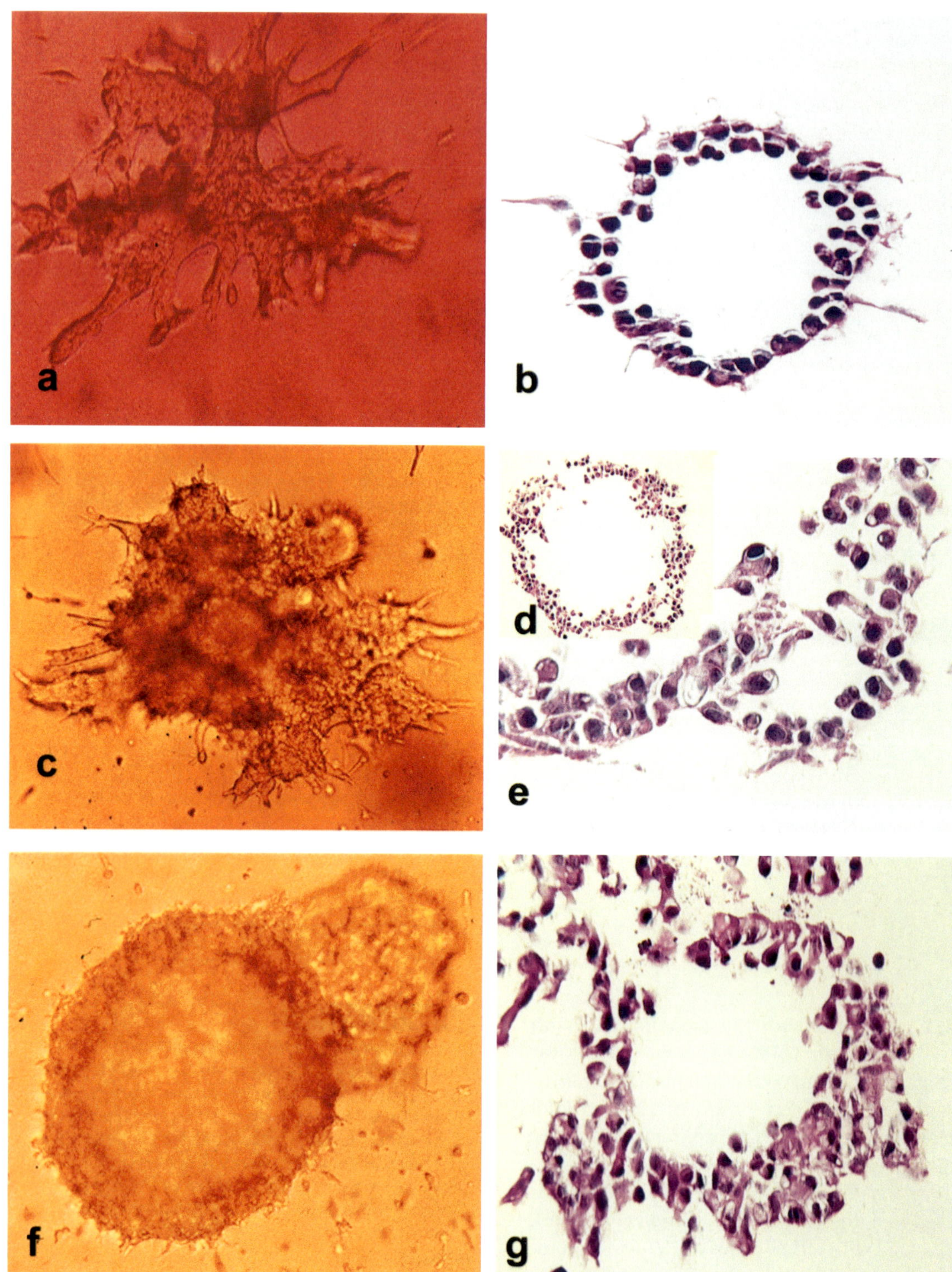

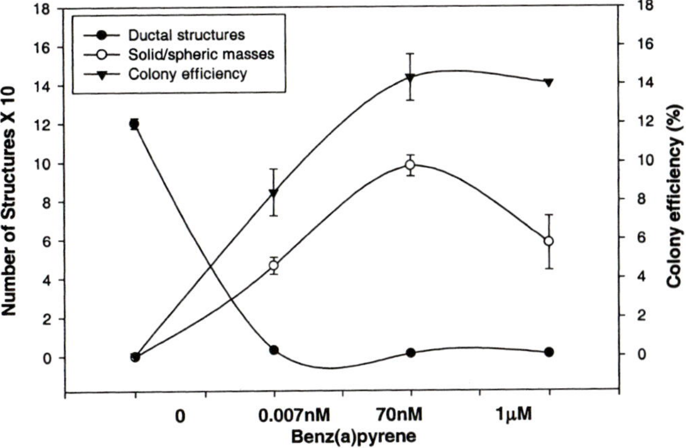

◀ Figure 4.13 a–g

MCF-10F cells treated with different doses of E$_2$ showing that the ductulogenic capacity is decreased with increasing doses. This in vitro technique evaluates the capacity of cells to differentiate by providing evidence of whether-treated cells form tridimensional structures when grown in a collagen matrix. Parental, control, and treated cells were suspended at a final density of 2×10^3 cells/ml in 89.3 % Vitrogen[100] collagen matrix (Collagen Co., Palo Alto, CA) and plated into four 24 well chambers pre-coated with agar base. The cells were fed with fresh feeding medium containing 20 % horse serum twice a week. The cells were examined under an inverted microscope for a period of 21 days or longer for determining whether they formed ductule-like structures or whether they grew as unorganized clumps. a MCF-10F cells in collagen matrix phase contrast microscope (× 10); b cross section of the same structure showed in a after fixation in 10 % neutral buffered formalin, embedded in paraffin, sectioned, and stained with hematoxylin-eosin (H&E) for histological examination (H&E (× 4); c MCF-10F cells treated with 0.007 nM of 17β-estradiol; d cross section of the same structure showed in c prepared as indicated in b; e Higher magnification of d (× 40); f MCF-10F cells treated with 70 nM of 17β-estradiol. Phase contrast microscope (× 40); g histological section of f prepared as indicated in b (× 40)

Figure 4.14

Curves showing the dose response effect of MCF-10F cells to the transforming effect of benzo(a)pyrene, (nomenclature as described in Fig. 4.12)

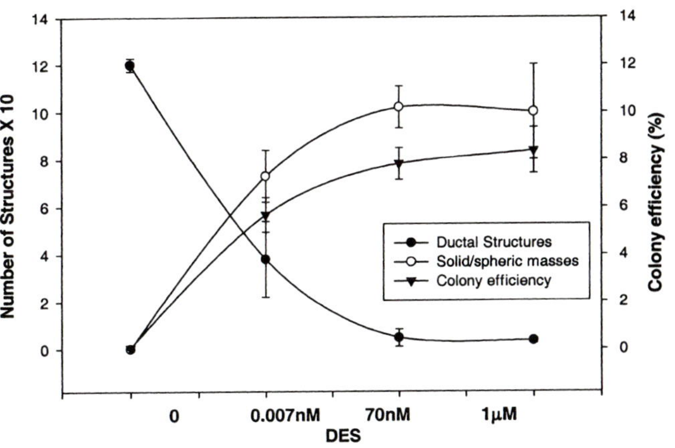

Figure 4.15 ▶

Curves showing the dose response effect of MCF-10F cells to the transforming effect of diethylstilbestrol (*DES*), (nomenclature as described in Fig. 4.12)

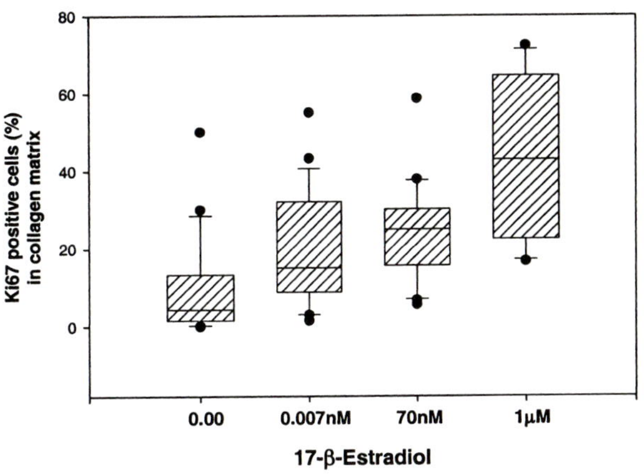

Figure 4.16 ▶

Dose response effect of 17β-estradiol-transformed cells growing in collagen matrix. The proliferative activity was determined by counting the number Ki67 positive cells in histological sections of paraffin embedded cells growing in collagen different among them, however, the CE increased from 0 in controls to 6.1, 9.2, and 8.7 with increasing E_2 doses (Fig. 4.12).

Ductulogenesis was quantitatively evaluated by estimating the ability of the cell plated in collagen to form tubules or spherical masses (SM) (Fig. 4.13). Non-transformed cells produce ductules like structure and transformed cells produce spherical or solid masses of cells. Cells treated with DMSO, cholesterol or progesterone at different concentrations were unable to alter the ductular pattern. E_2, BP and DES treated cells induces the loss of MCF-10F cells to produce ductules in a dose dependent fashion and the number of solid masses paralleled the formation of colonies in agar methocel (Figs. 4.14, 4.15). Histological analysis shows that MCF10-F cells form ductules in collagen matrix that are lined by a single layer of cuboidal epithelial cells (Fig. 4.13a), this pattern was not disturbed by cholesterol or progesterone treatment. Most of the cells growing in the collagen matrix are actively proliferating as detected by immunostaining with Ki67 (Fig. 4.16).

4.5.2.2 Transformation Effect of the Estrogen Metabolites

2-OH-E_2 (Fig. 4.17), 4-OH-E_2 (Fig. 4.18), and 16α-OH-E_2 (Fig. 4.19) induce the formation of colonies in agar methocel. Cells treated with cholesterol were unable to produce colonies. The size of the colonies was significantly smaller in those cells treated with 2-OH-E_2 or progesterone. Whereas the number of colonies was dose dependent reaching its maximum efficiency at the concentration of 70 nM for most of the compounds, 4-OH-E_2 was the most efficient in inducing larger colonies and number at a dose of 0.007 nM (Fig. 4.18). E_2 (Fig. 4.12), and BP (Fig. 4.14) behave very similar and are more transforming agents than DES and 2-OH-E_2 (Figs. 4.15, 4.17).

The metabolites of estrogen significantly impair the formation of ductules replacing them by structures filled by large cuboidal cells. Some of the cells present cytoplasmic vacuolization and pyknosis. Cells treated with 2-OH E_2 or 16-α-OH-E_2 is less efficient in altering the ductulogenic capacity (Figs. 4.17,

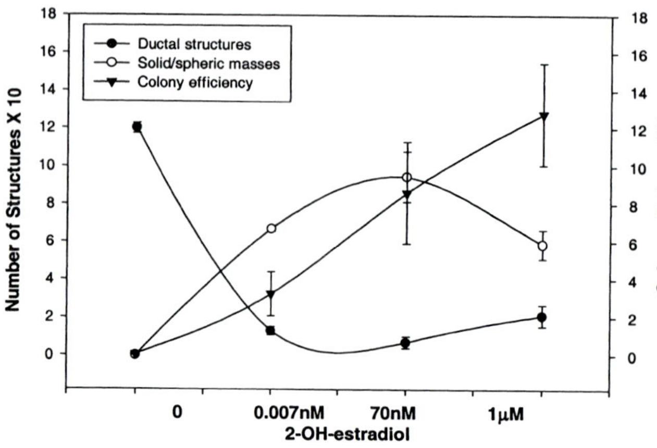

Figure 4.17

Curves showing the dose response effect of MCF-10F cells to the transforming effect of 2-OH-E_2, (nomenclature as described in Fig. 4.12)

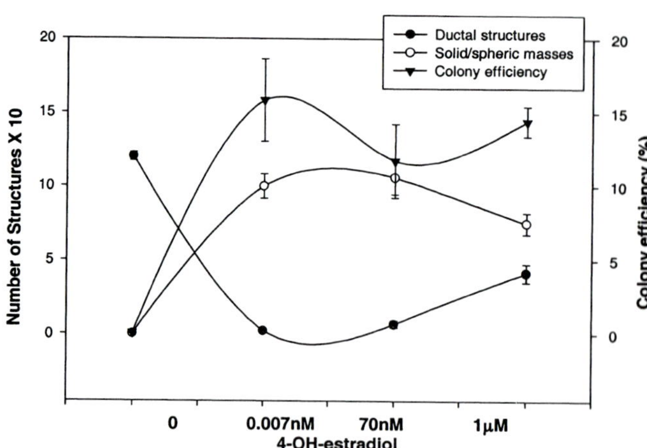

Figure 4.18

Curves showing the dose response effect of MCF-10F cells to the transforming effect of 4-0H-E_2, (nomenclature as described in Fig. 4.12)

4.19). Importantly 4-OH-E_2 at a dose of 0.007 nM induces significant changes in the ductulogenic capacity with a maximal number of solid masses (Fig. 4.18). These structures also have a high proliferative index (Fig. 4.20).

Figure 4.19

Curves showing the dose response effect of MCF-10F cells to the transforming effect of 16-α-OH-E$_2$, (nomenclature as described in Fig. 4.12)

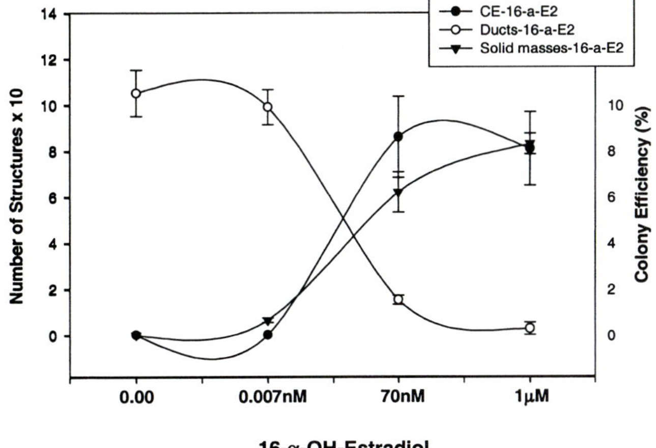

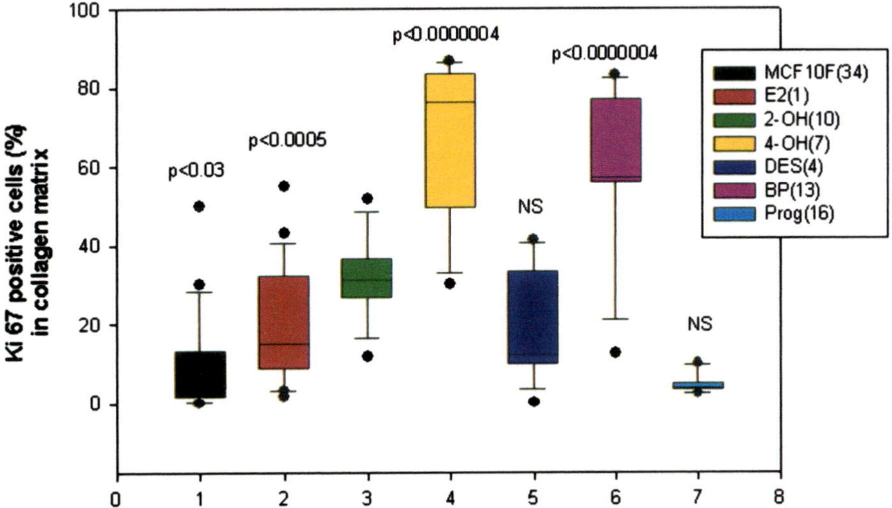

Figure 4.20

Histogram depicting the proliferative activity of MCF-10F cells treated as indicated in Fig. 4.9 with different compounds at 70 nM concentration and growing in a collagen matrix. The values are expressing the percentage of positive cells immunoreacted with antibody Ki67. 4-OH-E$_2$ transformed cells are the ones with the highest number of proliferating cells. Progesterone do not stimulate the proliferation of MCF-10F cells

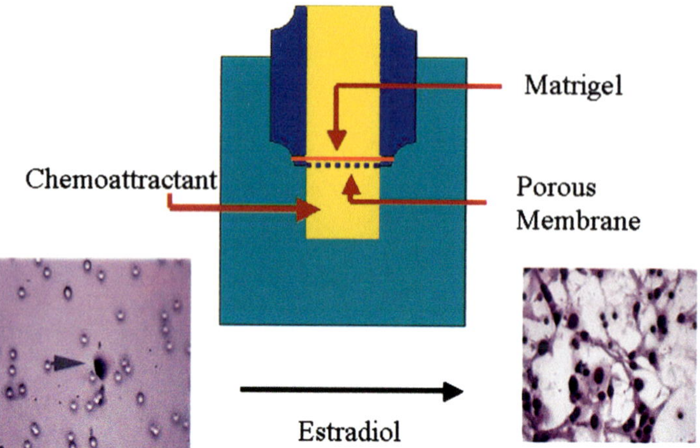

Figure 4.21

Schematic representation of the invasiveness assay using the Boyden-type chambers (Transwell, Coastar, Cambridge, MA) separated by a porous polycarbonate filter (8 μm pore size) (Nucleopore, Pleasanton, CA), coated with reconstituted basement membrane material (Matrigel; Collaborative Research, Bedford, MA). For the chemoinvasion assay, filters were coated with Matrigel, which was prepared by reconstituting Matrigel with 100 μM of MEM with 0.1 % BSA. The filters were coated and dried overnight. Fibronectin (Collaborative Research, Bedford, MA) at a concentration of 1 μg/ml in 0.5 ml of MEM with 0.1 % BSA was used as chemoattractant and placed in the lower chamber. Trypsinized cells (3×10^5) were seeded in the upper chamber and incubated for 12 h at 37°C in a carbon dioxide incubator. Then the filters were fixed, stained by Diff Quick (Sigma), cut out and mounted onto glass slides. The total number of cells that crossed the membrane was counted under a light microscope. The values were expressed as chemoinvasion index. Values of chemoinvasion were expressed as the number of cells that migrated to the lower chamber. The experiments were repeated three times and results expressed as the mean ± SE of the three experiments. The *lower left panel* shows a single MCF-10F cell (*arrow*) on a background of membrane pores; that migrated after treatment with cholesterol as indicated in Fig. 4.9; the *lower right panel* shows numerous cells that migrated after treatment with 70 nM of 17β-E$_2$

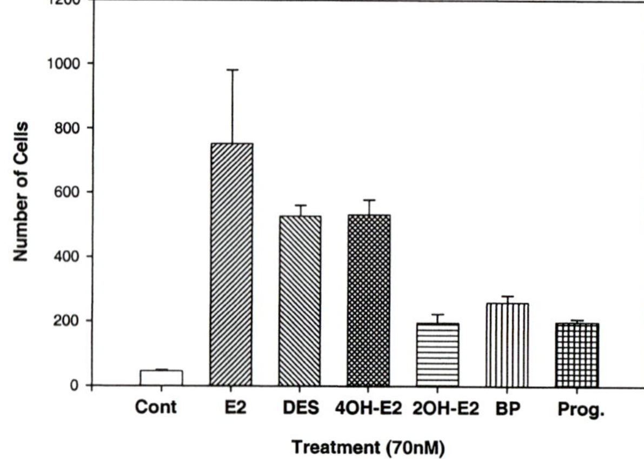

Figure 4.22

Histogram depicting the invasive capacity of MCF-10F cells treated with different compounds (abscissa) as indicated in Fig. 4.9. The ordinate shows the numbers of cells that have crossed the Matrigel membrane

The invasive capacity of E$_2$, DES, 4OH-E$_2$ and BP transformed cells measured in the Boyden chamber (Fig. 4.21), was very high when compared with the control or those treated with DMSO, P, or 2OH-E$_2$ (Fig. 4.22).

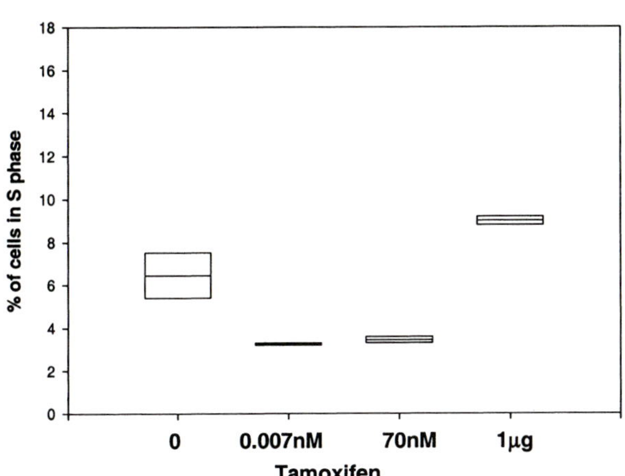

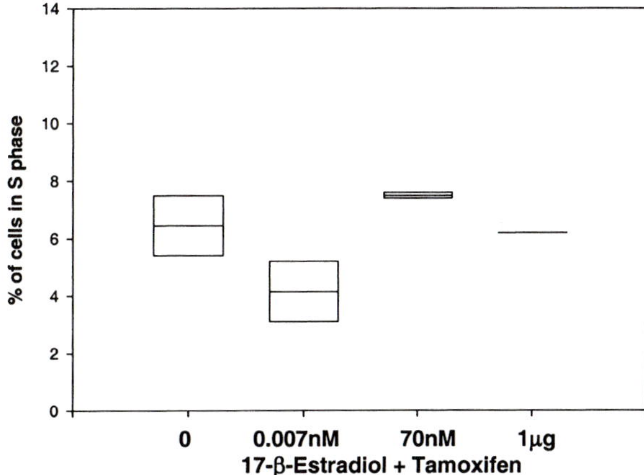

Figure 4.23

Box plot showing the effect of tamoxifen treated cells as explained in Fig. 4.9, on the S-phase of the cell cycle

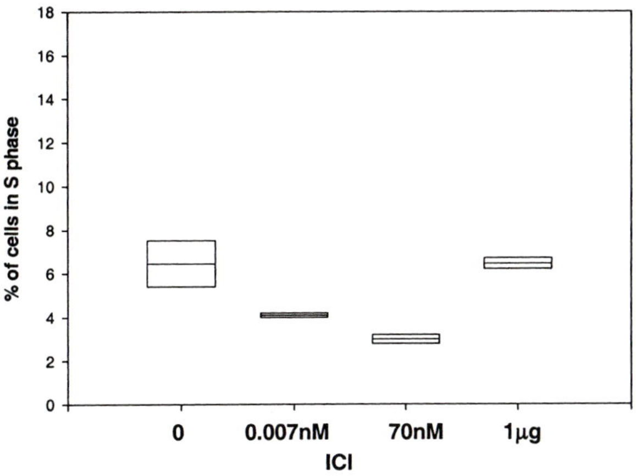

Figure 4.24

Box plot showing the effect of ICI treated cells as explained in Fig. 4.9, on the S-phase of the cell cycle

4.5.2.3 Role of Antiestrogens in the Expression of the Transformation Phenotype

The proliferative activity of the MCF-10F cells that had been treated with tamoxifen alone (Fig. 4.23) or ICI-182,780 (Fig. 4.24) was not modified when compared with the control. Those cells that were treated with 17β-estradiol in presence of tamoxifen (Fig. 4.25) or ICI-182,780 (Fig. 4.26) showed no increment of the proliferative activity neither in monolayer nor in collagen matrix. Instead, colony formation in agar methocel was abrogated and the ductulogenic capacity was maintained (Fig. 4.27). The proliferative activity of these cells in collagen matrix was also abrogated (Fig. 4.28). 4-OH-E$_2$ transforming efficiency was not abrogated by ICI neither in the colony efficiency assay nor in the loss of ductulogenic capacity (Fig. 4.29). The histology of the solid masses induced by 4-OH estradiol in collagen matrix was not modified by ICI, even the number of cells was significantly higher. ICI-182,780 was unable to abrogate the invasive phenotype induced by estrogen (Fig. 4.30) and tamoxifen even exacerbated the invasive phenotype.

Figure 4.25

Box plot showing the effect of 17β-E$_2$ + tamoxifen treated cells as explained in Fig. 4.9 on the S-phase of the cell cycle

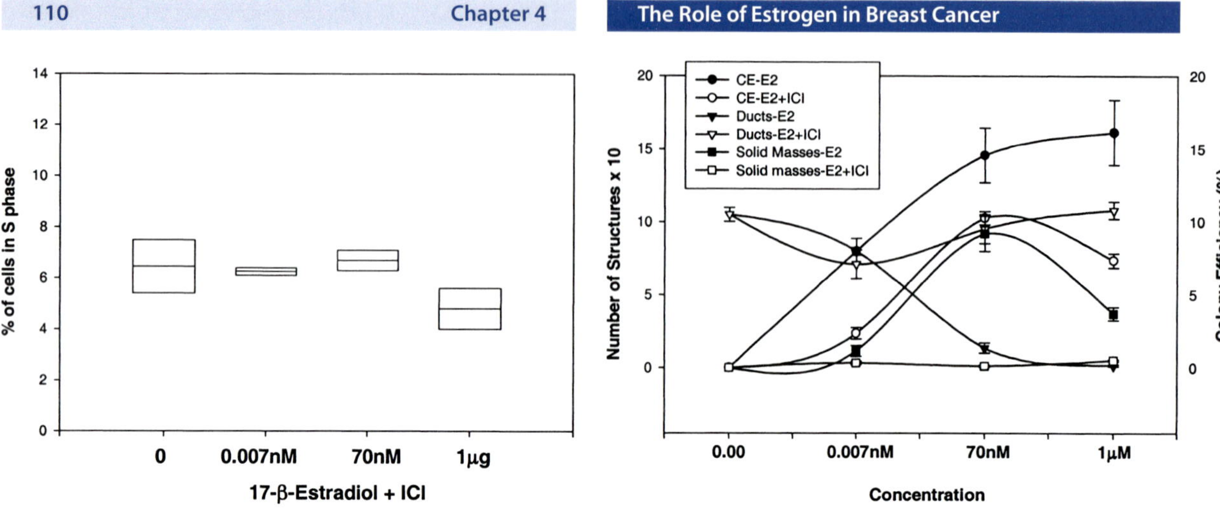

Figure 4.26

Box plot show showing the effect of 17β-estradiol + ICI treated cells as is explained in Fig. 4.9 on the S-phase of the cell cycle

Figure 4.27

Curves depicting the transforming affect of $17\beta\text{-}E_2$ alone or in combination with ICI, (nomenclature as described in Fig. 4.13)

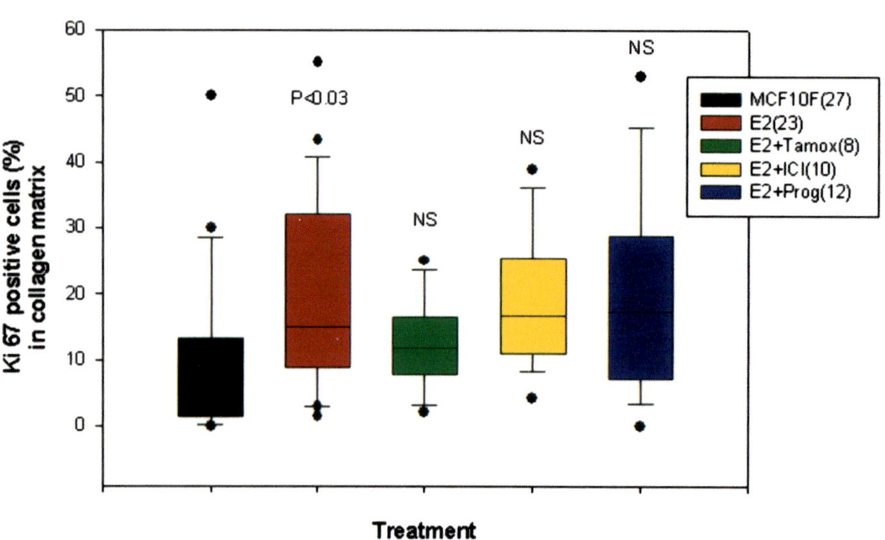

Figure 4.28

Histogram depicting the proliferative activity of MCF-10F cells treated as indicated in Fig. 4.9 with combination of 17β-estradiol + tamoxifen, $(E_2 + Tamox)$ or plus ICI $(E_2 + ICI)$ or plus progesterone $(E_2 + Prog)$. The *number in parenthesis* indicates the number of ductules or structures counted

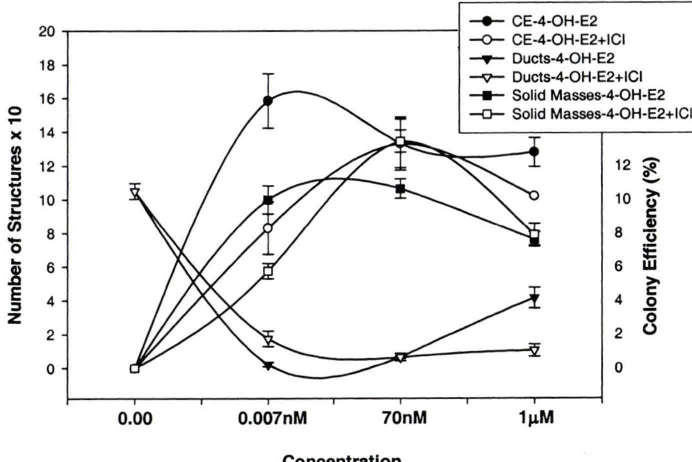

Figure 4.29

Curves depicting the transforming effect of 4-OH-E$_2$ alone and in combination with ICI (*4-OH-E$_2$ + ICI*), (nomenclature as described in Fig. 4.13)

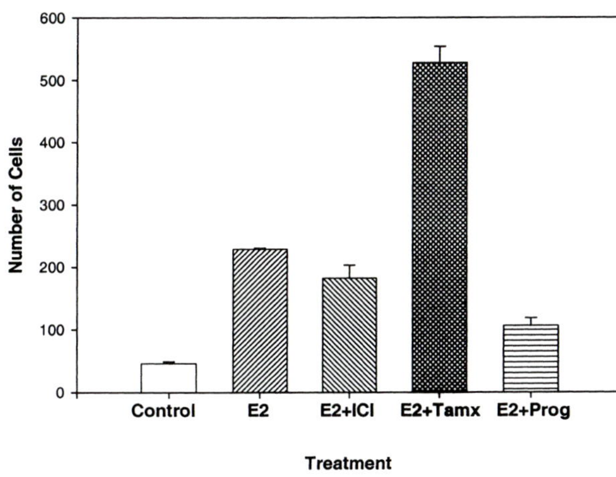

Figure 4.30

Fig. 4.30. Invasiveness phenotype in MCF-10F cells treated with 17β-estradiol (*E$_2$*) and in combination with ICI (*E$_2$ + ICI*), tamoxifen (*E$_2$ + Tamox*) and with progesterone (*E$_2$ + Prog*)

4.5.2.4 Detection of Estrogen Receptors in MCF-10F Cells

The ER α was not detected in the MCF-10F cells or in those transformed by estrogens or their metabolites (Fig. 4.31). The positive control MCF-7 cells was positive for ERα showing by Western blot the specific band corresponding to a 67 kDa, instead the band was absent in the negative control MDA-MB-235 cell line (Fig. 4.31).

The ERβ protein expression analysis showed two bands 68 and 53 kDa of molecular weight corresponding to ERβ long and short form, respectively. Both bands were present in the MCF-10F cells and in the transformed cells (Fig. 4.31). Those cells transformed by 17β-estradiol as well as those treated with progesterone significantly overexpressed the long form of ERβ. Instead, MCF-7 cells showed the short form of the ERβ (Fig. 4.31).

The progesterone receptor (PR) expression was negative in the MCF-10F cells when compared with MCF-7 cells that was used a positive control presenting the 186 and 82 kDa PR long and short form respectively. The estrogen-transformed cells also expressed PR (Fig. 4.31).

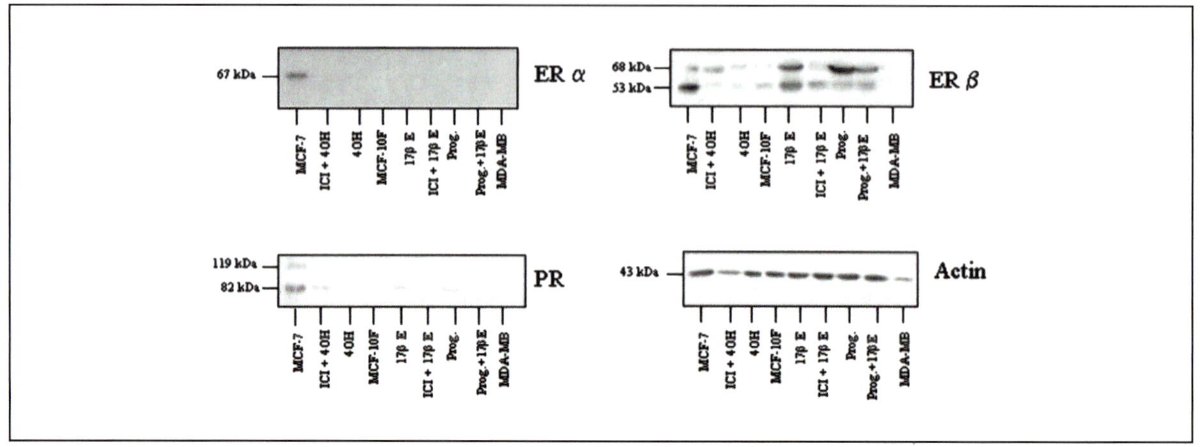

Figure 4.31

Western Blots of ERα, ERβ and progesterone receptors. Proteins were isolated from MCF-10F cells transformed with 70 nM, ICI+4-OH-E₂, 4-OH-E₂, 17β-estradiol, ICI + 17β-estradiol, progesterone and progesterone + 17β-estradiol as indicated in Fig. 4.9. MCF-7 and MDA-MB-235 cell lines were used as control. The medium was removed and the cells were rinsed with PBS at room temperature. The cells were lysed using a syringe with a 21-gauge needle followed by microcentrifugation of the cell lysate at 2,000 × G for 10 min at 4°C. The proteins were electrophoretically separated in a SDS-PAGE polyacrylamide gel 10% running at 90 V during 8 h at room temperature. The proteins were transferred to nitrocellulose membranes (Amersham Arlington Heights, IL.). Membranes were blocked using 5% of non-fat dried milk during 1 h at room temperature and hybridized to anti-ER monoclonal antibody against the full length alpha form of the estrogen receptor (San Cruz Biotech, Santa Cruz, CA) at a concentration of 1/50, anti-ER (Clone ER-7G5) beta polyclonal antibody against 19 aac synthetic peptide derived from human ER-β protein (Zymed Lab, Inc., San Francisco, CA), at a concentration 1/50 (60 µg/ml), anti-PR Clone PR-2C5) monoclonal antibody against peptide representing N-terminal of human PR conjugates to carrier protein (Zymed Lab., Inc., San Francisco, CA), at a concentration 1/50 (20 µg/ml) overnight at 4°C. Horseradish peroxidase-conjugated anti-mouse, anti-rabbit (Amersham, Arlington Heights, IL) were used as secondary antibodies in a concentration 1/2,500 and incubated during 1 h at room temperature. Enhanced chemiluminescence system (Amersham, Arlington Heights, IL) was used for final immunoblot detection

4.5.2.5 Evidence for a Role of ERβ and Metabolic Activation of Estrogen in the Transformation of Human Breast Epithelial Cells

Short-term treatment of HBEC with physiological doses of 17β-estradiol induces anchorage independent growth, colony formation in agar methocel, and reduced ductulogenic capacity in collagen gel, all phenotypes whose expression is indicative of neoplastic transformation, and that are induced by BP under the same culture conditions. Progesterone was unable to induce significant increase in colony formation, although small colonies less than 50 µm in diameter were observed, whereas none were found in the MCF-10F cells treated with DMSO or cholesterol. The ductulogenic pattern was not impaired by progesterone but the luminal size was smaller than those found in the MCF-10F cells treated with DMSO or cholesterol. Altogether, these data clearly indicate that HBEC when treated with 17β-estradiol produces significant morphogenetic changes. The fact that MCF-10F cells are ERα-negative, indicates that this receptor pathway is not involved in the carcinogenic process. Although the presence of ERβ may indicate that the response of the cells to grow and form colonies in agar methocel could be mediated by this receptor. The biological role of the ERβ has been in part explained by gene knockout studies, in which the presence of ERα but not ERβ was necessary for the development of the mouse mammary gland [169]. ERβ may be acting as an antagonist of ERα, thus, by removing ERβ the suppressive effect of the receptor is lost. If that were the case in our HBEC, the presence of ERβ will abrogate the emergence of transformation. Alternatively, the downstream signaling pathway may dictate the putative suppressive effects of ERβ. Both ER subtypes can signal via classic estrogen response elements or via AP-1 enhancers. The downstream effects of signaling through AP-1 are both receptor and ligand specific [170]. In the model described above, it seems that the presence of ERβ is the pathway used by estrogen to induce cell proliferation in MCF-10F cells. This is supported by the fact that either tamoxifen or a pure antiestrogen like ICI abrogated these phenotypes. However, the Invasion phenotype, an important marker of tumorigenesis is not modified when the cells are treated in presence of tamoxifen or ICI, suggesting that other pathways may be involved. Although we cannot rule out the possibility that 4-OH-E$_2$ may interact with other receptors still not identified, with the data presently available the direct effect of 4-OH-E$_2$ at so low doses support the concept that metabolic activation of estrogens mediated by various cytochrome P450 (CYP) complexes, generate through this pathway reactive intermediates that elicit direct genotoxic effects leading to transformation. An increase in catechol estrogen (4-OH-E$_2$) due to either elevated rates of synthesis or reduced rates of monomethylation will easily lead to their autoxidation to semiquinones and subsequently quinones, both of which are electrophiles capable of covalently binding to nucleophilic groups on DNA. Through this pathway estrogen metabolites exert direct genotoxic effects that might increase mutation rates, or compromise the DNA repair system, leading to the accumulation of genomic alterations essential to tumorigenesis. This assumption was confirmed when we found that none of the transformation phenotypes induced by 4-OH-E$_2$ were not abrogated when this compound was used in presence of the pure antiestrogenic ICI. The novelty of these observation lies in the role of ERβ in transformation and that this pathway can be successfully bypassed by the estrogen metabolite 4-OH-E$_2$.

4.5.3 Genomic Changes Induced by Estrogen and Its Metabolites in Human Breast Epithelial Cells

From the E$_2$-treated cells six clones out the 24 colonies formed were expanded and maintained in culture. These clones were designated E$_2$-1 to E$_2$-6 (Table 4.1). From DES treated MCF-10F cells seven clones were selected, from 24 colonies, expanded and maintained in culture, being designated DES-1 to DES-7 (Table 4.1). These clones were selected for genomic analysis. DNA fingerprint analysis of parent, E$_2$-, DES-, and BP-treated cells and their derived clones revealed that their allelic pattern was identical in all the cell lines analyzed (Fig. 4.32). These results confirmed that all the cells tested had the same HBEC origin, and that they were free of contamination from other cell lines maintained in our laboratory. Among 67 markers tested, which were selected based on chromosomal changes reported to be present in breast and other cancers, only clones DES-5, E$_2$-1 and E$_2$-2, exhibited LOH in chromosomes 3 and 11, respectively. LOH in chromosome 3 was detected at three different loci, which were detected with five different markers, 3p21.3–21.2 (marker D3S1478 and D3S2384), 3p21.1–14.2 (marker D3S1450), and 3p21 (marker D3S1217 and D3S1447) (Figs. 4.33, 4.34). It was of interest that clone DES-5, in addition to exhibiting LOH in chromosome 3, was the one exhibiting the most marked expression of transformation phenotypes, i. e., larger colony size and absent ductulogenic ability in collagen gel. The expression of LOH in chromosome 3 in DES-transformed breast epithelial cells acquired relevance in view of the light that frequent homozygous deletions, rearrangements, and hypermethylation at 3p21 loci have been reported to be present in spontaneously occurring breast lesions, such as ductal hyperplasia, carcinoma in situ, and invasive carcinoma [171–176]. The existence of suppressor genes on 3p has also been suggested by transfection studies in which 3p DNA fragments inhibited

Table 4.1. Phenotypic markers of cell transformation induced in MCF-10F cells by 17β-estradiol (E_2), and benzo(a)pyrene (*BP*)

Cell type	Number of passages	Doubling time	Colony number	Colony efficiency (%)	Colony size (diameter in μm)
MCF-10F	113	93±5.6	0.0	0.0	0.0
BP	4	42±3.8	89	18±4.5	670±46
E_2	4	78±16.0	24*	4.8±0.9	170±34
E_2-1	4	81±3.0	36	7.2±3.7	180±12
E_2-2	4	68±10	45	9.0±2.0	150±6
E_2-3	5	66±8.0	39	7.9±5.6	190±9
E_2-4	3	82±6.0	20	3.5±1.1	134±5
E_2-5	6	61±5.6	63	12.6±3.0	193±12
E_2-6	4	73±3.0	54	10.8±4.9	189±5

* From these 24 colonies clones E_2-1 to E_2-6 were recovered and expanded

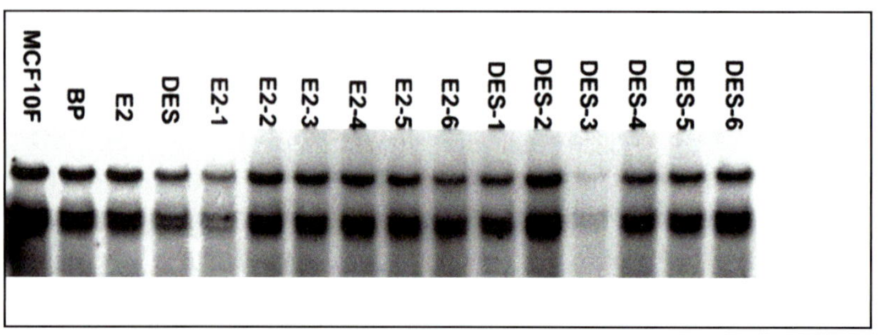

Figure 4.32

Fingerprint analysis of genomic DNA obtained from the MCF-10F cells listed in Table 4.1 and of DES-treated and its derived clones DES-1 to DES-6. The identity of these cells was confirmed by Southern blot hybridization of genomic DNA with a cocktail of the three minisatellite probes D2S44, D14S13 and D17S74. Genomic DNAs were digested in HifI, and hybridized with probes (reprinted from: Russo, et al, J. Steroid Biochem. Mol. Bio. 80:149–162, 2002, with permission)

tumorigenesis in nude mice [177, 178]. We have observed LOH at 3p21 using markers D3S1217 and D3S1447, and in the region 3p21.1-p21.2 with markers D3S1478 and D3S2384. LOH in this region has been reported in nearly all-small cell lung carcinomas [179]. Even though deletion in these regions is not considered to be specific for breast cancer, the present observations might indicate that they represent a genetic event triggered by estrogens, which could play a key role in the development and progression of tumors originated from this type of epithelium. LOH in 3p21.3 has been found more frequently in breast cancer metastases than in primary tumors. Several putative "metastasis-related genes" are located in this region, such as 37LRP [180–183], CTNNB1, that encodes β catenin [149], and the αRLC gene, that encodes a new integrin subunit, identified by positional cloning, that shows homology with the α1 integrin involved in the metastatic process [184]. We have also found LOH in the 3p21.1–14.2 (marker

Figure 4.33

LOH analysis of MCF-10F, and of clones E_2-1, E_2-2, and DES-1, DES-3, DES-4, and DES-5, derived from E_2 and DES-treated cells. *Arrows* indicate the loss of alleles in E_2-2, and DES-5 clones. To obtain DNA, treated and control cells were lysed in 5 ml of TNE (0.5 M Tris pH 8.9, 10 mM NaCl, 15-mM EDTA) with 500 Dg/ml proteinase K and 1% sodium dodecyl sulfate (SDS), and incubated at 48°C for 24 h. Following two extractions with phenol (equilibrated with 0.1 M Tris pH 8.0), the DNA was spooled from 2 volumes of 100% ethanol, air dried and resuspended in 20 mM EDTA. The DNA was then treated sequentially with RNase A (100 µg/ml) for 1 h at 37°C and 100 µg/ml proteinase K, I % SDS, at 48°C for 3 h, followed by two extractions with saturated phenol. The DNA was again retrieved from the aqueous phase by ethanol precipitation, washed extensively in 70% ethanol, and after air-drying suspended in TE (I0 mM Tris, pH8.0), 1 mM EDTA. The allelic losses were evaluated at the regions of chromosomes 1, 2, 3, 6, 8, 9, 11, 12, 13, 16, 17, and 18 most frequently reported to exhibit loss of heterozygosity (LOH) in spontaneous breast tumors. DNA amplification of microsatellite length polymorphisms was utilized for detecting allelic losses present in the transformed clones. Microsatellites are polymorphic markers used primarily for gene mapping which can be broadly defined as relatively short (<l00 bp) runs of tandem repeated di- to tetranucleotide sequence motifs. The origin and nature of these polymorphism sequences is not well established, but they may result from errors of the polymerase during replication and/or from slightly unequal recombination between homologous chromatids during meiosis. These microsatellites have proven to be useful markers for investigating LOH and could be applicable to allelotyping as well as regional mapping of deletions in specific chromosomal regions. They are highly polymorphic, very common (between 10^5 and 10^6 per genome), and are flanked by unique sequences that can serve as primers for polymerase chain reaction (PCR) amplification. Detection of Allelic Loss: LOH was defined as a total loss of or a 50%, or more reduction in density in one of the heterozygous alleles. All experiments were repeated at least three times to avoid false positive or false negative results. To control for possible DNA degradation, the same blots used to assess allelic loss were analyzed with additional DNA gene probes that detect large fragments. The bands were quantitated using a Ultra-Scan XL laser densitometry (Pharmacia LKB Biotechnology Inc.) within the linear range of the film (reprinted from: Russo, et al, J. of Steroid. Biochem. Mol. Biol. 80:149–162, 2002, with permission)

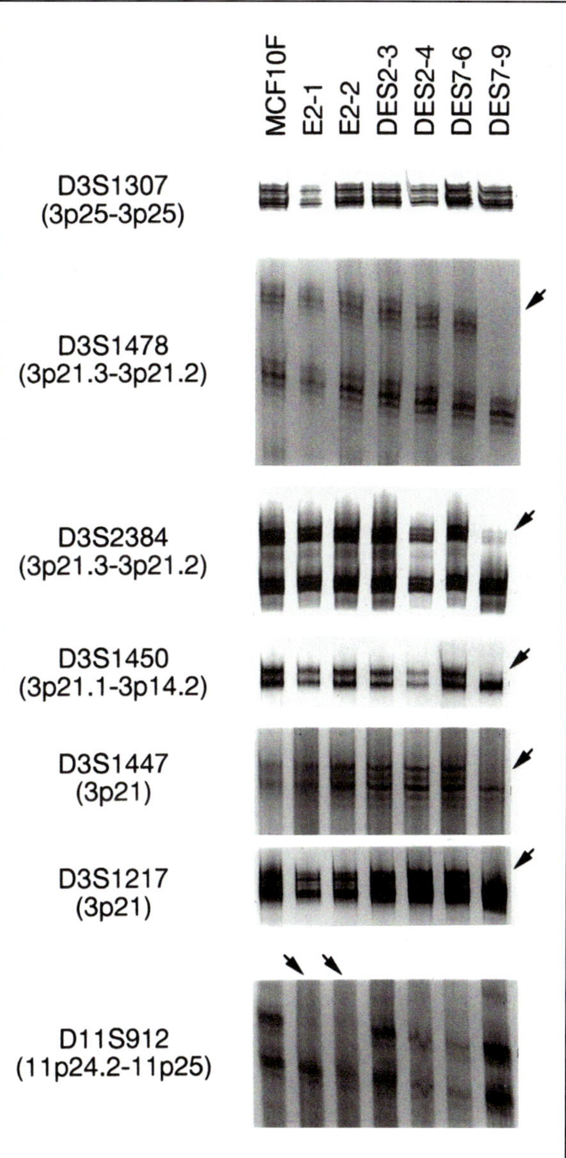

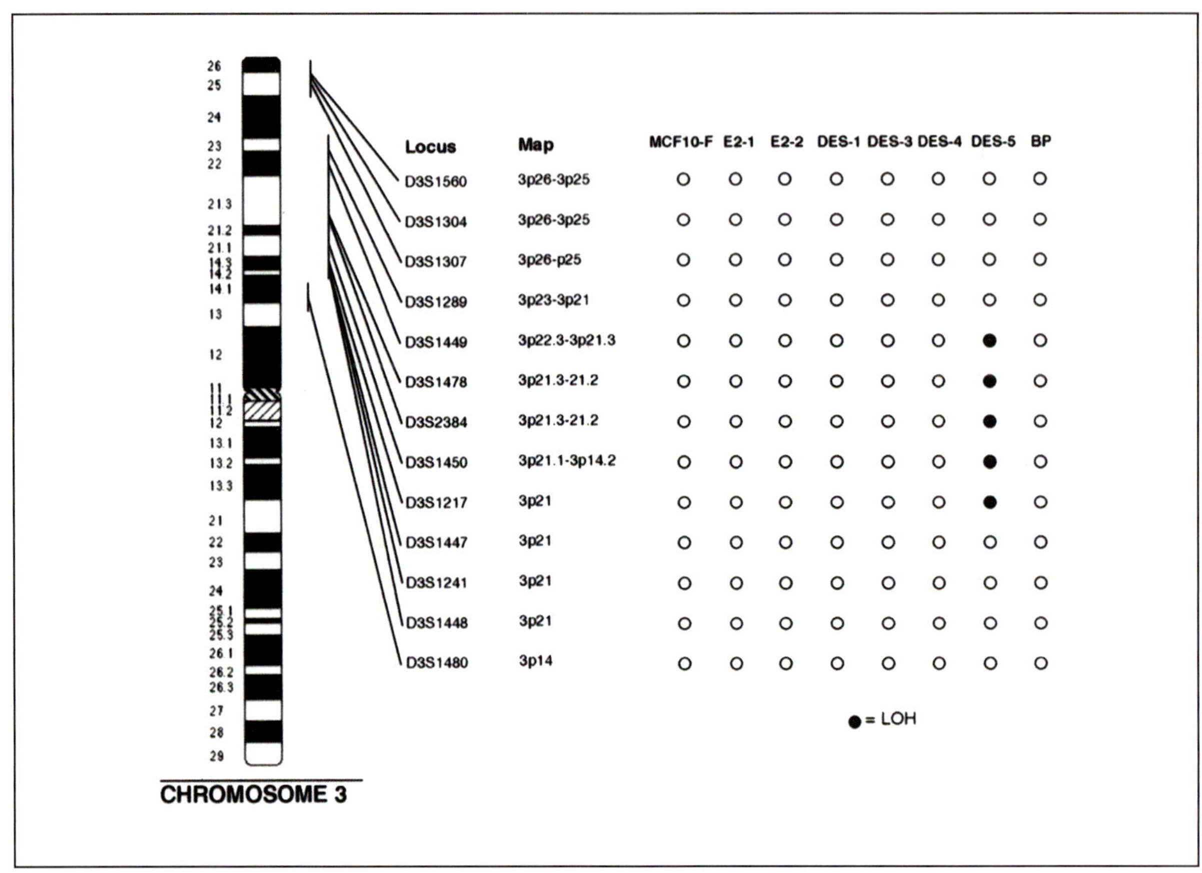

Locus	Map	MCF10-F	E2-1	E2-2	DES-1	DES-3	DES-4	DES-5	BP
D3S1560	3p26-3p25	○	○	○	○	○	○	○	○
D3S1304	3p26-3p25	○	○	○	○	○	○	○	○
D3S1307	3p26-p25	○	○	○	○	○	○	○	○
D3S1289	3p23-3p21	○	○	○	○	○	○	○	○
D3S1449	3p22.3-3p21.3	○	○	○	○	○	○	●	○
D3S1478	3p21.3-21.2	○	○	○	○	○	○	●	○
D3S2384	3p21.3-21.2	○	○	○	○	○	○	●	○
D3S1450	3p21.1-3p14.2	○	○	○	○	○	○	●	○
D3S1217	3p21	○	○	○	○	○	○	●	○
D3S1447	3p21	○	○	○	○	○	○	○	○
D3S1241	3p21	○	○	○	○	○	○	○	○
D3S1448	3p21	○	○	○	○	○	○	○	○
D3S1480	3p14	○	○	○	○	○	○	○	○

Figure 4.34

Ideogram of chromosome 3 showing LOH in clone DES-5 derived from DES transformed MCF-10F cells

D3S1450). This region has been found to be associated with dysregulated cell proliferation rather than with tumor progression [175]. It is also frequently deleted in in situ carcinoma, benign tumors, and familial breast cancers [150, 151, 176]. The 3p14.2 region contains a fragile site known as FRA3B, from which the FHIT gene has recently been cloned. It encodes a protein showing homology with a yeast hydrolase, and its transcripts show rearrangements in different cell lines and tumors [149–151, 185–190]. A telomerase-regulating genes have been located in 3p21.3-p22 and 3p12–21.1 using the microcell monochromosome transfer technique [152].

Clones E_2-1 and E_2-2 identically expressed LOH in chromosome 11 at 11q23.3 (marker D11S29), and 11q24.2-q25 (marker D11S912) (Figs. 4.32, 4.35). BP-treated cells did not exhibit LOH at any of the loci

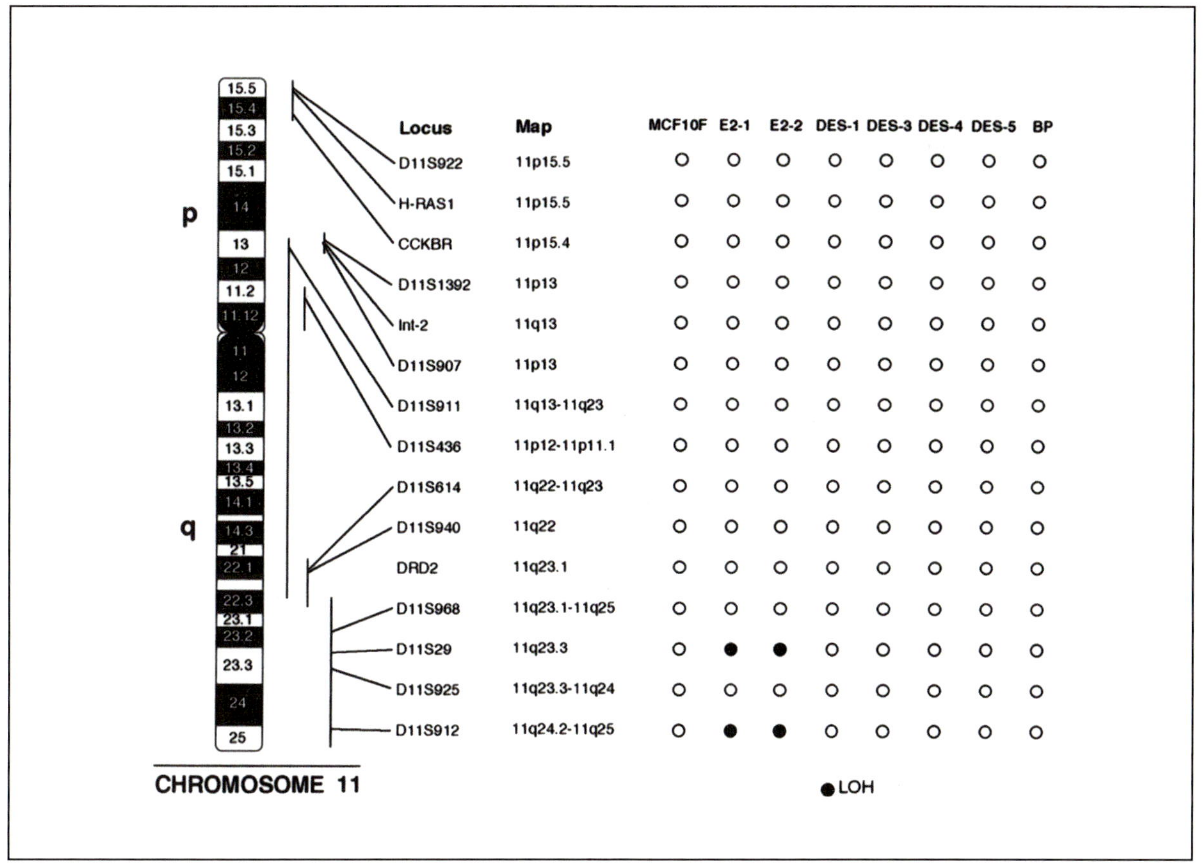

Locus	Map	MCF10F	E2-1	E2-2	DES-1	DES-3	DES-4	DES-5	BP
D11S922	11p15.5	○	○	○	○	○	○	○	○
H-RAS1	11p15.5	○	○	○	○	○	○	○	○
CCKBR	11p15.4	○	○	○	○	○	○	○	○
D11S1392	11p13	○	○	○	○	○	○	○	○
Int-2	11q13	○	○	○	○	○	○	○	○
D11S907	11p13	○	○	○	○	○	○	○	○
D11S911	11q13-11q23	○	○	○	○	○	○	○	○
D11S436	11p12-11p11.1	○	○	○	○	○	○	○	○
D11S614	11q22-11q23	○	○	○	○	○	○	○	○
D11S940	11q22	○	○	○	○	○	○	○	○
DRD2	11q23.1	○	○	○	○	○	○	○	○
D11S968	11q23.1-11q25	○	○	○	○	○	○	○	○
D11S29	11q23.3	○	●	●	○	○	○	○	○
D11S925	11q23.3-11q24	○	○	○	○	○	○	○	○
D11S912	11q24.2-11q25	○	●	●	○	○	○	○	○

Figure 4.35

Ideogram of chromosome 11 showing LOH in clones E_2-1 and E_2-2 derived from E_2 transformed MCF-10F cells

tested. Interestingly, we have found that all the clones of the cells transformed with either E_2, DES or BP presented microsatellite instability (MSI), expressed as an allelic expansion at 3p21 locus (marker D3S1447). It has been reported that both arms of chromosome 11 contain several regions of LOH in cancers of the breast and of other organs, and that transfer of chromosome 11 to mammary cell lines suppresses tumorigenicity in athymic mice [153]. Several genes, such as HRAs, CTSD, ILK, TSG101 and KI1 have been reported to be located on the short arm of chromosome 11 [153–158, 186, 187]. A region of deletion on 11q22–23 has been described on the long arm of chromosome 11 in 40 to 60% of breast tumors [162, 176, 191–193]. The ataxia telangiectasia susceptibility gene (ATM) is the most widely studied candidate gene in this region [165]. ATM may act up-

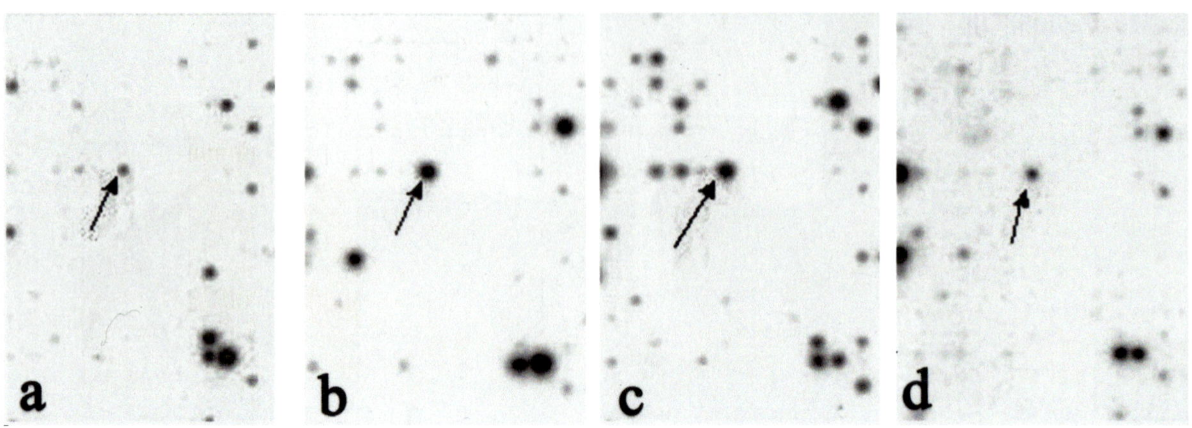

Figure 4.36 a–d

cDNA Array (Clonetech human Cancer 1.2) of MCF-10F cells treated with **a** cholesterol, **b** 17β-estradiol, **c** 4-OH-E$_2$, and **d** benzo(a)pyrene, as explained in Fig. 4.9. The *arrow* points to the spot containing the gene CENP-F

stream of the TP53 gene in cell cycle regulation [166, 194] and its heterozygous mutation is associated with high incidence of early-onset breast cancer. This region has been reported to contain several tumor suppressor genes and genes involved in the metastatic process. In this latter group, the MMP genes encoding matrix metalloproteases involved in invasion, ETS1 encoding a transcription factor involved in angiogenesis, and VACM-1, encoding a protein probably involved in cell cycle regulation have been identified [195]. Although some of these genes might be affected during the transformation of HBEC induced by estrogens, a more detailed allelotyping using multiple markers is required for better defining the significance of LOH in these cells. Approximately 35% of breast cancers show LOH at the D11S29 and NCAM loci [196], and a higher frequency of LOH at this locus has also been found in melanomas [197]. LOH has been found at frequencies of 25% and 29% at the distal D11S968 (11qter) and D11S29 (11q23.3 locus), slightly above the accepted baseline of 0–20% in colorectal cancer. The fact that breast cancer, melanoma, and colorectal cancer have been found to be influenced by estrogens [198], give relevance to our data that treatment of MCF-10F cells with estrogens induces LOH in this specific locus. LOH at 11q23-qter occurs frequently in ovarian and other cancers [199, 200].

4.5.4 Other Genomic Changes Induced by Estrogen and Its Metabolites in the Transformation of Human Breast Epithelial Cells

In order to determine if the gene expression profile induced by E$_2$, 4-OH estradiol and BP were the same or whether they are divergent in their pattern of expression, mRNA from these transformed cells was extracted and hybridized to cDNA array membranes that contained 1,176 human genes (Clontech Human Cancer 1,2 array). The genomic signature of the three transformed cells present a cluster of genes that are commonly upregulated (Table 4.2), indicating that a similar mechanism is involved in the transformation pathway. Interestingly there are genes that are upregulated in the E$_2$ and 4-OH-E$_2$ transformed cells such as the CENP-E (Figs. 4.36, 4.37; Tables 4.3, 4.4) that are not modified in the BP transformed cells (Table 4.5). The same occurs for several genes that are downregulated differentially in the three transformed cells (Table 4.6).

Figure 4.37

Histogram depicting the amplification of CENP-F in the four cell types studied (see also Fig. 4.36)

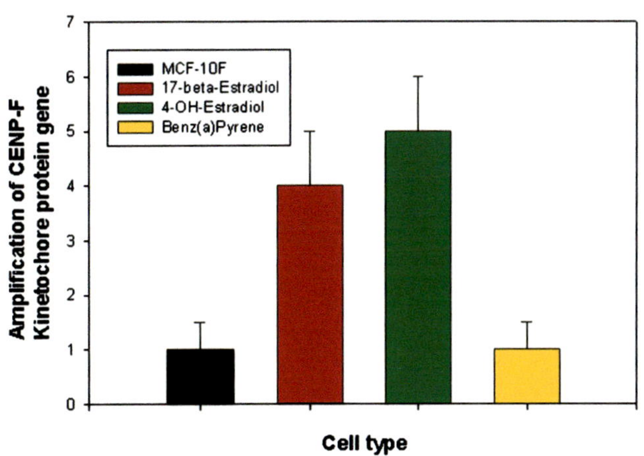

Table 4.2. Common up-regulated genes in MCF-10F cells transformed by BP, E_2 and 4OH using cDNA array

Gene description	Swissprot #	Function	BP/10F	E_2/10F	4OH/10F
c-myc oncogene	P01106	Oncogene	3.24	3.66	6.21
fos-related antigen	P15407	Oncogene	10.25	2.31	15.04
HER3	P21860	Oncogene	2.09	3.32	7.95
SRF accessory protein 2	P41970	Transcription	3.61	2.46	9.11
hEGR1	P18146	Transcription	3.2	6.49	2.91
Splicing factor 9G8	Q16629	mRNA processing	2.23	2.93	4.42
Antigen KI-67	P46013	Cell proliferation	3.2	2.7	5.97
HMG-I	P17096	Chromatin	2.36	3.26	7.95
nm23-H4	O00746	Kinase	2.02	2	2.24
Cytokeratin 2E	P35908	Keratin	43.09	2.38	4.37

Table 4.3. Specific up-regulated genes in E_2-transformed cells by cDNA array

Array location	Gene description	Swissprot #	Function	E_2/10F
A02g	Neurogenic locus notch protein	Q04721	Oncogene	2.2
A03g	c-myc binding protein MM-1	Q99471	Oncogene	2.19
B14n	Retinoic acid receptor beta	P28702	Transcription	4.76
C05l	Retinoic acid receptor gamma 1	P13631	Transcription	4.59
C10m	TAX1-binding protein 151	Q13311	Transcription	4.57
D14a	CENP-F kinetochore protein	P49454	Transcription	2.33
C04b	TRAP1	Q12931	Signaling	3.06
E13j	GDNPF	None	Signaling	3.16
B04n	hBAP	Q99623	Transducer	2.15
C05d	GADD153	P35638	Apoptosis	6.34
B06e	KIAA0175	Q14680	Kinase	2.24
B09d	Casein kinase I gamma 2	P78368	Kinase	2.88
A11k	CKS2	P33552	Kinase	2.24
B02d	PCTK1	Q00536	Kinase	2.51
B14k	51C protein	Q13577	Phospholipase	4.14
E10j	TIMP1	P01033	Protease inhibitor	2.8
D02d	Cadherin 5	P33151	Cell adhesion	2.14
F14c	Adenylosuccinate lyase	P30566	Nucleotide metabolism	2.13
C04h	HHR23A	P54725	Stress response	2.37
F06d	LDHB	P07195	Carbohydrate metabolism	3.16
D06c	Mesothelin precursor	Q13421	Surface antigen	6.46
D06e	Integrin beta 4	P16144	Cell adhesion	3.23
D08e	Integrin alpha 7B precursor	Q13683	Cell adhesion	2.59
E07f	Interleukin-1 beta precursor	P01584	Interleukin	2.09
F08f	Cytokeratin 18	P05783	Keratin	2.34
F13l	RI58	Q13325	Unclassified	2.48

Table 4.4. Specific up-regulated genes in 4OH-E$_2$ transformed cells by cDNA array

Array location	Gene description	Swissprot #	Function	4OH/10F
A01i	Leukemia-associated gene 1	O43261	Oncogene	2.74
A02b	EB1 protein	Q15691	Oncogene	5.45
A03b	Ezrin	P15311	Oncogene	3.5
A04e	Tyrosine-protein kinase receptor tyro3	Q06418	Oncogene	2.84
A02g	Neurogenic locus notch protein	Q04721	Oncogene	2.75
A03e	VEGFR1	P17948	Oncogene	2.64
A03g	c-myc binding protein MM-1	Q99471	Oncogene	4.06
B03m	14–3-3 protein sigma	P31947	Oncogene	2.96
A08n	HG4–1	O43846	Cell cycle	8.92
A10m	CDC10 protein homolog	Q16181	Cell cycle	3.89
A12n	GTP-binding protein GST1-HS	P15170	Cell cycle	8.66
C05f	KIAA0030	P49736	Cell cycle	3.88
C06f	MCM4 DNA replication licensing factor	P33991	Cell cycle	14.74
C07h	KIAA0078	O60216	Cell cycle	3.54
C13e	Proliferating cyclic nuclear antigen	P12004	Cyclin	10.1
A05i	G2/mitotic-specific cyclin B1	P14635	Cyclin	3.69
D03b	DNA-binding protein CPBP	Q99612	Transcription	4.19
A01c	AP-1	P05412	Transcription	11.47
E04e	Interferon gamma antagonist	None	Growth factor	2.65
E12b	Heparin-binding EGF-like growth factor	Q99075	Growth factor	3.26
E14d	Fibroblast growth factor 8	P55075	Growth factor	2.79
B12a	GRB3–3	P29354	Signaling	2.74
B14j	Rho GDP dissociation inhibitor 1	P52565	Signaling	2.66
C04b	TRAP1	Q12931	Signaling	4.05
B04k	Caveolin-1	Q03135	Signaling	2.54
C02i	TDG	Q13569	DNA repair	7.74
A13b	p78 putative serine/threonine-protein kinase	P27448	Kinase	3.67
B06e	KIAA0175	Q14680	Kinase	15.24
A05j	Cell division protein kinase 6	Q00534	Kinase	3.19
D09m	Glutathione-S-transferase (GST) homolog	P78417	Stress response	6.55
D07b	High mobility group protein HMG2	P26583	Chromatin	9.7
D11a	Heterochromatin protein homolog 1	P45973	Chromatin	3.47
D08a	High mobility group protein I&Y	P17096	Chromatin	7.95
D14a	CENP-F kinetochore protein	P49454	Chromatin	4.13

Table 4.4. (continued)

Array location	Gene description	Swissprot #	Function	4OH/10F
D08b	Histone H4	None	Histone	11.06
F03d	Thymidylate synthase	P04818	Nucleotide metabolism	2.83
F04d	Purine nucleoside phosphorylase	P00491	Nucleotide metabolism	2.63
F07e	Ribonucleotide reductase	P31350	Nucleotide metabolism	5.19
F08b	UMK	Q92528	Nucleotide metabolism	3.65
F09c	Uridine phosphorylase	Q16831	Nucleotide metabolism	3.82
F12d	Uridine 5'-monophosphate synthase	P11172	Nucleotide metabolism	6.34
F05e	Ornithine decarboxylase	P11926	Metabolism	12.9
F06d	L-lactate dehydrogenase H subunit	P07195	Metabolism	5.93
B05l	Calmodulin 1	P02593	Calcium-binding	5.41
D02d	Cadherin 5 (CDH5)	P33151	Cell adhesion	2.77
D03e	Integrin alpha 3 (ITGA3)	P26006	Cell adhesion	3.89
E04k	PRSM1 metallopeptidase	Q15779	Metalloproteinase	2.58
E10j	TIMP1	P01033	Protease inhibitor	3.07
F06f	Cytokeratin 14	P02533	Keratin	4.29
F08j	HSC70-interacting protein	P50502	Chaperone	3.37
F03n	KIAA0204	Q92603	Unclassified	3.69

Table 4.5. Specific up-regulated genes in BP-transformed cells by cDNA array

Array location	Gene description	Swissprot #	Function	BP/10F
C05l	RAR-gamma 1	P13631	Transcription	3.77
B04k	Caveolin-1	Q03135	Signaling	3.35
A03b	Ezrin	P15311	Oncogene	2.01
C04h	HHR23A	P54725	Stress response	2.04
C08g	mutL protein homolog	P40692	Stress response	4.31
E07h	Glycosylation-inhibiting factor	P14174	Cell communication	4.44
D06e	Integrin beta 4	P16144	Cell adhesion	4.24
D08e	Integrin alpha 7B precursor	Q13683	Cell adhesion	3.06
D05e	Integrin alpha 6 precursor	P23229	Cell adhesion	2.24
D07e	Integrin alpha 1	P56199	Cell adhesion	2.31
F05d	LDHA	P00338	Carbohydrate metabolism	6.25
F08f	Cytokeratin 18	P05783	Cytokeratin	3.04
F14e	BIGH3	Q15582	Microfilament	6.73

Table 4.6. Common down-regulated genes in MCF-10F cells transformed by Bp, E$_2$ and 4OH using cDNA array

Array loc.	Gene description	Swissprot #	Function	Bp/10F	E$_2$/10F	4OH/10F
A11g	PIG7	Q99732	Tumor suppressor	0.02	0.04	0.19
A14h	CD82 antigen	P27701	Tumor suppressor	0	0.18	0
B06k	Rho GDP dissociation inhibitor 2	P52566	Tumor suppressor	0	0	0.21
A02g	Neurogenic locus notch protein	Q04721	Transcription	0.29	0.47	0.38
A13h	Active breakpoint cluster region-related protein	Q12979	Transcription	0.13	0.25	0.46
A14c	Ets-related protein tel	P41212	Transcription	0	0.08	0.08
C06m	B4–2 protein	Q12796	Transcription	0	0	0
B03n	T3 receptor-associating cofactor 1	O00613	Intracellular transducers	0.48	0.41	0.22
E04b	HDGF	P51858	Growth factor	0.34	0.1	0.24
F07i	HNRNPK	Q07244	mRNA processing	0	0	0.17
B02j	RalB GTP-binding protein	P11234	G protein	0	0.24	0
B04j	RhoC	P08134	G protein	0.09	0.06	0.48
B12j	p21-rac2	P15153	G protein	0.12	0.2	0.49
B13i	p21-rac1	P15154	G protein	0	0	0.33
A06j	CDK5	Q00535	Kinase	0.18	0	0.41
B05h	NDR protein kinase	Q15208	Kinase	0	0	0
B08c	Tissue-specific extinguisher 1	P10644	Kinase	0	0	0.19
A09l	CDKN1A	P38936	Kinase inhibitor	0.09	0.03	0.08
A10d	HGF-SF receptor	P08581	Kinase inhibitor	0	0	0.31
B02m	Hint protein	P49773	Kinase inhibitor	0	0	0.37
B07l	Calvasculin	P26447	Calcium-binding	0	0.11	0.46
B09n	CD27 ligand	P32970	Death receptor ligand	0.37	0	0
C02c	BAG-1	Q99933	BCL family protein	0	0	0.19
C09m	AH receptor	P35869	Nuclear receptor	0.06	0.12	0
F04i	Lipocalin 2	P80188	Trafficking	0	0	0
F09h	TRAM protein	Q15629	Trafficking	0	0	0.29
F10h	Dual-specificity A-kinase anchoring protein 1	Q92667	Targeting	0	0.19	0.24
D01d	Cadherin 3	P22223	Cell adhesion	0.32	0.14	0.08
D02e	Integrin beta 6 precursor	P18564	Cell adhesion	0.16	0.11	0.22
E02f	IGF-binding protein 3	P17936	Hormone	0	0	0
E02m	HLA-C	Q30182	Immune	0.19	0.17	0
E02n	GRP 78	P11021	Immune	0	0	0
F03b	Fibronectin precursor	P02751	Extracellular matrix	0.32	0.13	0.09
F13n	Insulin-induced protein 1	O15503	Unclassified	0.13	0.33	0.35
F08m	PM5 protein	Q15155	Unclassified	0.17	0.34	0

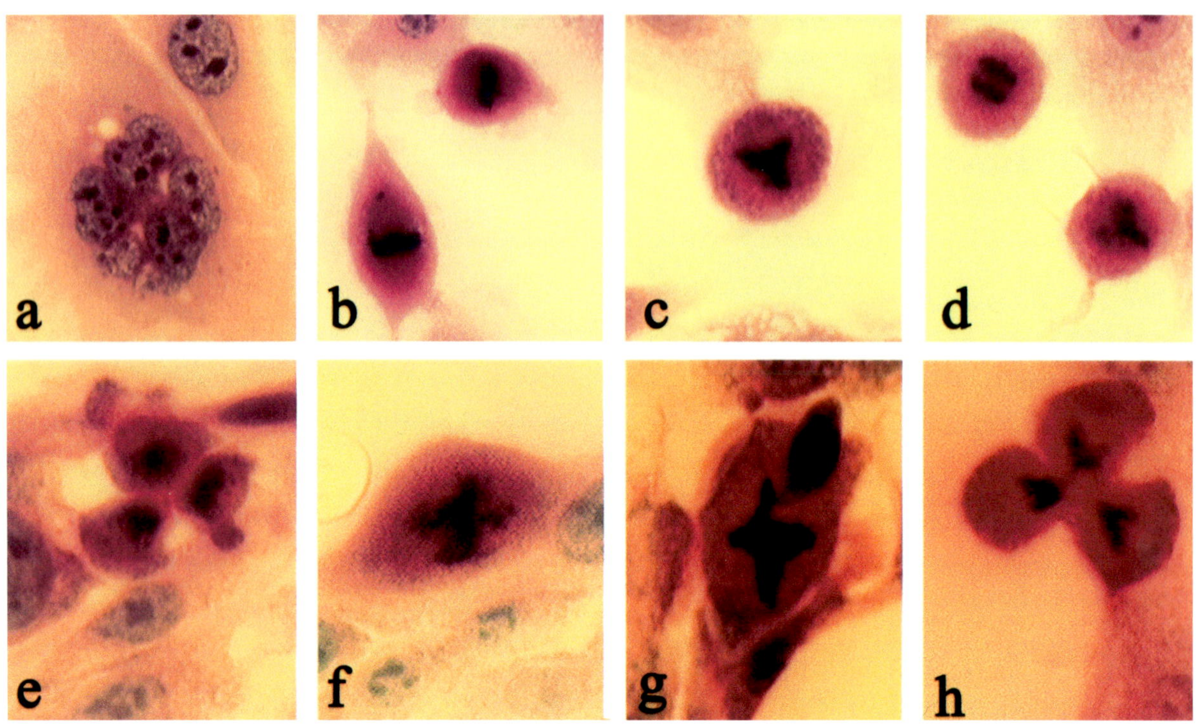

Figure 4.38 a–h

Cytospin preparation stained with H&E. **a** Multinucleated E$_2$-MCF-10F-transformed cells; **b** normal mitosis of MCF-10F cells; **c, d** abnormal mitosis of E$_2$-transformed cells; **e, f** 2-OH E$_2$-transformed cells; **g, h** 4-OH-E$_2$-transformed cells (×40)

4.5.5 Chromosomal Alterations Induced by Estrogen and Its Metabolites

Our laboratory has discovered than during the process of cell transformation induced by estrogen and its metabolites there is an increase in the number of multinucleated cells and abnormal mitoses (Figs. 4.38–4.40) that is associated with the overexpression of one component of the centromere–kinetochore complex CENP-F (Figs. 4.36, 4.37). It is important to emphasize that the percentage of these abnormal mitoses is less than 1% (Fig. 4.41). The movements that chromosomes undergo during mitosis are facilitated by the mitotic spindle, an apparatus composed principally of microtubule fibers that attach to a pair of kinetochores located on opposite sides of the centromere region of chromosomes. The microtubule-kinetochore interaction is essential for chromosome segregation. Disruptions of this interaction will lead to unequal distribution of chromosomes in daughter cells [201]. We have found that the CENP-F, a ca.

300 kDa protein that has been recently identified to be a novel member of the kinesin superfamily of microtubule-based motor proteins [201] is overexpressed in MCF-10F transformed cells by estrogens and metabolites but not in the BP transformed cells (Figs. 4.36, 4.37). CENP-F staining appeared only in mitotic cells, suggesting that it is a mitosis-specific motor. Its association with kinetochores suggests that it transports chromosomes along the spindle microtubules. This phenomenon, however, was not observed in the BP transformed cells, indicating that whereas aneuploidy is part of the neoplastic transformation process, it is depending on the nature of the

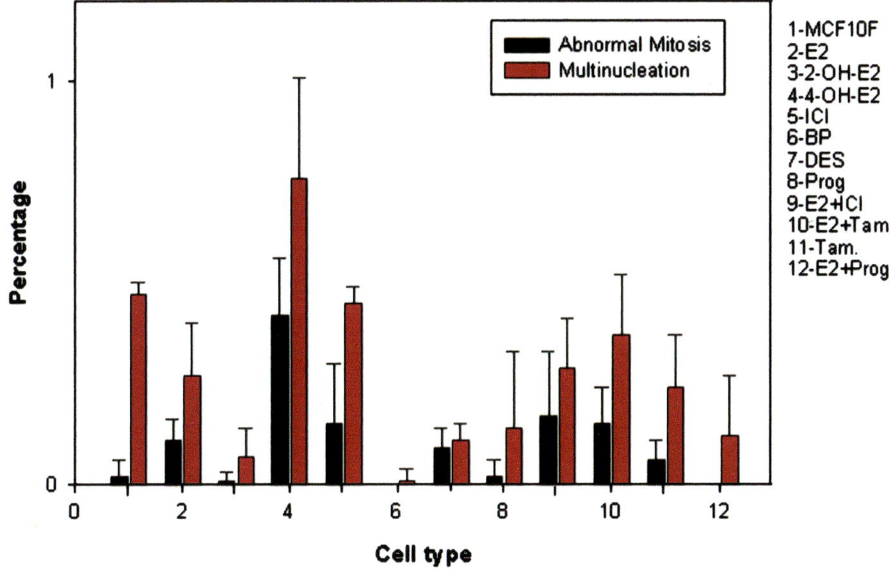

Figure 4.39

Histogram showing the percentage of abnormal mitoses and multinucleated cells

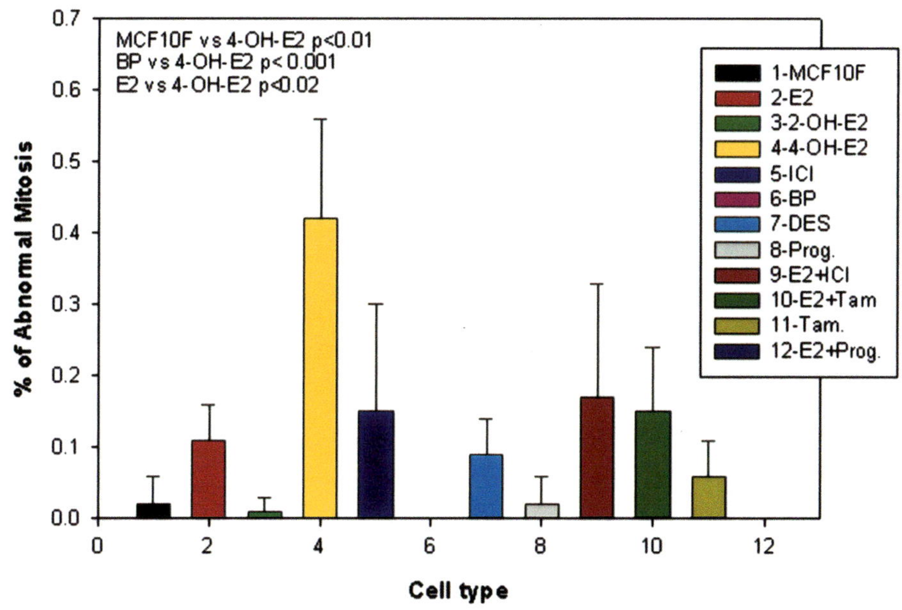

Figure 4.40

Histogram showing the percentage of abnormal mitosis

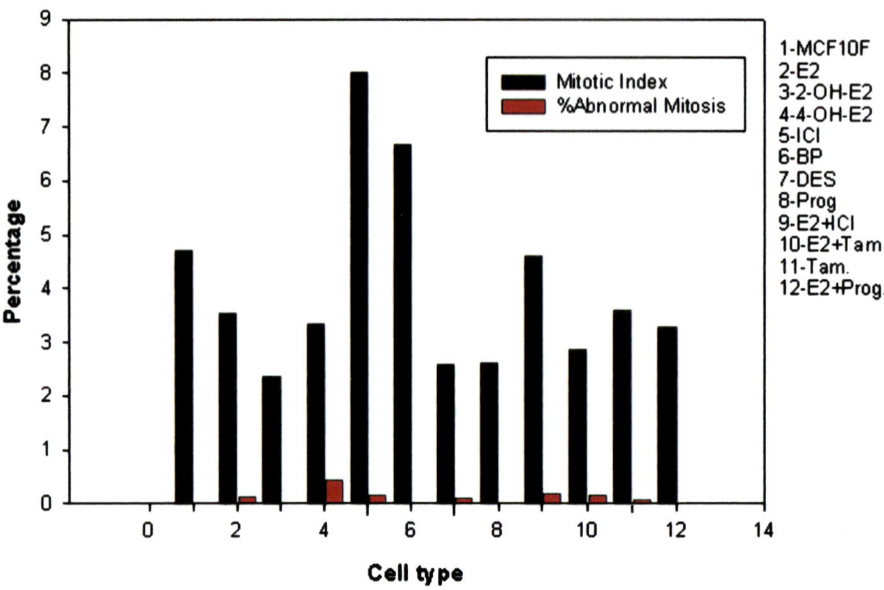

Figure 4.41

Histogram showing a comparative value of the percentage of mitosis of mitotic index, and the percentage of abnormal mitosis

carcinogenic insult and probably not the main driving force to cause genomic instability. This concept was further confirmed by the lack of significant karyotypic changes detected in these transformed cells (Fig. 4.42) and by the fact that the same clusters of genes were overexpressed in cells transformed with E_2, 4-OH-E_2 and BP (Table 4.2), indicating that there is a common pathway of transformation that may be responsible for driving the normal cell to neoplasia. The data also point toward the concept that certain compounds like steroid hormones or their metabolites may affect certain genes more readily than others, inducing the expression of genes that alter the mitotic spindle and therefore making the cell aneuploide. However, they do not support the concept that aneuploidy is the driving force of transformation but a consequence of it.

Figure 4.42 ▶

Karyotypic analysis of MCF-10F control cells, 17β-E_2, and 4-OH-E_2-transformed cells. Twenty cells were counted and analyzed per group. The model chromosome number was 46 and all the cells had a 46, xx, add (1) (:p36.3), t(3;9) (p13, p22)

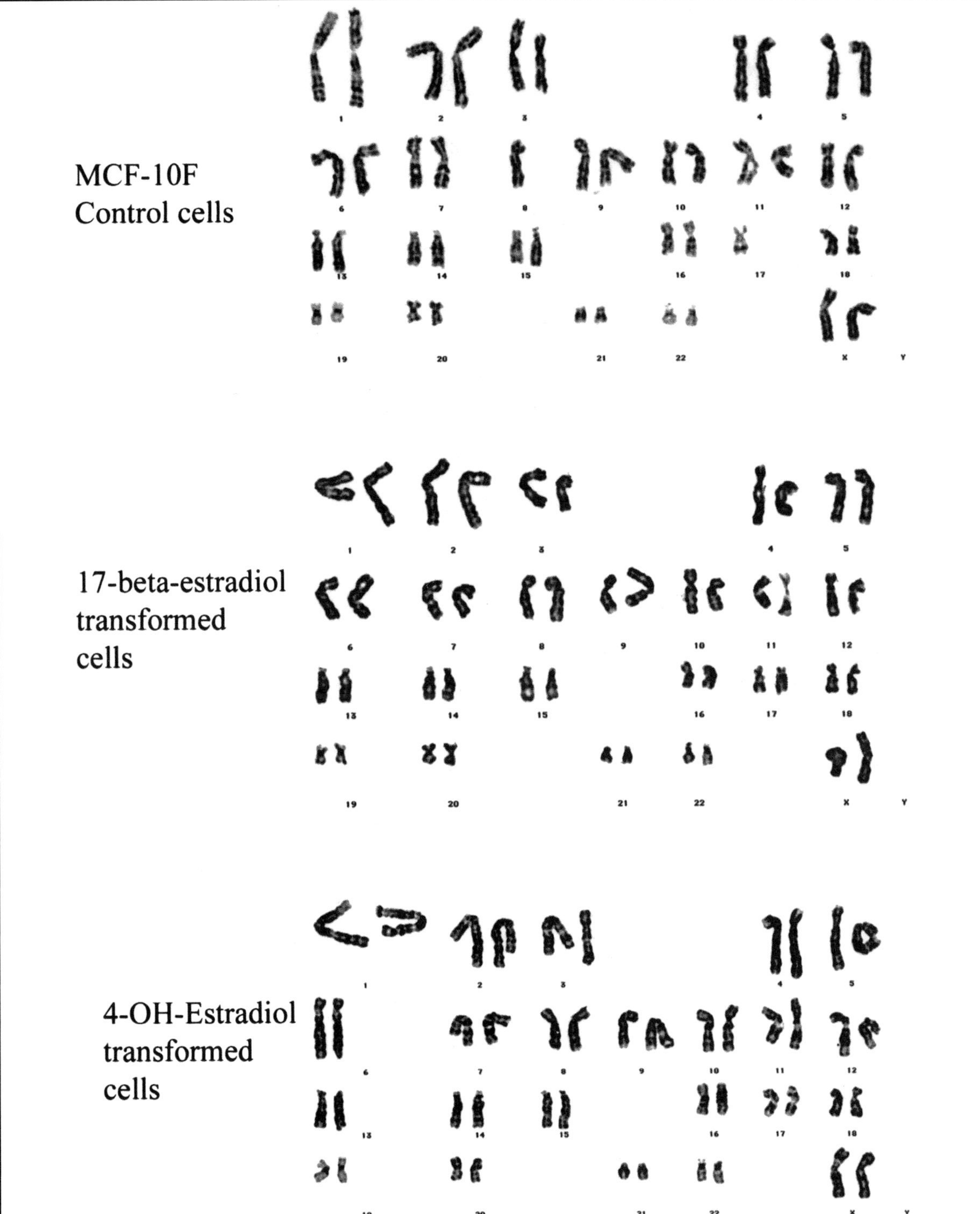

MCF-10F
Control cells
17-beta-estradiol
transformed
cells
4-OH-Estradiol
transformed
cells

4.6 A Unified Concept in the Role of Estrogen in Breast Cancer

Prolonged exposure to estrogen has long been identified as a risk factor for human breast cancer, but the role of estrogen in the development of human breast cancer has been difficult to ascertain. One of the difficulties is to relate breast cancer development to circulating levels of estrogens. The levels of free estrogens are significantly higher in the primary breast cancer tissues than those in the circulation, highlighting the importance of in situ metabolism of estrogens by estrone sulfatase and aromatase. There are three mechanisms that have been considered responsible for the carcinogenicity of estrogens: a receptor-mediated hormonal activity, cytochrome P450-mediated metabolic activation, and induction of aneuploidy. The receptor-mediated hormonal activity of estrogen has generally been related to stimulation of cellular proliferation, resulting in more opportunities for accumulation of genetic damages leading to carcinogenesis. Since local synthesis of estrogen in the stromal component can increase the estrogen levels and growth rate of breast carcinoma, a paracrine mechanism is likely to account for interactions between aromatase-containing stromal cells and ER-containing breast tumor epithelial cells. Further studies are warranted to investigate the regulatory mechanisms that are involved in the control of expression of aromatase, type I 17β-HSD and ER. In addition, expression of the ER occurs in cells other than the proliferating cells, suggesting that another paracrine mechanism is operative to mediate the biological response to estrogens. More importantly, estrogen may not need to activate nuclear receptors alpha to initiate or promote breast carcinogenesis. We have evidence that ERβ may be also involved in this process and that oxidative catabolism of estrogens mediated by various CYP complexes constitutes a pathway of their metabolic activation and generates reactive free radicals and intermediate metabolites reactive intermediates that can cause oxidative stress and genomic damage directly. Estrogen-induced genotoxic effects include increased mutation rates, MSI and LOH in chromosomes 3, and 11. Compromised DNA repair system that allows accumulation of genomic lesions essential to estrogen-induced tumorigenesis. Metabolic biotransformation of estrogen does occur in human mammary explant culture. Increased formation of catechol estrogens as a result of elevated hydroxylations of 17β-estradiol at C-4 and C-16α positions has been observed in human breast cancer patients and in women at a higher risk of developing this disease. There is also evidence that formation of superoxide and hydrogen peroxide as a result of the metabolism of estrogen might also be involved in estrogen-mediated oxidative stress. In fact, a substantial increase in base lesions observed in the DNA of invasive ductal carcinoma of the breast has been postulated to result from the oxidative stress associated with metabolism of 17β-estradiol. Altogether the data thus far accumulated indicate that more than one pathway may be necessary to initiate neoplastic transformation and maintaining of the transformation phenotypes leading to tumorigenesis.

References

1. Landis, S.H., Murray, T., Bolden, S., Wingo, P.A. CA Cancer J. Clin. 49:8, 1999.
2. Pike, M.C. Spicer, D.V., Dahmoush, L. Press, M.F. Estrogens, progesterone, normal breast cell proliferation and breast cancer risk, Epidemiol. Rev. 15:17–35, 1993.
3. Kelsey, J.L., Gammon, M.D., John, E.M. Reproductive factors and breast cancer, Epidemiol. Rev. 15:36–47, 1993.
4. Bernstein, L., Ross, R.K. Endogenous hormones and breast cancer risk, Epidemiol. Rev. 15:48–65, 1993.
5. Henderson, B.E., Ross, R., Bernstein, L. Estrogens as a cause of human cancer: the Richard, Estrogens as a cause of human cancer: the Richard & Hinda Rosenthal Foundation Award Lecture, Cancer Res. 48:246–253, 1988.
6. Topper, Y.J., Sankaran, L., Chomczynski, P., Prosser, P., Qasba, P. Three stages of responsiveness to hormones in the mammary cell, In: A. Angeli, H.L. Bradlow, L. Dogliotti (Eds.), Endocrinology of the Breast: Basic and Clinical Aspects, Ann. New York Acad. Sci. 464:1–10, 1986.
7. Lippman, M.E., Huff, K.K., Jakesz, R., Hecht, T., Kasid, A., Bates, S., Dickson, R.B. Estrogens regulate production of specific growth factors in hormone-dependent human breast cancer, In: A. Angeli, H.L., Bradlow, L. Dogliotti (Eds.), Endocrinology of the Breast: Basic and Clinical Aspects, Ann. New York Acad. Sci. 464:11–6, 1986.
8. Dupont, W.D., Page, D.L. Menopausal estrogen replacement therapy and breast cancer. Arch. Int. Med. 151:67–72, 1991.

9. Toniolo, P.G. Endogenous estrogens and breast cancer risk: the case for prospective cohort studies. Environ Health Perspect. 105 Suppl 3:587–92, 1997

10. Greenwald, P., Barolom, J., Nasca, P., Burnett, W. Vaginal cancer after maternal treatment with synthetic estrogens. N. Engl. J. Med. 12:285(7): 390–240, 1971.

11. Beral, V., Hannaford, P., Kay, C. Oral contraceptive use and malignancies of the genital tract. Results from the Royal College of General Practitioners' Oral Contraception Study. Lancet 2:1331–1335, 1988.

12. Hilakivi-Clarke, L. Estrogen-regulated non-reproductive behaviors and breast cancer risk: animal models and human studies. Breast Cancer Res. Treat. 46:143, 1997.

13. Davis, D.L., Telang, N.T., Osborne, M.P., Bradlow, H.I. Medical hypothesis: bifunctional genetic-hormonal pathways to breast cancer. Environ Health Perspect. 105 suppl 3:571–576, 1997.

14. Sonnenschein, C., Soto, A.M. An updated review of environmental estrogen and androgen mimics and antagonists. J. Steroid Biochem. Mol. Biol. 65:143–150, 1998.

15. Price, M.A., Tennant, C.C., Smith, R.C., Kennedy, S.J., Butow, P.N., Kossoff, M.B., Dunn, S.M. Predictors of breast cancer in women recall following screening, Aust. New Zealand J. Surg. 69:639–646, 1999.

16. Couse, J.F., Korach, K.S. Estrogen receptor null mice: what have we learned and where will they lead us? Endocr. Rev. 20:358–417, 1999.

17. Shiau, A.K., Barstad, D., Loria, P.M., Cheng, L., Kushner, P.J., Agard, D.A., Greene, G.L. The structural basis of estrogen receptor/ coactivator recognition and the antagonism of this interaction by tamoxifen. Cell 95:927–937, 1998.

18. McDonnell, D.P. The molecular pharmacology of SERMs. TEM 10:301–311, 1999.

19. Tsai, M.J., O'Malley, B.W. Molecular mechanisms of steroid/thyroid receptor superfamily members. Annu. Rev. Biochem. 63:451–486, 1994.

20. Katzenellenbogen, B.S. Dynamics of steroid hormone receptor action, Annu. Rev. Physiol. 42:17–35, 1980.

21. Mosselman, S., Polma, J., Dijkema, R. ER-: identification and characterization of a novel human estrogen receptor, FEBS Lett. 392:49–53, 1996.

22. Kuiper, G.G.J.M., Carlsson, B., Grandien, K., Enmark, E., et al., Comparison of the ligand binding specificity and transcript tissue distribution of estrogen receptors or and, Endocrinology 138:863–870, 1997.

23. Paech, K., Webb, P., Kuiper, G.G., Nilsson, S., Gustatsson, J., Kushner, P.J., Scanlan, T.S. Differential ligand activation of estrogen receptors ER-alpha and ER-beta at API sites, Science 277:150:8–1510, 1997.

24. Rao, B.R. Isolation and characterization of an estrogen binding protein which may integrate the plethora of estrogenic actions in non-reproductive organs J. Steroid Biochem. Mol. Biol. 65:3–41, 1998.

25. Bhat, R.A., Harnish, D.C., Stevis, P.E., Lyttle, C.R., Komm, B.S. A novel human estrogen receptor beta: identification and functional analysis of additional N-terminal amino acids. J. Steroid Biochem. Mol. Biol. 67:233–240, 1998.

26. Hu, Y-F., Russo, I.H., and Russo, J. Estrogen and Human Breast Cancer. In: Endocrine disruptors (M. Matzler Ed.) Springer Verlag, Heidelberg 2001 pp 1–26.

27. van Landeghem, A.A.J., Poortman, J., Nabuurs, M., Thijssen, J.H.H. Endogenous concentration and subcellular distribution of estrogens in normal and malignant human breast tissue. Cancer Res. 45:2900–2906, 1985.

28. Labrie, F. Intracrinology, Mol. Cell Endocrinol. 78:C113–118, 1991.

29. Labrie, F., Simard, J., Luu-The, V., Pelletier, G., Belghmi, K., Belanger, A. Structure, regulation and role of 3 beta-hydroxysteroid dehydrogenase, 17 beta-hydroxysteroid dehydrogenase and aromatase enzymes in the formation of sex steroids in classical and peripheral intracrine tissues. Baillie-re's Clin. Endocrinol. Metab. 8:451–474, 1994.

30. Pasqualini, J.R., Chetrite, G., Nguyen, B.L., Maloche, C., Talbi, M., Feinstein, M.C., Blacker, C., Botella, J., Paris, J. Estrone sulfate-sulfatase and 17 beta-hydroxysteroid dehydrogenase activities: a hypothesis for their role in the evolution of human breast cancer from hormone-dependence to hormone-independence. J. Steroid. Biochem. Mol. Biol. 53:407–412, 1995.

31. Reed, M.J., Purohit, A. Breast cancer and the role of cytokines in regulating estrogen synthesis: An emerging hypothesis. Endocrine Review 18, 701–715, 1997.

32. Simpson, E.R., Mahendroo, M.S., Means, G.D., Kilgore, M.W., Hinshelwood, M.M., Graham-Lorence, S., Amarneh, B., Ito, Y., Fisher, C.R., Michael, M.D. et al. Aromatase cytochrome P450, the enzyme responsible for estrogen biosynthesis. Endocrine Rev. 15:342–355, 1994.

33. Santen, R.J., Santner, S.J., Pauley, R.J., Tait, L., Kaseta, J., Demers, L.M., Hamilton, C., Yue, W., Wang, J.P. Estrogen production via the aromatase enzyme in breast carcinoma: which cell type is responsible? J. Steroid Biochem. Mol. Biol. 61:267–271, 1997.

34. Brodie, A., Lu, Q., Nakamura, J. Aromatase in the normal breast and breast cancer. J. Steroid Biochem. Mol. Biol. 61:281–286, 1997.

35. Koh, J.I., Kubota, T., Sasano, H., Hashimotom, M., Hosoda, Y., Kitajima, M. Stimulation of human tumor xenograft growth by local estrogen biosynthesis in stromal cells. AntiCancer Res. 18:2375–2380, 1998.

36. Mor, G., Yue, W., Santen, R.J., Gutierrez, L., Eliza, M., Berstein, L.M., Harada, N., Wang, J., Lysiak, J., Diano, S., Naftolin, F. J. Steroid Biochem. Mol. Biol. 67:403, 1998.

37. Miller, W.R, O'Neill, J. The importance of local synthesis of estrogen within the breast. Steroids 50:537–548, 1987.

38. Dowsett, M. Future uses for aromatase inhibitors in breast cancer. J. Steroid Biochem. Mol. Biol. 61:261–266, 1997.

39. Sasano, H., Ozaki, M. Aromatase expression and its localization in human breast cancer. J. Steroid Biochem. Mol. Biol. 61:293–298, 1997.

40. Orentreich, N., Brind, J.L., Rizer, R.L. Age changes and sex

differences in serum dehydroepiandrosterone sulfate concentrations throughout adulthood. J. Clin. Endocrinol. Metab. 59:551–555, 1984.

41. Falany, J.L., Falany, C.N. Regulation of estrogen activity by sulfation in human MCF-7 breast cancer cells. Oncol. Res. 9:589–596, 1997.

42. Utsumi, T., Yoshimura, N., Takeuchi, S., Ando, J., Maruta, M., Maeda, K., Harada, N. Steroid sulfatase expression is an independent predictor of recurrence in human breast cancer. Cancer Res. 59:377–381, 1999.

43. Martel, C., Rheaume, E., Takahashi, M., Trudel, C., Couet, J., Luu-The, V., Simard, J., Labrie, F. Distribution of 17 beta-hydroxysteroid dehydrogenase gene expression and activity in rat and human tissues. J. Steroid Biochem. Mol. Biol. 41:597–603, 1992.

44. Luu-The, V., Zhang, Y., Poirier, D., Labrie, F. Characteristics of human types 1, 2 and 3 17 beta-hydroxysteroid dehydrogenase activities: oxidation/reduction and inhibition. J. Steroid Biochem. Mol. Biol. 55:581–587, 1995.

45. Simard, J., Durocher, F., Mebarki, F., Turgeon, C., Sanchez, R., Labrie, Y., Couet, J., Trudel, C., Rheaume, E., Morel, Y., Luu-The, V., Labrie, F. Molecular biology and genetics of the 3 beta-hydroxysteroid dehydrogenase/delta5-delta4 isomerase gene family. J. Endocrinol. 50:189–207, 1996.

46. Sasano, H., Frost, A.R., Saitoh, R., Harada, N., Poutanen, M., Vihko, R., Bulun, S.E., Silverberg, S.G., Nagura, H. Aromatase and 17 beta-hydroxysteroid dehydrogenase type 1 in human breast carcinoma. J. Clin. Endocr. Metab. 81:4042–4046, 1996.

47. Miller, W.R., Anderson, T.J., Lack, W.J.L. Relationship between tumour aromatase activity, tumour characteristics and response to therapy. J. Steroid Biochem. Mol. Biol. 37:1055–1059, 1990.

48. Esteban, J.M., Warsi, Z., Haniu, M., Hall, P., Shively, J.E., Chen, S. Detection of intratumoral aromatase in breast carcinomas. An immunohistochemical study with clinicopathologic correlation Am. J. Pathol. 940:337–343, 1992.

49. Russo, J., Russo, I.H. Role of hormones in human breast development: The menopausal breast. In: Wren BG (ed) Progress in the management of menopause. Parthenon Publishing 1997 New York. P 184

50. Russo, I.H., Russo, J. Role of hormones in cancer initiation and progression. J. Mammary Gland Biol. Neoplasia 3:49–61, 1998.

51. Russo, J., Russo, I.H. Role of differentiation in the pathogenesis and prevention of breast cancer. Endocr. Related Cancer 4:7, 1997.

52. Calaf, G., Alvarado, M.E., Bonney, G.E., Amfoh, K.K., Russo, J. Influence of lobular development on breast epithelial cell proliferation and steroid hormone receptor content. Int. J. Oncol. 7:1285, 1997.

53. Russo, J., Russo, I.H. Influence of differentiation and cell kinetics on the susceptibility of the rat mammary gland to carcinogenesis. Cancer Res. 40:2677, 1980.

54. Russo, J., Russo, I.H. Biological and molecular bases of mammary carcinogenesis. Lab Invest. 57:112, 1987.

55. Russo, J., Rivera, R., Russo, I.H. Influence of age and parity on the development of the human breast. Breast Cancer Res. Treat. 23:211–218, 1992.

56. Russo, J., Grill, C., Ao, X., Russo, I.H. Pattern of distribution for estrogen receptor α and progesterone receptor in relation to proliferating cells in the mammary gland. Breast Cancer Res. Treat. 53:217–227, 1999.

57. Clark, R.B.k, Howell, A. Potten, C.S., Anderson E., Dissociation between steroid receptor expression and cell proliferation in the human breast. Cancer Res. 57:4987–4991, 1997.

58. Foster, J.S., Wimalasena, J. Evidence that transforming growth factor-beta is a hormonally regulated negative growth factor in human breast cancer cells. Mol. Endocrinol. 10:488–98, 1996.

59. Wang, W., Smith, R., Burghardt, R., Safe, S.H. 17 beta-Estradiol-mediated growth inhibition of MDA-MB-468 cells stably transfected with the estrogen receptor: cell cycle effects. Mol. Cell Endocrinol. 133:49–62, 1997.

60. Zajchowski, D.A., Sager, R., Webster, L. Estrogen inhibits the growth of estrogen receptor-negative, but not estrogen receptor-positive, human mammary epithelial cells expressing a recombinant estrogen receptor. Cancer Res. 53:5004–5011, 1993.

61. Calaf, G., Tahin, Q., Alvarado, M.E., Estrada, S., Cox, T. and Russo, J. Hormone receptors and cathepsin D levels in human breast epithelial cells transformed by chemical carcinogens. Breast Cancer Res. and Treat. 29:169–177, 1993.

62. Santen, R. J. Symposium overview. J. Natl. Cancer Institute Monograph 27, 2000, pp 15–16.

63. Adlercreutz, H., Gorbach, S.L., Goldin, B.R., Woods, M.N., Hamalainen, E. Estrogen metabolism and excretion in Oriental and Caucasian women. J. Natl. Cancer Inst. 86:1076–1082, 1994.

64. Roy, D., Liehr, J.G. Temporary decrease in renal quinone and reductase activity induced by chronic administration of estradiol to male Syrian hamsters- increased superoxide formation by redox cycling of estrogen. J. Biol. Chem. 263:3646–3651, 1988.

65. Meads, T., Schroer, T. A. Polarity and nucleation of microtubules in polarized epithelial cells. Cell Motil. Cytoskeleton, 32:273–288, 1995.

66. Whitehead, C. M., Salisbury, J. L. Regulation and regulatory activities of centrosomes. J. Cell. Biochem. Suppl., 32–33: 192–199, 1999.

67. Sluder, G., Hinchcliffe, E H. Control of centrosome reproduction: the right number at the right time. Biol. Cell, 91:413–427, 1999.

68. Pihan, G.A., Doxsey, S.J. The mitotic machinery as a source of genetic instability in cancer. Semin. Cancer Biol. 9:289–302, 1999.

69. Brinkley, B.R., Goepfert, T.M. Supernumerary centrosomes and cancer: Boveri's hypothesis resurrected. Cell Motil. Cytoskeleton, 41:281–288, 1998.

70. Lingle, W.L., Lutz, W.H., Ingle, J.N., Maihle, N.J., Salisbury, J.L. Centrosome hypertrophy in human breast tumors: im-

plications for genomic stability and cell polarity. Proc. Natl. Acad. Sci. USA, 95:2950–2955, 1998.

71. Mendelin, J., Grayson, M., Wallis, T., Visscher, D. W. Analysis of chromosome aneuploidy in breast cancer progression using fluorescence in situ hybridization. Lab. Invest. 79:387–393, 1999.

72. Lengauer, C., Kinzler, K.W., Vogelstein, B. Genetic instabilities in human cancers. Nature (London) 396:643–648, 1998.

73. Chakravarti, D., Mailander P., Cavalieri, E.L., and Rogan, E.G. Evidence that error-prone DNA repair converts dibenzo[a,l]pyrene-induced depurinating lesions into mutations: Formation, clonal proliferation and regression of initiated cells carrying H-ras oncogene mutations in early preneoplasia. Mutation Res. 456:17–32, 2000.

74. Khan, S.A., Rogers, M.A., Khurana, K.K., Meguid, M.M., Numann, P.J. Estrogen receptor expression in benign breast epithelium and breast cancer risk. J. Natl. Cancer Inst. 89:3742, 1997.

75. Russo, J., Reina, D., Frederick, J., Russo, I.H. Expression of phenotypical changes by human breast epithelial cells treated with carcinogens in vitro. Cancer Research, 48:2837–2857. 1988.

76. Russo, J., Calaf, G., and Russo, I.H. A critical approach to the malignant transformation of human breast epithelial cells. CRC Critical Reviews in Oncogenesis 4:403–417, 1993.

77. Russo, J., Gusterson, B.A., Rogers, A.E., Russo, I.H., Wellings, S.R. and Van Zwieten, M.J. Comparative Study of Human and Rat Mammary Tumorigenesis. Lab. Invest. 62:1–32, 1990.

78. Harlan, L.C., Coates, R.J., Block, G. Estrogen receptor status and dietary intakes in breast cancer patients. Epidemiology 4:25–31, 1993.

79. Habel, L.A., Stanford, J.L. Hormone receptors and breast cancer. Epidemiol. Rev. 15:209–219, 1993.

80. Moolgavkar, S.H., Day, N.E., Stevens, R.G. Two-stage model for carcinogenesis: Epidemiology of breast cancer in females. J. Natl. Cancer Inst. 65:559–569, 1980.

81. Hu, Y.F., Lau, K.M., Ho, S.M. and Russo, J. Increased expression of estrogen receptor beta in chemically transformed human breast epithelial cells. Int. J. Oncol. 12:1225–1228, 1998.

82. Lau, K.M., Leav, I., Ho, S.M. Rat estrogen receptor α and β, and progesterone receptor mRNA expression in various prostatic lobes and microdissected normal and dysplastic epithelial tissues of the Noble rats. Endocrinology 139:424–427, 1998.

83. Brandenberger, A.W., Tee, M.K., Jaffe, R.B. Estrogen receptor alpha (ER-alpha) and beta (ER-beta) mRNAs in normal ovary, ovarian serous cystadenocarcinoma and ovarian cancer cell lines: down-regulation of ER-beta in neoplastic tissues. J. Clin. Endocrinol. Metab. 83:1025–1028, 1998.

84. Aronica, S.M., Kraus, W.L., Katzenellenbogen, B.S. Estrogen action via the cAMP signaling pathway: stimulation of adenylate cyclase and cAMP-regulated gene transcription. Proc. Natl. Acad. Sci. USA 91:8517–8521, 1994.

85. Rosen, J.M., Humphreys, R., Krnacik, S., Juo, P., Raught, B. The regulation of mammary gland development by hormones, growth factors, and oncogenes. Prog. Clin. Biol. Res. 387:95–110, 1994.

86. Murphy, L.C., Dotzlaw, H., Leygue, E., Coutts, A., Watson, P. The regulation of mammary gland development by hormones, growth factors, and oncogenes. J. Steroid Biochem. Mol. Biol. 65:175–180, 1998.

87. Ball, P., Knuppen, R. Catecholestrogens (2- and 4-hydroxyoestrogens). Chemistry, biosynthesis, metabolism, occurrence and physiological significance. Acta Endocrinol. (Copenh.) 232(suppl): 1:127, 1980.

88. Zhu, B.T., Bui, Q.D., Weisz, J., Liehr, J.G. Conversion of estrone to 2- and 4- hydroxyestrone by hamster kidney and liver microsomes: Implications for the mechanism of estrogen-induced carcinogenesis. Endocrinology 135:1772–1779, 1994.

89. Ashburn, S.P., Han, X., Liehr, J.G. Microsomal hydroxylation of 2- and 4-fluoroestradiol to catechol metabolites and their conversion to methyl ethers: Catechol estrogens as possible mediators of hormonal carcinogenesis. Mol. Pharmacol. 43:534–541, 1993.

90. Knuppen, R., Ball, P., Emons, G. Importance of A-ring substitution of estrogens for the physiology and pharmacology of reproduction. J. Steroid Biochem. 24:193–198, 1986.

91. Osborne, M.P., Bradlow, H.L, Wong, G.Y.C., Telang, N.T. Upregulation of estradiol C16 alpha-hydroxylation in human breast tissue: a potential biomarker of breast cancer risk. J. Natl. Cancer Inst. 85:1917–1920, 1993.

92. Sipe, H.J. Jr., Jordan, S.J., Hanna, P.M., Mason, R.P. The metabolism of 17 beta-estradiol by lactoperoxidase: a possible source of oxidative stress in breast cancer. Carcinogenesis 15:2637–2643, 1994.

93. Malins, D.C., Holmes, E.H., Polissar, N.L., Gunselman, S.J. The etiology of breast cancer. Characteristic alteration in hydroxyl radical-induced DNA base lesions during oncogenesis with potential for evaluating incidence risk. Cancer 71, 3036–3043, 1993.

94. Cavalieri, E.L., Stack, D.E., Devanesan, P.D., Todorovic, R., Dwivedy, I., Higginbotham, S., Johansson, S.L., Patil, K.D., Gross, M.L., Gooden, J.K., Ramanathan, R., Cerny, R.L., and Rogan, E.G. Molecular origin of cancer: Catechol estrogen-3,4-quinones as endogenous tumor initiators. Proc. Natl. Acad. Sci. USA 99:10937–10942, 1997.

95. Li, J.J. and Li, S.A. Estrogen carcinogenesis in Syrian hamster tissue: role of metabolism. Fed. Proc. 46:1858–1863, 1987.

96. Furth, J. Hormones as etiological agents in neoplasia. In: Becker FF (ed) Cancer. A Comprehensive Treatise. 1. Etiology: Chemical and Physical Carcinogenesis. Plenum Press, New York, Chapt. 4, 1982, pp 89–134.

97. Li, J.J. and Li, S.A. Estrogen carcinogenesis in hamster tissues: A critical review. Endocr. Rev.11, 524–531,1990.

98. Li, J.J. Estrogen carcinogenesis in hamster tissues: Update. Endocr. Rev. 1:94–95, 1993.

99. Liehr, J.G. Is estradiol a genotoxic mutagenic carcinogen? Endocr. Rev. 21: 40–54, 2000.

100. Cavalieri, E., Frenkel, K., Liehr, J.G., Rogan, E., Roy, D. Estrogens as endogenous genotoxic agents-DNA adducts and mutations. J. Natl. Cancer Inst. Monograph 27:75-93, 2000.

101. Liehr, J.G. Genotoxicity of estrogens: A role in cancer development? Human reproduction Update 7:1–9, 2001.

102. Rajah, T.T. and Pento, J.T. The mutagenic potential of anti-estrogens at the HPRT locus in V79 cells. Res. Comm. Molecul. Pathol. & Pharmacol. 89:85–92, 1995.

103. Kong, L-Y., Szaniszlo, P., Albrecht, T. and Liehr, J.G. Frequency and molecular analysis of HPRT mutations induced by estradiol in Chinese hamster V79 cells. Intl. J. Oncol. 17, 1141–1149, 2000.

104. Tsutsui, T., Tamura, Y., Yagi, E. Involvement of genotoxic effects in the initiation of estrogen-induced cellular transformation: studies using Syrian hamster embryo cells treated with 17β-estradiol and eight of its metabolites. Int. J. Cancer 86:8–14, 2000.

105. Russo, J., Hu, Y.F., Tahin, Q., Mihaila, D., Slater, C., Lareef, M.H. and Russo, I.H. Carcinogenicity of Estrogens in Human breast epithelial cells. Acta Pathologica, Microbiologica Immunologica Scandinavica (APMIS) 109:39–52, 2001.

106. Thibodeau, P.A., Bissonnette, N., Bedard, S.K., et al. Induction by estrogens of methotrexate resistance in MCF-7 breast cancer cells. Carcinogenesis 19:1545–1552, 1998.

107. Hodgson, A.V., Ayala-Torres, S. and Thompson, E.B. and Liehr, J.G. Estrogen-induced microsatellite DNA alterations are associated with Syrian hamster kidney tumorigenesis. Carcinogenesis, 19:2169–2172, 1888.

108. Loeb, L.A. A Mutator Phenotype in Cancer. Perspec. In Can. Res. 61:3230–3239, 2001.

109. Boyd, J., Takahashi, H., Waggoner, S.E., Jones, L.A., Hajek, R.A., Wharton, J.T., Liu, F.S., Fujino, T., McLachlan, J.A. Molecular genetics analysis of clear cell adenocarcinomas of the vagina associated and unassociated with diethylstilbestrol exposure in utero. Cancer 77:507–513, 1996.

110. Richard, S.M., Bailliet, G., Paez, G.L., Bianchi, M.S., Peltomaki, P., Bianchi, N.O. Nuclear and mitochondrial genome instability in human breast cancer. Cancer. Res. 60:4231–4237, 2000.

111. Forgacs, E., Wren, J.D., Kamibayashi, C., Kondo, M., Xu, X.L., Markowitz, S., Tomlinson, G.E., Muller, C.Y., Gazdar, A.F., Garner, H.R., Minna, J.D. Searching for microsatellite mutations in coding regions in lung, breast, ovarian and colorectal cancers. Oncogene 20, 1005–1009, 2001.

112. Piao, Z., Lee, K.S., Kim, H., Perucho, M., Malkhosyan, S. Identification of novel deletion regions of chromosome arms 2q and 6p in breast carcinomas by amplotype analysis. Genes, Chromosomes & Cancer 30:113–122, 2001.

113. Caldes, T., Perez-Segura, P., Tosar, A., de La Hoya, M., Diaz-Rubio, E. Microsatellite instability correlates with negative expression of estrogen and progesterone receptors in sporadic breast cancer. Teratogenesis, Carcinogenesis, & Mutagenesis. 20: 283–291, 2000.

114. Miyazaki, M., Tamaki, Y., Sakita, I., Fujiwara, Y., Kodta, M., Masuda, N., Ooka, M., et al. Detection of microsatellite alterations in nipple discharge accompanied by breast cancer. Breast Cancer Research & Treatment 60:35–41, 2000.

115. Ando, Y., Iwase, H., Ichihara, S., Toyoshima, S., Nakamura, T., Yamashita, H., et al. Loss of heterozygosity and microsatellite instability in ductal carcinoma in situ of the breast. Cancer Letters. 156:207–214, 2000.

116. Tokunaga, E., Oki, E., Oda, S., Kataoka, A., Kitamura, K., Ohno, S., Maehara, Y., Sugimachi, K. Frequency of microsatellite instability in breast cancer determined by high-resolution fluorescent microsatellite analysis. Oncology 59:44–49, 2000.

117. Shaw, J.A., Smith, B.M., Walsh, T., Johnson, S., Promrose, L., Slade, M.J., Walker, R.A., Coombes, R.C. Microsatellite alterations plasma DNA of primary breast cancer patients. Clinical Cancer Research. 6:1119–1124, 2000.

118. Cavalieri, E.L., and Rogan, E.G. The approach to understanding aromatic hydrocarbon carcinogenesis. The central role of radical cations in metabolic activation. Pharmacol. Ther. 55:183–99, 1992.

119. Cavalieri, E.L., and Rogan, E.G. Mechanisms of tumor initiation by polycyclic aromatic hydrocarbons in mammals. In: The Handbook of Environmental Chemistry: PAHs and Related Compounds (Neilson, A.H., Ed.) 1998, Vol. 3 J, pp 81–117, Springer, Heidelberg, Germany.

120. Chakravarti, D., Pelling, J.C., Cavalieri, E.L. and Rogan, E.G. Relating aromatic hydrocarbon-induced DNA adducts and c-Harvey-ras mutations in mouse skin papillomas: The role of apurinic sites. Proc. Natl. Acad. Sci. USA 92:10422–10426, 1995.

121. Liehr, J.G., Fang, W.F., Sirbasku, D.A. and Ari-Ulubelen, A. Carcinogenicity of catecholestrogens in Syrian hamsters. J. Steroid Biochem. 24:353–356, 1986.

122. Li, K.M., Devanesan, P.D., Rogan, E.G., and Cavalieri, E.L. Formation of the depurinating 4-hydroxyestradiol (4-OHE$_2$)-1-N7Gua and 4-OHE$_2$-1-N3Ade adducts by reaction of E$_2$-3,4-quinone with DNA. Proc. Am. Assoc. Cancer Res. 39:636, 1998.

123. Chakravarti, D., Mailander, P., Franzen, J., Higginbotham, S., Cavalieri, E. and Rogan, E. Detection of dibenzo[a,l]pyrene-induced H-ras codon 61 mutant genes in preneoplastic SENCAR mouse skin using a new PCR-RFLP method. Oncogene, 16:3203–3210, 1998.

124. Miller, W.R. and O'Neill, J. The importance of local synthesis of estrogen within the breast. Steroids 50:537–548, 1987.

125. Simpson, E.R., Mahendroo, M.S., Means, G.D., Kilgore, M.W., Hinshelwood, M.M., Graham-Lorence, S., et al. Aromatase cytochrome P450, the enzyme responsible for estrogen biosynthesis. Endocrine Rev. 15:342–355, 1994.

126. Yue, W., Wang, J.P., Hamilton, C.J., Demers, L.M., and Santen, R.J. In situ aromatization enhances breast tumor estra-

diol levels and cellular proliferation. Cancer Research 58:927–932, 1998.

127. Yue, W., Santen, R.J., Wang, J.P., Hamilton, C.J., and Demers, L.M.. Aromatase within the breast. Endocrine-Related Cancer 6:157–164, 1999.

128. Jefcoate, C.R., Liehr, J.G., Santen, R.J., Sutter, T.R., Yager, J.D., Yue, W., Santner, S.J., Tekmal, R., Demers, L., Pauley, R., Naftolin, F., Mor, G., and Berstein, L. Tissue-specific synthesis and oxidative metabolism of estrogens. In: JNCI Monograph 27: Estrogens as Endogenous Carcinogens in the Breast and Prostate (E. Cavalieri and E. Rogan, Eds.), Oxford Press, 2000, 95–112.

129. Reed, M.J., and Purohit, A. Breast cancer and the role of cytokines in regulating estrogen synthesis: An emerging hypothesis. Endocrine Review 18:701–715, 1997.

130. Spink, D.C., Hayes, C.L., Young, N.R., Christou, M., Sutter, T.R., Jefcoate, C.R., et al. The effects of 2,3,7,8-tetrachlorodibenzo-p-dioxin on estrogen metabolism in MCF-7 breast cancer cells: Evidence for induction of a novel 17ß-estradiol 4-hydroxylase. J. Steroid Biochem. Mol. Biol. 51:251–258, 1994.

131. Hayes, C.L., Spink, D.C., Spink, B.C., Cao, J.Q., Walker, N.J., and Sutter, T.R. 17ß-Estradiol hydroxylation catalyzed by human cytochrome P450 1B1. Proc. Natl. Acad. Sci. USA 93:9776–9781, 1996.

132. Spink, D.C., Spink, B.C., Cao, J.Q., DePasquale, J.A., Pentecost, B.T., Fasco, M.J., et al. Differential expression of CYP1A1 and CYP1B1 in human breast epithelial cells and breast tumor cells. Carcinogenesis 19:291–298, 1998.

133. Badawi, A.F., Devanesan, P.D., Edney, J.A., West, W.W., Higginbotham, S., Rogan, E.G., and Cavalieri, E.L. Estrogen metabolites and conjugates: Biomarkers of susceptibility to human breast cancer. Proc. Amer. Assoc. Cancer Res. 42, 664, 2001.

134. Visscher, D. W., Micale, M. A., Crissman, J. D. Pathological and biological relevance of cytophotometric DNA content to breast carcinoma genetic progression. J. Cell. Biochem. Suppl. 17:114–122, 1993

135. Berado, M. D., O'Connell, P., Allred, D. C. Biological characteristics of premalignant and preinvasive breast disease. Pasqualine, J. R. Katzenellenbogen, B.S. eds. Hormone-Dependent Cancer 1996, 1–23 Marcel Dekker, Inc. New York.

136. Oshimura, M., Barrett, J. C. Chemically-induced aneuploidy in mammalian cells: mechanisms and biological significance in cancer. Environ. Mutagen. 8:129–159, 1986.

137. Aardema, M. J., Crosby, L. L., Gibson, D. P., Kerckaert, G. A., LeBoeuf, R. A. Aneuploidy and consistent structural chromosome changes associated with transformation of Syrian hamster embryo cells. Cancer Genet. Cytogenet. 96:140–150, 1997.

138. Aldaz, C. M., Chen, T., Sohin, A., Cunningham, J., Bondy, M. Comparative allelotypes of in situ and invasive human breast cancer: high frequency of micro-satellite instability in lobular breast carcinomas. Cancer Res. 55:3976–3981, 1995.

139. Pihan, G. A., Doxsey, S. J. The mitotic machinery as a source of genetic instability in cancer. Semin. Cancer Biol. 9:289–302, 1999.

140. Mitelman, F., Levan, G. Clustering of aberrations on specific chromosomes in human neoplasms. A survey of 1871 cases. Hereditas 95:79–139, 1981.

141. Goepfert, T.M., McCarthy, M., Kittrell, F.S., Stephens, C., Ullrich, R.L., Brinkley B.R., and Medina, D. Progesterone facilitates chromosome instability (aneuploidy) in p53 null normal mammary epithelial cells. The FASEB Journal 14:221–2229, 2000.

142. Greendale, G. A., Reboussin, B. A., Sie, A., Singh, R., Olsen, L. K., Gateswood, O., Bassett, L. W., Wasilauskas, C., Bush, T., Barrett-Connor, E. Effects of estrogen and estrogen-progestin on mammographic parenchymal density. Ann Int. Med. 130:262–269, 1999.

143. Schairer, C., Lubin, J., Troisi, R., Sturgeon, S., Brinton, L., Hoover, R. Menopausal estrogen and estrogen-progestin replacement therapy and breast cancer risk. J. Am. Med. Assoc. 283:485–491, 2000.

144. Ross, R. K., Paganini-Hill, A., Wan, P. C., Pike, M. C. Effect of hormone replacement therapy on breast cancer risk: estrogen versus estrogen plus progestin. J. Natl. Cancer Inst. 92:328–332, 2000.

145. Fukasawa, K., Choi, T., Kuriyama, R., Rulong, S., Vande Woude, G. F. Abnormal centrosome amplification in the absence of p53. Science 271:1744–1747, 1996

146. Pihan, G. A., Purohit, A., Wallace, J., Knecht, H., Woda, B., Quesenberry, P., Doxsey, S.J. Centrosome defects and genetic instability in malignant tumors. Cancer Res. 58:3974–3985, 1998.

147. Zhou, H., Kuang, J., Zhong, L., Juo, W.-L., Gray, J. W., Sahin, A., Brinkley, B. R., Sen, S. Tumour amplified kinase STK15/BRAK induces centrosome amplification, aneuploidy and transformation. Nature (London) Genetics 20:189–193, 1998.

148. Lingle, W. L., Salisbury, J. L. Altered centrosome structure is associated with abnormal mitoses in human breast tumors. Am. J. Pathol. 155:1941–1951, 1999.

149. Trent, J.M., Wiltshire, R., Su, L., Nicolaides, N.C., Vogelstein, B., Kinzler, K.W. The gene for the APC-binding protein beta-catenin (CTNNB1) maps to chromosome 3p22, a region frequently altered in human malignancies. Cytogenet. Cell Genet. 71:343–344, 1995.

150. Dietrich, C.U., Pandis, N., Teixeira, M.R, Bardi, G., Gerdes, A.M., Andersen, J.A., Heim, S. Chromosome abnormalities in benign hyper-proliferative disorders of epithelial and stromal breast tissue. Int. J. Cancer 60:49–53, 1995.

151. Pennisi, E. New gene forges link between fragile site and many cancers. Science 272:649, 1996.

152. Cuthbert, A.P., Bond, J., Trott. D.A., Gill, S., Broni, J., Marriott, A., Khoudoli, G., Parkinson, E.K., Cooper, C.S., Newbold, R.F. Telomerase repressor sequences on chromosome 3 and induction of permanent growth arrest in human breast cancer cells. J. Natl. Cancer Inst. 91:37–45, 1999.

153. Negrini, M., Sabbioni, S., Haldar, S., Possati, L., Castagnoli, A., Corallini, A., Barbanti-Brodano, G., Croce, C.M. Tumor and growth suppression of breast cancer cells by chromosome 17-associated functions. Cancer Res. 54:1818–1824, 1994.

154. Borresen, A.L., Andersen, T.I., Garber, J., Barbier-Piraux, N., Thorlacius, S., Eyfjord, J, Ottestad L, Smith-Sorensen B, Hovig E, Malkin D. Screening for germ line TP53 mutations in breast cancer patients. Cancer Res. 52:3234–3236, 1992.

155. Puech, A., Henry, I., Jeanpierre, C., Junien, C. A highly polymorphic probe on 11p15.5: L22.5.2 (D11S774). Nucleic Acids Research 19:5095–5099, 1991.

156. Hannigan, G.E., Bayani, J., Weksberg, R., Beatty, B., Pandita, A., Dedhar, S., Squire, J. Mapping of the gene encoding the integrin-linked kinase, ILK, to human chromosome 11pl5.5-pl5.4. Genomics 42:177–179, 1997.

157. Wang, H., Shao, N., Ding, Q.M., Cui, J., Reddy, E.S., Rao, V.N. BRCA1 proteins arc transported to the nucleus in the absence of serum and splice variants BRCA1a, BRCA1b are tyrosine phosphoproteins that associate with E2F, cyclins and cyclin dependent kinases. Oncogene 15:143–157, 1997.

158. Dong, J-T., Lamb, P.W, Rinker-Schaeffer, C.W., Vukanovic, J., Ichikawa, T., Isaacs, J.T., Barrett, J. KA/1, a metastasis suppressor gene for prostate cancer on human chromosome 11p11.2. Science 268:884–886, 1995.

159. Wei, Y., Lukashev, M., Simon, D., et al. Regulation of integrin function by the urokinase receptor. Science 273:1551–1555, 1996.

160. Hampton, G.M., Mannermaa, A., Winquist, R., Alavaikko, M., Blanco, G., Taskinen, P.G., Kiviniemi, H., Newsham, I., Cavenee, W.K., Evans, G.A. Losses of heterozygosity in sporadic human breast carcinoma: A common region between 11q22 and 11q23.3. Cancer Res. 54:4586–4589, 1994.

161. Negrini, M., Rasio, D., Hampton, G.M., Sabbioni, S., Rattan, S., Carter, S.M., Rosenberg, A.L., Schwartz, G.F., Shiloh, Y., Cavenee, W.K., Croce, C.M. Definition and refinement of chromosome 11 regions of loss of heterozygosity in breast cancer: Identification of a new region at 11 q23.3. Cancer Res. 55:3003–3007, 1995.

162. Winqvist, R., Hampton, G.M., Mannermaa, A., Blanco, G., Alavaiko, M., Kiviniemi, H., Taskinen, P.J., Evans, G.A., Wright, F.A., Newsham, I., Cavenee, W.K. Loss of heterozygosity for chromosome 11 in primary human breast tumors is associated with poor survival after metastasis. Cancer Res. 55:2660–2664, 1995.

163. Elson, A., Wang, Y., Daugherty, C.J., Morton, C.C., Zhou, F., Campos-Torres, J., Leder, P. Pleiotropic defects in ataxia-telangiectasia protein-deficient mice. Proc. Natl. Acad. Sci. USA 93:13084–13089, 1996.

164. Westphal, C.H., Schmaltz, C., Rowan, S., Elson, A., Fisher, D.E., Leder, P. Genetic interactions between atm and p53 influence cellular proliferation and irradiation-induced cell cycle checkpoints. Cancer Res. 57:1664–1667, 1997.

165. Soule, H.D., Maloney, T.M., Wolman, S.R., Peterson, Jr. W.D., Brenz, R., McGrath, C.M., Russo, J., Pauley, R., Jones, R.F., Brooks, S.C. Isolation and characterization of a spontaneously immortalized human breast epithelial cell line, MCF-10. Cancer Res. 50:6075–6086, 1990.

166. Tait, L., Soule, H., and Russo, J. Ultrastructural and immunocytochemical characterizations of an immortalized human breast epithelial cell line MCF-10. Cancer Res. 50:6087–6099, 1990.

167. Calaf, G., Russo, J. Transformation of human breast epithelial cells by chemical carcinogens. Carcinogenesis 14:483–492, 1993.

168. Russo, J., Calaf, G., Russo, I.H. A critical approach to the malignant transformation of human breast epithelial cells. CRC Critical Reviews in Oncogenesis 4:403–417, 1993.

169. Krege, J.H., Hodgin, J.B., Couse, J.F., et al. Generation and reproductive phenotypes of mice lacking oestrogen receptor β. Proc. Natl. Acad. Sci. U.S.A. 95:15677–15682, 1998.

170. Paech, K., Webb, P., Kuiper, G.G., Nilsson, S., Gustafsson, J., Kushner, P.J., Scanlan, T.S. Differential ligand activation of estrogen receptors ERalpha and ERbeta at AP1 sites. Science 277:1508–1510, 1997.

171. Ali, I.U., Lidereau, R., Callahan, R. Presence of two members of c-erbAB and c-erbA2 in smallest region of somatic homozygosity on chromosome 3p2l-p25 in human breast carcinoma. J. Natl. Cancer Inst. 81:1815–1820, 1989.

172. Chen, L-C., Matsumura, K., Deng, G., Kurisu, W., Ljung, B-M., Lerman, M.I., Waldman, F.M., Smith, H.S. Deletion of two separate regions on chromosome 3p in breast cancers. Cancer Res. 54:3021–3024, 1994.

173. Bergthorsson, J.T., Eiriksdottir, G., Barkardottir, R.B., Egilsson, V., Arason, A., Ingvarsson, S. Linkage analysis and allelic imbalance in human breast cancer kindreds using microsatellite markers from the short arm of chromosome 3. Human Genetics 96:437–443, 1995.

174. Kerangueven, F., Noguchi, T., Wargniez, V. Multiple sites of loss of heterozygosity on chromosome arms 3p and 3q in human breast carcinomas. Oncology Reports 3:313–316, 1996.

175. Pandis, N., Bardi, G., Mitelman, F., and Heim, S. Deletion of the short arm of chromosome 3 in breast tumors. Genes Chrom. Cancer 18:241–245, 1997.

176. Man, S., Ellis, I., Sibbering, M., Blarney, R., and Brook, J. Highs level of allele loss at the FHIT and ATM genes in non-comedo ductal carcinoma in situ and grade I tubular invasive breast cancers. Cancer Res. 56:5484–5489, 1996.

177. Sanchez, Y., el-Naggar, A., Pathak, S., and Killary, A.M. A tumor suppressor locus within 3pl4-pl2 mediates rapid cell death of renal cell carcinoma in vivo. Proc. Natl. Acad. Sci. USA 91:3383–3387, 1994.

178. Killary, A., Wolf, M., Giambernardi, T., and Naylor, S. Definition of a tumor suppressor locus within human chromosome 3p21 -p22. Proc. Natl. Acad. Sci. USA 89:10877–10881, 1992.

179. Hibi, Y., Yamakawa, I.C., Ueda, R., Horio, Y. Aberrant upregulation of a novel integrin α subunit gene at 3p2 l.3 in small cell lung cancer. Oncogene 9:611–619, 1994.

180. Jackers, P., Minoletti, F., Belotti, D., Clausse, N., Sozzi, G., Sobel, M.E., Castronovo, V. Isolation from a multigene family of the active human gene of the metastasis-associated multifunctional protein 37LRP/p40 at chromosome 3p2 l.3. Oncogene 13:495–503, 1996.

181. Wewer, U.M., Taraboletti, G., Sobel, M.E., Albrechtsen. R., Liotta, L.A. Role of laminin receptor in tumor cell migration. Cancer Res. 47:5691–5698, 1987.

182. Martignone, S., Menard, S., Bufalino, R., et al. Prognostic significance of the 67-kilodalton laminin receptor expression in human breast carcinomas. J. Natl. Cancer Inst. 85: 398–402, 1993.

183. Maemura, M., and Dickson, R.B. Are cellular adhesion molecules involved in metastasis of breast cancer. Breast Cancer Res. Treat. 32:239–260, 1994.

184. Ben Cheickh, M., Rouanet, P., Louason, G., Jeanteur, P., and Theillet, C. An attempt to define sets of cooperating genetic alterations in human breast cancer. Int. J. Cancer 51:542–547, 1992.

185. Negrini, M., Monaco, C., Vorechovsky, I., Ohta, M., Druck, T., Baffa, R., Huebner, K., Croce, C.M. The FHIT gene at 3pl4.2 is abnormal in breast carcinomas. Cancer Res. 56:3173–3179, 1996.

186. Theillet, C., Lidereau, R., Escot, C., Hutzell, P., Brunet, M., Gest, J., Schlom, J., Callahan, R. Loss of a c-H-ras-I allele and aggressive human primary breast carcinomas. Cancer Res. 46:4776–4781, 1986.

187. Mackay, J., Elder, P., Porteous, D.I., et al. Partial deletion of chromosome 11p in breast cancer correlates with size of primary turnout and estrogen receptor level. Br. J. Cancer 58:710–714, 1988.

188. Takita, K-I., Sato, T., Miyagi, M., Watatani, M., Akiyama, F., Sakamoto, G., Kasumi, F., Abe, R., Nakamura, Y. Correlation of loss of alleles on the short arms of chromosomes 11 and 17 with metastasis of primary breast cancer to lymph nodes. Cancer Res. 52:3914–3917, 1992.

189. Winqvist, R., Mannermaa, A., Alavaikko, M., Blanco, G., Taskinen, P.J., Kiviniemi, H., Newsham, I., Cavenee, W. Refinement of regional loss of heterozygosity for chromosome 11pl5.5 in human breast tumors. Cancer Res. 53:4486–4488, 1993.

190. Gudmundsson, J., Barkardottir, R.B., Eiriksdottir, G., Baldursson, T., Arason, A., Egilsson, V., Ingvarsson, S. Loss of heterozygosity at chromosome 11 in breast cancer: association of prognostic factors with genetic alterations. Br. J. Cancer 72:696–701, 1995.

191. Deng, G., Chen, L.C., Schott, D.R., Thor, A., Bhargava, V., Ljung, B.M., Chew, K., Smith, H.S. Loss of heterozygosity and p53 gene mutations in breast cancer. Cancer Res. 54:499–505, 1994.

192. Negrini, M., Sabbioni, S., Ohta, M., Veronese, M.L., Rattan, S., Junien, C., Croce, C.M. Seven-megabase yeast artificial chromosome contig at region 11pl5:Identification of a yeast artificial chromosome spanning the breakpoint of a chromosomal translocation found in a case of Beckwith-Wiedmann syndrome. Cancer Res. 55:2904–2909, 1995.

193. Carter, S., Negrini, M., Baffa, R., Gillum, D.R., Rosenberg, A.L., Schwartz, G.F., Croce, C.M. Loss of heterozygosity at 11 q22-q23 in breast cancer. Cancer Res. 54:6270–6274, 1994.

194. Swift, M., Morrel, D., Massey, R., Chase, C. Incidence of cancer in 161 families affected by ataxia-telangiectasia. New Eng. J. Med. 325:1831–1836, 1991.

195. Byrd, P.J., Stankovic, T., McConville, C. M., Smith, A.D., Cooper, P.R., Taylor, A.M. Identification and analysis of expression of human VACM-1, a cullin gene family member located on chromosome 11 q22-23. Genome Res. 7:71–75, 1997.

196. Tomlinson, I.P., Nicolai, H., Solomon, E., Bodmer, W.F. The frequency and mechanism of loss of heterozygosity on chromosome 1lq in breast cancer. Journal of Pathology 180:38–43, 1996.

197. Tomlinson, I.P., Beck, N.E., Bodmer, W.F. Allele loss on chromosome 1lq and microsatellite instability in malignant melanoma. European Journal of Cancer 32A:1797–802, 1996.

198. Connolly, K.C., Gabra, H., Millwater, C.J., Taylor, K.J., Rabiasz, G.J., Watson, J.E., Smyth, J.F., Wvllie, A.H., Jodrell, D.I. Identification of a region of frequent loss of heterozygosity at 11 q24 in colorectal cancer. Cancer Res. 59:2806–2809, 1999.

199. Launonen, V, Stenback, F., Puistola, U., Bloiu, R., Huusko, P., Kytola, S., Kauppila, A., Winqvist, R. Chromosome 11q22.3-q25 LOH in ovarian cancer: association with a more aggressive disease course and involved subregions. Gynecol. Oncol. 71:299–304, 1998.

200. Dahiva, R., McCarville, J., Lee, C., Hu, W., Kaur, G., Carroll, P., Deng, G. Deletion of chromosome 1 lpl5, pl2, q22, q23–24 loci in human prostate cancer. International Journal of Cancer 72:283–288, 1997.

201. Yen, T.J., Li, G., Schaar, B., Szilak, I., and Cleveland, D.W. CENP-E is a putative kinetochore motor that accumulates just prior to mitosis. Nature 359:536–539, 1992.

Pathogenesis of Breast Cancer

5.1 Introduction

It is not known when in the lifetime of a woman the initiation of breast cancer takes place, or whether a specific agent causes it. The fact that late menarche and a full-term pregnancy completed before age 24, or early full-term pregnancy, reduces the risk of breast cancer development, whereas early menarche, nulliparity and exposure to ionizing radiations at ages younger than 19 are associated with a higher breast cancer incidence [1, 2], indicates that the period encompassed between menarche and first full-term pregnancy represents a window of high susceptibility for the initiation of breast cancer.

5.2 The Site of Origin of Breast Cancer

An important concept that emerged from the study of breast development is that the TDLU, which had been identified as the site of origin of the most common breast malignancy, the ductal carcinoma [1, 3, 4], corresponds to a specific stage of development of the mammary parenchyma, the lobule type 1 (Figs. 5.1, 5.2). This observation is supported by comparative studies of normal and cancer-bearing breasts ob-

▼ **Figure 5.1 a–c**

a Lobule type 1; b Mild ductal hyperplasia originating in lob 1; c Ductal carcinoma in situ (H&E, ×4, ×4 and ×10 respectively)

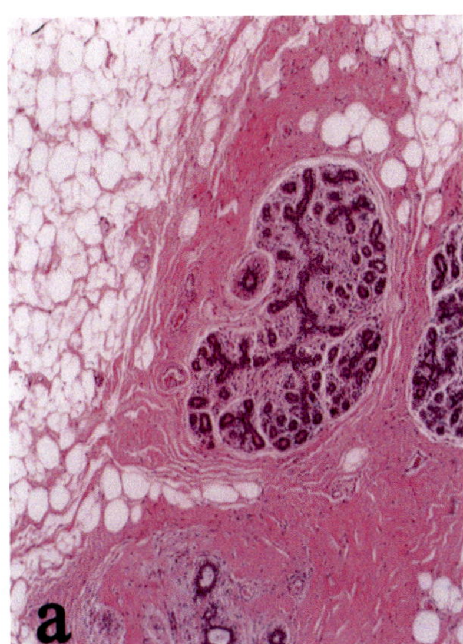
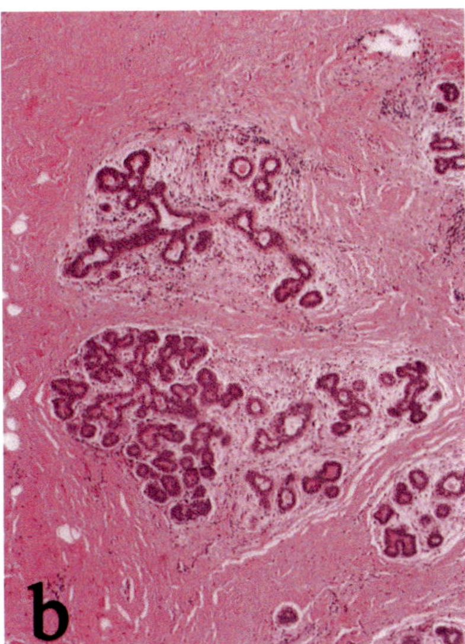
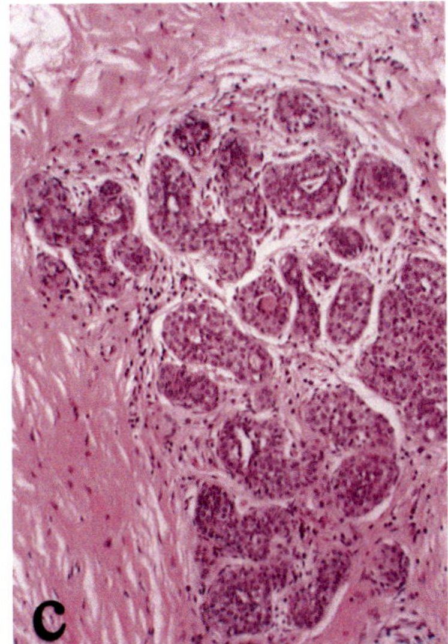

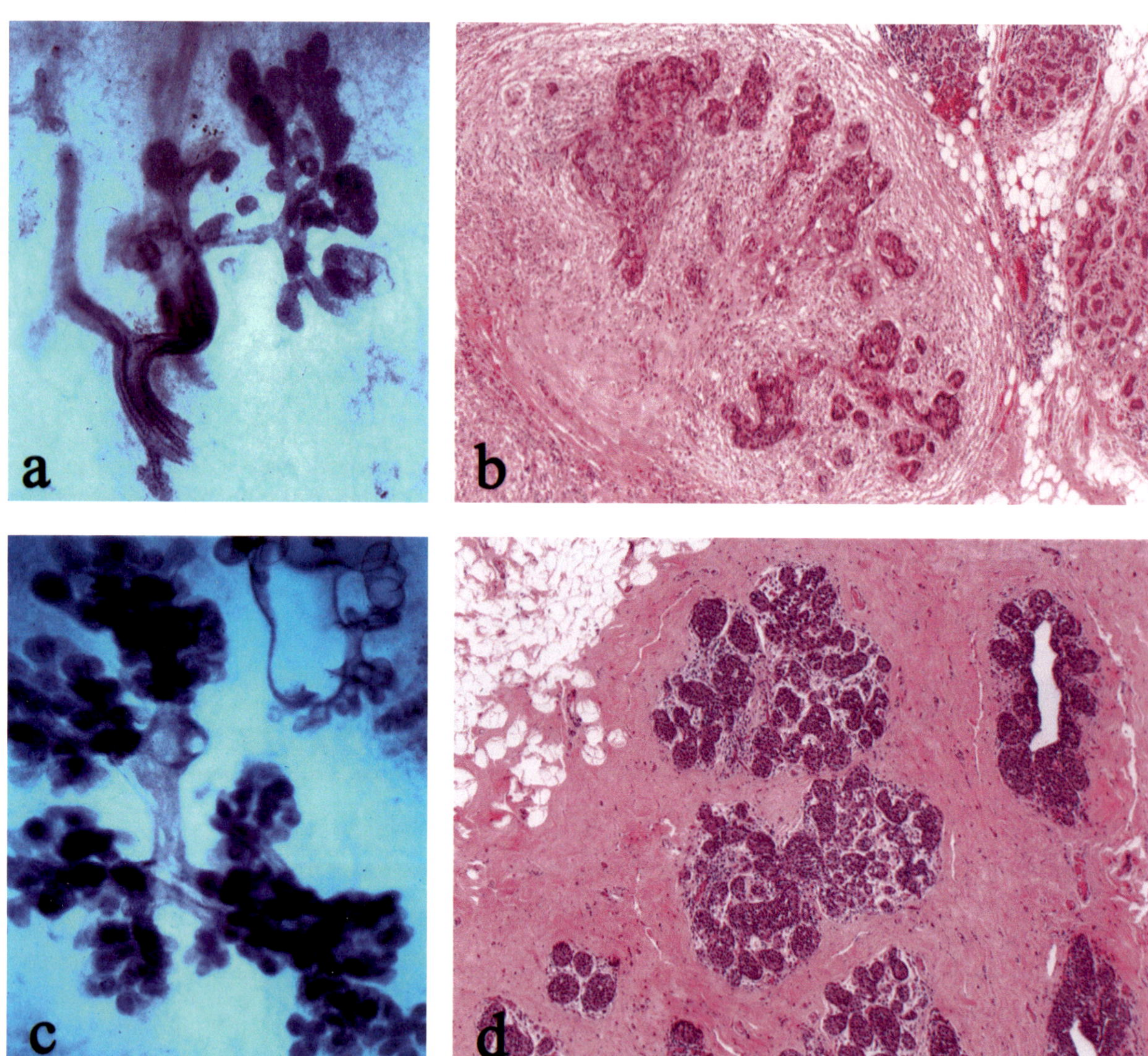

tained at autopsy. It was found that the non tumoral parenchyma in cancer associated breasts contained a significantly higher number of hyperplastic terminal ducts, atypical Lobule 1 and ductal carcinomas in situ originated in Lobule 1 than those breasts of women free of breast cancer (Table 5.1). These observations indicate that the Lobule 1 is affected by preneoplastic as well as by neoplastic processes [5, 6]. The finding that the lobules type 1 that are undifferentiated struc-

Figure 5.2 a–d

a Whole mount showing ductal carcinoma in situ in lobule type 1 (toluidine blue, × 4). **b** Histological section of **a**, depicting ductal carcinoma in situ (H&E, × 4). **c** Whole mount showing a lobular carcinoma in situ emerging from lobule type 2 (toluidine blue, × 4). **d** Histological section of **c**, depicting a lobular carcinoma in situ, H&E, × 4

Table 5.1. Average number of selected lesions/breast. *DCIS* ductal carcinoma in situ

Lesion	Random autopsy breasts (n=185)	Cancer associated breasts (n=10)	p value for different populations (Students t-test)
Hyperplastic terminal duct	0.08	1.82	<0.01
Lobule type 1 (TDLU) with atypia	10.31	44.50	<0.01
DCIS arising in lobule type 1	0.08	5.47	<0.001

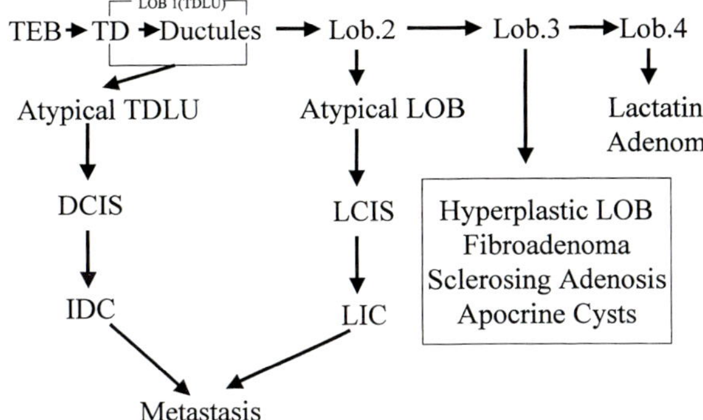

Figure 5.3

Pathogenetic pathway of human breast cancer. *TEB* terminal end buds, *TD* terminal ducts, *TDLU* terminal ductal lobular unit, *DCIS* ductal carcinoma in situ, *LCIS* lobular carcinoma in situ, *IDC* invasive ductal carcinoma, *LIC* lobular invasive carcinoma

tures originate the most undifferentiated and aggressive neoplasm acquires relevance to the light that these structures are more numerous in the breast of nulliparous women, who are, in turn, at a higher risk of developing breast cancer. The Lobule 1 found in the breast of nulliparous women never went through the process of differentiation, whereas the same structures, when found in the breast of postmenopausal parous women did [5] (see Chapter 2).

More differentiated lobular structures have been found to be affected by neoplastic lesions as well, although they originate tumors whose malignancy is inversely related to the degree of differentiation of the parent structure, i.e., Lobule 2 originate lobular carcinomas in situ, (Fig. 5.2), whereas Lobule 3 give

rise to more benign breast lesions, such as hyperplastic lobules, cysts, fibroadenomas and adenomas, and Lobule 4 to lactating adenomas [1]. We concluded from these observations that each specific compartment of the breast gives origin to a specific type of lesion (Fig. 5.3), and also provides the basis for a new biological concept that the differentiation of the breast determines the susceptibility to neoplastic transformation.

5.3 Supporting Evidence for the Site of Origin of Breast Cancer

5.3.1 In Vitro Studies

In the previous section it has been indicated that ductal carcinomas originate in TDLU (Lobule 1) and lobular carcinomas in Lobule 2, whereas the Lobule 3 is not associated with the development of malignancies [1, 3]. To ascertain whether Lobule 1 and Lobule 2 are more susceptible than Lobule 3 to undergo neoplastic transformation, an in vitro system that reproduces the in vivo conditions of the breast epithelium have been developed. For these purposes, normal breast tissues, obtained fresh and sterile from reduction mammoplasties, have been utilized. Upon digestion of the tissues with collagenase and hyaluronidase, epithelial cells in aggregates, or organoids, are separated by micromanipulation (Fig. 5.4). Organoids are classified as Lobule 1, Lobule 2 or Lobule 3 by applying the same criteria developed for classifying these structures in whole mount and histopathological preparations (see Chapter 2). Plating of each lobular type separately allows one to evaluate wheth-

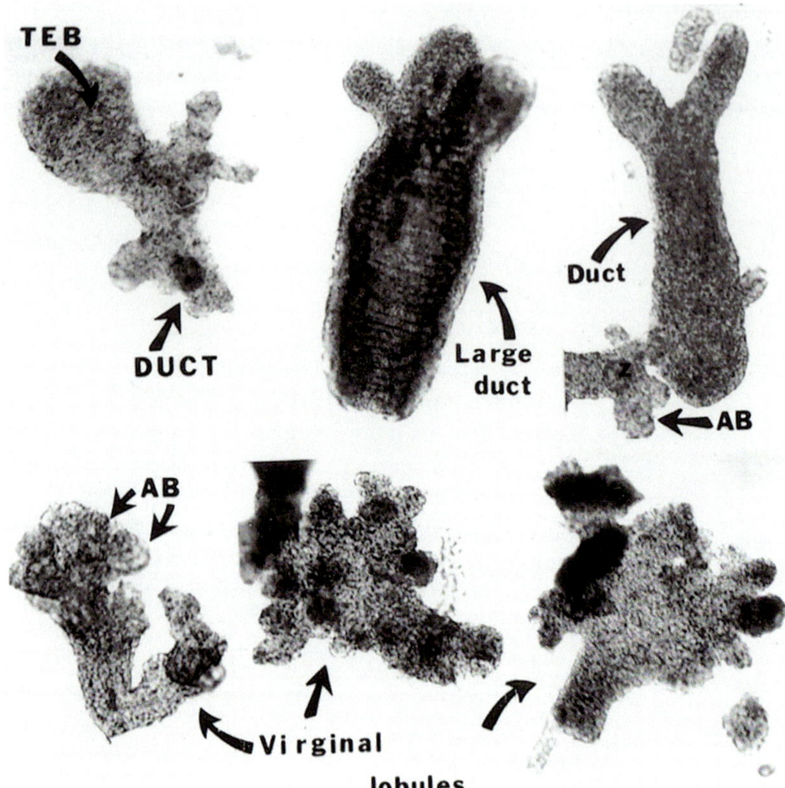

er the behavior of cells in culture correlates with the specific type of lobule that originated them. Cells from Lobule 1 and Lobule 2, which in organ culture have shown to exhibit a higher DNA-LI, attach to the dishes promptly and start growing logarithmically, whereas cells from Lobule 3, which have a lower DNA-LI, have a long lag phase before they attach to the dish and start growing. The number of doublings per lobular unit of time was also higher in Lobule 1 and Lobule 2 than in Lobule 3 [7] (Figs. 5.5, 5.6). The susceptibility of the different lobule types to be transformed by chemical carcinogens in vitro has been tested in 52 human breast samples. Organoids representing Lobule 1, Lobule 2 and Lobule 3 were plated, and when the cells reached their logarithmic phase of growth they were treated with the chemical carcinogens N-methyl-N-nitrosourea (NMU), 7,12-dimethylbenz(a)anthracene (DMBA), methyl-N- nitro-

nitroso-guanidine (MNNG) or benzo(a)pyrene (BP) for 24 h. The cells were followed up for several passages until they exhibited changes indicative of neoplastic transformation, such as variations in cell morphology, loss of contact inhibition, and anchorage independent growth. The changes in cell shape induced by the carcinogens were the result of increased number of surface microvilli and decreased cell-cell interaction. The property to form domes when plated in plastic flasks (Fig. 5.7), which is characteristic of normal breast epithelial cells, was lost in carcinogen treated cells; this phenomenon was interpreted to be the result of an abnormal pattern of growth caused by altered contact inhibition. Treated cells showed increased ability to survive and to form colonies in agar methocel, and to exhibit multinucleation [7, 8]. These types of responses, however, were observed only in the epithelial cells derived from breast tissues con-

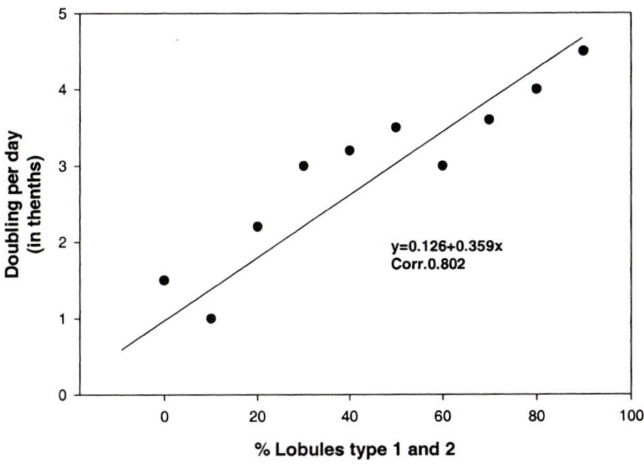

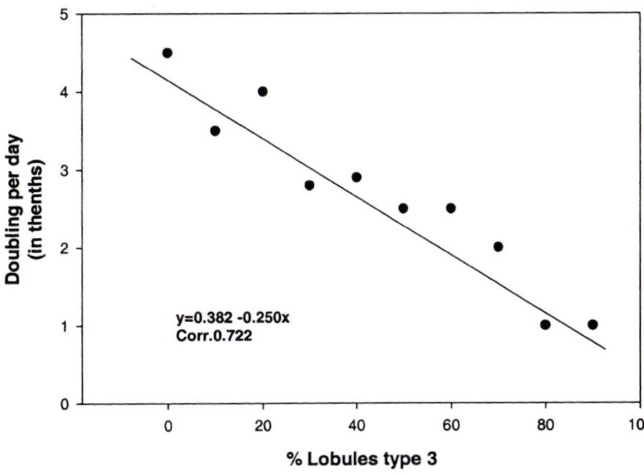

Figure 5.5

Correlation of doublings per day in type 1 and type 2 lobular structures

Figure 5.6

Fig. 5.6. Correlation of doublings per day and type 3 lobular structures

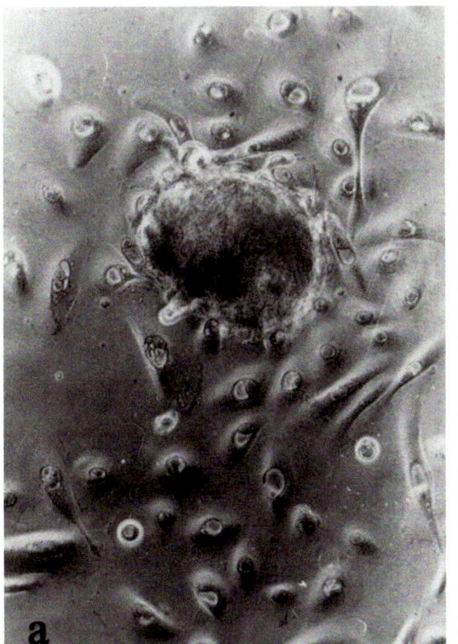

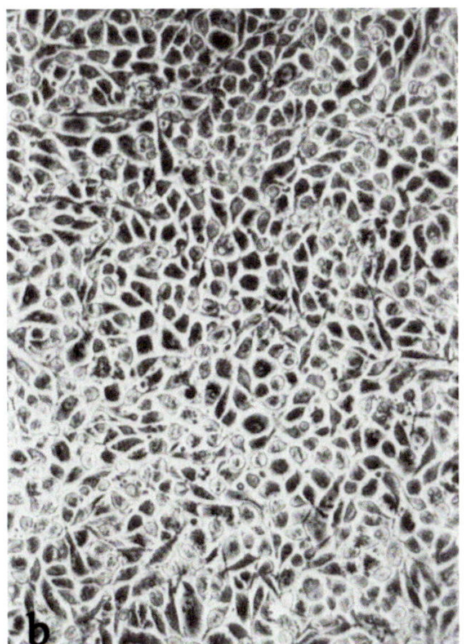

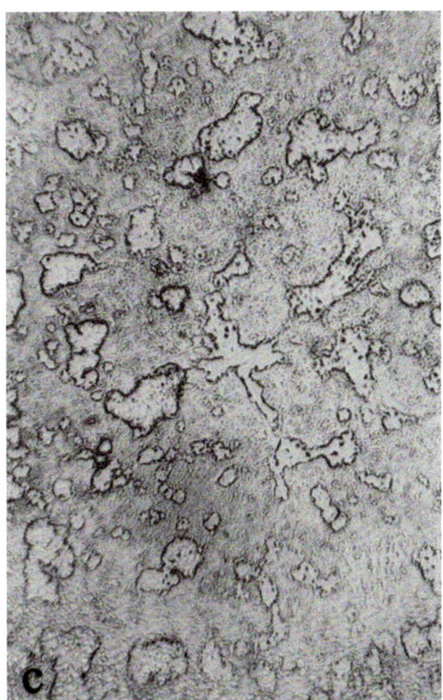

Figure 5.7 a–c

Organoids of lobule type 1 growing in plastic (phase contrast, ×40). b Confluent monolayer of lobule type 1 before the formation of domes (phase contrast, ×10). c Dome formation (phase contrast, ×10)

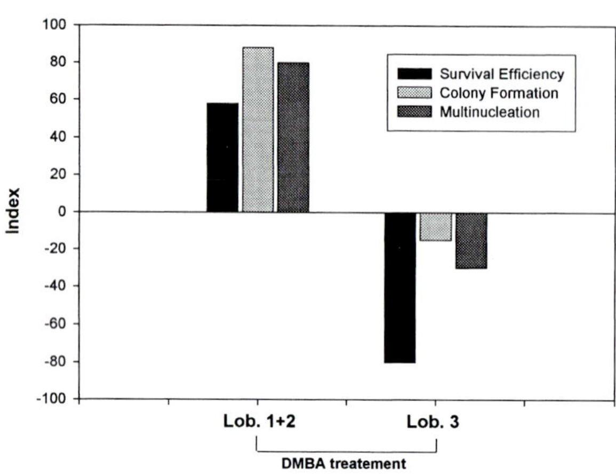

Figure 5.8

Histogram showing the expression of transformation phenotypes in primary culture of lobules type 1,2, and 3 treated with DMBA by 24 h and followed up over several weeks. (3–9 weeks)

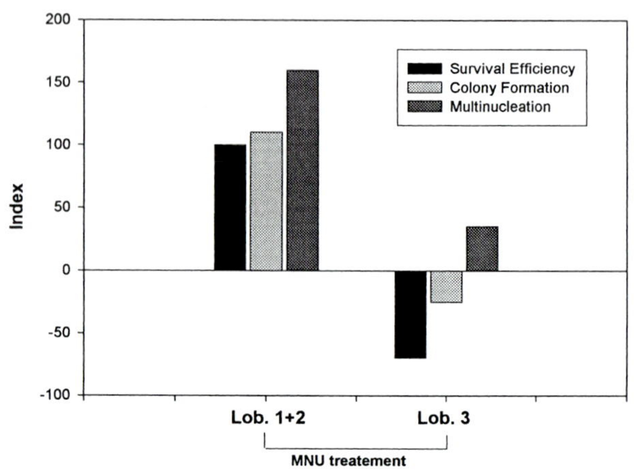

Figure 5.9

Histogram showing the expression of transformation phenotypes in primary culture of lobules type 1,2, and 3 treated with MNU (N-methyl-nitrosourea) for 24 h and followed up over several weeks (3–9 weeks)

taining Lobule 1 and Lobule 2. The phenomena were not observed in the breast cells derived from Lobule 3 [7, 8] (Figs. 5.8, 5.9).

These observations led to conclude that primary cultures of human breast epithelial cells are susceptible to be transformed in vitro by chemical carcinogens, however, the expression of phenotypes indicative of neoplastic transformation depends upon the stage of development of the breast and of the in vivo cell proliferation rate [7, 8]. The finding that Lobule 1 and Lobule 2 express more readily changes indicative of neoplastic transformation in vitro indicates that these structures are more susceptible to the transforming effect of genotoxic agents, thus supporting the observations that they are the site of origin of mammary carcinomas; it also correlates with the lack of association of the Lobule 3 with the development of malignant neoplasms [1, 4–6]. Of greater relevance is the observation that the breast of nulliparous women contains more numerous Lobule 1 and Lobule 2 than the breast of parous women, in which predominates the Lobule 3, further emphasizing the protective effect of gland differentiation, which modulates the response of breast epithelial cells to carcinogens under in vitro conditions.

5.3.2 Breast Architecture as a Determining Factor in the Susceptibility of the Human Breast to Cancer

The breast of women that underwent reduction mammoplasty contains the three types of lobules described previously (Fig. 2.4, 2.5, 2.6) [9, 10]. The three lobular structures are in general surrounded by a loose stroma that demarcate them from the interlobular stroma that may have different ratio of connective and fat tissue (Fig. 5.10a). All the lobules were very well demarcated and not fibrous tissue was observed (Fig. 5.11a, Table 5.2). Quantitation of the three lobular structures in the overall population of breast tissue studied indicated that lobules type 1 represented 22.5% of the structures, whereas Lobule 2 were 37.3% and Lobule 3, 38.4% of the total number of structures. The differences are statistically significant (Table 5.3). The separation of the breast sam-

Table 5.2. Profile of the lobular structures in the breast tissues obtained from reduction mammoplasty (RM), prophylactic mastectomy for familial breast cancer (FAM) and modified radical mastectomy for invasive cancer (MRM)

Group	Number of cases	Well-defined lobules – n (%)	Not well-defined lobules – n (%)	Fibrosis		
				None – n (%)	Mild to moderate – n (%)	Marked – n (%)
RM	33	33 (100)	0 (0)	33 (100)	0	0
FAM	17	8 (47.0)	9 (53)	0	3 (17.6)	14 (82.4)
MRM	43	40 (93)	3 (7.0)	1 (2.3)	39 (90.3)	3.0 (7.4)

Table 5.3. Lobular architecture of the breast tissue from reduction mammoplasty (*RM*), prophylactic mastectomy for familial breast cancer (*FAM*), and modified radical mastectomy (*MRM*)

Group	Number of cases	Age $\overline{X}\pm SD$	Lob 1 $\overline{X}\pm SD$ (%)	Lob 2 $\overline{X}\pm SD$ (%)	Lob 3 $\overline{X}\pm SD$ (%)
RM (all)	33	29.4±8.2	22.5±23.7	37.3±28.6	38.4±34.2
– RM (nulliparous)	9	22.9±6.7	45.9±27.4	47.2±22.0	6.9±7.0
– RM (parous)	24	31.9±2.3	16.9±8.3	35.5±3.1	47.9±33.4
FAM (all)	17	37.0±2.9	47.9±37.3	39.9±31.3	9.91±4.41
– FAM (nulliparous)	8	37.6±3.2	51.3±34.4	39.9±26.2	8.83±8.39
– FAM (parous)	9	36.5±2.6	44.0±42.00	40.0±38.1	16.10±9.9
MRM (all)	43	35.4±3.9	74.3±25.8	22.3±22.1	3.35±10.0
– MRM (nulliparous)	7	36.0±3.6	80.0±19.0	16.8±15.0	1.74±4.6
– MRM (parous)	36	35.2±4.3	70.4±26.4	25.4±22.7	3.80±12.48

ples, based on the pregnancy history of the host, such as nulliparity and parity, showed a different pattern of lobular development. The breast of nulliparous women contained a significantly higher number of lobules type 1 and 2, with 45.9% and 47.2% respectively and a highly significantly lower number of lobules type 3, (6.9%) (Table 5.3). In the breast of parous women, the pattern was inverse, being the lobules type 2 and 3 the most abundant, 35.5% and 47.9% respectively, whereas, lobule type 1 comprised only 16.9% of the total.

The breast of women with familial breast cancer (verified to be either BRCA+, or carrier of genetic abnormalities) (Table 5.4) was obtained from prophylactic mastectomies. The average age of these women was 37.0±2.9 years of age (Table 5.3). The whole mount, as well as the histological appearance of the lobular structures was different to the observed in the breast tissue of women that underwent reduction mammoplasty (Fig. 5.10). Eight out of 17 breast samples presented a well-demarcated lobular structure but all of them have moderate or marked fibrous of the intralobular stroma (Fig. 5.11, Table 2). Ductal hyperplasia (mild to severe) in the Lobules 1 or 2 was observed in 7 cases, carcinoma in situ (solid, cribriform and papillary) in 1 case and invasive carcinomas ipsilaterally or contralaterally was observed in 9 cases (Table 5.5).

The distribution of lobules type 1,2 and 3 in the breast tissue derived from women with BRCA+, or being carriers of genetic abnormalities by linked analysis was 47.9, 39.9 and 9.9% respectively (Table

Table 5.4. Profile of the breast tissue obtained from prophylactic mastectomy in BRCA1 positive or carrier of familial breast cancer

Sample number	Pedigree number	BRCA1	Age	Parity	Breast with cancer	Breast studied
217	1973–11	Positive	33	Yes	Right	Right and left
231	3312–18	Carriers	33	No	Left	Left
234	1234–68	Positive	33	Yes	–	Right and left
222	3703–1	Carriers	34	No	–	Right and left
221	3300–1	Carriers	35	Yes	–	Right and left
230	3619–5	Carriers	36	No	–	Right
205	2850–19	Carriers	36	No	Left	Right
203	3481–1	Carriers	37	Yes	Right	Right and left
202	3481–10	Carriers	37	Yes	Right	Left
232	2887–3	Unlinked	38	No	–	Right and left
229	1816–62	Positive	38	No	Left	Left
206	1815–1	Carriers	38	Yes	Right	Left
228	2552–13	Carriers	39	Yes	Right	Left
210	1086–28	Carriers	40	Yes	Right	Right
218	1816–680	Positive	40	No	Left	Right
223	1816–680	Positive	40	No	–	Right and left
212	3386–1	Carriers	43	No	–	Right and left

Table 5.5. Type of lesions found in the breast tissue studied from reduction mammoplasty (*RM*), prophylactic mastectomy for familial breast cancer (*FAM*), and modified radical mastectomy (*MRM*)

Group	Number of Cases	Lobules counted (number)	Ductal hyperplasia		DCIS	
			n	%	n	%
RM	33	31,220	0	0	0	0
FAM	17	3,162	7	41.2	1	5.9
MRM	43	2,901	27	63.0	5	11.4

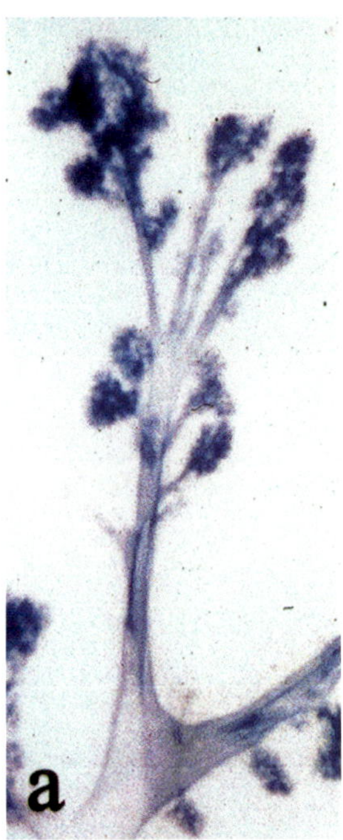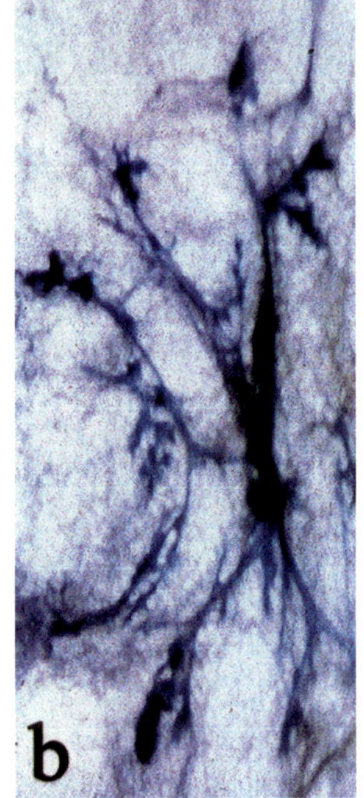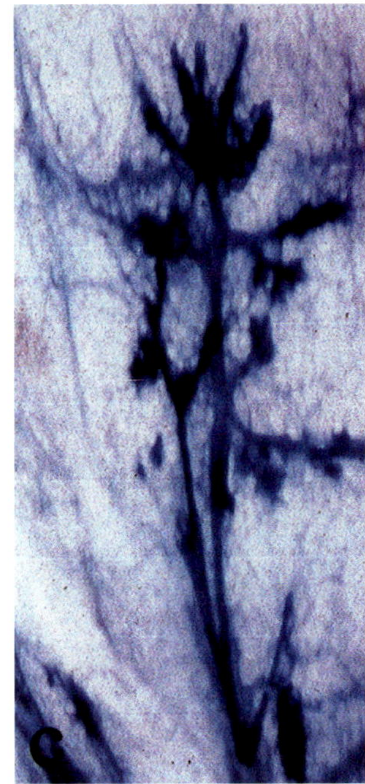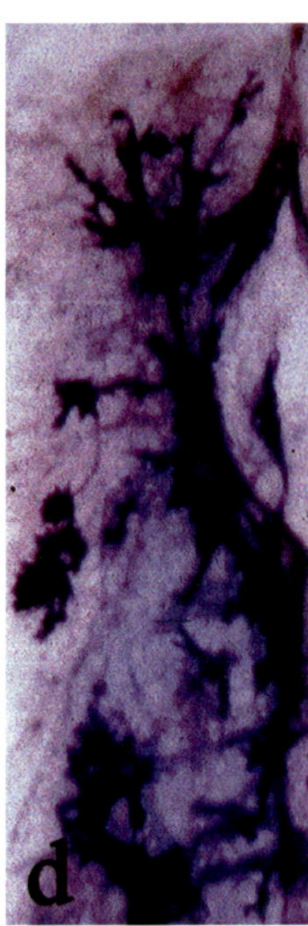

Figure 5.10 a–d

a Whole mount of normal breast tissue of a nulliparous woman. b–d Lobules type 1 of parous women with familial breast cancer (toluidine blue, ×4)

5.2). This pattern was significantly different than that observed in the RM group I, containing a higher percentage of lobules type 1 ($p < 0.0008$) whereas lobules type 3 were significantly lower ($p < 0.00004$) (Table 5.2).

The separation of the breast samples, based on the pregnancy history of the host, such as nulliparity and parity, indicated that in both subgroups the percentage of lobules type 1 was significantly higher than lobules type 3 (Table 5.3), and that the differences between nulliparous and parous observed in the control or RM group were not present in the breast tissue derived from women with familial breast cancer (Table 5.3). Lobule type 1 represents 51.3% and 44.0% in the nulliparous and parous women respectively. This indicates a reversion of the pattern observed in the parous in which the lobules type 1 are less frequent. In the familial cases, the comparison of the nulliparous

from the RM group with those of the prophylactic mastectomy for familial breast cancer (FAM) group is not statistically different. Instead, the parous breast tissue of the reduction mammoplasty (RM) group was significantly different from those of the FAM group (Table 5.3).

In order to determine if those breast tissue with BRCA+ were different from those designated to be carrier, but in which not BRCA was determined yet (Table 5.4), these two groups (BRCA+ and carriers) were separated and it was found that the percentage of lobular structures were not significantly different.

The age of women from RM group was different from those of the FAM group, the average was 29.4 for the first group and 37.0 years of age for the second group. This difference is significant. In order to determine if age may be contributory to the differences observed, the data were retabulated for the RM Group

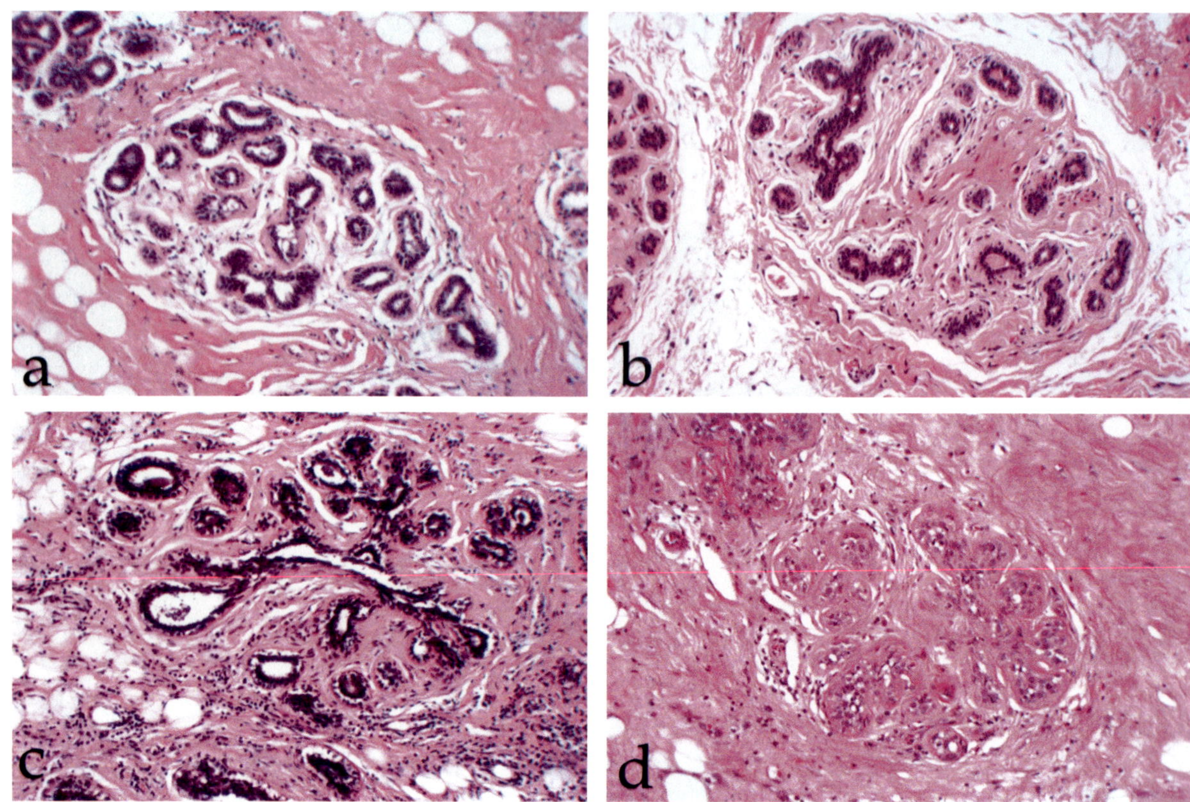

Figure 5.11 a–d

Histological section of a lobule type 1. **a** Lob 1 with a good demarcation between the intralobular and inter-lobular stroma. **b, c** Lob 1 with increase density in the intralobular stroma. **d** Lob 1 with marked fibrosis in the intra-lobular stroma and lack of demarcation from the extra-lobular stroma (H&E, × 25)

for those women with matching age to those of FAM Group, and it was found that the difference between both groups still persists, indicating that the familial factor could be in itself a deterrent in the pattern of architectural development of the breast.

The architectural pattern of the breast tissue obtained from modified radical mastectomy was from forty-three breast samples. The average age for this group is 35.4 years with not significant difference between the age for the nulliparous and parous women (Table 5.3). Quantitation of the three lobular structures in the overall population of breast tissue studied indicated that lobules type 1 represented 74.25% of the structures, whereas lob.2 were 22.3% and lobules 3, 3.4% of the total number of structures. The differences are statistically significant (Table 5.3).

The separation of the breast samples, based on the pregnancy history of the host, such as nulliparity and parity, showed no different pattern of lobular devel-

opment. The breast of nulliparous women contained a significantly higher number of lobules type 1 and 2, with 80.0% and 16.8% respectively and a highly significantly lower number of lobules type 3, (1.7%) (Table 5.3). In the breast of parous women, the pattern was similar, being the lobule type 1 and 2 the most abundant, 70.4% and 25.4% respectively, whereas, lobules type 3 comprised only 3.8% of the total. The differences between nulliparous and parous were not statistically significant (Table 5.3).

The histological appearance of the MRM group lobular structures was not different from that observed in the breast tissue of women that underwent reduction mammoplasty (RM), but it was different from the FAM group. In the former 92.8% of the lobules were well defined whereas only 47.0% in the FAM group were. In the MRM group 3 out of 40 breast samples had marked fibrosis in the intralobular stroma (Table 5.2); it was significantly lower than in the FAM group, in which most of the lobules presented marked intralobular fibrosis. Ductal hyperplasia in the lobules 1 or 2 was observed in 62.9% and carcinoma in situ in 11.4% of MRM cases (Table 5.5). The age of women from MRM group was not different from those of the FAM group, (Table 5.3).

Altogether these results show that the breast of parous women from the FAM and the MRM group exhibited a different architectural pattern from those of parous women of the RM group, that can be considered the normal or control population [5]. The observation that the lobular type 1 of the breast of both nulliparous and parous women of the FAM and MRM group are the most frequent structure is in agreement with the knowledge that the cancer in the breast starts in the lobules type 1, [1, 3, 11]. The greater proportion of lobules type 1 found in the breast of nulliparous and parous women of the FAM and MRM groups suggest that these breasts were at higher risk of developing malignancies due to the fact that each lob 1 is the target of carcinogenic insult [1, 3].

5.3.3 Specific Considerations on the Relation Between Lobular Development and Familial Breast Cancer-Related Genes

At the present time we do not know which is or are the genes that are controlling the differentiating pattern of the human breast [5, 9, 12]. It has been postulated that BRCA1 and/or BRCA2 may serve to control cell proliferation and differentiation during developmental stages characterized by rapid growth [13]. This model predicts that individuals possessing germline mutations in BRCA1 and/or BRCA2 may be particularly susceptible to early events in mammary carcinogenesis during pregnancy [13]. Recent epidemiological observation suggest that women with a positive family history of breast cancer may experience a significantly greater increase in breast cancer risk associated with their first pregnancy relative to women without a family history of breast cancer [14]. How BRCA1 and/or BRCA2 control breast differentiation is unknown. In both sporadic and familial breast cancer, the pattern of lobular development is very similar. In rodents as well as in the breast tissue of women that underwent plastic surgery for cosmetic reasons, parity is associated with lobular differentiation [11, 15]. In both cases, lobular differentiation makes the mammary tissue refractory to neoplastic transformation by chemical carcinogens [16]. Moreover, the relation of the differentiation effect induced by pregnancy and the induced protection against breast cancer in women who have undergone this first full-term pregnancy early in life [17] is an indication that the same operational events are modified in both familial and sporadic cases of breast cancer.

In addition to the overall architectural differences described above, the breast tissues from women with hereditary breast cancer present histological differences in the intralobular stroma. The intralobular stroma at difference of the more dense collagenized interlobular stroma is a dynamic compartment of the breast composed of loosely arranged connective tissue, containing cells such as fibroblasts, blood vessels and inflammatory cells such as lymphocytes, mast cells, and macrophages [18, 19]. The intralobular stroma contrast with the interlobular stroma that has fewer cells separated by larger quantities of more compact collagen. The role of intralobular stroma during breast development from adolescence to premenopausal maturity, pregnancy and lactation, involution, and postmenopausal changes has been implicated, however, how the interaction with the epithelial cells takes place is unknown. Most of our understanding of the interaction between epithelial and stroma in the breast are from the experiments of Sakakura et al. [20]. In the present work, we indicate that the intralobular stroma of the lobules type 1 of the breast of women with familial breast cancer has lost the loosely arranged connective tissue for a more dense stroma that erase its demarcation from the intralobular stroma (Fig. 5.11d). The intralobular stroma of the breast tissue from the FAM group was more fibrotic and dense. These findings suggest either that in the breast cancer families, the development of the breast parenchyma has failed to respond to the normal physiological stimuli that determine the formation of lobular structures, indicative of differentiation, or that the involution pattern of the lobular structures type 3 after pregnancy is more rapid in these women than in those in the control. It is noteworthy that early pregnancies influence breast cancer risk by altering the structure of the mammary parenchyma [1, 5]. It has been hypothesized that late pregnancies could likewise influence breast cancer risk via alterations in the mammary parenchyma, by delaying or interrupting the normal process of involution of glandular tissue of the breast [21]. In the mouse it has been observed that BRCA1 is induced during puberty, pregnancy, and following treatment of ovariectomized animals with 17β-estradiol and progesterone. Therefore it is not surprising that in the human breast alteration of this gene may explain the morphological pattern observed. The findings that the intralobular stroma is more fibrotic in the FAM group than in the MRM and RM groups, may explain in part, the increased mammographic density in women with familial breast cancer. Although the intralobular stroma is only a small component of all the factors that determine the mammographic pattern, the mammographic breast density reflects proliferation of breast stroma through collagen formation and fibrosis. The factors that determine breast densities depend on the interplay of hormones, namely, estrogen and growth factors, such as epidermal growth factor, transforming growth factor, and insulin growth factors I and II. How all these factors and the genes related to familial breast cancer interrelate in the biology of the intralobular stroma is not known [22–26].

The development of mammary ductal structures involves a complex interplay between epithelium and mesenchyme [20, 27–32]. The branching of the mammary ducts depends upon circulating hormones for stimulation and synchronization with reproductive events, but is also influenced by local factors to provide signals that modulate glandular growth, differentiation and morphogenesis. The matrix-degrading metallo-proteinase stromelysin-1, stromelysin-3, and gelatinase A are expressed during ductal branching morphogenesis of the murine mammary gland [33]. Although, the role of metalloproteinases in the branching pattern of the mammary gland and its relation with BRCA1, requires further investigation, on the basis of these data it is possible to postulate that the breast tissue from women with hereditary breast cancer suffers from an alteration of the interaction between the epithelium and the stroma.

It has been reported in the literature [34] that breast tissue of women from sporadic breast cancer contained higher numbers of ductal carcinoma in situ and ductal hyperplasias than those from the familial breast cancer. The data shown above indicate that BRCA1 or related genes associated with familial breast cancer play a role in the lobular pattern of the breast mainly by altering the rate of involution after pregnancy, with the consistent increase in the lobules type 1 as compared with the control population [10]. More specific to the role of familial breast cancer genes is the alteration in the epithelial-stromal relationship, by increasing the percentage of lobular structures with marked intralobular fibrosis. These observations indicate that more studies in this direction are needed. Genetic influences are responsible of at least 5 % of the breast cancer cases; they also seem to influence the pattern of breast development and differentiation, as evidenced by the study of prophylactic mastectomy specimens obtained from women with familial breast and breast/ovarian cancer, or proven to be carriers of the BRCA1 gene, as determined by linkage analysis. The study of prophylactic mastectomy specimens obtained from both nulliparous and parous women revealed that the morphology and architecture of the breast were similar in these two groups of women [10]. Their breast tissues were predominately composed of Lob 1, and only a few specimens contained Lob 2 and Lob 3, in frank contrast with the predominance of Lob 3 found in parous women without familial history of breast cancer [5, 6, 10]. The developmental pattern of the breast of parous women of the familial breast cancer group was similar to that of nulliparous women of the same group, and less developed than the breast of parous women without history of familial breast cancer. The breast of women belonging to the familial breast cancer group also presented differences in the branching pattern of the ductal epithelium, observations that suggested that the genes that control lobular development might have been affected in those women belonging to families with a history of breast and breast/ovarian cancer [5, 6, 10]. Supporting evidence to this fact is the poor milk production reported in carriers of the BRCA1 mutation compared with female relatives without mutation [35] and the poor differentiation of the mammary gland of mice with BRCA1 mutations [36].

5.3.4 Unifying Concepts

Breast cancer originates in undifferentiated terminal structures of the mammary gland. The terminal ducts of the Lob 1 of the human female breast, that are the sites of origin of ductal carcinomas, are at their peak of cell replication during early adulthood, a period during which the breast is more susceptible to carcinogenesis. The susceptibility of Lob 1 to undergo neoplastic transformation has been confirmed by in vitro studies, which have shown that this structure has the highest proliferative activity and rate of carcinogen binding to the DNA. More importantly, when treated with carcinogens in vitro its epithelial cells express phenotypes indicative of cell transformation [7, 8]. These studies indicate that in the human breast the target cell of carcinogens is found in specific compartment whose characteristics are the determinant factors in the initiation event. These target cells will become the stem cells of the neoplastic event, depending upon:

1. Topographic location within the mammary gland tree
2. Age at exposure to a known or putative genotoxic agent
3. Reproductive history of the host

The higher incidence of breast cancer observed in nulliparous women supports this concept, because it parallels the higher cancer incidence elicited by carcinogens in rodents when exposure occurs at a young age.

In addition, it has been shown that an increase in parity is associated with a pronounced decrease in the risk of breast cancer, each additional live birth conferring a 10% risk reduction [17]. Thus, the protection afforded by early full-term pregnancy in women could be explained by the higher degree of differentiation of the mammary gland at the time in which an etiologic agent or agents act. Even though differentiation significantly reduces cell proliferation in the mammary gland, the mammary epithelium remains capable of responding with proliferation to given stimuli, such as a new pregnancy. Under these circumstances, however, the cells that are stimulated to proliferate are from structures that have already been primed by the first cycle of differentiation, thus creating a second type of stem cells that are able to metabolize the carcinogen and repair the DNA damage induced more efficiently than the cells of the virginal gland, and are less susceptible to carcinogenesis, as it has been demonstrated in the rodent experimental system [37]. However, a carcinogenic stimulus powerful enough may overburden the system, successfully initiating a neoplastic process. These conditions might explain the small fraction of women developing breast cancer after an early first full-term pregnancy, meaning completion of the first cycle of differentiation. The relevance of this work lies in the vis-à-vis comparison of in vivo and in vitro studies in the human breast that validate experimental data for extrapolation to the human situation. The finding that differentiation is an important inhibitor of cancer initiation provides a powerful rationale to identify the genes controlling this process for breast cancer prevention.

5.4 Molecular Changes in the Initiation and Progression of Breast Cancer

Normal and differentiated human breast epithelial cells (HBEC), both in vivo and in vitro, have a limited ability to divide [8, 28, 39]. Cellular mortality of these cells is characterized by a progressive cessation of cell growth manifested in cell culture as senescence [38, 40]. Whereas immortality in vitro may not have a definitive step in the process of transformation, it has been postulated that it may represent ductal hyperplasia or the preneoplastic stage occurring in vivo [39]. A suitable in vitro model of immortal HBECs has been lacking, till the establishment of an immortal HBEC line MCF-10F, that arose spontaneously without chemical or viral intervention, from mortal human mammary epithelial cells S-130, thereby providing an ideal in vitro model for isolating genes that may be critical to the process of immortalization [40, 41]. Among the changes that occurred in MCF-10F cells during the process of immortalization, were a balanced reciprocal chromosomal translocation t(3;9) (3p13:9p22) [40], calcium-independent growth in culture [41], insertional mutation of p53 in exon 7 [12], and stabilization of telomere length [12]. Defining molecular mechanisms involved in HBEC immortalization may be crucial to understanding the early events in the development of breast cancer [39]. Using differential display techniques by comparing total RNA from the spontaneously immortalized HBEC line MCF-10F with total RNA from its mortal parental counterpart S130, two genes emerged as important players in the early stages of cell immortalization. One of them is ferritin H chain and the other is S100p [42, 43].

5.4.1 Differential Expression of Human Ferritin H Chain Gene and Breast Cancer

The cDNA clone (233 bp) isolated by subtractive hybridization between the mortal HBEC S-130 and its mortal counter part MCF-10F was cloned, purified and sequenced. Sequence comparison in the GenBank database revealed it to be 100 % homologous at

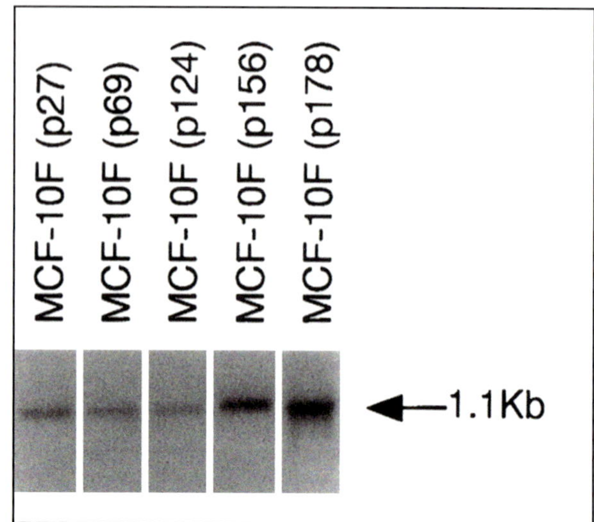

Figure 5.12

Northern analysis showing increased message signal of ferritin H chain with increase in passage number of MCF-10F cells

the nucleotide level to the coding sequence (exon 4) of human ferritin H chain gene (accession M11146) [43]. The underlined sequence shows 100 % homology at the amino acid translation level to the terminal portion of the mature peptide (nucleotides 584–626) [44, 45].

The expression of ferritin H chain increased with the progression of cell immortalization (Fig. 5.12) and it is highly expressed in the neoplastic cells (Figs. 5.13, 5.14). In situ hybridization using an antisense ribo probe for ferritin H chain showed no signal in normal breast lobules (Fig. 5.15); an increased localized signal was observed in areas with ductal hyperplasia (Fig. 5.15), The same information was obtained by Northern blot (Fig. 5.14). Breast biopsies containing areas with carcinoma in situ (Fig. 5.15), and areas with infiltrating duct carcinoma (Fig. 5.15) highly expressed ferritin H. No signal was detected using a sense ribo probe. Normal breast tissue (lobules type 1, 2 and 3) had no detectable signal for ferritin H. One case with mild ductal hyperplasia, 2 moderate ductal hyperplasia and 4 cases of severe

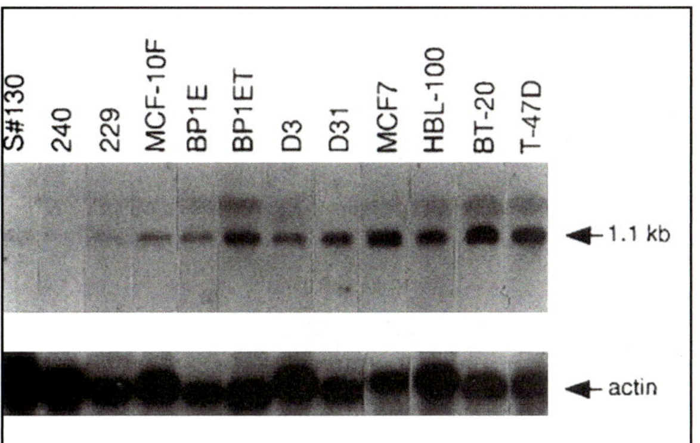

Figure 5.13

Northern analysis of primary, immortal, chemical carcinogen-treated, and cancer human breast epithelial cells (HBECs), showing an increased signal for ferritin H chain mRNA in immortal MCF-10F cells, a much higher signal intensity in MCF-10F cells treated with chemical carcinogens (BP1E, BP1ET, D3, and D3–1), and highest signal intensity in breast cancer cell lines (MCF7, HBL-100, BT-20, and T-47D) (reprinted with permission from: Higgy, N.A., Salicioni, A.M., Russo, I.H., Zhang, P.L. and Russo, J. Differential expression of human ferritin H chain gene in immortal human breast epithelial MCF-10F cells. Molecular Carcinogenesis, 20:332–339,1997)

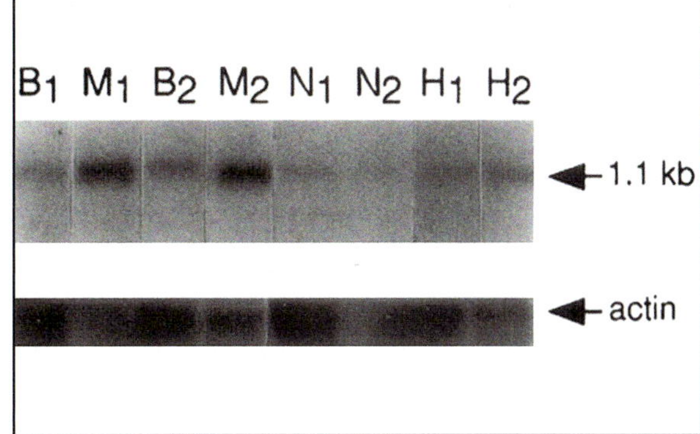

Figure 5.14

Fig. 5.14. Northern analysis of total RNA from breast cancer tissue (M1 and M2), normal tissue from the same patient (B1 and B2), normal control breast tissue (N1 and N2), and tissue with ductal hyperplasia (H1 and H2). High signal intensity is seen in the malignant tissue, very low levels are detected in normal tissue samples, and an increase in signal above normal levels is seen in tissue showing ductal hyperplasia (reprinted with permission from: Higgy, N.A., Salicioni, A.M., Russo, I.H., Zhang, P.L. and Russo, J. Differential expression of human ferritin H chain gene in immortal human breast epithelial MCF-10F cells. Molecular Carcinogenesis, 20:332–339,1997)

ductal hyperplasia showed an increase in signal intensity correlating with the degree of hyperplasia. Ductal carcinoma in situ had more intense labeling signal while invasive ductal and lobular carcinoma showed the highest levels of reactivity.

The increase of ferritin H chain gene may provide iron necessary for the clonal selection and uncontrolled growth of cells (Fig. 5.16). It has been shown that iron and its binding proteins participate in a variety of reactions required for cell proliferation [46, 47], it is critical for the activity of the enzyme ribonucleotide reductase, a rate-limiting step in DNA synthesis [48, 49].

Ferritin has been shown to have an immunosuppressive effect on host immune response in cancer patients [43, 50]. Placental isoferritin (PLF), an acidic form of ferritin, and its p43 super heavy chain were described to be synthesized by breast cancer cells but

absent in normal breast epithelium [51]. Breast cancer associated p43 induces alterations of the expression of cell surface molecules in breast cancer cells that could have an effect on the modulation of cancer cell adhesive interactions [52]. Cytokines such as TNF, interleukin 1α, and NF-κB family of transcription factors specifically induce synthesis of ferritin H, by selective increase in ferritin H transcription (Fig. 5.16) [52, 53].

Increased ferritin H chain gene transcription may contribute to immortalization of HBECs through several possible mechanisms; it may be a source of iron required by rapidly dividing cells for clonal expansion; it may provide iron capable of participating in free radical reactions leading to oxidative DNA damage and mutation; or it may affect immune surface antigens and provide immortal cells with growth advantage by escaping immune surveillance. Ferritin

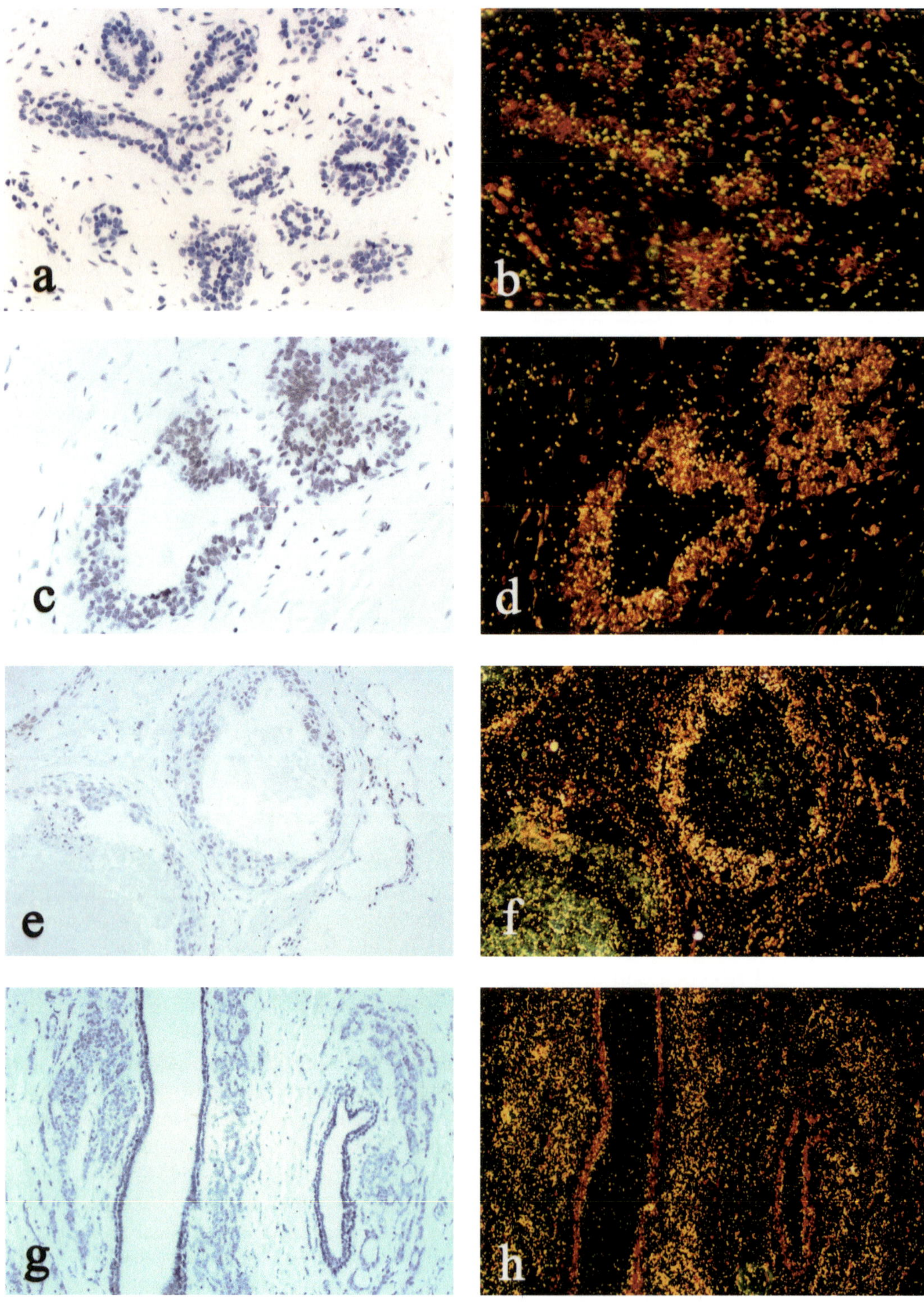

Figure 5.16

The possible role of increased ferritin H chain gene in HBEC immortalization and malignancy (reprinted with permission from: Higgy, N.A., Salicioni, A.M., Russo, I.H., Zhang, P.L. and Russo, J. Differential expression of human ferritin H chain gene in immortal human breast epithelial MCF-10F cells. Molecular Carcinogenesis, 20:332–339, 1997)

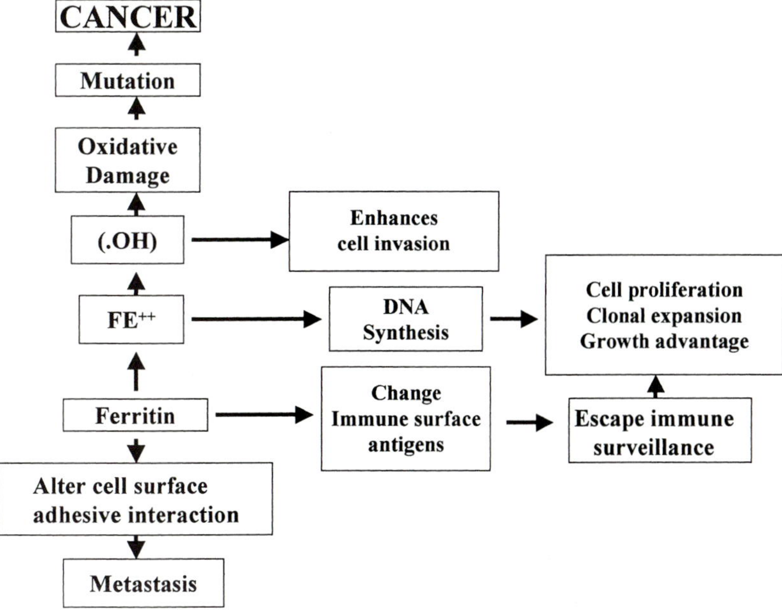

Normal breast lobules. **a** Hematoxylin staining, ×100. **b** In situ hybridization showing low background signal, ×100. **c** Hematoxylin staining. **d** In situ hybridization showing an increase in labeling for ferritin H chain mRNA, ×100. **e** Hematoxylin staining, ×100. **f** In situ hybridization, ×100. **g** Hematoxylin staining, ×100. **h** In situ hybridization showing a marked increase in labeling intensity, ×100 (reprinted with permission from: Higgy, N.A., Salicioni, A.M., Russo, I.H., Zhang, P.L. and Russo, J. Differential expression of human ferritin H chain gene in immortal human breast epithelial MCF-10F cells. Molecular Carcinogenesis, 20:332–339, 1997)

H chain gene induction may either be a consequence of, or an inducer of cell immortalization. In either instance, it may prove to become a valuable marker of cell immortalization and/or an early indicator of malignant transformation (Fig. 5.16).

5.4.2 S100P Calcium-Binding Protein as a Marker of Cancer Initiation

Differential display techniques identified a band called 10F-D, which was differentially amplified using the primers $HT_{11}C$ and HAP-6 in the immortal cell line MCF-10F as compared to its mortal parental counterpart S130 cells (Fig. 5.17). After the search for homologies in gene-bank databases (GenBank + EMBL + DDBJ + PDB) was completed, the cDNA band 10F-D (439 bp) showed very high homology (99%) to the *H. sapiens* mRNA encoding for the calcium-binding protein S100P (Fig. 5.18) [4].

The Northern analysis confirmed the differential expression of S100P. The level of S100P expression was increased 9–10-fold in the immortal cells including MCF-10F (spontaneously immortalized), BP1E (BP-transformed) [54], D3.1 (7,12-dimethyl-benz(a) anthracene (DMBA)-transformed; [54] and T47D (tumor cell line) as compared to the S130 mortal cells and two primary cultures 244 and 248 (Fig. 5.19).

The expression of S100P was also clearly upregulated (2–20-fold) in ductal invasive carcinomas when compared to their normal adjacent tissues (Figs. 5.20,

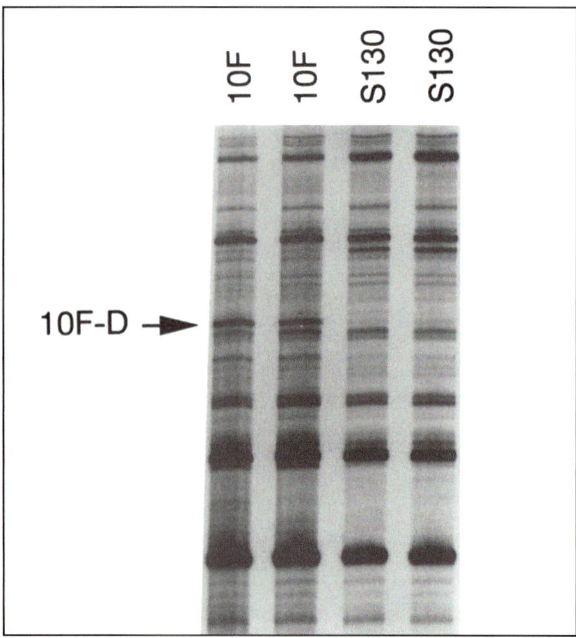

Figure 5.17

Differential display gel, in duplicate, using total RNA from the spontaneously immortalized HBECs MCF-10F (*10F lanes*) and its mortal parental counterpart S130 cells (*S130 lanes*). The *arrow* shows the band called 10F-D displayed only in the immortal cells (reprinted with permission from: Ismael D.C.G. Silva, Yun Fu Hu, Irma H. Russo, Xiang Ao, Ana M. Salicioni, Xiaoqi Yang and Jose Russo[3]. S100P Ca[+2]-binding Protein Overexpression is Associated with Immortalization and Neoplastic Transformation of Human Breast Epithelial Cells in vitro and Tumor Progression in vivo. International Journal of Oncology 16:231–240, 2000)

Figure 5.18

Nucleotide and amino acid sequence of 10F-D. The underlined bases represent the start and stop codons from S100P calcium-binding protein

S100 P (10F-D) sequence, the ORF is highlighted, start and stop codons underlined.

AAGCTTGCACC**ATG**AGGAACTAGAGACAGCCATGGGCATGATCATAGACGT

CTTTTCCCGATATTCGGGCAGCGAGGGCAGCACGCAGACCTGACCAAGGGG

GAGCTCAAGGTGCTGATGGAGAAGGAGCTACCAGGCTTCCTGCAGAGTGGA

AAAGACAAGGATGCCGTGGATAAATTGCTCAAGGACCTGGACGCCAATGGA

GATGCCCAGGTGGACTTCAGTGAGTTCATCGTGTTCGTGGCTGCAATCACG

TCTGCCTGTCACAAGTACTTTGAAGAAGGCAGGACTCAAATGATGCCCTGG

AGATGTCACAGATCCTGCAGAGCCATGGTCCCAGGCTTCCCAAAAGTGTTT

GTTGGCAATTATTCCCCTAGGCTGAGCCTGCTCATATACCGCTGATTAATA

AATGCTTATGAAAAAAAAAAAAAAAAAAA

S100 P (10F-D) amino acid sequence

MTELETAMGMIIDVFSRYSGSEGSTQTLTKGELKVLMEKELPGFLQSGKDK

DAVDKLLKDLDANGDAQVDFSEFIVFVAAITSACHKYFFEKAGL

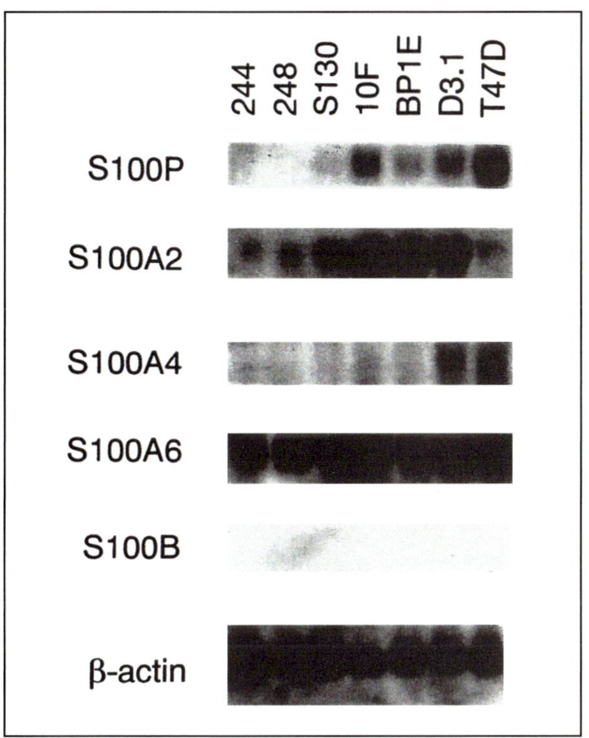

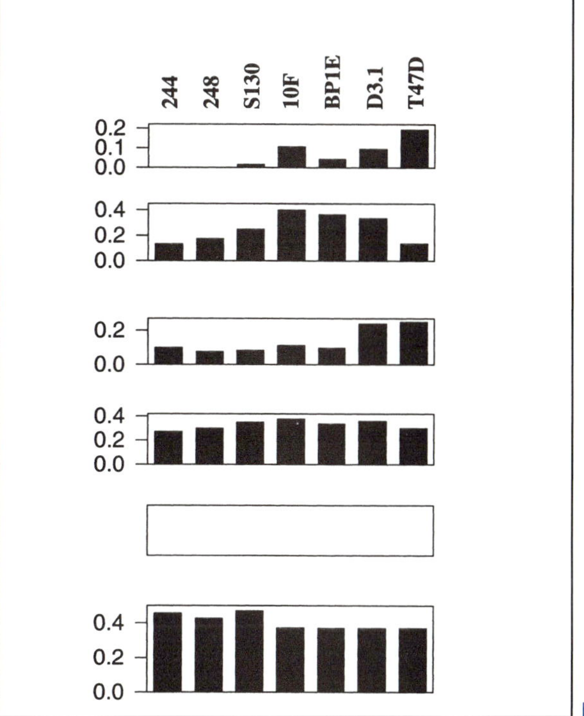

Figure 5.19 a, b

a Northern blot hybridization using ^{32}P labeled S100P, S100A2, S100A4, S100A6, and S100B cDNA as probes. The blot contained 30 µg of total RNA from samples 244 and 248 (primary culture cells); S130 and MCF-10F (mortal and immortal cell lines. respectively), BPIE and D3.1 (benzo(a)pyrene and DMBA transformed cell lines, respectively) and T47D (breast cancer cell line). S100P started being expressed only when the cells became spontaneously immortalized (10F), and became also expressed in transformed (BPIE and D3.1) and breast cancer cell lines (T47D). S100A2 and S100AG were expressed in all cell lines with the difference that S100A2 seemed downregulated in primary and mortal cells as well as in T47D. S100A4 was present only in DMBA transformed cells (D3.1) and in the breast cancer cell line T47D. S100B was not expressed in these cells. β-actin mRNA detection was used as a control for verifying the loading of RNA samples. **b** Histogram showing relative mRNA expression of S100P, S100A2, S100A4, S100A6 and S100B in primaries (samples 244 and 243), mortal (S130). Immortal (MCF-10F), benzo(a)pyrene transformed (BPIE), DMBA transformed (D3.1) and breast cancer (T47D) cells. S100P expression was increased 9–10-fold in the spontaneously immortalized HBEC MCF-10F when compared to its mortal parental counterpart S130 or primary cultures (samples 244 and 243). The S100P gene was kept activated in the chemical transformed (BPIE and D3 1) and breast cancer (T47D) cell lines, S100A1 was 10–20 times upregulated in D3.1 and T47D cells. S100A6 seemed equally expressed while S100A2 expression was 1–2-fold increased in MCF-10F, BPIE and D3.1 (reprinted with permission from: Ismael D.C.G. Silva, Yun Fu Hu, Irma H. Russo, Xiang Ao, Ana M. Salicioni, Xiaoqi Yang and Jose Russo. S100P Ca[+2]-binding Protein Overexpression is Associated with Immortalization and Neoplastic Transformation of Human Breast Epithelial Cells in vitro and Tumor Progression in vivo. International Journal of Oncology 16:231–240, 2000)

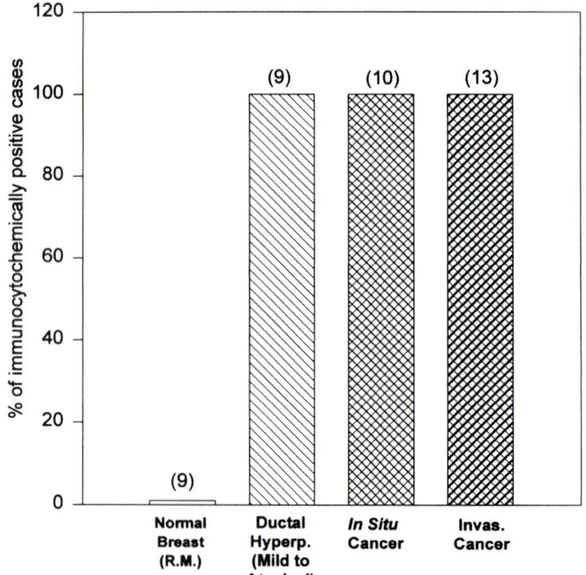

Figure 5.20

Histogram depicting the percentage of breast tissue reaction with S100P by immunocytochemistry. The *numbers in parenthesis* are the total numbers of cases studied

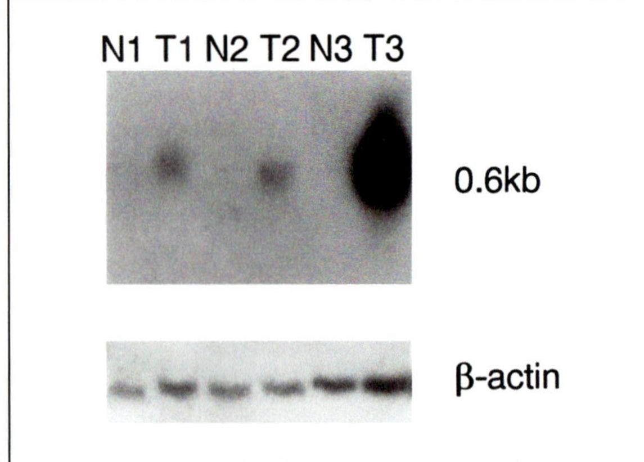

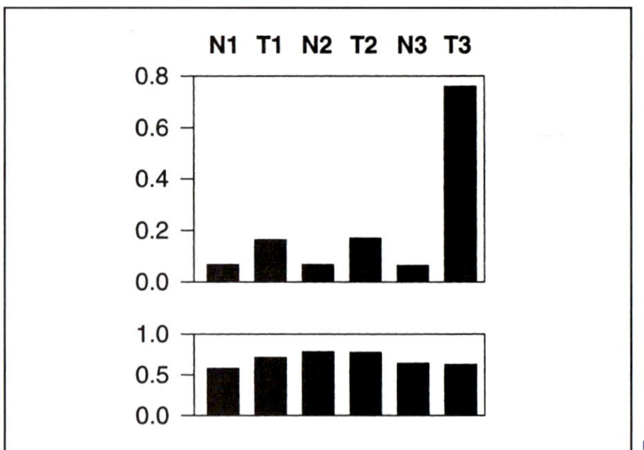

Figure 5.21 a, b

a Northern blot analysis of 30 µg of total RNA from ductal invasive carcinoma samples (Tl–T3) and its respective adjacent normal breast tissue (Nl–N3) S100P labeled probe were used. One transcript with 0.6 kb was detected only in the tumor samples. T3 contains RNA from a poor differentiated, lymph node positive ductal invasive carcinoma. b Histogram showing that relative S100P expression was increased 2–20-fold in the tumor samples Tl, T2 and T3 when compared to their normal adjacent tissues N1, N2 and N3. In the lane containing RNA from a poorly differentiated, lymph node positive ductal invasive carcinoma (T3), the S100P expression was increased 20 times as compared to the other two tumors Tl and T2

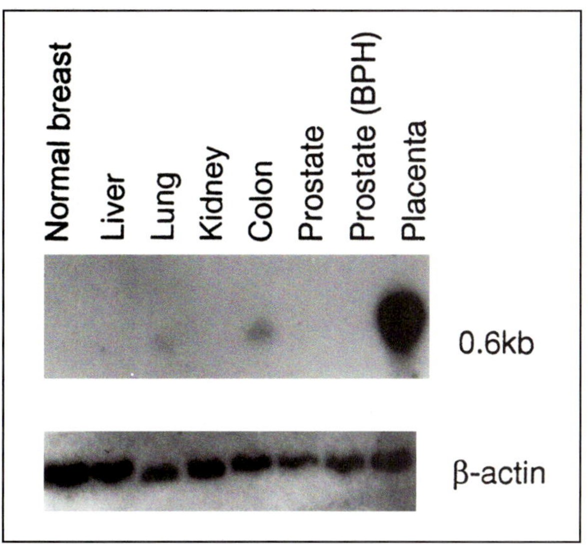

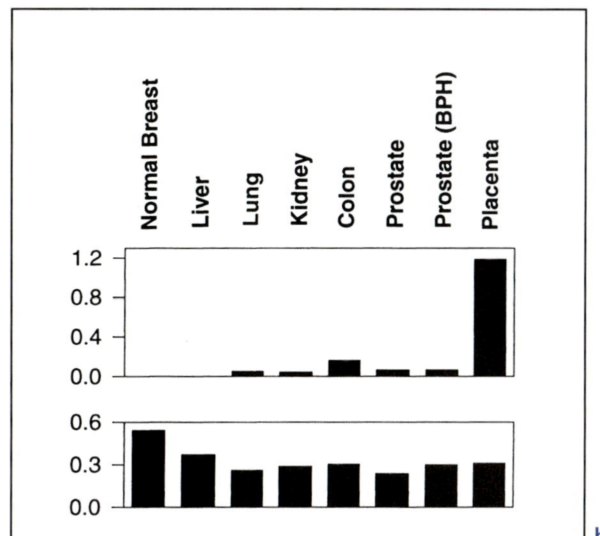

Figure 5.22 a, b

a Northern blot analysis of 30 µg of total RNA from human liver, lung, kidney, colon, prostate, benign prostatic hyperplasia and full-term placenta, after hybridization with S100P labeled probe. S100P expression was present in very low amount in lung and colon when compared to the amount of expression seen in full-term placenta. β-actin labeled probes were used to assess the RNA loading in each lane. **b** Histogram showing that relative S100P expression was increased 20-fold in placenta when compared to other tissues such as prostate, benign prostatic hyperplasia, kidney, liver and normal, breast. A 0.5–1-fold increase in expression was found in colon and lung (reprinted with permission from: Ismael D.C.G. Silva, Yun Fu Hu, Irma H. Russo, Xiang Ao, Ana M. Salicioni, Xiaoqi Yang and Jose Russo[3]. S100P Ca^{+2}-binding Protein Overexpression is Associated with Immortalization and Neoplastic Transformation of Human Breast Epithelial Cells in vitro and Tumor Progression in vivo. International Journal of Oncology 16:231– 240, 2000)

5.21). Notably, a much higher increase in S100P overexpression (20-fold) was observed in breast cancer. RNA from a poorly differentiated, lymph node-positive, ductal invasive carcinoma sample. In various normal tissues we examined, the expression of S100P was high (10–15-fold) in full-term placenta, low in lung, breast and colon and essentially absent in other tissues (Fig. 5.22).

Immunocytochemical localization of S100P with monoclonal antibodies was absent in all the normal breast tissue analyzed. All the ductal hyperplasias, typical and atypical, ductal carcinomas in situ and invasive carcinomas were positive (Fig. 5.23). Interestingly, cases of morphologically normal breast tissues adjacent to five ductal hyperplasias, two of the carcinomas in situ and three of the invasive carcinomas

were slightly positive for S100P. The S100P protein was localized in the cytoplasm of the epithelial cells and tended to accumulate at high concentrations in the apical and supranuclear regions (Fig. 5.24).

The S100P calcium-binding protein, first isolated from human placenta [55, 56], belongs to the family of S100 calcium-binding proteins initially characterized as a group of abundant low molecular weight acidic proteins (10–12 kDa) highly enriched in nervous tissue [57]. S100 proteins are characterized by a common structural motif, the EF-hand domain, which consists of 12 amino acid residues and binds to calcium with high affinity and specificity [58]. Calcium is not only an essential component of cell membrane structures influencing their viscosity and permeability, but also a major second messenger in the

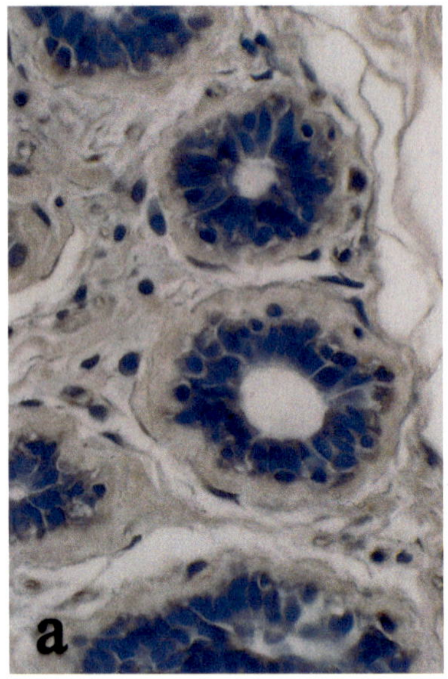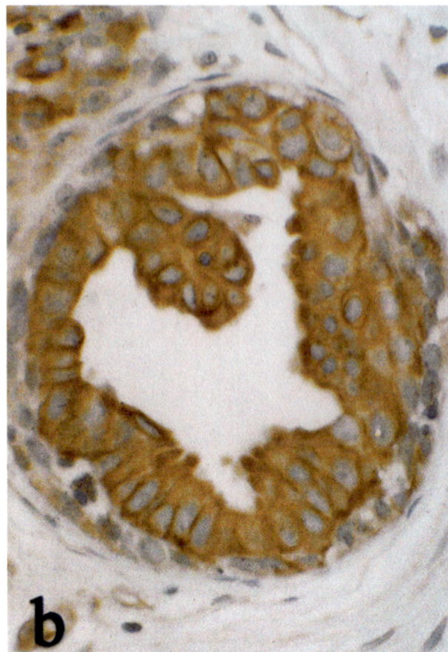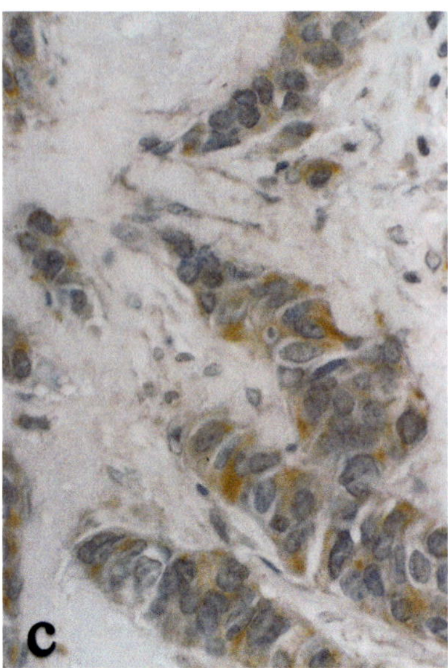

Figure 5.23 a–c

Immunocytochemical localization of S100P in paraffin sections of formalin fixed tissue. **a** Normal breast epithelial and myoepithelial cells of the ductules of a lobule type 1, ×60. **b** Carcinoma in situ. **c** Invasive ductal carcinoma, ×60

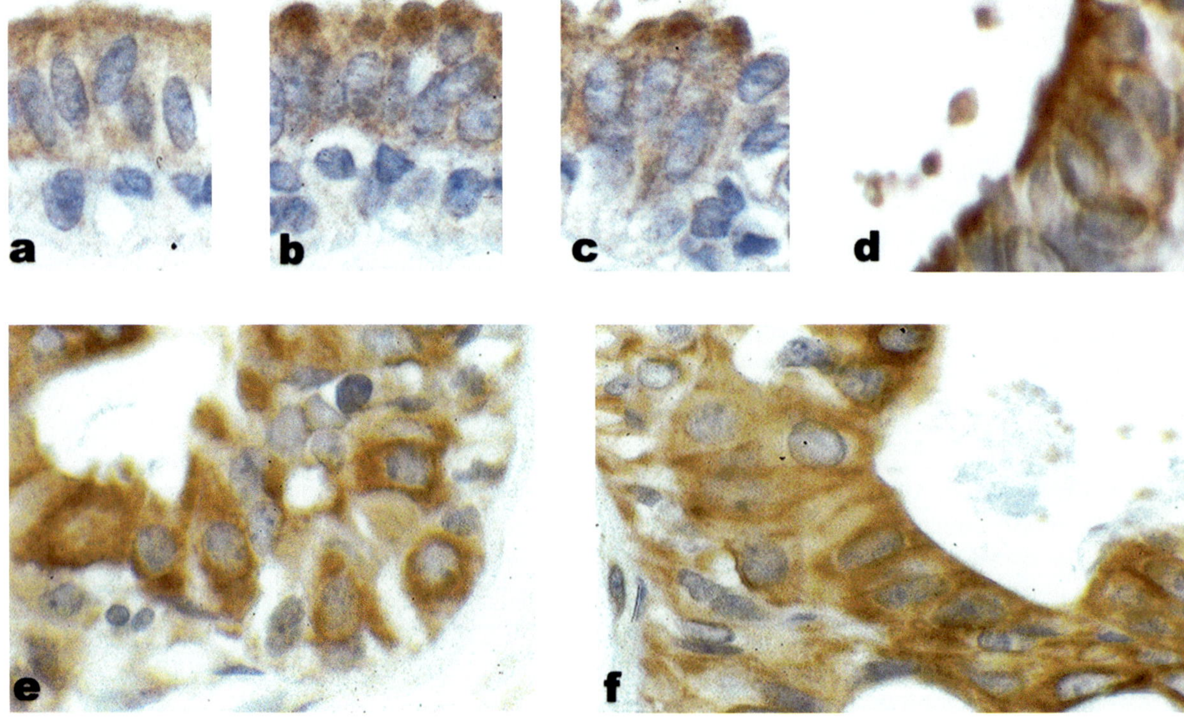

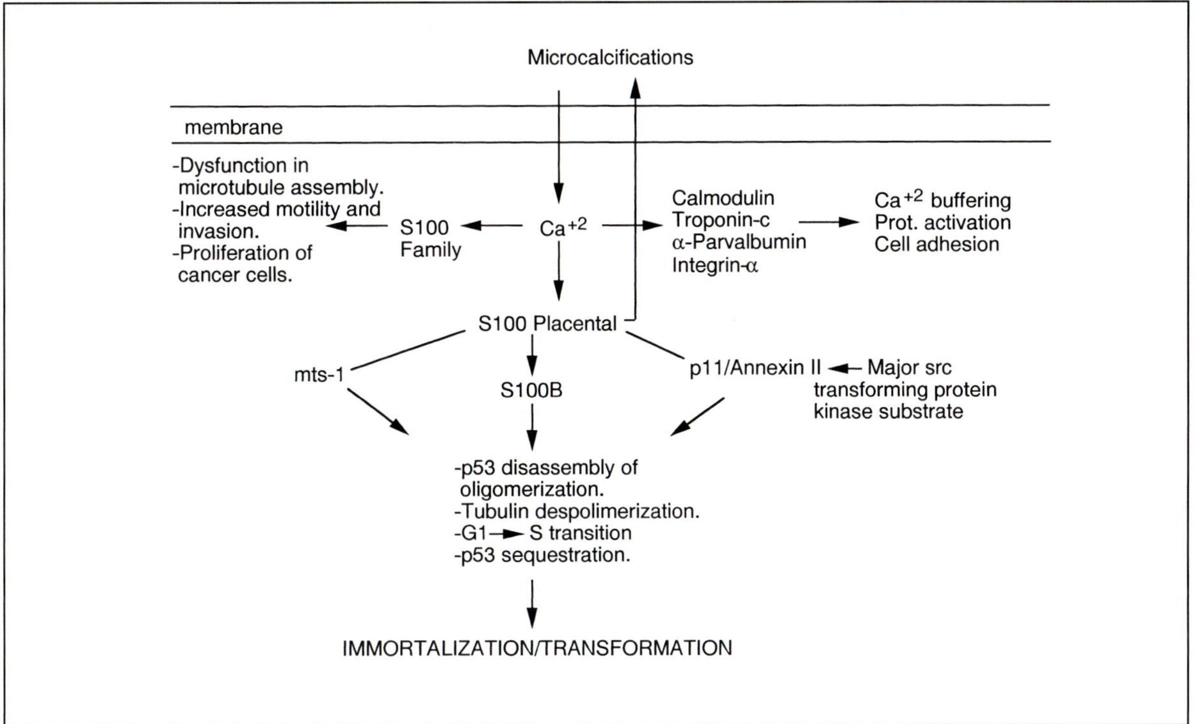

◄ Figure 5.24 a–f

a Immunocytochemical localization of S100P in the cytoplasm of epithelial cells from a ductal hyperplasia of the breast. **b, c** show the immunoreacted protein migrating toward the apical portion of the cells and extruding in the lumen (**d**); **e, f** strong reactivity in the cytoplasm of invasive ductal carcinoma, × 40

Figure 5.25

Hypothetical model explaining how S100P could be involved in the mechanisms of immortalization and transformation of HBEC. S100P shares considerable homology with the mts-1 gene (metastasis-associated gene), which was postulated to be involved in p53 sequestration, tubulin depolymerization, and G1–S transition. S100P is also very similar to p11, the regulatory subunit of annexin 11, and the major cytoplasmic avian sarcoma viruses (src) transforming protein kinases substrate. At the amino acid level, S100P shares 50.6% homology with S100B that binds P53 and not only induces total inhibition of P53 oligomerization but also promotes disassembly of the P53 oligomerization making this protein a cellular target for the S100 family members involved in cell cycle control at the GO-GI/S boundary. Because S100P calcium-binding protein overexpression is a very early event in the carcinogenic process we also postulate that this imbalance in the calcium metabolism might explain the micro-calcification phenomena, a very important signal found in the early stages of malignancy. Other functions of the EF-hand calcium-binding proteins, other than S100P, proteins are also shown

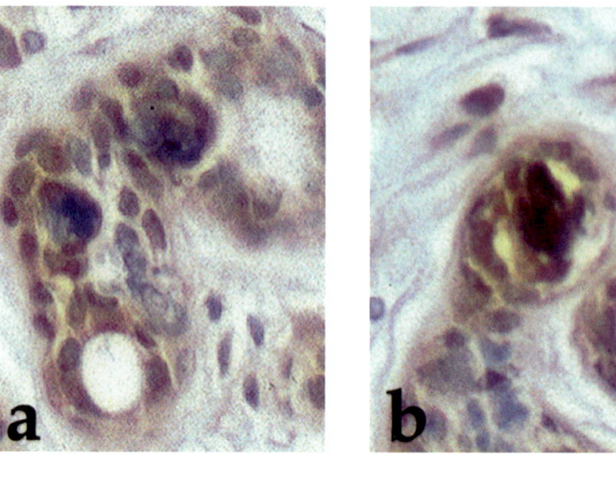
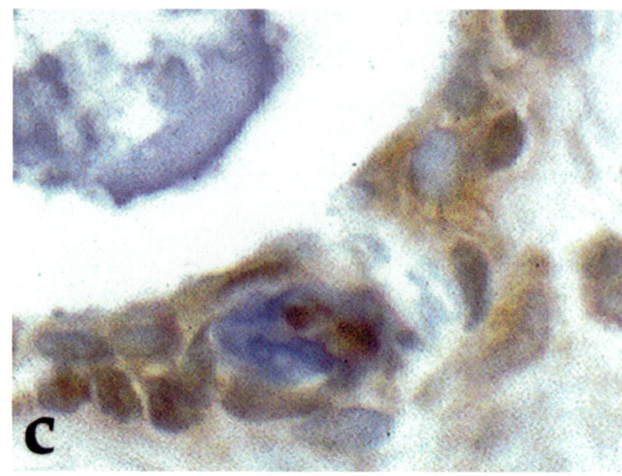
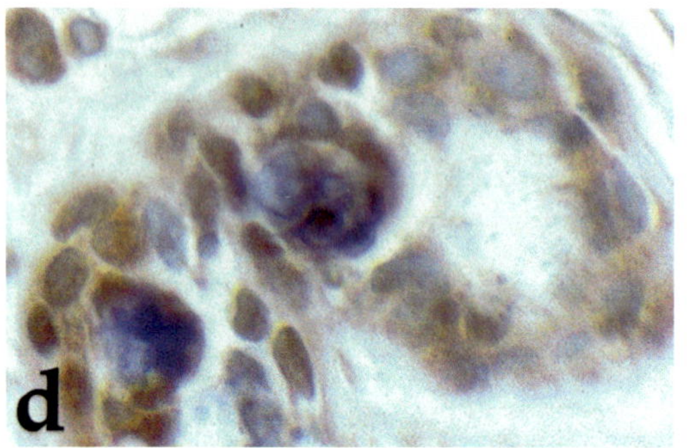
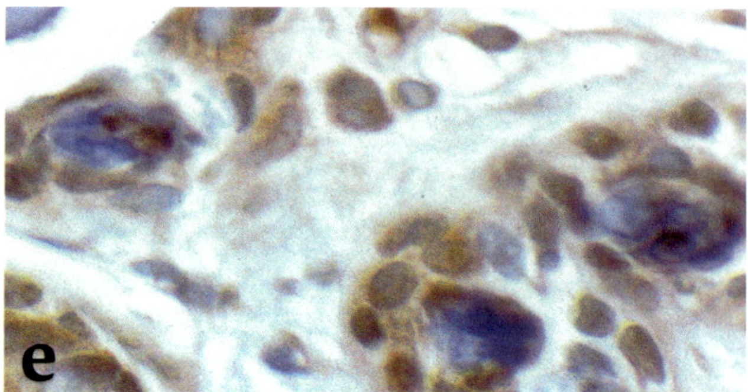

control of a variety of biological processes, such as cell cycle progression, differentiation and cell death [59]. An increase in the concentration of calcium in culture media decreases cell proliferation and induces cell differentiation in HBEC [60, 61], whereas lowering concentration of calcium in the culture media extends the lifespan of primary cultures and mortal HBEC [40, 41]. Intracellular concentration of calcium is tightly controlled by a number of calcium-binding proteins and an increase in calcium-binding proteins could conceivably diminish the intracellular pool of free calcium [59]. In this regard, our current finding that S100P is overexpressed during the process of cell immortalization appears to provide an explanation for our previous observation that the intracellular concentration of free calcium is higher in the mortal cells as compared to the immortal cells [62]. It should be noted, however, that preferential expression of S100P mRNA occurs in immortal cells, but not their

Figure 5.26 a–e

Immunocytochemical localization of S100P in relation with micro-calcification of ductal hyperplasia, ×40

mortal parental counterparts or primary HBEC cultures, regardless of different calcium concentrations. These results suggest that the S100P protein might be one of the molecules involved in specific pathways of cell cycle control whose imbalance might enable cells to escape from senescence reaching therefore the immortal cell status (Fig. 5.25). Although it is important to correlate the expression of S100 during the process of cell immortalization and with the ability of these cells to pump the Ca^{2+} out of the cells more efficiently and also be implicated with the formation of micro calcifications (Fig. 5.26).

5.4.3 Role of Intracellular Ca^{2+} During Cell Immortalization and Cell Transformation

The growth of HBECs cells in culture is strongly regulated by the concentration of calcium in the culture medium [60]. These cells grow and can be subcultured for up to 1 year if the Ca^{2+} concentrations in the culture medium ranges from 0.03 to 0.06 mM [40, 62]. In this culture condition, the majority of the cells assume a spherical morphology (Figs. 5.27, 5.28), produce duct-like structures in collagen, display all the ultrastructural features of breast epithelial cells, and maintain their normal diploid karyotype [40]. If the calcium concentration in the medium is elevated to 1.05 mM or above, the cells change their morphology to mainly elongated and flattened cells which form tight junctions and domes at confluence (Figs. 5.27. 5.28) [41, 62]. This change takes place as early as 5 h after the switch from low to high calcium medium and the cells finally undergo terminal differentiation and stop dividing [40, 62]. The calcium-induced changes in growth properties have also been reported in other epithelial cells derived from epidermis, bronchus, and esophagus [63, 64].

The relative calcium concentration maps using indo-1 fluorescence dye revealed that the mortal human breast epithelial cells do not effectively buffer their intracellular calcium (Ca$_i$) against elevated levels of extracellular calcium (Ca$_o$), as shown in Fig. 5.29. Elevation of Ca$_o$ from 0.04 to 1.05 mM resulted in elevated and sustained increases in Ca$_i$ for at least 30 min, as evidenced by Fig. 5.29. The immortal and transformed HBECs, on the other hand, did not show observable increases in their Ca$_i$ subsequent to the elevation of Ca$_o$ to 1.05 mM. Ca$_i$ of both mortal and immortal HBECs growing in medium containing

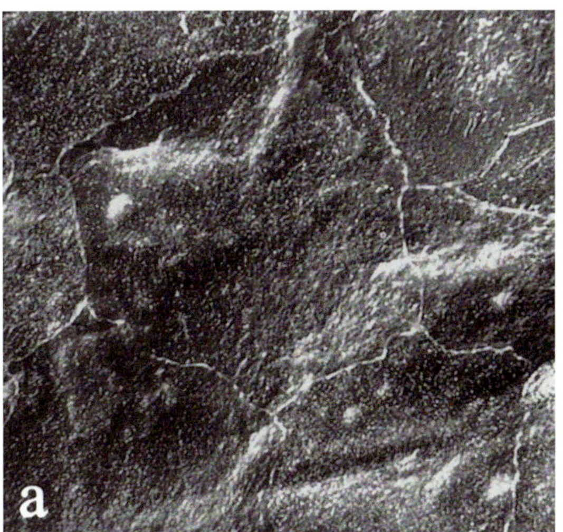

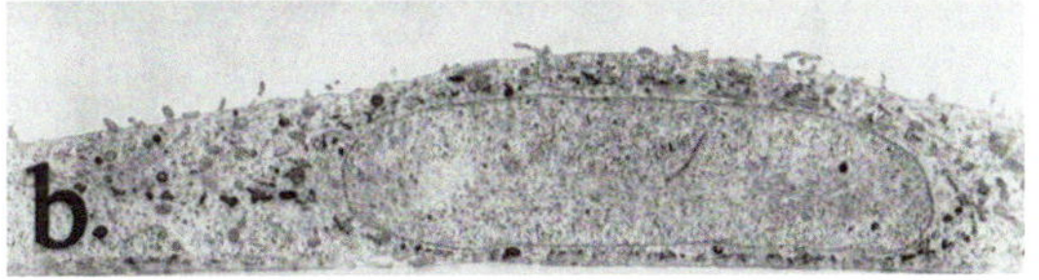

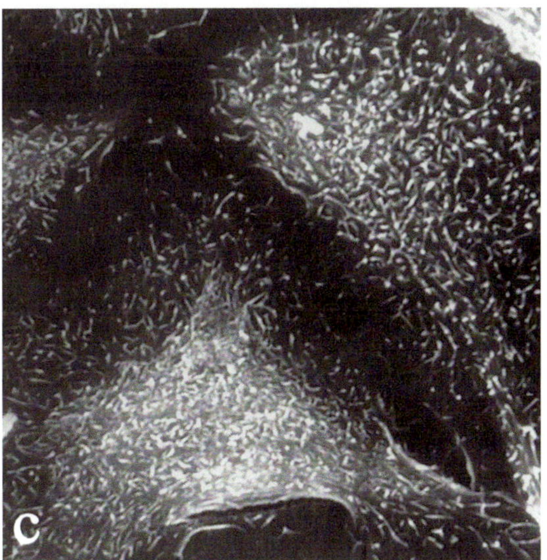

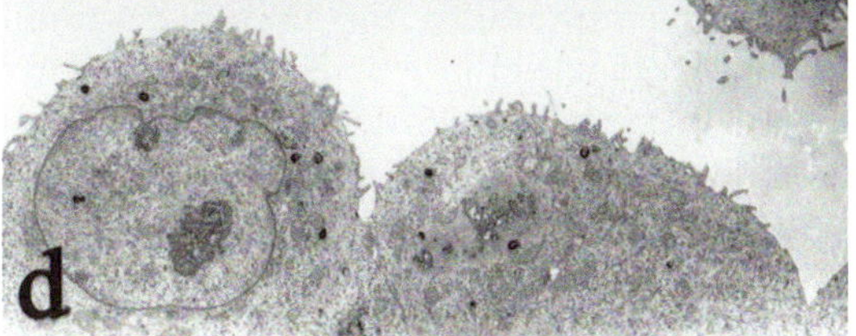

a Scanning electron micrograph of MCF-10F cells growing in high calcium covered with short microvilli and closely attached with a ridge between cells, ×2,000. b Electron micrograph of a cross section of a, ×2,000. c MCF-10F cells growing in monolayer in low calcium. The cells are round and covered by long microvilli ×2,000. d Electron micrograph of c, ×2,000

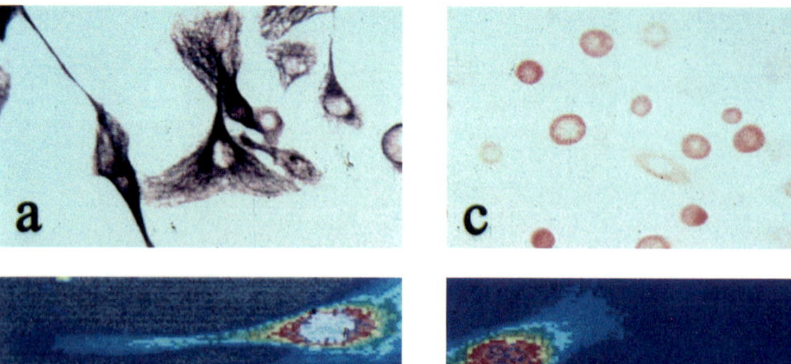

Figure 5.28 a–d

a Monolayer cultures of HBEC in chamber slides stained for immunocytochemistry with antibodies against tubulin and growing in high Ca^{2+} medium, ×40. **b** Cells stained with fura-2A. **c** Cells growing in low Ca^{2+} medium, ×40. **d** Cell stained with fura-2A. The cells growing in high calcium concentrate more intra-cellular Ca^{2+} (**b**) than those growing in low Ca^{2+} (**d**)

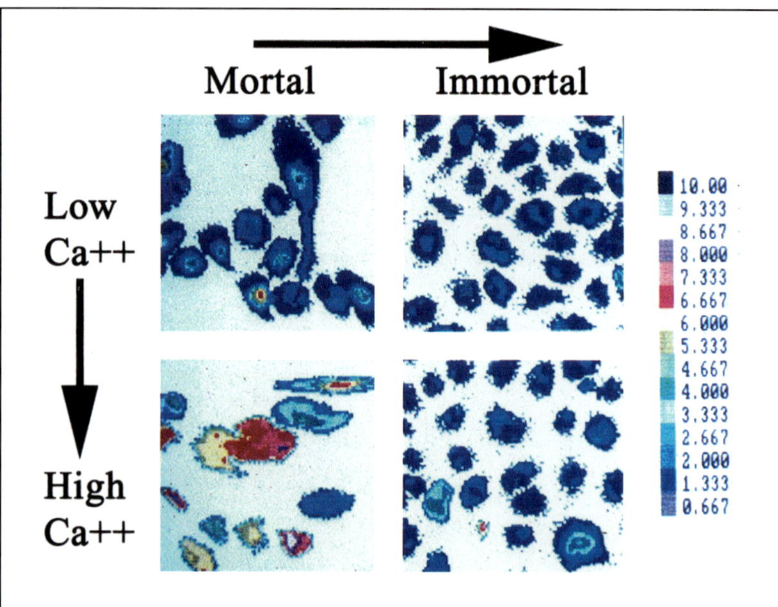

Figure 5.29

Relative levels of Ca in HBEC expressed as a function of Ca levels of Ca_i. Levels of Ca_i in mortal and immortal cells in medium containing 0.04 mM Ca are shown in *upper panel*, whereas Ca_i levels 30 min after the switch to medium containing 1.05 mM Ca are shown in *lower panel*

0.04 mM was maintained at a very low concentration (approximately 20 nM). However, if the extracellular calcium was increased to 1.05 mM, the Ca^{2+} increased 2–3-fold in the mortal cells, as depicted in Fig. 5.30. The immortal and oncogene transformed cell lines on the other hand did not show significant changes in their Ca_i following the elevation of Ca_o from 0.04 to 1.05 mM, as shown in Fig. 5.30. The Ca_i of both MCF-10A and MCF-l0AneoT was maintained at around 20 nM regardless of the Ca_o levels. To test whether or not the increased Ca_i in the mortal cells was reversible, cells that had been grown in high calcium medium for 3 days were switched back to low calcium for 24 h. Ca_i in MCF-10 M cells dropped precipitously

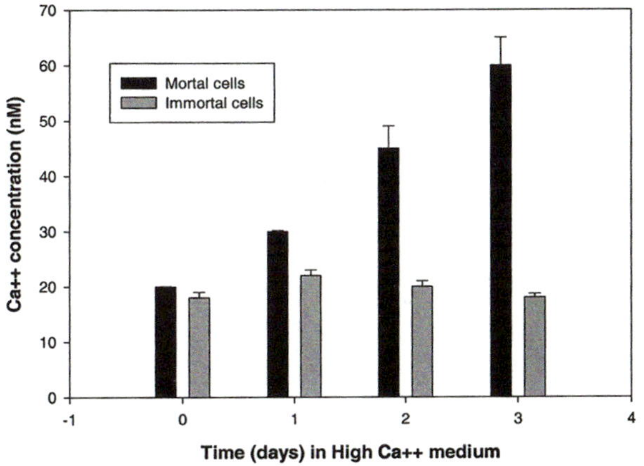

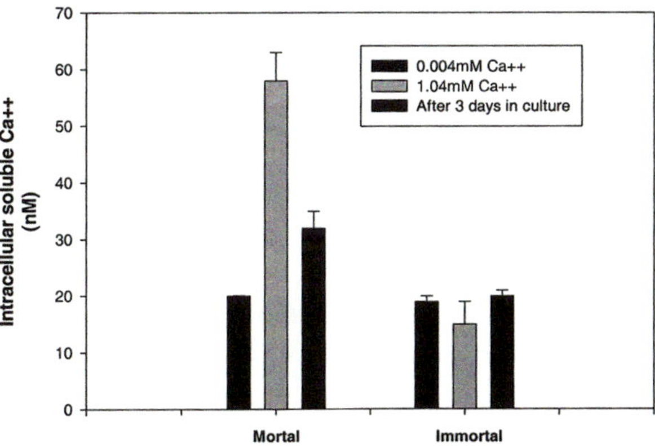

Figure 5.30

Quantitation of Ca in mortal and immortal cells. The cells were grown in medium containing 0.04 mM calcium and then switched to medium containing 1.05 mM Ca^{2+} for the specified periods. The cells were trypsinized, washed, and loaded with fura-2A for Ca_i ($p < 0.001$)

Figure 5.31

Reversibility of Ca_i increases in mortal and immortal cells in response to low and high Ca. The cells were grown in medium containing 0.04 mM Ca^{2+} (*solid bars*) or 1.05 mM Ca^{2+} (*gray bars*) for 3 days before harvesting. Part of the cells that had been grown in medium containing 1.05 mM Ca^{2+} for 3 days were replated in 0.04 mM Ca^{2+} medium for 24 h, trypsinized, washed, and Ca, was determined (*dark bars*) ($p < 0.001$ and $p < 0.001$ respectively)

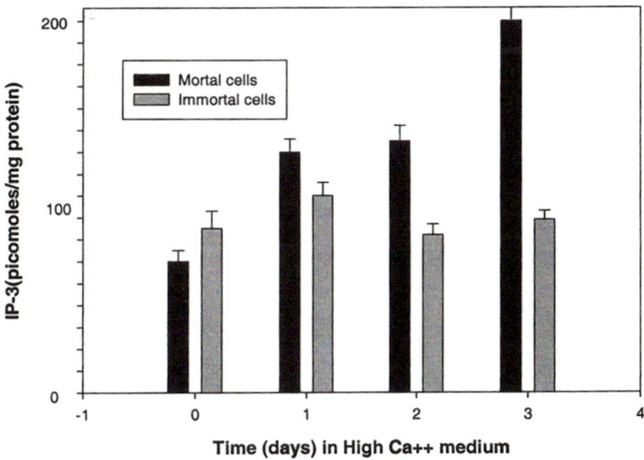

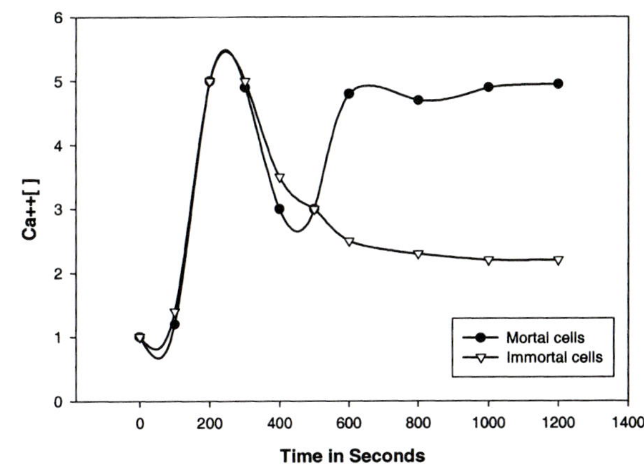

Figure 5.32

Quantitation of intracellular IP_3 in MCF-10 M, MCF-10A, and MCF-10AneoT. The cells were grown in medium containing 0.04 mM Ca^{2+} and then switched to medium containing 1.05 mM Ca^{2+} for the specified periods. The cells were then trypsinized, washed with PBS, and IP3 was determined as described in the text ($p < 0.001$)

Figure 5.33

Curves showing the mobilization of Ca^{2+} in mortal and immortal cells after the switch of medium from low to high Ca^{2+}

subsequent to a switch back to low calcium medium, as shown in Fig. 5.31. The immortal and transformed cells, on the other hand, did not show a significant difference in their Ca_i levels after the switch back to low calcium medium as expected.

Switching of the mortal cells from low to high calcium medium resulted not only in substantial and significant increase in Ca, but also in significant increases in inositol triphosphate, as depicted in Fig. 5.32. The sustained increases in intracellular IP3 closely matched Ca increases over the 3-day period subsequent to the switch to high calcium medium. The intracellular levels of IP3 in the immortal and transformed HBE cells, on the other hand, did not change significantly, but remained more or less at the basal level (Fig. 5.32).

There is a marked difference in the manner in which mortal HBE cells maintain Ca_i compared with their immortal counterpart when Ca_o is increased. It is well established that nearly all cell types maintain their Ca at a very low concentration compared with Ca_o [65]. To do this, cells have evolved elaborate calcium buffering systems. These include high affinity calcium binding proteins such as calmodulin [66] and Ca-ATPase pump, which actively pumps calcium out from the cells against a calcium concentration gradient [67]. Opposed to these calcium buffering and export systems are the calcium influx pathways which increase intracellular calcium such as the putative calcium channels [65, 68], Na^+/Ca^{2+} exchanger which drives Ca^{2+} into the cells as Na+ is driven out [69] and second messenger molecules such as IP3, which mobilize calcium from its intracellular stores [70].

Any of these calcium buffering or influx pathways may be modified in either the mortal or immortal human breast epithelial cells to account for the differential calcium buffering capacity in these cells. Calcium efflux studies indicated difference in the rate at which Ca^{2+} is extruded from MCF-10 M and MCF-10A cells subsequent to increasing extracellular calcium (Fig. 5.33). The data tend to favor the calcium influx pathways as the ones crucial for the significant increases in Ca_i in the mortal cells. The fact that Ca_i increases in mortal cells is closely correlated to increases in IP3, raises the possibility that increases in extracellular calcium activate phospholipase C, resulting in the hy-

drolysis of phosphoinositol 4,5 bisphosphate phosphate (PIP2) to diacylglycerol and IP3 [70, 71]. The increased IP3 may, in turn, activate the so-called second messenger operated Ca^{2+} channels resulting in calcium influx from the external milieu [72]. It has been shown that the bombesin induced mobilization of IP3 and calcium in the human breast cancer cell line MCF-7 partly depends on the extracellular calcium since the calcium increases could be inhibited by the calcium channel blocker Ni^{2+} [73].

These data show that the ability of calcium to influence in a negative way the growth of normal human breast and other cells of epithelial origin may be solely due to their inability to buffer Ca_i against increases in extracellular calcium. The calcium-mediated induction of terminal differentiation of MCF-10 M requires sustained increases in Ca_i. The increased Ca_i may then activate a series of enzymes, which have been implicated in terminal differentiation such as protein kinase C. The increased intracellular calcium may also activate Ca^{2+}/Mg^{2+} dependent endonuclease, the enzyme system responsible for the fragmentation of cellular DNA leading to programmed cell death [74, 75]. A detailed knowledge of these mechanisms will lead to a better understanding of growth regulation of human breast epithelial cells both in vitro and in vivo.

5.4.4 The Role of Intracellular Calcium and S100 Protein Expression in the Formation of Microcalcifications in Preneoplastic and Neoplastic Lesions of the Breast

The expression of S100P during the process of cell immortalization is closely associated with the alterations in the mobilization of calcium as shown above. The clinical relevance of this finding is that calcium deposits (or microcalcifications) take place in ductal hyperplasia and ductal carcinoma in situ (Figs. 5.26, 5.34, 5.35) is also associated with the overexpression of S100P and ferritin H. The inability of the immortal cells of retaining the Ca_i (Figs. 5.33, 5.36), whereas the mortal cells do, could indicate that this process is linked to the overexpression of S100P. Supporting this explanation is data from electron microscopic

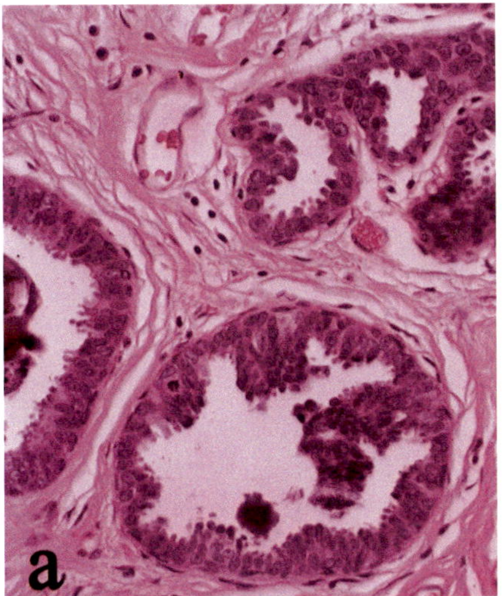
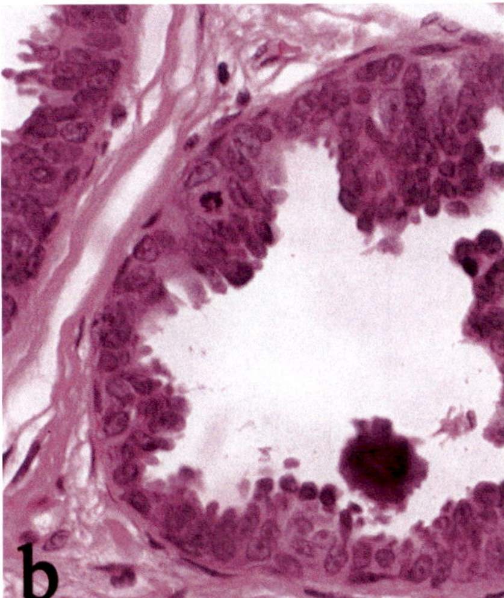
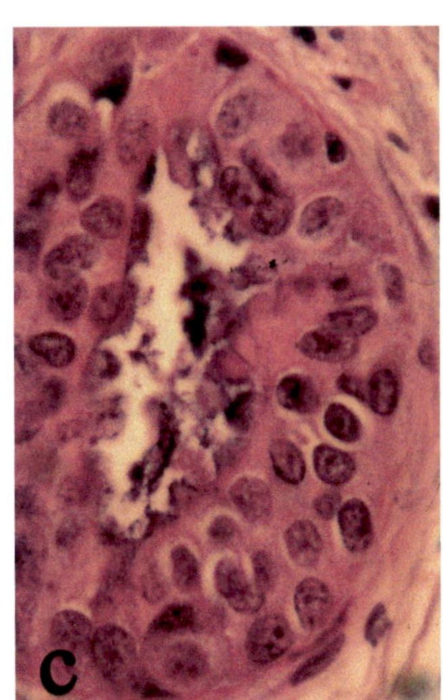

Figure 5.34 a–c

Histological section of ductal carcinoma in situ showing severe microcalcifications (H&E, **a** ×10, **b** ×20, and **c** ×40)

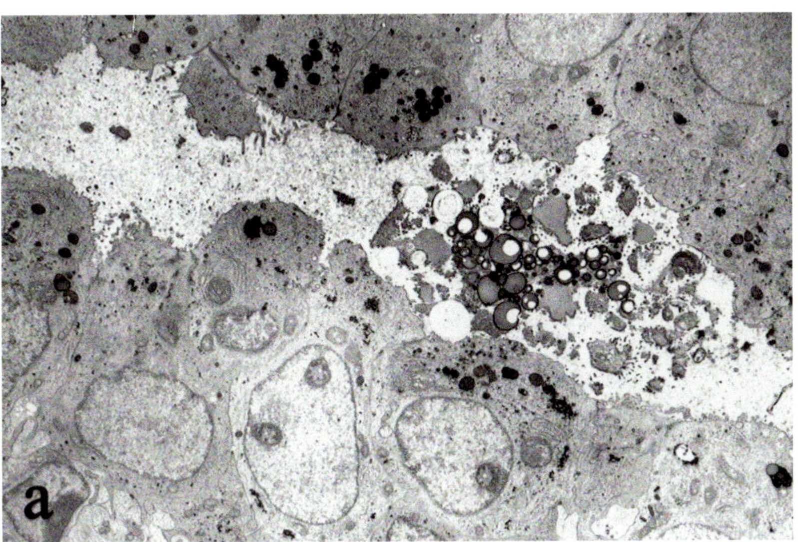
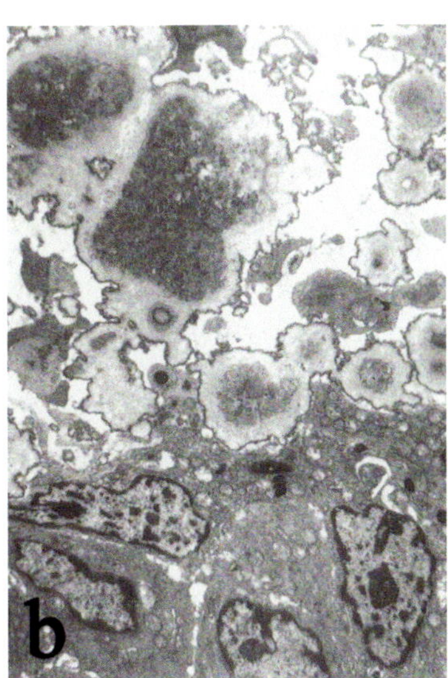

Figure 5.35 a, b

Electron micrograph of ductal hyperplasia showing micro-calcification, ×2,000. **b** Electron micrograph showing the halo of proteinaceous material surrounding the calcium core, ×2,000

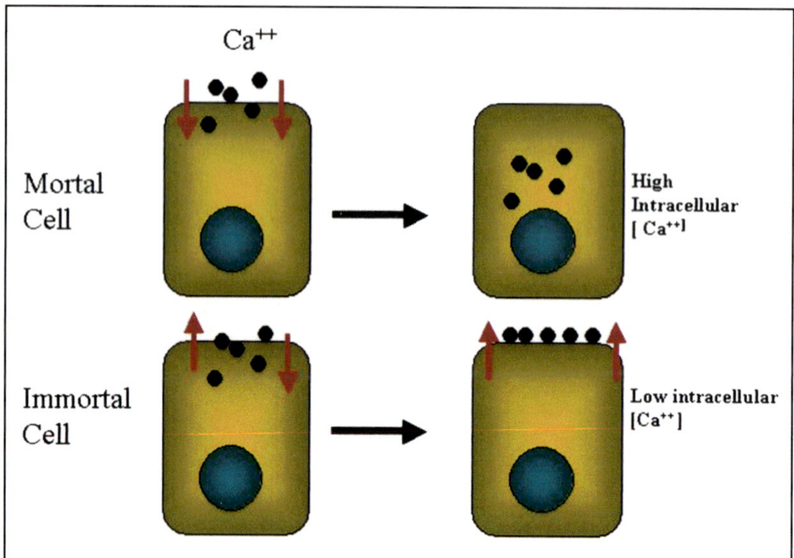

Figure 5.36

Schematic representation of Ca2+ mobilization and formation of microcalcifications

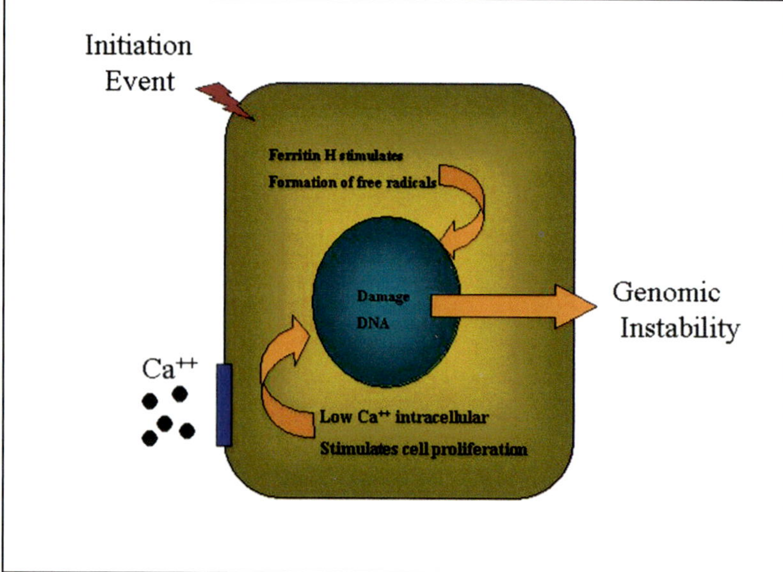

Figure 5.37

Schematic drawing showing the effect of an initiation event in the levels of ferritin H and Ca++ levels in the HBEC. This overexpression of ferritin H may result in the increased formation of free radicals that may be responsible for DNA damage. The low pH concentration may facilitate cell proliferation and both effects may help in genomic instability studies (Fig. 5.35) that show that the accumulation of Ca^{2+} deposits outside the apical portion of the epithelial cells in both atypical ductal hyperplasia and ductal carcinoma in situ, correlate with a proteinaceous material that has been confirmed by immunocytochemistry to be S100P protein (Fig. 5.26). Therefore, it is possible that the phenotypic alterations induced by the immortalization process that is associated with a lack of calcium buffering system, overexpression of S100p protein and ferritin H are all linked. The low Ca_i may result in stimulation of cell proliferation that associated with the high level of ferritin H will increase the formation of more free radicals, resulting in DNA damage that explain the formation of microsatellite instability (MSI), as it has been demonstrated in breast cells in culture [76, 77] as well as in early lesions of the breast (Fig. 5.37) [78].

5.5 Genetic Changes Associated with Initiation and Progression of Breast Cancer

Human neoplasms arise through a progressive accumulation of genetic alterations, such as amplification of different oncogenes and mutation or loss of tumor suppressor genes [79]. Invasive ductal carcinoma of the breast, the most commonly diagnosed malignancy in women, is considered to be the result of a histopathologically defined multistep process that progressively develops through stages of ductal hyperplasia (DH), atypical ductal hyperplasia (ADH), ductal carcinoma in situ (DCIS), invasive ductal carcinoma (IDC), and metastatic disease [79–81]. However, it is not known whether the expression of genetic changes correlates with defined histopathological stages of cancer progression [82–85].

Microsatellites, which are short repetitive sequences of DNA scattered throughout the genome [86, 87] have been used to detect genomic alterations in various human cancers through the identification of loss of heterozygosity (LOH) or MSI [88, 89] (Fig. 5.38). Studies using this approach provided direct evidence for the involvement of chromosomes 13 in human breast carcinomas, and led to the identification of the well-known tumor suppressor gene *RB1*

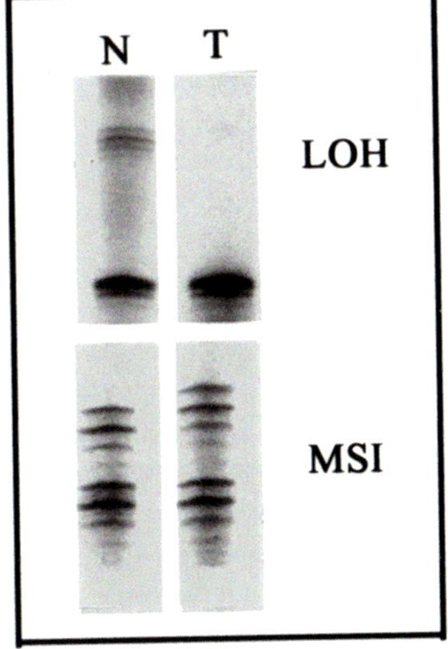

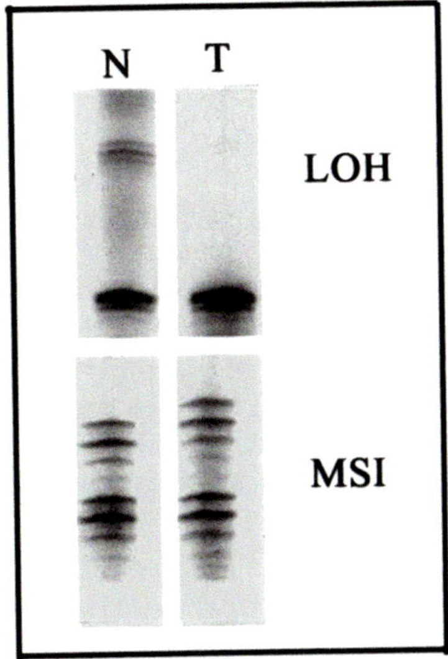

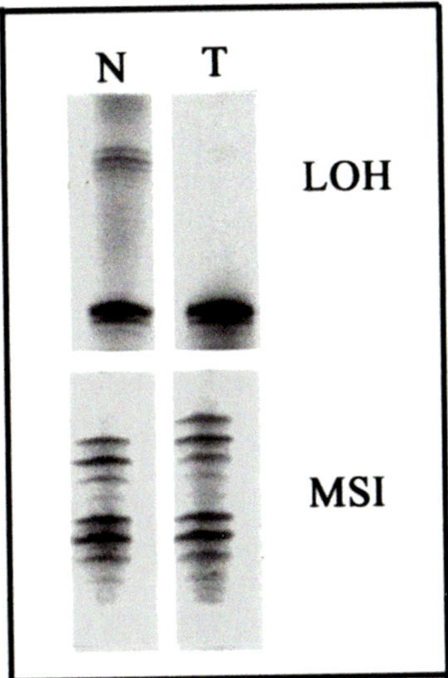

(13q14), and breast cancer susceptibility gene *BRCA2* (13q12–13) [90].

The completion of the genomic project provided unlimited possibilities to understand the role of genes in breast cancer (see Chapter 8). Of significant importance is also the development of new techniques like cDNA array, proteomic, tissue microarray and laser capture microdissection that alone or in combination has broadened our perspectives in breast cancer research.

5.5.1 Laser Capture Microdissection

For decades, paraffin-embedded tissue (PET) has been used by pathologists to examine microscopic sections of pathologic conditions [91]. Pathology and molecular biology merged when DNA within PET became valuable material for molecular analysis [92]. With the ability to extract DNA from PET, cellular phenotype and genotype within tissue sections could be correlated. The possibility also exists to analyze archived PET sections stored for years to decades [91]. A shortcoming in the utilization of PET for molecular analysis is the heterogeneous nature of the sample. To resolve this, various microdissection techniques have been employed to obtain homogenous cells from PET, such as manual scraping of tissue with scalpel blades, needles, or other probes to positively select cells of interest [93–95]. These techniques are limited because of poor delineation of tissue and high susceptibility to contamination from dissimilar cells. Infrared laser capture microdissection (LCM), developed at the National Institute of Health, became commercially available [96–98]. Laser capture microdissection yields homogenous populations of targeted cells from specific microscopic regions of PET sections [97]. Using LCM on PET, it is possible to obtain a homogenous supply of nuclei from which DNA could be extracted.

DNA from PET can serve as substrate for in vitro amplification using polymerase chain reaction (PCR) [99]. The efficiency of PCR amplification is related to the purity and total quantity of DNA in a sample [94]. Lack of amplification can be attributed to insufficient DNA or the presence of PCR inhibitors in the DNA

extract. Knowing the quantity of DNA in a sample can help distinguish between these two possible causes [94]. Knowledge about the quantity of DNA also allows the researcher to maximize the number of PCR tests performed on a sample by consuming only as much DNA as necessary [94]. However, there is limited information on the amount of DNA obtained by LCM as well as information on the number of cells and DNA concentration per capture. We have quantified the number of nuclei and the concentration of DNA obtained from microdissected paraffin embedded cancer tissue using a novel photographic and fluorescent technique. Tissue samples were exclusively obtained from the epithelial component of carcinomas in situ. Those cells recovered in the thermoplastic membrane each time the laser was fired was considered as one "capture." The samples were divided in three groups based upon the number of captures obtained in each one of them: samples containing 40, 20, or 10 captures. The DNA from each one of these groups was diluted 50 times by combining 40 μl of the DNA sample with 960 μl of TE and 1,000 μl of working PicoGreen reagent.

To determine the number of nuclei per field, a focus of carcinoma in situ was selected and photographed (Fig. 5.39). Thirty-two captures were obtained from the epithelial component of the tumor and photographed again (Fig. 5.39). The capsule was placed on the microscope stage and each capture was photographed with a ×40 objective. On average, each capture contained 21 ± 5.4 nuclei within a diameter of 33 ± 6.4 μm.

To determine the amount of DNA found in each capture, 3 groups of 5 samples with each group containing 40, 20, and 10 captures were utilized. This method of grouping also enabled to determine whether a relationship existed between the number of captures and concentration of DNA. DNA was extracted from each sample using a digestion buffer described previously and its relative absorption was measured by a fluorometer. Fluorescence (235 RFU) of negative controls (digestion buffer + PicoGreen) was subtracted from the average RFU of each sample. DNA concentration was determined by using the linear regression equation of the DNA standard ($y = 1.9948x + 136.08$), where y represents the average ab-

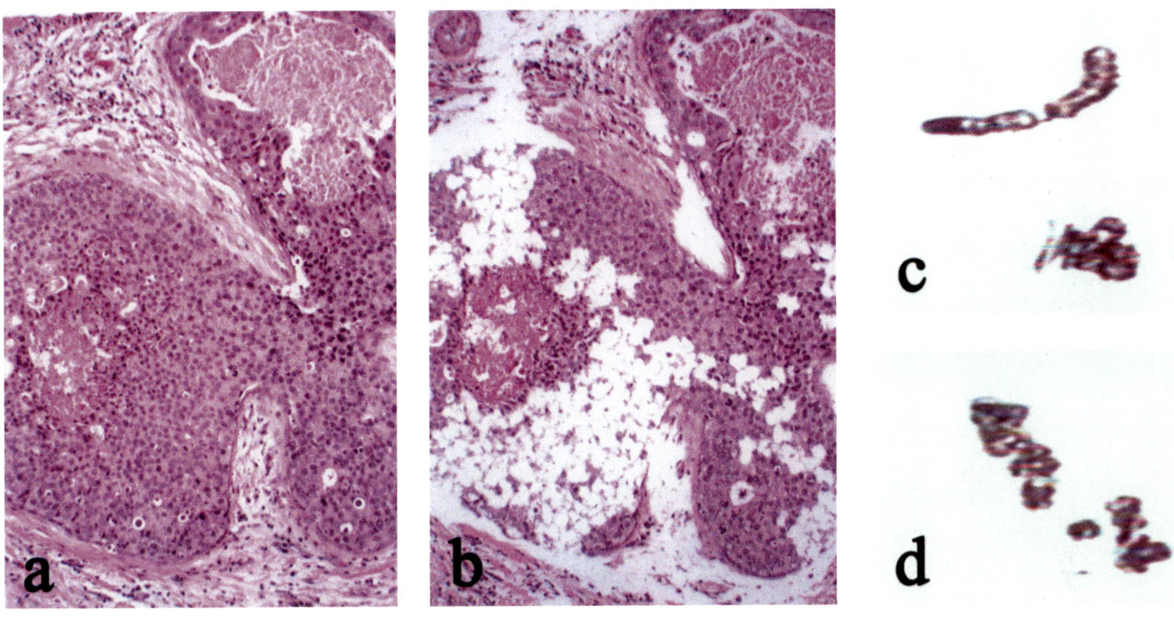

Figure 5.39 a–d

Light micrograph ([T] 10) of ductal carcinoma in situ. An example of laser capture microdissection of **a** a locus of ductal carcinoma in situ prior to and **b** following laser capture microdissection. Sample was taken from archived tissue of patient diagnosed with breast cancer. **c, d** The size of the captures were approximately 30 µm with an amplitude of 40 mw and a pulse width of 40 ms

Table 5.6. Conversion of total DNA concentration obtained from the standard regression line to total DNA per cell

Number of captures	Total number of cells	Mean relative fluorescent units	[DNA] standard plot (1:50 dilution) pg/ml	[DNA] prior to (1:50 dilution) pg/ml	Total DNA in 50 µl of digestion buffer pg	Total DNA/ capture pg	Total DNA/ cell pg
40	840	3,992	1,933	96,650	4,833	120.8	5.75
20	420	1,992	880	44,000	2,200	110.0	5.24
10	210	1,055	460	23,000	1,150	115.0	5.48

sorption of each sample and x the DNA concentration. The concentration of each group was also demonstrated graphically in Fig. 5.40 by drawing a perpendicular line from the intersection of the absorption (y) with the regression line to the x-axis. Table 5.6 summarizes the results and indicates the concentration of DNA per capture and per cell is approximately 115.3 pg and 5.5 pg respectively. This is lower than the 400 pg/capture suggested previously [100], however, no information on the diameter, amplitude, and pulse duration of the microbeam was available for comparisons.

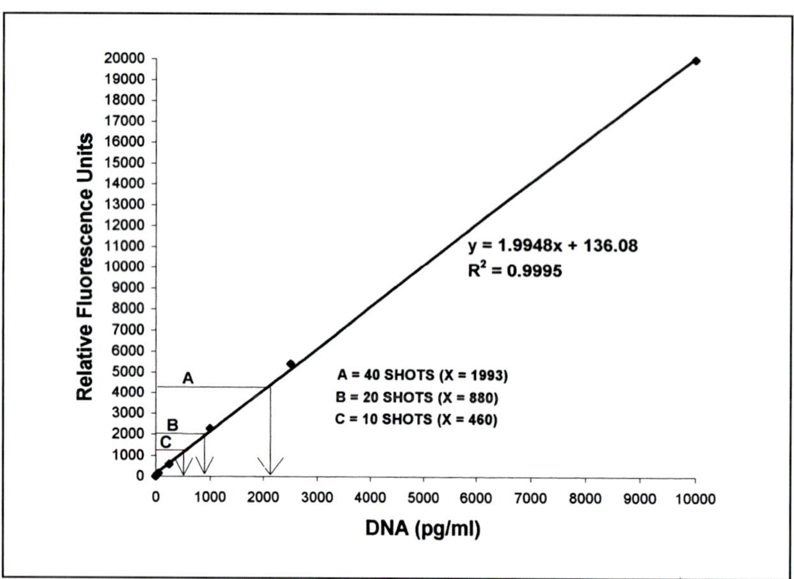

Figure 5.40

Dynamic range and sensitivity of the PicoGreen dsDNA quantification assay. Lambda DNA was serially diluted and assayed for linearity. The total amount of DNA (*pg*) was plotted against relative fluorescent units. The fluorescence was linear over the range of 25 pg to 10 ng with a correlation coefficient of 0.9995. Added to the linear regression line is the placement of the relative fluorescent units obtained from the DNA contained within 40, 20, and 10 captures (reprinted with permission from: Blumenstein R., Dias M., Russo I.H., Tahin Q. and Russo, J. DNA content and cell number determination in microdissected samples of breast carcinoma in situ. Int. J. of Oncology 21:447–450, 2002)

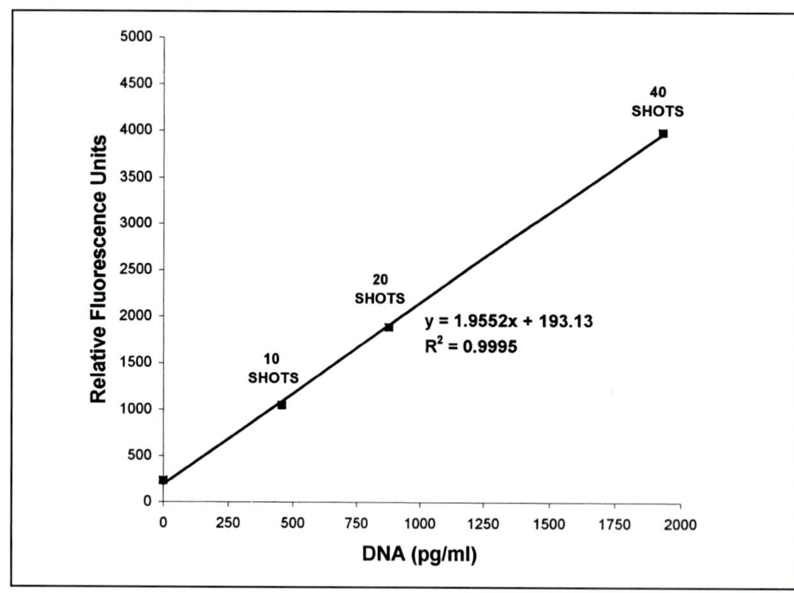

Figure 5.41

Relationship between the number of captures and the concentration of DNA. A linear relationship between the concentration of DNA and the number of captures was observed with a regression line having a correlation coefficient of 0.9995 (R^2) (reprinted with permission from: Blumenstein R., Dias M., Russo I.H., Tahin Q. and Russo, J. DNA content and cell number determination in microdissected samples of breast carcinoma in situ. Int. J. of Oncology 21:447–450, 2002)

To demonstrate graphically the relationship between the number of captures and the concentration of DNA, each group containing 40, 20, and 10 captures was plotted relative to its respective fluorescence absorption. These results are demonstrated in Fig. 5.41, which shows a linear relationship with a regression line having a correlation coefficient of 0.9995 (R^2). This is in agreement with others [100] that have found a high degree of linearity between the amount of DNA and the number of cells captured. This protocol utilizing PicoGreen overcame the difficulties encountered when using UV spectrophotometry for detection of sub-nanogram amounts of DNA. This technique is expected contribute significantly to studies using small amounts of homogenous DNA obtained by LCM, especially for detection of genomic changes in lesions representing progressive stages of cancer evolution by comparison with normal cells and possibly with different population of tumor cells within the same tissue section.

5.5.2 Microsatellite Instability and Loss of Heterozygosity in Microdissected Lesions of the Breast

It has been previously reported MSI at the chromosomal regions of 13q12–13, 11q25 and 16q12.1 in the early stages of chemical transformation of HBEC (see Chapter 8) [76, 77]. In order to test the hypothesis that if MSI represents an early event in breast carcinogenesis in vivo a relationship would exist between microsatellite alteration and the progression of cancer, a polymorphic studies in ductal carcinoma *in situ* of the breast using three microsatellite DNA polymorphic markers, *D13S289*, *D13S260*, and *D13S267*, that flank the BRCA2 region at 13q12–13 have been performed. Microscopically identifiable populations of epithelial cells from normal ducts and ductal carcinoma in situ (DCIS) were collected by microdissection from 10-µm-thick serial paraffin sections [100–102]. Of 35 informative DCIS, MSI was found to be present in 5 (14%) and LOH in 4 (11%) of the cases with marker *D13S260*. At locus *D13S267*, which is more distal to *D13S260*, MSI was seen in 3 (9%), and LOH in 8 (24%) of a total of 33 informative cases. Marker *D13S289*, the most distal of those flanking the *BRCA2* locus had 23 informative cases, 5 of which were affected by MSI (22%), and 2 by LOH (9%) (Table 5.7). Nine (30%) of these cases exhibited MSI and LOH at loci *D13S260*, 9 (26%) at *D13S267*, and 7 (30%) at *D13S289*, indicating that these three markers reflected approximately the same incidence of genomic alterations at the *BRCA2* region (Table 5.7).

The application of microsatellite DNA polymorphic analysis provided evidence that MSI and LOH in chromosomal region of 13q12–13 are associated with the development of pre-invasive breast cancers, thus indicating the involvement of DNA repair defects and/or gene inactivation in breast carcinogenesis. For further testing the pattern of expression of genomic changes in the progression of breast cancer, DNA extracted by microdissection from breast tissues of 21 breast cancer patients that contained three different types of breast lesions: ductal hyperplasia (DHP), ductal carcinoma in situ (DCIS), and invasive ductal carcinoma (INV) (Table 5.8) were analyzed. Specific loci at chromosomes 11, 13, 16, and 17 using an array of seven markers, *D11S912*, *D11S940*,

Table 5.7. Microsatellite instability (MSI) and loss of heterozygosity (LOH) in ductal carcinoma in situ of the breast

Markers	Map	Total cases[a]	MSI (%)	LOH (%)	MSI and LOH (%)
D13S260	13q12–13	35	5 (14)	4 (11)	9 (26)
D13S267	13q12–13	33	3 (9)	8 (24)	11 (30)
D13S289	13q12–13	23	5 (22)	2 (9)	7 (30)

[a] Including both informative and uninformative cases

Table 5.8. Microsatellite instability (*MSI*) and loss of heterozygosity (*LOH*) in ductal hyperplasia (*DHP*), carcinoma in situ (*CIS*), and invasive carcinoma (*INV*)

Markers	Location	Histopathological type of breast lesions					
		DHP[a]		CIS*		INV**	
		MSI	LOH	MSI	LOH	MSI	LOH
Int2	11q13.3	2/24 (8.3)	0/24 (0)	4/35 (11.4)	2/35 (5.7)	2/14 (14.3)	0/14 (0)
D11S614	11q21–23.3	2/33 (6.1)	0/30 (0)	3/38 (7.9)	0/38 (0)	2/16 (12.5)	0/16 (0)
D11S912	11q25	3/37 (5.4)*	1/33 (3.03)**	15/54 (27.8)*	5/54 (9.2)**	3/22 (13.6)*	8/22 (36.4)**
D11S940	11q21–23.3	1/27 (3.7)	0/37 (0)	2/39 (5.1)	1/39 (2.6)	2/16 (12.5)	0/16 (0)
D13S260	13q12–13	0/14 (0)	0/14 (0)	3/23 (13)	3/23 (13)	2/13 (15)	4/13 (31)
D13S267	13q12–13	0/11 (0)	0/11 (0)	3/21 (14)	7/21 (33)	1/12 (8)	2/12 (17)
D13S289	13q12–13	0/7 (0)	0/7 (0)	3/11 (27)	2/11(18)	1/5 (20)	3/5 (60)

[a] Number of lesions affected/number of informative cases (%)
* Fisher's exact test $p<0.05$
** Fisher's exact test $p<0.01$

D13S260, *D13S289*, *D13S267*, *D16S285* and *D17S855* were tested. Among these markers, D11S912 showed MSI in 10/19 (53%) of all samples including 2/8 of the preneoplastic lesion DHP, 8/15 DCIS, and 3/5 of INV (Table 5.8). MSI was detected in chromosome 13 with marker *D13S260* in 5/16 (31%) DCIS and 3/4 (75%) INV (Table 5.3), but was absent in DHP, suggesting a correlation with the progression of the disease, and consistent with its alteration in more advances phases of in vitro transformation, such as in BP1E cells. In addition, the high MSI incidence in all samples for markers *D11S912* (53%), *D13S260* (23%), *D13S289* (36%), and *D13S267* (45%), as compared to lower rates of *D11S940* (10%), *D16S285* (6%) and *D17S855* (9%) may suggest that instability preferentially occurs in specific loci during breast carcinogenesis, also in good agreement with the data from the transformed HBEC system (see Chapter 8).

5.5.3 Example of Breast Cancer Genetic Heterogeneity Revealed by Laser Capture Microdissection Technique

It has been found that alterations in the p arm of chromosome 9 may be a common denominator in human neoplasia, playing an important role in growth promotion and clonal expansion of various tumors [103–105]. Some of these alterations may play a role in the development of precursor conditions such as hyperplasia and carcinoma in situ of the breast [106]. Genetic alterations such as deletions and/or mutations in 9p have been more frequently reported in breast cancer cell lines than in primary breast cancers [107–109]. However, a high level of allelic losses and homozygous deletions have been recently reported in the p arm of chromosome 9, suggesting that loss or inactivation of one or more putative tumor suppressor genes located in this region may be involved in the pathogenesis of breast cancer [110–114]. One question that emerged from our study is whether the p arm of chromosome 9 exhibited allelic losses in invasive ductal carcinomas of the

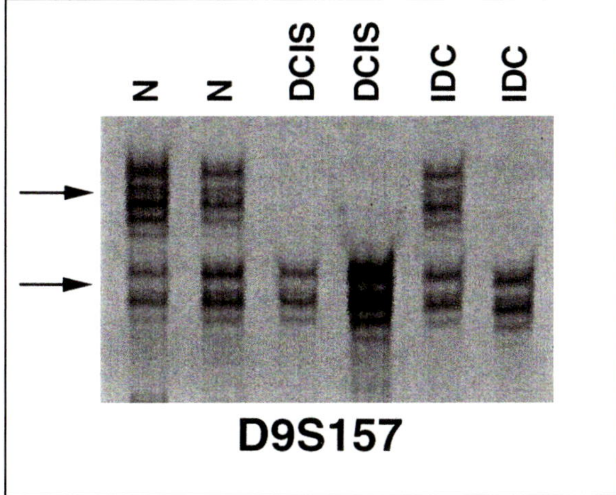

Figure 5.42

Representative microsatellite amplification (D9S157) in normal breast (*N*), ductal carcinoma in situ (*DCIS*) and invasive carcinoma (*IDC*)

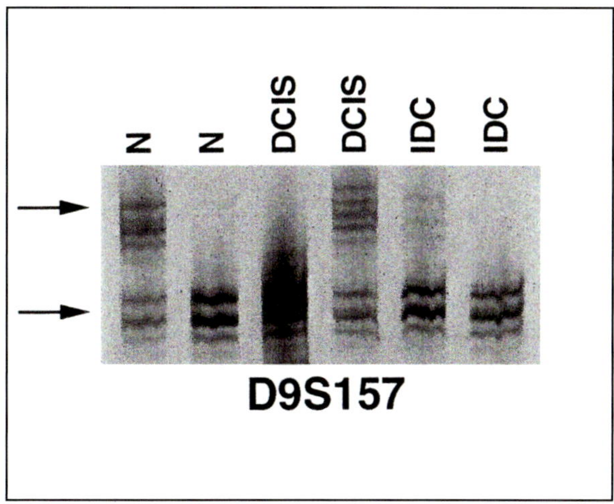

Figure 5.43

Representative microsatellite amplification (D9S157) in normal breast (*N*), DCIS and IDC, taken at different areas of the same specimen

breast, and if so, to determine when these lesions emerged during the process of neoplastic progression. For this purpose we analyzed archival paraffin-embedded tissues of sporadic breast cancer patients by comparing normal lobular structures, DCIS and IDC using five highly informative microsatellite markers (D9S199, D9S157, D9S171, D9S265, and D9S270). Because molecular analysis requires a high degree of purity in the phenotype of tissues or cells to be studied, we employed the newly described technique of laser capture microdissection (LCM) [115–117] to obtain selected cells without contamination of stromal, inflammatory or other cells that could interfere with final results of molecular analysis.

Microsatellite DNA polymorphism analysis of chromosome 9p markers revealed that invasive ductal carcinomas exhibited LOH with the five markers tested, although the frequency varied with each specific marker. The highest one was observed at 9p22–23 (D9S157), with lower frequencies for markers D9S171, D9S199, D9S265, and D9S270. DCIS lesions presented LOH with 4 of the 5 markers tested, being the highest frequency at 9p22–23 (D9S157)

(Fig. 5.42), followed by 9p21 (D9S171), D9S199, and D9S265, which were similar to the frequencies observed in IDC. LOH at various loci of chromosome 9p has been shown in several tumors and tumor-derived cell lines. Although the most common loci studied encompass the p16INK4 locus, recent studies indicate that another tumor suppressor gene(s) could reside within different 9p loci, namely 9p22–23 [103, 110, 112, 118–120]. Interestingly, phenotypically normal breast tissues adjacent to carcinomas either invasive or in situ also exhibited LOH at D9S157 and/or D9S171 (Fig. 5.43). These findings indicated that LOH at these loci was an early event in breast cancer progression, confirming that genetic alterations at specific loci of 9p occur much earlier than recognized before and even earlier than discernable morphological or histopathological alterations. In order to confirm this observation we performed LOH analyses in microdissected normal skin and lymphocytes from lymph nodes free of metastatic disease from seven of the patients. It was observed that the pattern of LOH displayed in some histologically normal appearing breast tissue was not present in genomic DNA from

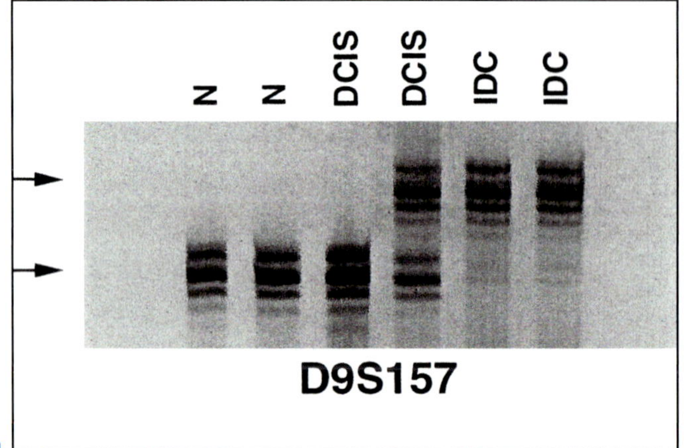

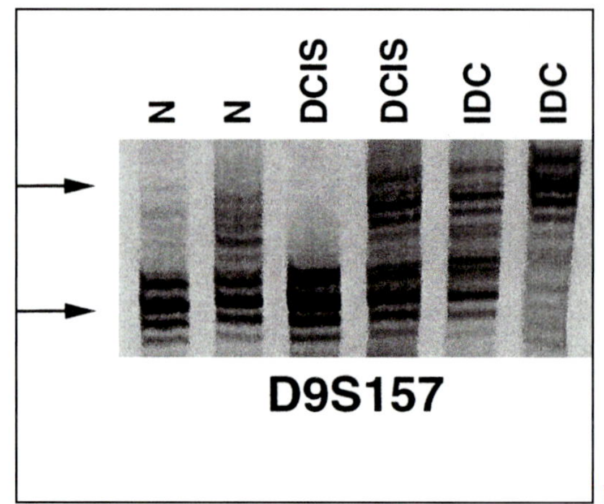

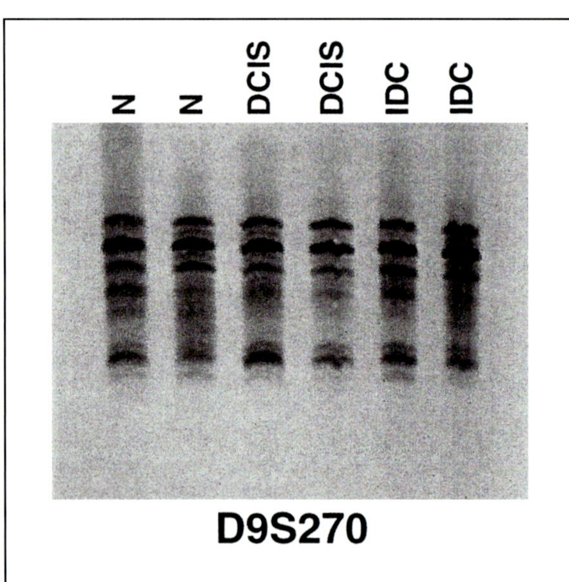

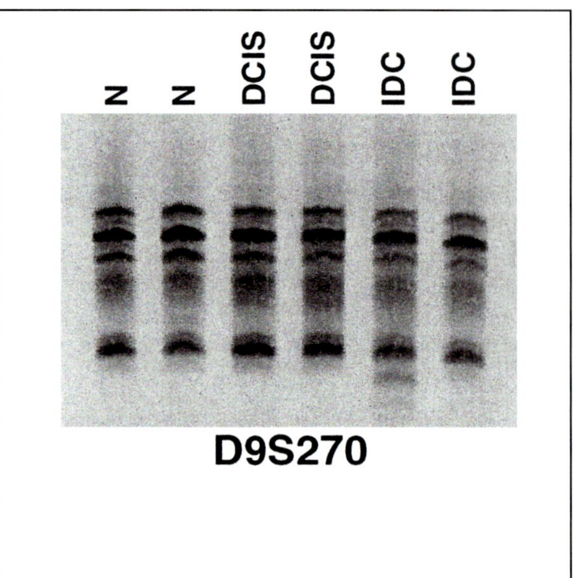

normal skin of the same patient (compare Fig. 5.44a with 5.44b). None of the seven cases of matched skin/lymphocyte DNA displayed LOH or other genetic alterations in any of the five markers tested (Fig. 5.44c,d). The presence of genetic alterations within morphologically normal breast tissue adjacent to carcinoma foci confirms previously reported observations [121]. These findings have significant practical implications for the evaluation of what has to be considered the "free margin" of a tumor when performing breast conserving surgical therapeutic

Figure 5.44 a–d

Representative microsatellite amplification (D9S157) in normal breast (*N*), DCIS and IDC. Two foci of cells were analyzed in each case: **a** no LOH was observed in DNA from skin microdissection but **b** LOH was present in one foci of breast tissue's DNA. **c, d** The LOH is not observed when other marker (D9S270) is used procedures. Therefore, the use of genetic markers should be taken into consideration for their use in addition to the histopathological evaluation of the resected margins.

An unexpected finding was the intralesional heterogeneity with respect to allelic loss also found in in situ and invasive carcinomas, since LOH was observed in some, but not in all the tumor foci studied. For example, in patient number 1 LOH was present at 9p22–23 (marker D9S157) in 6 out of 10 foci of invasive carcinoma, in 3 out of 9 foci of DCIS, and in 4 out of 10 foci of normal tissue analyzed. These observations suggest the coexistence in the same lesion of clones of cells that differ in their genetic composition. It is possible that clusters of cells within a tumor that contain 9p LOH might be at a more advanced stage of genetic progression than adjacent tumor foci without this allelic loss.

Altogether, these data are supportive of a model whereby LOH of chromosome arm 9p, particularly at locus 9p22–23, namely with marker D9S157 and in a lesser scale marker D9S171 (9p21), occurs very early in the progression of cancer, even when cells still are phenotypically normal. Furthermore, we observed that different populations of cells exist within a single tumor, an indication that they do not share clonal origin.

Although the monoclonal origin of breast cancer and other solid tumors has been suggested by multiple genetic studies [122–124], recent cytogenetic analyses of breast cancer have suggested that up to 70 % of primary breast carcinomas are cytogenetically polyclonal [125–127]. Confirmation of these findings can be achieved by isolating homogeneous population of cells utilizing the laser capture microdissection technique [128–130]. Laser microdissected samples show more chromosomal aberrations than DNA isolated from tumor sections, a phenomenon that has been attributed to the fact that chromosomal imbalances might be masked by non-tumoral components within the tumor mass [131]. In studies that have compared allelic loss in synchronous in situ and invasive breast cancers [85, 132, 133], the maintenance of LOH in the invasive tumor has been interpreted as an evidence of clonal derivation from the in situ cancer. Our data are supported by those of Fujii

et al. [85], who found substantial allelic heterogeneity among multiple foci of individual DCIS lesions.

The study demonstrated that more than one clone of neoplastic cells exists within a single tumor, a phenomenon that could explain variations in the biological behavior of tumors that appear morphologically similar. The heterogeneity within different foci of similar lesions as well as in normal tissues suggests that significant genetic divergence also occurs during cancer initiation and progression. This diversity is likely to result from genetic instability of both breast cancer cells and normal cells that might be prone to become transformed.

5.6 Summary and Conclusions

The fact that lobules type 1 have the highest proliferative index, concentration of estrogen receptors, and number of blood vessels per lobular structure, clearly indicate that this type or structure is the natural target of malignancy. The early genomic alterations observed in ductal hyperplasia are the activation of ferritin H that is associated with oxidative damage and the S100P protein that may be involved in the transport of calcium and therefore as regulator of cell proliferation in breast epithelial cells. Both genes are expressed in immortal cells in vitro and they are expressed in the early preneoplastic lesions such as ductal hyperplasia and remain activated in atypical hyperplasia, ductal carcinoma and invasive carcinoma of the breast. This intracellular milieu could provide the adequate environment for genomic changes at the level of mismatch repair originating lesions such as MSI and/or other genomic changes like LOH providing a new paradigm of the initiation of breast cancer.

References

1. Russo, J., Gusterson, B.A., Rogers, A.E., Russo, I.H., Wellings, S.R. and Van Zwieten, M.J. Comparative study of human and rat mammary tumorigenesis. Lab. Invest. 62:1–32, 1991.
2. McGregor, D.H., Land, C.E., Choi, K., Tokuoka, S., Liu, P.I., Wakabayashi, I., Beebe, G.W. Breast cancer incidence among atomic bomb survivors, Hiroshima and Nagasaki 1950–1989. J. Natl. Cancer Inst. 59:799–811, 1977.
3. Wellings, S.R. Development of human breast cancer. Adv. Cancer Res.. 31:287–299, 1980.
4. Wellings, S.R., Jensen, H.M. and Marcum, R.G. An atlas of subgross pathology of 16 human breasts with special reference to possible precancerous lesions. J. Natl. Cancer Inst. 55:231–275, 1975.
5. Russo, J., Rivera, R. and Russo, I.H. Influence of age and parity on the development of the human breast. Breast Cancer Res. Treat. 23:211–218, 1992.
6. Russo, J., Romero, A.L. and Russo, I.H. Architectural pattern of the normal and cancerous breast under the influence of parity. J. Cancer Epidemiol. Biomarkers & Prevention 3:219–224, 1994.
7. Russo, J., Reina, D., Frederick, J. and Russo, I.H. Expression of phenotypical changes by human breast epithelial cells treated with carcinogens in vitro. Cancer Res. 48:2837–2857, 1988.
8. Russo, J., Calaf, G, Russo, I.H. 1A critical approach to the malignant transformation of human breast epithelial cells. CRC Critical Rev. Oncogen. 4:403–417, 1993
9. Russo, J. and Russo, I.H. Development of Human Mammary Gland. In: The Mammary Gland Development, Regulation, and Function. (M.C. Neville and C.W. Daniel, eds Plenum Pub. Corp. 1987, pp. 67–93.
10. Russo, J., Lynch, H., and Russo, I.H. Mammary gland architecture as a determining factor in the susceptibility of the human breast to cancer. Breast Journal 7(5):278–291, 2001.
11. Russo, J., Russo, I.H. Toward a physiological approach to breast cancer prevention. Cancer Epidemiol, Biomarkers & Prevention 3:353–364, 1994.
12. Barnabas, N., Moraes, R., Calaf, G., Estrada, S., Russo, J. Role of p53 in MCF-10F cell immortalization and chemically-induced neoplastic transformation. Int. J. Oncol. 7:1289–1296, 1995.
13. Rajan, J.V., Marquis, S.T., Gardner, H.P., Chodosh, L.A. Developmental expression of BRCA2 co-localizes with BRCA1 and is associated with proliferation and differentiation in multiple tissues. Developmental Biology 184:385–401, 1997.
14. Colditz, G.A., Rosner, B.A., Speizer, E. Risk factors for breast cancer according to family history of breast cancer. J. Natl. Cancer Inst. 1996; 88:365–371.
15. Russo, I.H., Russo, J.. Developmental stage of the rat mammary gland as determinant of its susceptibility to 7,12-dimethylbenz(a)anthracene. J. Natl. Cancer Inst. 1978 61:1439–1449.
16. Hu, Y.F., Russo, I.H., Zalipsky, U., Lynch, H.T., Russo, J. Environmental chemical carcinogens induce transformation of breast epithelial cells from women with familial history of breast cancer. In vitro Cell Dev. Biol. 33:495–498, 1997.
17. Lambe, M, Hsieh, C.C., Trichopoulos, D, Ekbom A, Pavia M, Adami HO. Transient increase in the risk of breast cancer after giving birth. N. England J. Med. 331:5–9, 1994.
18. Eyden, B., Watson, R.J., Harris, M., Howell, A. Intralobular stromal fibroblasts in the resting human mammary gland: ultrastructural properties and intercellular relationship. J. Sub-microsc Cytol. 18:397–408, 1986.
19. Ozzello, L. Epithelial-stromal junction of normal and dysplastic mammary glands. Cancer 25:586–600, 1970.
20. Sakakura, T., Sakagami, Y., Nishizuka, Y. Persistence of responsiveness of adult mouse mammary gland to induction by embryonic mesenchyme. Dev. Biol. 72:201–210. 1979.
21. Henson, D.E., Tarone, R.E. On the possible role of involution in the natural history of breast cancer. Cancer 71:2154–2156, 1994.
22. Marquis, S.T., Rajan, J.V., Wynshaw-Boris, A., et al. The developmental pattern of BRCA1 expression implies a role in differentiation of the breast and other tissues. Nature Genet. 11:17–26, 1995.
23. Pankow, J.E., Vachon, C.M., Kuni, C.C., King, R.A., Anett, D.K., Grabrick, D.M., Rich, S.S., Anderson, V.E., Sellers, T.A. Genetic analysis of mammographic breast density in adult women: Evidence of a gene effect. J. Natl. Cancer Inst. 89:549–556, 1997.
24. Wilkinson, E., Clopton, C., Gordonson, J., Green, R., Hill, A., Pike, M.C. Mammographic parenchymal pattern and the risk of breast cancer. J. Natl. Cancer Inst. 59:1397–1400, 1977.
25. Wolfe, J.N., Albert, S., Belle, S., Salane, M. Familial influences on breast parenchymal patterns. Cancer 46:2433–2437, 1980.
26. Saftlas, A.F., Wolfe, J.N., Hoover, R.N., Brinton, L.A., et al. Mammographic parenchymal patterns as indicators of breast cancer risk. Am. J. Epidemiol. 129:518–526, 1089.
27. Oza, A.M., Boyd, N.F. Mammographic parenchymal patterns: a marker of breast cancer risk. Epidemiol. Rev. 15:196–208, 1993.
28. Russo, J., Hu, Y-F. Silva, I.D.C.G., and Russo, I.H. Cancer risk related to mammary gland structure and development. Microscopy Research and Technique 52:204–223,2001.
29. Propper, A. Role du mesenchyme dans la differenciation de la glande mammaire chez l'embryon de lapin. Bull. Soc. Zool. Fr. 97:505–512, 1972.
30. Sakakura, T., Nishizuka, Y., Dawe, C. Mesenchyme-dependent morphogenesis and epithelium specific cytodifferentiation in mouse mammary gland. Science 194:1439–1441, 1976.
31. Cunha, G.R., Young, P., Hamamoto, S., Guzman, R., Nandi, S. Developmental response of adult mammary epithelial cells to various fetal and neonatal mesenchymes. Epithelial Cell Biol. 1:105–118, 1992.

32. Kratochwil, K., Schwartz, P. Tissue interaction in androgen response of embryonic mammary rudiment of mouse: identification of target tissue of testosterone. Proc. Natl. Acad. Sci. USA 73:4041–4044, 1976.

33. Faulkin, J.L., DeOme, K.B. Regulation of growth and spacing of gland elements in the mammary fat pad of the C3H mouse. J. Natl. Cancer Inst. 24:953–969, 1960.

34. Sun, C., Lenair, G., Lynch, H., Narod, S. In situ Breast Cancer and BRCA1. Lancet 348:408, 1996.

35. Jernstrom, H., Johannsson, O., Borg, A., Olsson, H. Do BRCA1 mutations affect the ability to breast-feed? significantly shorter length of breast-feeding among BRCA1 mutation carriers compared with their unaffected relatives. Breast 7:320–324, 1998.

36. Xu X, Wagner KU, Larson D, et al. Conditional mutation of BRCA1 in mammary epithelial cells results in blunted ductal morphogenesis and tumour formation. Nat. Genet. 1999; 22:37–43 and tumour formation. Nat. Genet. 22:37–43, 1999.

37. Russo, I.H. and Russo, J. Mammary gland neoplasia in long-term rodent studies. Environ. Health Perspect. 104:938–967, 1996.

38. Russo, J., Calaf, G., Sohi, N., Tahin, Q., Zhang, P.L., Alvarado, M.E., Estrada, S., and Russo, I.H. Critical steps in breast carcinogenesis. Ann. NY Acad. Sci. 698:1–20, 1993.

39. Russo, J., Barnabas, N., Higgy, N., Salicioni, A.M., Wu, Y.L., Russo, I.H. Molecular basis of human breast epithelial cell transformation. In: Calvo F, Crepin M, Magdalenat H (eds,) Breast Cancer, Advances in Biology and Therapeutics, John Libbey Eurotext, 1996, pp. 33–43.

40. Soule, H.D., Maloney, T.M., Wolman, S.R., Peterson, W.D., Brenz, R., McGrath, C.M., Russo, J., Pauley, R.J., Jones, R.F., and Brooks, S.C. Isolation and characterization of a spontaneously immortalized human breast epithelial cell line MCF 10. Cancer Res. 50:6075–6086, 1991.

41. Tait, L., Soule, H.D., and Russo, J. Ultrastructural and immunocytochemical characterization of an immortalized human breast epithelial cell line, MCF10. Cancer Res. 50:6087–6094, 1991.

42. Silva, I.D.C.G., Hu, Y.F., Russo, I.H., Ao, X., Salicioni, A.M., Yang, X. and Russo, J. S100P Ca $^{+2}$-binding protein overexpression is associated with immortalization and neoplastic transformation of human breast epithelial cells in vitro and tumor progression in vivo. International Journal of Oncology 16:231–240, 2000.

43. Higgy, N.A., Salicioni, A.M., Russo, I.H., Zhang, P.I. and Russo, J. Differential expression of human ferritin H chain gene in immortal human breast epithelial MCF-10F cells Molecular Carcinogenesis 20:332–339, 1997.

44. Boyd, D., Vecoli, C., Belcher, D.M., Jain, S.K., Drysdale, J.W. Structural and functional relationships of human ferritin H and L chains deduced from cDNA clones. J. Biol. Chem. 260:11755–11761, 1985.

45. Costanzo, F., Santoro, C., Colantuoni, V. et al. Cloning and sequencing of a full length cDNA coding for a human apoferritin H chain: evidence for a multigene family. The EMBO J. 3:23–27, 1984.

46. Anison, P. Current concepts in iron metabolism. Clin. Haematol. 11:241–257, 1982.

47. Weinberg, E.D. Iron and neoplasia. Biol. Trace Elem. Res. 3:55–80, 1981.

48. Richard, P., Ehrenberg, A. Ribonucleotide reductase: a radical enzyme. Science 221:514–519, 1983.

49. Fan, H., Villegas, C., Wright, J.A. A link between ferritin gene expression and ribo-nucleotide reductase R2 protein, as demonstrated by retroviral vector mediated stable expression of R2 cDNA. FEBS Letters 382:145–148, 1996.

50. Keown, P., Descaps-Latscha, B. In vitro suppression of cell mediated immunity by ferro-proteins and ferric salts. Cellular Immunology 80:257–266, 1983.

51. Rosen, H.R., Moroz, C., Reiner, A., et al. Placental isoferritin associated p43 antigen correlates with features of high differentiation in breast cancer. Br. Cancer Res. & Treatment 24:17–26, 1992.

52. Rosen, H.R., Flex, D., Stierer, M., Moroz, C. Monoclonal antibody CM-H-9 detects placental isoferritin in the serum of patients with visceral metastases of breast cancer. Cancer Lett. 59:145–151, 1991.

53. Kwak, E.L., Larochelle, D.A., Blaumont, C., Torti, S.V., Torti, F.M. Role of NF-κB in the regulation of ferritin H by tumor necrosis factor-α. J. Biol. Chem. 270:15285–15293, 1995.

54. Calaf, G., and Russo, J. Transformation of breast epithelial cells by chemical carcinogens. Carcinogenesis 14:483–492, 1993.

55. Becker, T., Gerke, V., Kube, E., and Weber, K. S100P: a novel calcium-binding protein from human placenta. cDNA cloning, recombinant protein expression and calcium-binding properties. Eur. J. Biochem. 207:541–547, 1992.

56. Emoto, Y., Kobayashi, R., Akatsuba, H., and Hidaka, H. Purification and characterization of a new member of the S100 protein family from human placenta. Biochem. Biophys. Res. Comm. 182:1246–1253, 1992.

57. Moore, B.E. A soluble protein characteristic of the nervous system. Biochem. Biophys. Res. Commun. 19:739–744, 1965.

58. Sherbet, G.V., and Lakshmi, M.S. A100A4 (MTS1 calcium binding protein in cancer growth, invasion and metastasis. Anti Cancer Res. 18:2415–2422, 1998.

59. Schafer, B.W., and Heizmann, C.W. The S100 family of EF-hand calcium-binding proteins: functions and pathology. TIBS 21:134–140, 1996.

60. McGrath, C.M., and Soule, H.D. Calcium regulation of normal human mammary epithelial cell growth in culture. In vitro Cell Dev. Biol. 20:652–662, 1984.

61. Soule, H.D., and McGrath, C.M. A simplified method for passage and long-term growth of human mammary epithelial cells. In vitro 22:6–12, 1985.

62. Ochieng, J., Tahin, Q.S., Booth, C.C., and Russo, J. Buffering of intracellular calcium in response to increase levels in mortal, immortal and transformed human breast epithelial cells. J. Cell. Biochem. 46:250–254, 1993.

63. Hennings, H., Michael, D., Cheng, C., Steinert, P., Holbrook, K., Yuspa, S.H. Calcium regulation of growth and differentiation of mouse epidermal cells in culture. Cell 19:245–254, 1980.

64. Cristofalo VJ, Wallace JM, Rosma BA: In Sato SH, Ross R (eds): "Hormones and Cell Culture: Book B." Cold Spring Harbor, NY: Cold Spring Harbor Laboratory, 1979, pp 875–887.

65. Carafoli, E. Intracellular calcium homeostasis. Annu. Rev. Biochem. 56:395–433, 1987.

66. Babu, S.Y., Sack, J.S., Greenbough, T.J., Bagg, C.E., Means, A.R., Cook, W.J. Three-dimensional structure of calmodulin. Nature 315:37–40, 1985.

67. Schatzmann, H.J. ATP-dependent Ca^{2+}-extrusion from human red cells. Experientia 22:364–365, 1966.

68. Varecka, L., Carafoli, E. Vanadate-induced movements of Ca2+ and K+ in human red blood cells. J. Biol. Chem. 257:7414–7421, 1982.

69. Reuter, H., Seitz, N. The dependence of calcium efflux from cardiac muscle on temperature and external ion composition. J. Physiol. 195:451–470, 1968.

70. Berridge, M.J., Irvine, R.F. Inositol trisphosphate, a novel second messenger in cellular signal transduction. Nature 312:315–321,1984.

71. Hennings, H., Kruzewski, F.H., Yuspa, S.H., Tucker, R.W. Intracellular calcium alterations in response to increased external calcium in normal and neoplastic keratinocytes. Carcinogenesis 10:777–780, 1989.

72. Meldolesi, J., Pozzan, T. Pathways of Ca2+ influx at the plasma membrane: voltage-, receptor-, and second messenger-operated channels. Exp. Cell Res. 171:271–283, 1987.

73. Patel, K.V., Schrey, M.Y. Activation of inositol phospholipid signaling and Ca2+ efflux in human breast cancer cells by bombesin. Cancer Res. 50:235–239, 1990.

74. Kerr, J.F.R., Wyllie, A.H., Currie, A.R. Apoptosis: a basic biological phenomenon with wide-ranging implications in tissue kinetics. Br. J. Cancer 26:239–257, 1972.

75. Kyprianou, N., English, H.F., Davidson, N.E., Isaacs, J.T. Programmed cell death during regression of the MCF-7 human breast cancer following estrogen ablation. Cancer Res. 51:162–166, 1991.

76. Huang, Y., Bove, B., Wu, Y.L., Russo, I.H., Yang, X., Zekri, A., and Russo, J. Microsatellite instability during immortalization and transformation of human breast epithelial cells in vitro. Molecular Carcinogenesis 24:118–127, 1999

77. Wu, Y., Barnabas, N.; Russo, I.H., Yang, X. and Russo, J. Microsatellite Instability and Loss of heterozygosity in chromosomes 9 and 16 in human breast epithelial cells transformed by chemical carcinogens. Carcinogenesis 18:1069–1074, 1997

78. Russo, I.H., Tahin, Q., Huang, Y. and Russo, J. Cellular and molecular changes induced by the chemical carcinogen benzo(a)pyrene in human breast epithelial cells in association with smoking and breast cancer. J. of Women's Cancer 3:29–36, 2001.

79. Russo, J., Hu, Y.F., Yang, X., Huang, Y., Silva I., Bove, B., Higgy, N., Russo, I.H. Breast cancer multistage progression. Frontiers in Bio Science 3:944–960, 1998.

80. Harris, J.R., Hellmam, S. Natural history of breast cancer. In: Harris, J.R., Lippman, M.E., Morrow, M., Hellman, S. (eds), Diseases of the Breast, pp. 375–391. Philadelphia: Lippincott-Raven, 1996.

81. Lakhani, S.R. The transition from hyperplasia to invasive carcinoma of the breast. J. Pathol. 187:272–278, 1999.

82. Werner, M., Mattis, A., Aubele, M., Cummings, M., Zitzelsberger, HH., Hhutzler, P., Höfler, H. 20q13.2 amplification in intraductal hyperplasia adjacent to in situ and invasive ductal carcinoma of the breast. Virchows Arch. 435:469–472, 1999.

83. Eiriksdottir, G., Sigurdsson, A., Jonasson, J.G., Agnarsson, B.A., Sigurdsson, H., Gudmundsson, J., Bergthorsson, J.T., Barkardottir, R.B., Egilsson, V., Ingvarsson, S. Loss of heterozygosity on chromosome 9 in human breast cancer: association with clinical variables and genetic changes at other chromosome regions. Int. J. Cancer 64:378–382, 1995.

84. Kuukasjärvi, T., Karhu, R., Tanner, M., Kähkönen, M., Schäffer, A., Nupponen, N., Pennanen, S., Kallioniemi, A., Kallioniemi, O-P., Isola, J. Genetic heterogeneity and clonal evolution underlying development of asynchronous metastasis in human breast cancer. Cancer Res. 57:1597–1604, 1997.

85. Fujii, H., Marsh, C., Cairns, P., Sidransky, D., Gabrielson, E. Genetic divergence in the clonal evolution of breast cancer. Cancer Res. 56:1493–1497, 1996.

86. Weber, J.L., May, P.E. Abundant class of human DNA polymorphisms, which can be using the polymerase chain reaction. Am J Hum Genet 44:388–96, 1989.

87. Boyer, J.C., Umar, A., Risinger, J.L., et al. Microsatellite instability, mismatch repair deficiency, and genetic defects in human cancer cell lines. Cancer Res. 55:6063–6070, 1995.

88. Lonov, Y., Peinado, M.A., Malkhosyan, S., Shibata, D., Perucho, M. Ubiquitous somatic mutations in simple repeated sequences reveal a new mechanism for colonic carcinogenesis. Nature 363:558–61, 1993

89. Yee, C.J., Roodi, N., Verrier, C.S., Parl, F.F. Microsatellite instability and loss of heterozygosity in breast cancer. Cancer Res. 54:1641–1644, 1994.

90. Wooster, R., Cleton-Jansen, A.-M., Collins, N., Mangion, J., Cornelis, R.S., Cooper, C.S., Gusterson, B.A., Ponder, B.A.J., von Deimling, A., Wiestler, O.D., Cornelisse, C.J., Devilee, P., Stratton, M.R. Instability of short tandem repeats (microsatellite) in human cancers. Nature Genetics 6:152–156, 1994.

91. Sibata, D. Extraction of DNA from paraffin-embedded tissue for analysis by polymerase chain reaction: new tricks from an old friend. Human Pathology 25:461–563, 1994.

92. Honma, M., Ohara, Y., Murayama, H., Sako, K. and Iwasaki, Y. Effects of fixation and varying target length on the sensitivity of polymerase chain reaction for detection of human T-cell leukemia virus type I proviral DNA in formalin-fixed tissue sections. Journal of Clinical Microbiology 31:1799–1803, 1993.

93. Going, J.J. and Lamb, R.F. Practical histological microdissection for PCR analysis. Journal of Pathology 179:121–124, 1996.

94. Walsh, P.S., Varlaro, J., and Reynolds, R. A rapid chemiluminescent method for quantitation of human DNA. Nucleic Acids Research 20:5061–5065, 1992.

95. Whetsell, L., Maw, G.K, Nadon, N., Ringer, D. and Schafer, F.V. Polymerase chain reaction microanalysis of tumors from stained histological slides. Oncogene 7:2355–2361, 1992.

96. Emmert-Buck, M.R., R.F. Bonner, P.D. Smith, R.F. Chuaqui, Z. Zhuang, S.R. Goldstein, R.A. Weiss and L.A. Liotta. Laser capture microdissection. Science 274:998–1001, 1996.

97. Bonner, R.F., M.R. Emmert-Buck, K. Cole, T. Pohida, R.F. Chuaqui, S.R. Goldstein and L.A. Liotta. Laser capture microdissection: molecular analysis of tissue. Science 278:1481–1483, 1997.

98. Simone, N.L., R.F. Bonner, J.W. Gillespie, M.R. Emmert-Buck and L.A. Liotta. Laser- capture microdissection: opening the microscopic frontier to molecular analysis. Trends in Genetics 14:272–276, 1998.

99. Mies, C. Molecular biological analysis of paraffin-embedded tissues. Human Pathology 25:555–560, 1994.

100. Singer, V.L., I.J. Jones, S.T. Yue, R.P. Haugland. Characterization of PicoGreen reagent and development of a fluorescence-based solution assay for double-stranded DNA quantification. Analytical Biochemistry 249: 228–238, 1997.

101. Radford, D.M., Fair, K.L., Phillips, N.J., Ritter, J.H., Steinbrueck, T., Holt, M.S, Donis-Keller, H. Allelotyping of ductal carcinoma in situ of the breast: deletion of loci on 8p, 13q, 16p,17p and 17q. Cancer Research 55:3399–3405, 1995.

102. Aldaz, C.M., Chen, T., Sahin, A., Cunningham, J. Bondy, M. Comparative allelotype of in situ and invasive human breast cancer: high frequency of microsatellite instability in lobular breast carcinomas. Cancer Res. 55:3976–81, 1995.

103. Czerniak, B., Chatuverdi, V., Li, L., Hodges, S., Johnston, D., Ro, J., Luthra, R., Logothetis, C., Von Eschenbach, A.C., Grossman, H.B., Benedict, W.F., Batsakis, J.G. Superimposed histologic and genetic mapping of chromosome 9 in progression of human urinary bladder neoplasia: implications for a genetic model of multistep carcinogenesis and early detection of urinary bladder cancer. Oncogene 18:1185–1196, 1999.

104. Campbell, I.G., Beynon, G., Davis, M., Englefield, P. LOH and mutation analysis of CDKN2 in primary human ovarian cancers. Int. J. Cancer 63:222–225, 1995.

105. Nakanishi, H., Wang, X-L., Imai F.L., Kato J., Shiiba M., Myia, T., Imai, Y., Tanzawa, H. Localization of a novel tumor suppressor gene loci on chromosome 9p21–22 in oral cancer. Anti Cancer Res. 19:29–34, 1999.

106. Murphy, D.S., Hoare S.F., Going, J.J., Mallon, E.A., George W.D., Kaye, S.B. et al. Characterization of extensive genetic alterations in ductal carcinoma in situ by fluorescence in situ hybridization and molecular analysis. J. Natl. Cancer Inst. 87:1694–1704, 1995.

107. Berns, E.J., Klijn, J.M., Smid, M., Van Staveren, I., Gruis, N.A., Foekens, J.A. Infrequent CDKN2 (MTS1/p16 gene alterations in human primary breast cancer. Br. J. Cancer 72:964–967, 1995.

108. Quesnel, B., Fenaux, P., Philippe, N., Fournier, J., Bonneterre, J., Preudhomme, C., Peyrat, J.P. Analysis of p16 gene deletion and point mutation in breast carcinoma. Br. J. Cancer 72:351–353, 1995.

109. Xu, L., Sgroi, D., Christopher, J.S., Beauchamp, R.L., Pinney, D.M., Keel, S., Ueki, K., Rutter, J.L., Buckler, A.J., Louis, D.N., Gusella, J.F., Ramesh, V. Mutational analysis of CDKN2 (MTS1/p16INK4 in human breast carcinomas. Cancer Res. 54:5262–5264, 1994.

110. Brenner, A.J., Aldaz, M. Chromosome 9p allelic loss and p16/CDKN2 in breast cancer and evidence of p16 inactivation in immortal breast epithelial cells. Cancer Res. 55:2892–2895, 1995.

111. An, H-X., Niederacher, D., Picard, F., van Roeyen, C., Bender, H.G., Beckmann, M.W. Frequent allele loss on 9p21–22 defines a smallest common region in the vicinity of the CDKN2 gene in sporadic breast cancer. Genes Chrom. Cancer 17:14–20, 1996.

112. Minobe, K., Onda, M., Iida, A., Kasumi, F., Sakamoto, G., Nakamura, Y., Emi, M. Allelic loss in chromosome 9q is associated with lymph node metastasis of primary breast cancer. Jpn. J. Cancer Res. 89:916–922, 1998.

113. Cairns, P., Polascik, T.J., Eby, Y., Tokino, K., Califano, J., Merlo, A., Mao, L., Heath, J., Jenkins, R., Westra, W., Rutter, J., Buckler, A., Gabrielson, E., Tockman, M., Cho, K.R., Hedrick, L., Bova, G.S., Isaacs, W., Koc, W., Schwab, D., Sidransky, D. Frequency of homozygous deletion at p16/CDKN2 in primary human tumors. Nat. Genet 11:210–212, 1995.

114. Dutrilaux, B., Gerbault-Senreau, M., Zafrani, B. Characterization of chromosomal abnormalities in human breast cancer. Cancer Genet Cytogenet, 49:203–217, 1990.

115. Emmert-Buck, M.R., Bonner, R.F., Smith, P.D., Chuaqui, R.F., Zhuang, Z., Goldstein, S.R., Weiss, R.A., Liotta, L.A. Laser capture microdissection. Science 274:998–1001, 1996.

116. Bonner, R.F., Emmert-Buck, M., Cole, K., Pohida, T., Chuaqui, R., Goldstein, S., Liotta, L.A. Laser capture microdissection: molecular analysis of tissue. Science 278:1481–1483, 1997.

117. Simone, N.L., Bonner, R.F., Gillespie, J.W., Emmert-Buck, M.R., Liotta, L.A. Laser capture microdissection: opening the microscopic frontier to molecular analysis. Trends Genet. 14:272–276, 1998.

118. Wu, Y., Barnabas, N., Russo, I.H., Yang, X., Russo, J. Microsatellite instability and loss of heterozygosity in chromosomes 9 and 16 in human breast epithelial cells transformed by chemical carcinogens. Carcinogenesis 18:1069–1074, 1997.

119. Muzeau, F., Flejou, J.F., Thomas, G., Hamelin, R. Loss of heterozygosity on chromosome 9 and p16 (MTS1, CDKN2 gene mutations in esophageal cancers. Int. J. Cancer 72:27–30, 1997.

120. Morita, R., Fujimoto, A., Hatta, N., Takehara, K., Takata, M. Comparison of genetic profiles between primary melanomas and their metastases reveals genetic alterations and clonal evolution during progression. J Invest Dermat. 111:919–924, 1998.

121. Deng, G., Lu, Y., Zlotikov, G., Thor, A.D., Smith, H.S. Loss of heterozygosity in normal tissue adjacent to breast carcinomas. Science 274:2057–2059, 1996.

122. Nowell, P.C. The clonal origin of human tumors. Science 194:23–28, 1976.

123. Fialkow, P.J. Clonal origin of human tumors. Biochem Biophys Acta 458:283–321, 1976.

124. Noguchi, S., Motomura, K., Inaji, H., Imaoka, S., Koyamma, H. Clonal analysis of human breast cancer by means of the polymerase chain reaction. Cancer Res. 52:6594–6597, 1992.

125. Teixeira, M.R., Pandis, N., Bardi, G., Andersen, J.A., Mitelman, F., Heim, S. Clonal heterogeneity in breast cancer: karyotypic comparisons of multiple intra and extra-tumorous samples from 3 patients. Int. J. Cancer 63:63–68, 1995.

126. Teixeira, M.R. Pandis, N., Bardi, G., Andersen, J.A., Heim, S. Karyotypic comparisons of multiple tumors and macroscopically normal surrounding tissue samples from patients with breast cancer. Cancer Res. 56:855–859, 1996.

127. Pandis, N., Jin, Y., Gorunova, L., Petersson, C., Bardi, G., Idvall, I., Johansson, B., Ingvar, C., Mandahl, N., Mitelman, F., Heim, S. Chromosome analysis of 97 primary breast carcinomas: identification of eight karyotypic subgroups. Genes Chrom. Cancer, 12:173–185, 1995.

128. Böni, R., Matt, D., Voetmeyer, A., Burg, G., Zhuang, Z. Chromosomal allele loss in primary melanoma is heterogeneous and correlates with proliferation. J. Invest. Dermat. 110:215–217, 1998.

129. Ornstein, D.K., Englert, C., Gillespie, J.W., Paweletz, C.P., Linehan, W.M., Emmert-Buck, M.R., Petricoin III, E.F. Characterization of intracellular prostate-specific antigen from laser capture microdissected benign and malignant prostatic epithelium. Clin. Cancer Res. 6:353–356, 2000.

130. Milchgrub, S., Wistuba, I.I., Kim, B.K., Rutherford, C., Urban, J., Cruz Jr, P.D., Gazdar, A.F. Molecular identification of metastatic cancer to the skin using laser capture microdissection. Cancer, 88:749–754, 2000.

131. Aubele, M., Mattis, A., Zitzelsberger, H., Walch, A., Kremer, M., Hutzler, P., Höfler, H., Werner, M. Intratumoral heterogeneity in breast carcinoma revealed by laser microdissection and comparative genomic hybridization. Cancer Genet Cytogenet, 110:94–102, 1999.

132. Zhuang, Z., Merino, M.J., Chuaqui, R., Liotta, L.A., Emmert-Buck, M.R. Identical allelic loss on chromosome 11q13 in microdissected in situ and invasive breast cancer. Cancer Res. 55:467–471, 1995.

133. Radford, D.M., Phillips, N.J., Fair, K.L., Ritter, J.H., Holt, M., Donis-Keller, H. Allelic loss and the progression of breast cancer. Cancer Res. 55:5180–5183, 1995.

Animal Models for Human Breast Cancer

6.1 Introduction

From all experimental systems available for the study of mammary cancer, rodent models have been particularly useful, because these species develop spontaneous mammary tumors. The two models that will be discussed in this chapter are rodent models of mammary carcinogenesis and genetically engineered mice.

In several strains of female rats they are the most common hormone-dependent spontaneous neoplasms developed [1, 2]. The susceptibility of the rodent mammary gland to develop neoplasms has made this organ a unique target for testing the carcinogenic potential of specific chemicals. Several carcinogens, which induce mammary tumors in both mice and rats, have been extensively studied in both species [2, 3]. Tumors induced by administration of chemical carcinogens constitute useful tools for dissecting the multistep process of carcinogenesis, which involves initiation, promotion and progression, and serve as a baseline for testing the carcinogenic potential of chemicals in risk assessment. Chemically induced mammary tumors are, in general, hormone-dependent adenocarcinomas. Their incidence, number of tumors per animal, and even tumor type, are influenced by the age of the host at the time of carcinogen exposure, reproductive history, endocrinologic milieu, and diet, among other factors. These factors, in turn, influence the development and degree of mammary gland differentiation [4–6], which are subject to a multiplicity of endocrine stimulatory and inhibitory influences from embryogenesis onward [7]. If these influences are not exerted in proper temporal, sequential, and quantitative relationships, normal development, differentiation, and function are adversely affected. Mammary gland development, in turn, cannot be separated from its aging, a process that markedly influences the incidence of spontaneous tumors in all strains of rats, as well as in mice infected with the mammary tumor virus (MMTV).

The ideal animal tumor model should mimic the human disease. This means that the investigator should be able to ascertain the influence of host factors on the initiation of tumorigenesis, mimic the susceptibility of tumor response based on age and reproductive history, and determine the response of the tumors induced to chemotherapy. The utilization of experimental models of mammary carcinogenesis in risk assessment requires that the influence of ovarian, pituitary and placental hormones, among others, as well as overall reproductive events, and age at menarche and menopause, are taken into consideration, since they are important modifiers of the susceptibility of the organ to neoplastic development. Several species, such as rodents, dogs, cats, and monkeys, have been evaluated for these purposes; however, none of them fulfill all the criteria specified above. Rodents, however, are the most widely used models; therefore, this work will concentrate in discussing the rodent model.

6.2 General Concepts

The mammary gland, a specialized accessory gland of the skin that characterizes the mammalian species, is a frequent source of tumors, or neoplasms. The terms tumor or neoplasm are applied indistinctly to either benign or malignant lesions, since tumor (from the Latin *tumere*, to swell), means any pathological enlargement or new growth, also called neoplasm (from the Greek *neos* new + *plasma* formation), however, none of them defines the true nature of a given growth. Benign tumors are those that do not invade adjacent tissues, do not metastasize to distant sites, and can be cured by local excision. Malignant tumors, or cancer, are neoplasms characterized by their ability to invade, metastasize and ultimately cause the death of the host. They are called "carcinomas" when they are derived from epithelial cells or "sarcomas" if they are mesenchymal in origin.

Spontaneous mammary tumors are frequently observed in long-term rodent studies [8]. In mice the development of "spontaneous" mammary tumors is linked to the infection of female mice with either an exogenous mouse mammary tumor virus (MMTV), or a less virulent endogenous provirus. A third strain of MMTV transmitted through the milk and through the germ line has also been identified in the European mouse strain GR. The exogenous MMTV is an RNA virus first recognized to be transmitted through the milk of A and C3H strain mothers, the *Bittner factor*. DBA and RIII are also inbred strains of mice that harbor the highly oncogenic MMTV transmitted through the milk. Foster-nursed neonate mice (i.e., C3Hf or DBAf) become free of the milk-transmitted MMTV, although they retain the genetically transmitted MMTV, which induces mammary tumors late in life. In high incidence strains of mice, tumors develop as a multistep process initiated in preneoplastic lesions, the hyperplastic alveolar nodules, which evolve from pregnancy-dependent to pregnancy-independent adenocarcinomas. Nulliparous mice develop a low incidence of mammary tumors. Out of a total of 1,361 female B6Cf$_1$/CrlBR mice, only 5 adenomas (0.4%), 4 fibroadenomas (0.3%), 10 adenocarcinomas (0.9%), and 7 carcinomas (0.6%) developed by the end of a 24-month follow-up. Some mammary tumors that develop in females of susceptible strains, such as C3H, A, DBA, CBA and certain sub-strains of Balb/c, are strongly hormone-dependent in terms of their initiation. Multiple pregnancies enhance tumor development, and final tumorigenic response is greater in multiparous than in nulliparous animals. In RIII, BR6, DD, and GR mice mammary tumors develop during the first pregnancy, but they regress during lactation. In some strains of mice the growth of mammary tumors is stimulated by chronic administration of estrogens, certain steroidal contraceptives, progesterone, PRL and epidermal growth factor (EGF), whereas hormone deprivation, induced by hypophysectomy, ovariectomy, ovariectomy-adrenalectomy, and sialidectomy suppress mammary carcinogenesis [2].

In the rat, the majority of spontaneously developed tumors, with the exception of leukemia, are neoplasms of endocrine organs or of organs under endocrine control. Spontaneous mammary tumors develop in females of various strains of rats, such as August, Albany-Hooded, Copenhagen, Fisher, Lewis, Osborne-Mendel, Sprague-Dawley, Wistar and Wistar/Furth [2]. Spontaneous mammary tumors are third in incidence among spontaneous tumors found in the Fisher 344 rat used in the National Cancer Institute/National Toxicology Program (NCI/NTP) carcinogenicity bioassays [8]. They are predominantly benign tumors, i.e., fibroadenomas, fibromas and more rarely adenomas. Malignant tumors such as adenocarcinomas are rare, although they are the most frequent tumors induced by chemical carcinogens [9]. The development of spontaneous tumors varies as a function of strain, age and endocrine influences. Mammary gland tumors develop in older females; they are more frequent in multiparous than in nulliparous rats. As in the mice, hormone withdrawal inhibits tumor development, and hormone supplementation, such as chronic administration of estrogens, increases the incidence of adenocarcinomas, whereas chronic administration of prolactin or of growth hormone stimulates benign tumor growth [2]. The long latency period for spontaneous tumor development, up to 2 years in susceptible strains to develop a 50–70% tumor incidence, limits the usefulness of this model for experimental studies.

6.3 Chemically-Induced Mammary Tumorigenesis

The potential of chemicals to induce cancer was recognized almost two centuries ago as an occupational disease, when high incidence of skin cancer was linked to exposure to coal tar. Although it has not been proven that human breast cancer is caused by a given chemical or physical genotoxic agent, the human population is exposed to a large number of environmental chemicals, such as polycyclic aromatic hydrocarbons, nitrosoureas and aromatic amines that have been demonstrated to be carcinogenic in experimental animal models, and to induce mutagenesis and neoplastic transformation of human breast epithelial cells in vitro [10]. Although a specific etiologic agent or the conditions that might explain the initiation and progression of breast cancer in humans have not been identified, experimental animal models have proven to be useful tools for answering specific questions on the biology of mammary cancer relative to their validity to the human disease, as well as for assessing the risk for breast cancer posed by toxic chemicals. In vivo experimental animal models provide information not available in human populations; they are adequate for hazard identification, dose-response modeling, exposure assessment, and risk characterization, the four required steps for quantifying the estimated risk of cancer development associated with toxic chemical exposure. The utilization of experimental models of mammary carcinogenesis in risk assessment requires that the influence of ovarian, pituitary and placental hormones, among others, as well as overall reproductive events, are taken into consideration, since they are important modifiers of the susceptibility of the organ to undergo neoplastic transformation [6].

Chemically induced mammary tumors develop by a multistep process. The initial step is a biochemical lesion caused by the interaction of the carcinogen with cellular DNA. In this interaction the DNA is damaged, and if the damage is not repaired efficiently, the result is a mutation, chromosomal translocation, inactivation of regulatory genes or more subtle changes not well identified as yet. Neoplastic development requires that the lesion becomes fixed, aided by cell proliferation, progressing to a third stage of autonomous growth, resulting in cancer, when the lesion acquires the capacity to invade and metastasize [3]. Several carcinogens that induce mammary tumors in rodents have been identified and extensively studied for more than 50 years in mice and for more than 30 in rats [2]. Mammary carcinomas have been induced in strains of mice with low spontaneous mammary cancer incidence with 3,4-benzopyrene, 3-methylcholanthrene (MCA), 1,2,5,6-dibenzanthracene, 7,12-dimethylbenz(a)anthracene (DMBA) and urethane. Most of the mammary tumors induced in mice by chemical carcinogens are adenoacanthomas and type B adenocarcinomas. They develop after a relatively long period of time, and their induction requires multiple applications. Enhanced tumorigenicity has been obtained with prolonged hormonal stimulation. However, the hormone-responsiveness of chemically induced mammary tumors in mice has not been as thoroughly studied as it has been in the rat [3].

The most frequently utilized rat mammary carcinogens are DMBA and N-methyl-N-nitrosourea (MNU), although MCA, 2-acetylaminofluorene, 3,4-benzopyrene, ethylnitrosourea, and butylnitrosourea have also been extensively utilized as mammary cancer inducers [2, 3, 11]. The majority of rat mammary carcinomas induced by either DMBA or MNU are hormone-dependent. Maximal tumor incidence is elicited when the carcinogens are administered to young virgin females with an intact endocrine system. These models of hormone-dependent tumors constitute useful tools for dissecting the multistep process of carcinogenesis, and serve as a baseline for testing the carcinogenic potential of chemicals in risk assessment.

6.4 Radiation-Induced Mammary Tumorigenesis

Ionizing radiation is probably the most widely acknowledged and studied human carcinogen [11]. Exposure to radiation, either accidentally or for therapeutic reasons, has for long being associated with a greater incidence of neoplasms, namely hematopoietic, gonadal and of the breast. The female breast is one of the tissues with the highest sensitivity to radiation carcinogenesis. Breast cancer developed in irradiated women shows a strong association with young age at the time of exposure, an association not observed in irradiated rodents, but similar to what has been observed in chemically induced mammary carcinogenesis in rats [12, 13]. Since controversy exists concerning the shape of the dose-response curve, the effects of fractionated irradiation, and the effect of low levels of radiation, animal studies are necessary to address these issues. The rat model has been widely used in this regard, mainly since the demonstration in the early 1950s that a single supralethal dose of X-rays to female Holtzman rats (a Sprague-Dawley stock) maintained by temporary parabiosis induced an increased number of benign and malignant mammary tumors within 6 months of exposure. Sublethal doses of different types of radiation, including X-rays and neutrons, have been shown to induce mammary tumor development, often within a year, with linear dose-effect relationships for neutrons over the total dose range and for X-rays down to dose levels of 0.2 Gy. Irradiation of animals with fractionated doses of γ-radiation has resulted in linear-quadratic dose-response curves. Although most studies have utilized whole-body irradiation, localized irradiation also induces mammary tumors in the rat within the irradiated field. This effect occurs also in women, but reportedly not in several other animal species studied, e.g., mice, dogs and guinea pigs. In rats, mammary carcinomas can be induced by whole-body or segmental radiation with either X-rays, γ-rays or neutrons [11]. Several studies utilizing a variety of fractionated irradiation protocols, i.e., at 12-h intervals for 60 days, semi-weekly for up to 16 weeks, and monthly for up to 10 months, have shown in general, no increase in tumor latency, incidence or total number of mammary tumors, and no sparing or enhancing effect on mammary tumor development when compared with animals exposed to single doses of radiation. Some investigators, however, have reported an increased number of mammary carcinomas in animals receiving fractionated doses. Sprague-Dawley and Lewis rats are the most susceptible to radiation-induced tumorigenesis. AxC, Fisher, Long-Evans and Wistar/Furth are also susceptible, but to a lesser degree. The mammary tumors developed by irradiated rats are, in general, hormone-dependent adenocarcinomas or fibroadenomas. The hormonal status of the female rat is of paramount importance in determining the outcome of irradiation of the mammary gland. Ovariectomy completely prevents, and estrogen treatment enhances, radiation-induced mammary tumor formation. The latency period for tumor development is shortened and tumor incidence is increased considerably in estrogen-treated rats. The number of cribriform type adenocarcinomas, and the number of tumors/tumor-bearing rat are also increased. Radiation and estrogens, namely 17-β-estradiol (E_2) or diethylstilbestrol (DES), have been reported to exert either an additive or synergistic effect. The effect of E_2 administration and irradiation on mammary tumorigenesis has been reported to be equal for hormone administration 1 week before, or beginning 12 weeks after irradiation, but no additive effect has been observed when hormone administration was began 24 weeks after irradiation. The amplification of radiation-induced mammary tumorigenesis by estrogens has been attributed by several investigators to the effects of this hormone on the pituitary, an interpretation supported by the observations that DES-treatment of ACI rats, and E_2 treatment of rats of three different strains, for example, result in increased incidence of pituitary tumors, accompanied by marked increases in plasma prolactin (PRL) levels. The development of malignant mammary tumors in these rats appeared to be associated with the extent of increase in plasma PRL. Mammary tumor incidence and number or type of mammary tumors is not modified by irradiation during pregnancy, lactation, or postlactational regression in comparison with irradiation in the virginal state, at difference of what has been reported in chemically-induced mammary carcinogenesis [3]. Furthermore, radiation-induced mammary tumors developed in rats do not exhibit the age-dependency observed in women or in chemically-induced rat mammary carcinomas [12–15]. They do not exhibit topographic selectivity in their development, since they arise randomly in thoracic and abdomino-inguinal regions [2, 16]. Further studies are needed for clarifying these differences in tumor incidence between radiation- and chemically-induced mammary tumors in rats for validating this model for risk assessment. The reason for the differences in physiologic influences on the inductive action of chemicals and irradiation in rat mammary gland is not clear. It has been speculated that radiation-induced changes might occur in a specific stem cell population maintained throughout the reproductive life, while chemically induced changes depend upon the number and rate of turnover of other types of mammary gland cells [14].

6.5 Genetic Background and Mammary Carcinogenesis

Genetic differences among individuals may affect their susceptibility to the carcinogenic effect of chemicals. Inheritance may as well predispose an individual to develop certain specific types of cancer. These influences have been carefully dissected in rodent experimental animal models [17]. In carefully designed experiments, it has been demonstrated that the susceptibility of rats to the chemical carcinogens 2-acetylaminofluorene (AAF), DMBA and MNU is genetically determined [17]. Isaacs demonstrated that Buffalo, Lewis, Wistar/Furth and inbred Sprague-Dawley rats, all strains of Wistar genetic background are highly susceptible to chemically induced carcinogenesis, whereas the non-Wistar derived strains Fischer, August, ACI and Copenhagen are of low susceptibility [17]. However, there are exceptions to this rule, since the Wistar-derived inbred WN strain is of low susceptibility, and the non-Wistar derived Osborne-Mendel is highly susceptible. Of the commonly used strains, Sprague-Dawley and Wistar-Furth are the most susceptible and Fischer 344 and ACI rats show intermediate susceptibility. Copenhagen rats are essentially completely resistant even to the direct application of DMBA to the gland, although they do develop fibrosarcomas in response to parenteral DMBA. Extensive analyses comparing DMBA tumorigenesis, mammary gland growth rate, serum hormone levels, and DMBA toxicokinetics in female rats of several strains and F_1 hybrids between the strains, have not found major difference that correlated with susceptibility to tumorigenesis, since both susceptible and resistant strains develop similar percentages of malignant changes (60% in resistant, 80% in susceptible). However, macroscopically detectable tumors developed in 70% of susceptible and only in

10% of resistant glands. These findings have been confirmed by transplantation experiments between resistant or susceptible strains into F_1 hybrids, and between the two strains, and by direct exposure to DMBA. These observations indicate that genetic factors govern the progression from microscopic to macroscopic tumor, rather than from normal to histologically malignant epithelium, and furthermore, that resistant rat possess a dominant suppressor allele for the gene governing susceptibility. In contrast, tumor induction by DES is demonstrable in the ACI, but not in the Sprague-Dawley strain of rats, although a co-carcinogenic effect of DES with DMBA can be shown in these latter ones. Both malignant and benign tumors are increased by the combined treatment, but there is a relatively greater increase in benign tumors. The response of target organs other than the mammary gland to DES is also different in these two strains of rats, but the mechanisms are not known.

6.6 Pathogenesis of Rat Mammary Tumors

Chemical carcinogen induction of mammary tumors in rodents is one of the most widely studied and useful models of mammary carcinogenesis [11, 12, 14, 15, 18, 19]. For those reasons this section will focus mainly on that model. The two most widely utilized experimental systems of mammary tumorigenesis are the induction of rat mammary tumors by administration of either the indirect acting polycyclic hydrocarbon DMBA, given intragastrically (ig) to Sprague-Dawley rats [19], or the direct acting carcinogen NMU, given intravenously (iv) or subcutaneously (sc) to Sprague-Dawley or Fischer 344 rats, respectively [20]. A single ig dose of 80–100 mg DMBA/kg body weight induces tumors with latencies that generally range between 8 and 21 weeks. The final tumor incidence reaches 100% when the carcinogen is administered to intact virgin rats in their peak of maximal susceptibility, that in Sprague-Dawley rats occurs between the ages of 40 to 60 days of age. NMU, given in a single iv dose of 25 or 50 mg/kg body weight yields tumors with similar latency and incidence [20]. In a comparative study between the carcinogenic poten-

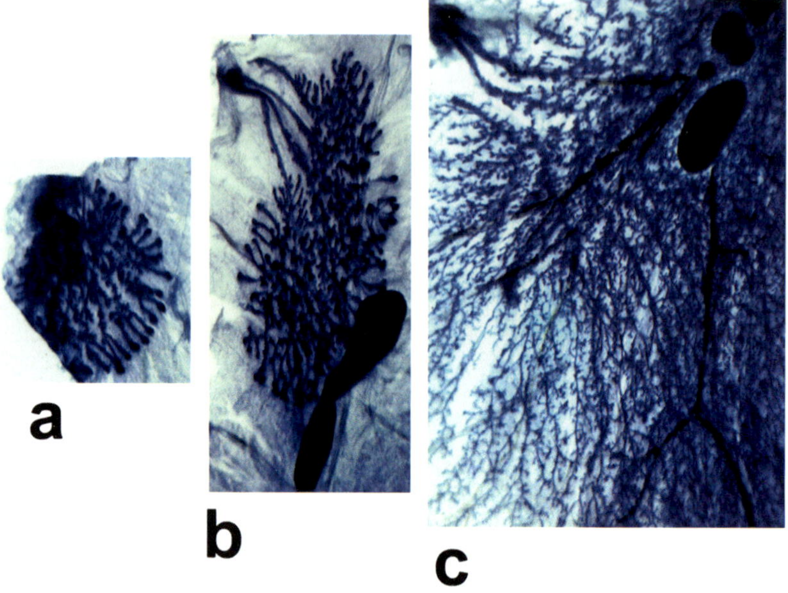

Figure 6.1 a–c

Whole mount preparation of the abdominal mammary gland **a** 21 days of age, **b** 35 days of age, **c** 55 days of age. Toluidine blue × 10. The procedure of whole mount preparation is a method of tissue fixation and staining, which takes advantage of the contrast between stainable parenchymal elements and the clear stroma, which should be composed mostly of fat. The ideal organ is the mammary gland, in which the parenchyma consists of epithelial-myoepithelial elements, which stain positively with either toluidine blue, alum carmin or hematoxylin. The stroma contains predominantly fat, which is cleared with acetone. Mammary glands in which the stroma is fibrous, such as in fetal and newborn stages, in adult breast tissue with fibrosis, or in parenchymal structures growing through muscular fibers, such as the rat thoracic glands, are less adequate for examination with this technique. The mammary gland was obtained from a deeply anesthetized animal that was placed on its back, with the four extremities stretched on a surgical board. The skin was opened by a longitudinal midline incision extending from the submaxillary to the pubic regions and separated from the muscle by blunt dissection with scissors. Ideal fixation for whole mount preparation was obtained by removing the skin pelt with all the mammary glands attached. The skin pelt was stretched and pinned to a corkboard and then immersed in 10% neutral buffered formalin for 24 h. After fixation, the mammary glands were identified by locating the corresponding nipple. Then they were dissected starting at the nipple and proceeding dorsolaterally. The mammary fat pad was lifted with forceps. It was separated from the subcutaneous tissue by dissection with iris scissors or a scalpel. Tissues were defatted by submersion in acetone and placed on a shaker bath under continuous agitation at approximately 80 rpm for 2 or more days. The acetone was changed when it became cloudy. Tissues were hydrated in 100%, 95% and 70% ethanol for 1 h each with continuous agitation in the shaker bath. After rehydration, the tissues were left in distilled water overnight, and stained in 0.025% toluidine blue solution for 2 h. The tissues were washed in distilled water for 30 min, immersed in pure methanol for 30 min, followed by 70% ethanol for 30 min, and then in distilled water. The tissue was then fixed in 4% ammonium molybdate for 30 min followed by washing and storing in distilled water overnight. The dehydration was performed in 70%, 95% and 100% ethanol for 1 h each, followed by xylene overnight. Small mammary glands or fragments of mammary tissue no larger than 4×2 cm and no thicker than 1–2 mm were mounted on slides and coverslipped with Permount (Fisher Scientific). These specimens are optimal for examination under the stereo microscope or a light microscope, and are adequate for obtaining photographs. Large mammary glands or thick fragments of tissue were placed in glycerin in plastic bags (Scotchpak heat sealable pouches) and sealed with a heat sealer (Kapak Corp., Bloomington, MN). The disadvantage of thick specimens is that they have to be observed under a stereo microscope focusing in different planes. They are difficult to photograph, and areas of interest have to be dissected into smaller fragments for mounting on slides

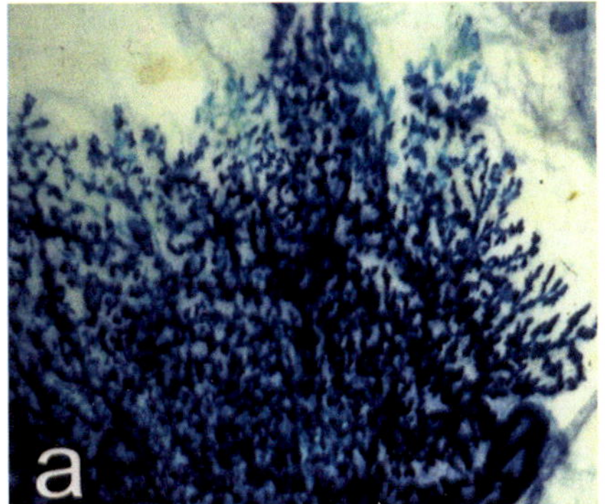
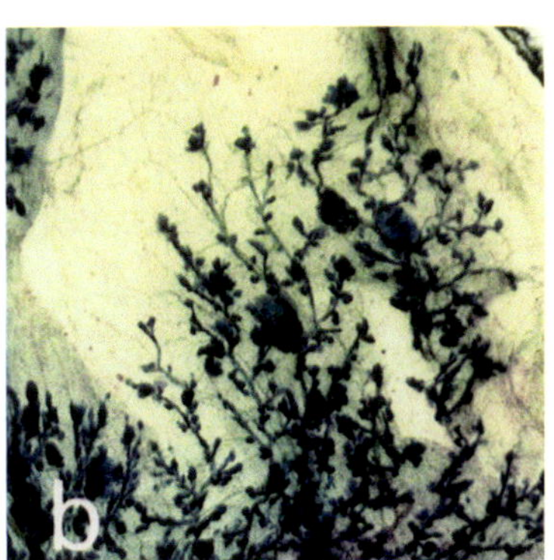

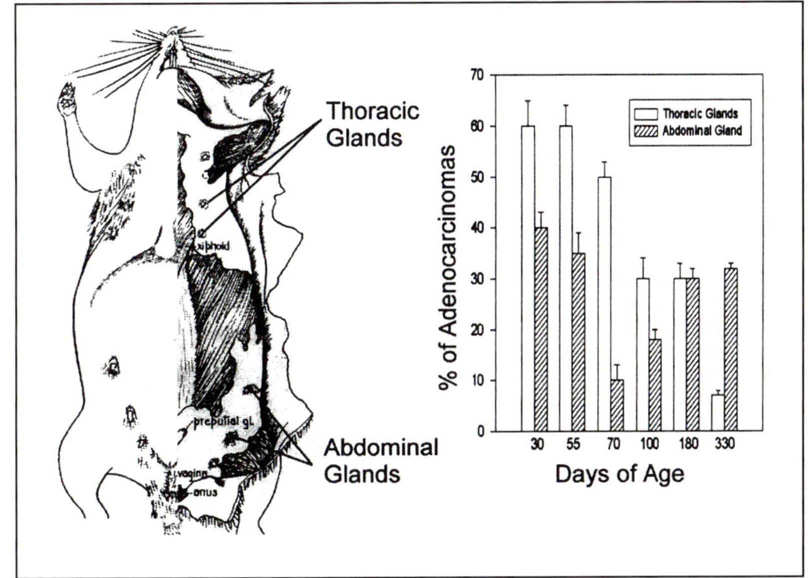

Figure 6.3

Drawing of a rat showing the distribution of the six pair of mammary glands. The fourth pair, or abdominal mammary gland, is the most frequently utilized for morphological, cell kinetics, and tumorigenic studies because of its large size and ease of access. However, they are less susceptible to be transformed by chemical carcinogens, as indicated in the histogram at the right hand side, which shows that the higher incidence of adenocarcinomas occurs in thoracic mammary glands in those animals inoculated with the carcinogen at ages younger than 100 days. These results were obtained by inoculating virgin Sprague Dawley rats intragastrically (ig) with a single dose of 8 mg 7, 12-dimethylbenz(a)anthracene (DMBA) (Sigma Chemical Co., St. Louis, MO) per 100 g body weight (bw). The carcinogen was dissolved in corn oil at a concentration of 16 mg DMBA/ml by heating in a water bath at 95°C for 30 min (reprinted with permission from: Russo, J. and Russo, I.H. Mammary tumor induction in animals as a model for human breast cancer. In: *Cancer Handbook* (J. Haier and G. L. Nicolson Eds.) Macmillan Publisher, N.Y. 2001, Chapter 59, pp 923–935)

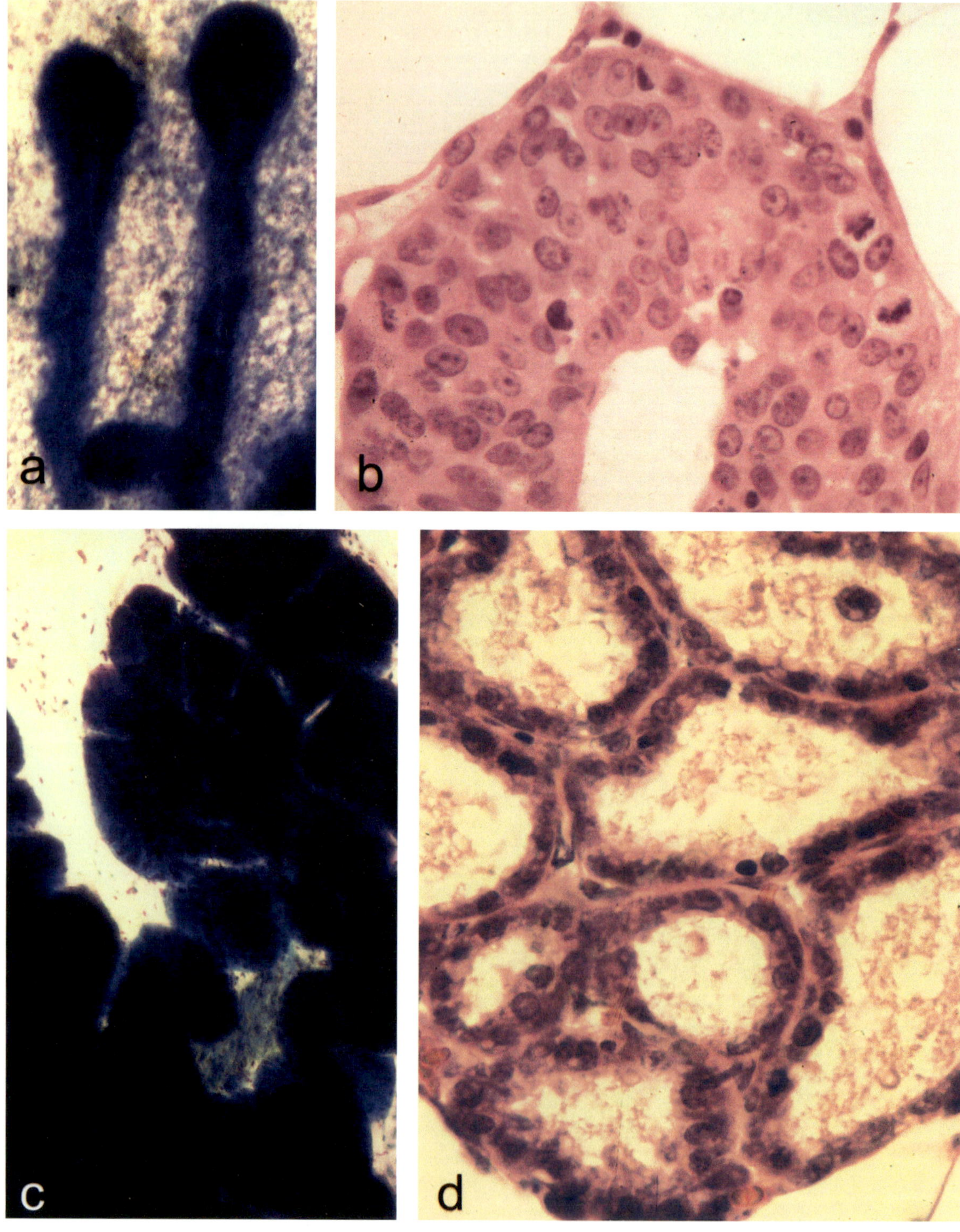

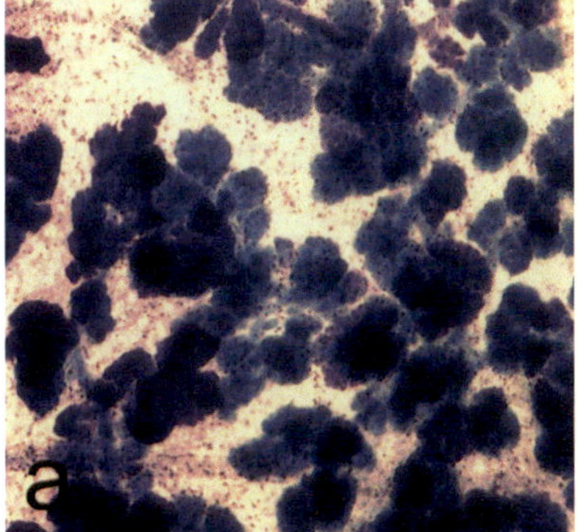
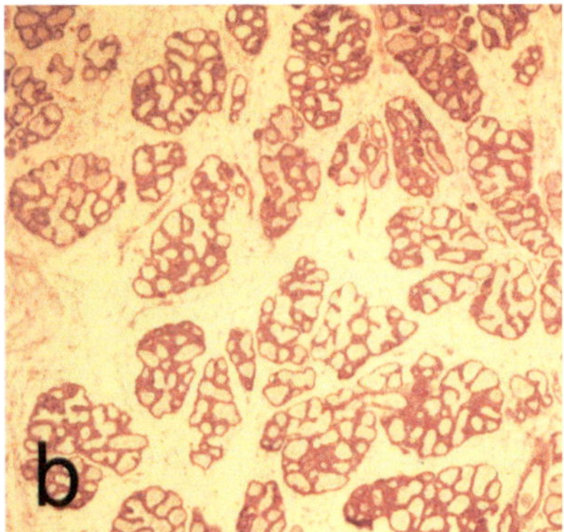
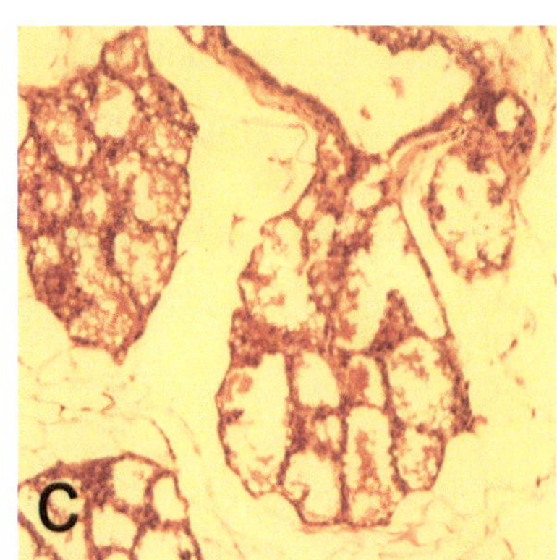

◀ **Figure 6.4 a–d**

a Whole mount of the TEB of the rat mammary gland at 45 days of age stained with toluidine blue, ×20. **b** Histological section at the tip of **a**, stained with H&E, ×40. **c** Lobule type 3 of a pregnant rat mammary gland stained with toluidine blue, ×20. **d** Histological section of **c** stained with H&E, ×40

Figure 6.5 a–c

a Whole mount of a 15 days pregnant rat mammary gland stained with toluidine blue, ×4. **b** Histological section of **a** showing the lobules type 3, stained with H&E, ×4. **c** Particular of a lobule type 3 stained with H&E, ×10

tial of DMBA, administered ig at a dose of 20 mg, and NMU, given iv at a dose of 50 mg/kg, it was demonstrated that both induce approximately equal tumor incidence and number of tumors per animal, with approximately equal latency, but a somewhat greater percentage of NMU-induced tumors were histologically malignant.

The analysis of the factors that modulate the tumorigenic response of the mammary gland, especially in short-term studies, have revealed that the most sensitive and reliable end points are both tumor latency and tumor histological type. Tumor latency is, in general, inversely related to carcinogen dose, whereas overall tumor incidence and number of malignant tumors per animal are directly related, especially when relatively early end points are used. No such a relationship has been found for benign tumors. The number of tumors per rat or per group, and the number or incidence of malignant tumors is an additional end point useful in analysis of data. Comparison of data among laboratories requires strict standardization of the experimental conditions, since considerable variations in tumor incidence and latencies between laboratories and between experiments in the same laboratory are frequently seen.

The induction of mammary carcinomas in the rat requires that the carcinogen act on a specific compartment of the mammary gland, the terminal end bud (TEB), a club-shaped undifferentiated structure found at the peripheral margins of the developing mammary parenchyma in young virgin rats (Figs. 6.1, 6.2). Although TEBs are present in the six pairs of mammary glands, tumor development does not occur as a random event. Tumor incidence in animals treated with the carcinogen between the ages of 20 and 180 days is greater in those glands located in the thoracic region, whereas glands located in the abdominal and inguinal areas develop a lower number of tumors (Fig. 6.3). In addition to differences in tumor incidence as a consequence of the topographic location of the gland, there are differences in tumor type, which seem to vary with the age of the animal at the time of carcinogen treatment. Ductal and papillary adenocarcinomas are more frequent in both thoracic and abdominal glands of younger animals,

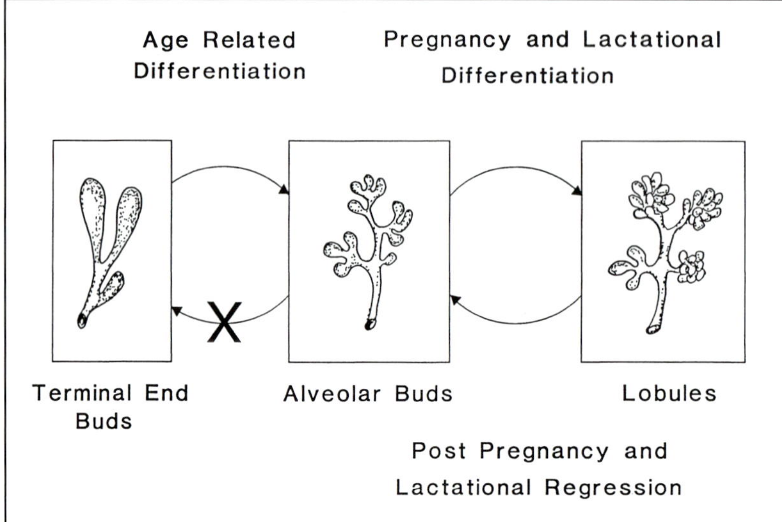

Figure 6.6

Terminal end buds, alveolar buds and lobules. *Arrows* indicate differentiation of terminal end buds into alveolar buds and lobular structures. After weaning neither alveolar buds nor lobules regress to terminal end buds (reprinted with permission from: Russo, J and Russo, IH, Cancer Epidemiol Biomarkers & Prevention, 3, 353–364, 1994)

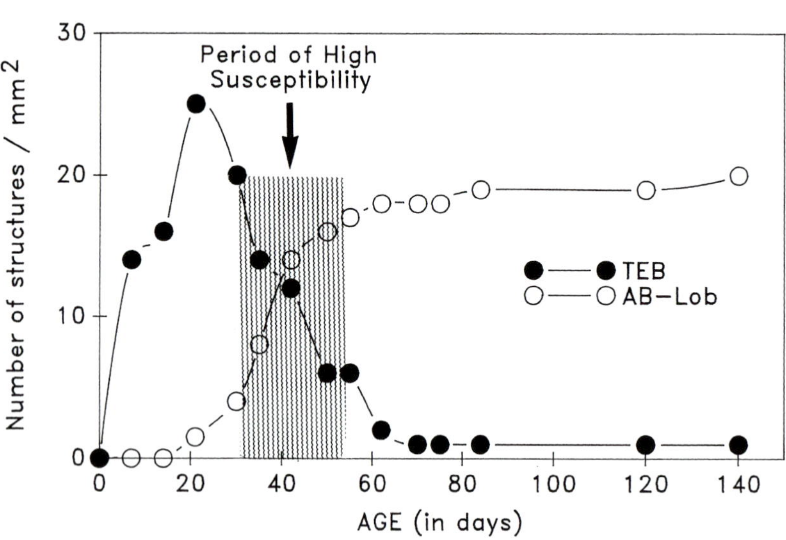

Figure 6.7

Histogram representing the number of structures /mm2 (ordinate) of the rat mammary gland in relation to age (abscissa). *Hatched area*, period of highest susceptibility of the mammary gland to neoplastic transformation by chemical carcinogens (reprinted with permission from: Russo, J and Russo, IH, Cancer Epidemiol Biomarkers & Prevention, 3, 353–364, 1994)

whereas adenocarcinomas with tubular pattern are found mostly in abdominal glands and in older animals. The development of the rat mammary gland occurs through a combined process of branching and differentiation of the parenchyma, mainly in those ducts ending in TEBs that progressively divide and differentiate into alveolar buds (ABs) (Figs. 6.1, 6.4–6.8). These structures in turn differentiate into lobules. Although this pattern of development is common to the six pairs of mammary glands, it does not occur simultaneously in all of them, but varies in relation to the topographic location of each specific pair. Individual structures, i.e., TEBs, ABs, and lobules, appear similar in morphology in all the glands, however, their relative number and the general architecture of the organ vary notably from one pair of glands to another (Fig. 6.8). The most notable ones are the thoracic mammary glands, since each single

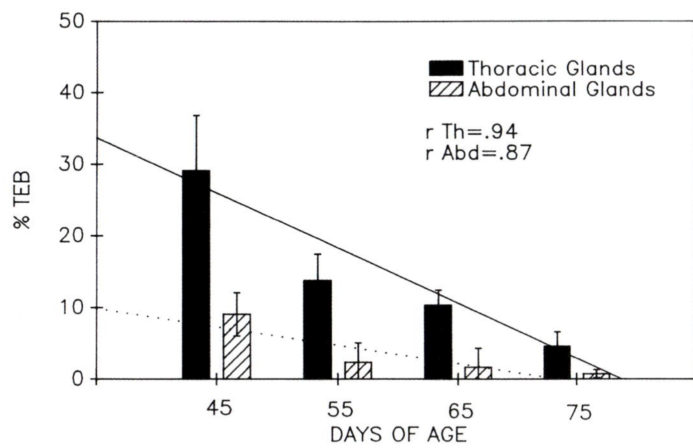

Figure 6.8

Age-dependence variations in percentage of TEB in thoracic and abdominal mammary glands of virgin rats. *r* correlation coefficient for *Th* thoracic, *Abd* abdominal mammary glands (reprinted with permission from: I.H. Russo and J. Russo Anticancer Res. 8:1247, 1988)

gland is composed of two different layers separated by connective and muscular tissue; one layer is composed of more numerous ABs and small lobules, whereas the adjacent one is more extensive and contains thin long ducts ending in prominent TEBs. The abdominal glands have a markedly reduced number of TEBs, which are located exclusively in the most distal portion of the gland, whereas the middle and proximal portions show a much more differentiated appearance. The difference in number of TEBs in thoracic versus abdominal mammary glands is significant (Fig. 6.8). With aging, TEBs decrease progressively and their reduction is proportional in all the glands. This reduction is mostly due to either their regression to TDs or to a greater differentiation to ABs and lobules (Fig. 6.7). The higher incidence in ductal carcinomas observed in thoracic glands is attributed to the difference in degree of development of the undifferentiated layer of this gland in comparison with the glands located in other topographic areas [14, 15].

6.7 Mammary Gland Differentiation as a Modulator of Carcinogenic Response

Mammary cancer in experimental models is the result of the interaction of a carcinogen with the target organ, the mammary gland. This target, however, is extremely complex, since the mammary gland does not respond to the carcinogen as whole, but only specific structures within the gland are affected by given genotoxic agents. The knowledge of the architecture and cell kinetic characteristics of the mammary gland at the time of carcinogen administration constitutes a necessary initial step for understanding the pathogenesis of the disease. It is also required for distinguishing those changes induced by the carcinogen from changes reflecting normal gland development, especially when evaluating early tumorigenic response in short term studies [1, 12, 18, 22].

The susceptibility of the mammary gland to DMBA- or NMU-induced carcinogenesis is strongly age-dependent; it is maximal when the carcinogens are administered to virgin females between the ages of 40 and 60 days, that is, soon after vaginal opening and during early sexual maturity (Fig. 6.7) [12]. Active organogenesis and high rate of proliferation of the glandular epithelium are characteristics of that period, in which there is also high DMBA activation (Figs. 6.9, 6.10) [14, 15, 18, 21]. Its significance, however, is uncertain, since NMU, which is also most effec-

Structure	DNA-LI	T_C	Cell cycle	GF_5	^{3}H-DMBA	Lesions
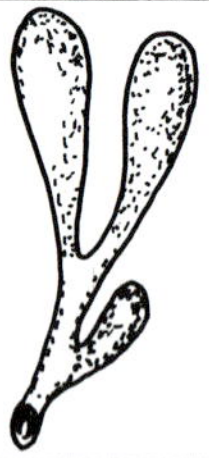 TEB	34%	11.65 h	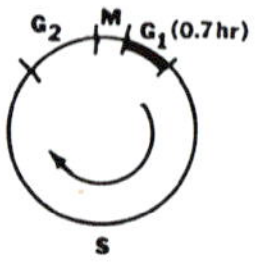	0.55	6.8 ± 2.8	Carcinoma
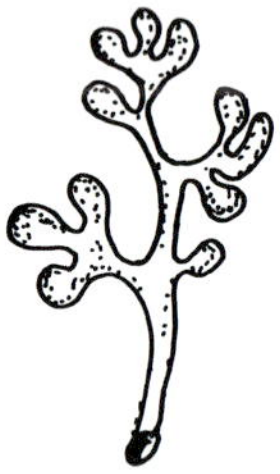 AB	4%	28.18 h	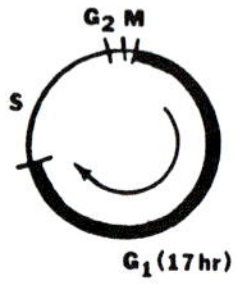	0.13	1.3 ± 0.8	Cysts HAN Adenomas Fibro-Ad.
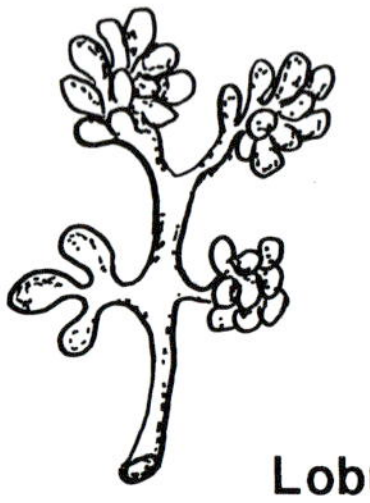 Lobule	0.1%	49.63 h	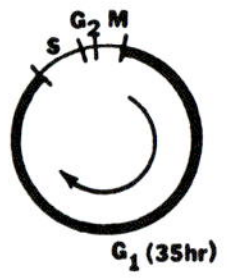	0.0049	0.9 ± 0.5	None

tive at that age, does not require activation. The incidence of DMBA-induced tumors reaches 100 % when the carcinogen is administered to rats aged 30 to 55 days, but the highest number of tumors/animal is observed when the carcinogen is given to animals between the ages of 40 and 46 days, coincident with the period in which the mammary gland exhibits a high density of highly proliferating TEBs (Figs. 6.7, 6.9). This high susceptibility is attributed to the specific characteristics of the mammary gland prevailing during that period of life. Administration of DMBA to virgin rats induces the largest number of transformed foci when TEBs are decreasing in number due to their differentiation into ABs (Figs. 6.7, 6.10). These structures, instead of differentiating into ABs, become progressively larger due to epithelial proliferation, with multilayering, secondary lumen forma-

Figure 6.9

Correlation between type of structure, terminal end bud (*TEB*), alveolar bud (*AB*), and lobule with their rate of ^{3}H-thymidine incorporation, or DNA-labeling index (DNA-LI), length of the cell cycle in hours (*Tc*) cell cycle, and growth fraction (GF_5), or rate of ^{3}H-thymidine incorporation after 5 days of continuous infusion. Nuclear uptake of ^{3}H-DMBA, detected by autoradiography and expressed as the number of grains/nucleus, is directly proportional to the DNA-LI and GF_5 and inversely proportional to the T_c of each specific structure. The development of carcinomas also correlated with high DNA-LI, Tc, and DMBA binding, whereas benign lesions or the absence of neoplasms were inversely related (reprinted with permission from: Russo, J and Russo, IH, Cancer Epidemiol Biomarkers & Prevention, 3, 353–364, 1994)

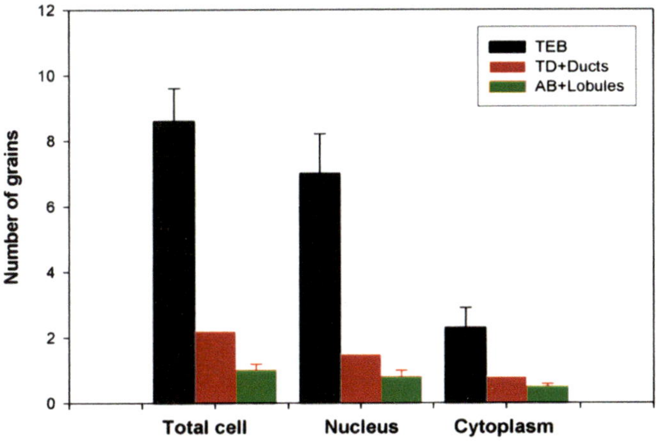
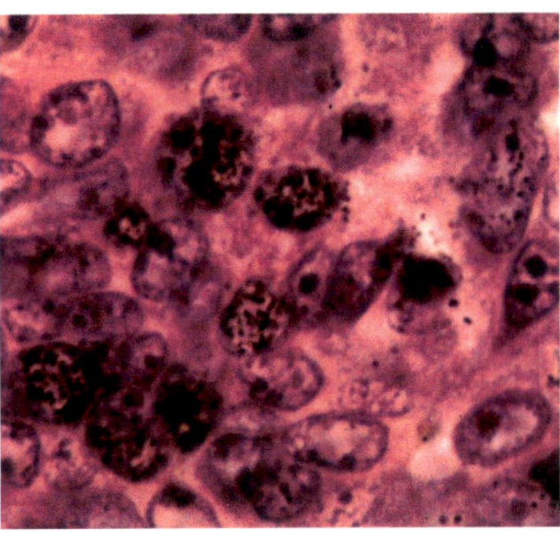

Figure 6.10

Left panel, histogram depicting the number of silver grains in the terminal end buds (*TEB*), terminal ducts and ducts (*TD + Ducts*) and alveolar buds and lobules (*AB + Lobules*) in the rat mammary gland of a Sprague-Dawley rat inoculated with 1 μCi of [³H]-DMBA intraperitoneally. The animal was sacrificed 24 h later and processed for autoradiographic studies. The *right panel* shows the silver grains in the TEB. Counterstained with H&E, × 40

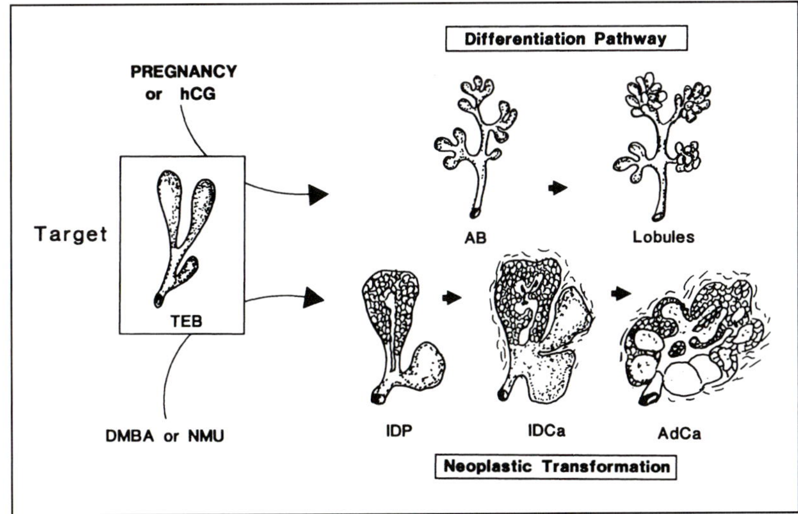

Figure 6.11

Pathogenesis of chemically-induced rat mammary tumors. The undifferentiated terminal end bud (*TEB*) affected by the carcinogen progresses to intraductal proliferation (*IDP*), and in situ ductal carcinoma (*IDCa*) that exhibits various histo-pathological types. Further tumoral growth and coalescence of neighboring lesions originate invasive adenocarcinomas (*AdCa*), which might become metastatic. (reprinted with permission from: Russo, J and Russo, IH, Cancer Epidemiol Bio-markers & Prevention, 3, 353–364, 1994)

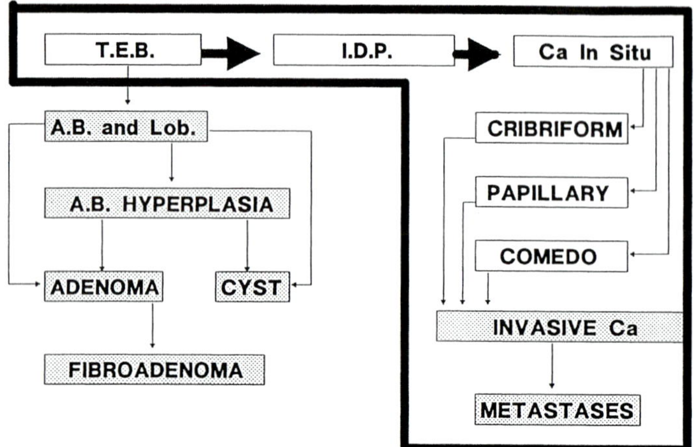

Figure 6.12

Chart representing two different pathogenetic pathways fro benign and malignant lesions. Malignant lesions originate from TEB and appear earlier than benign lesions originated from AB. The earliest lesion detected after DMBA administration is the IDP

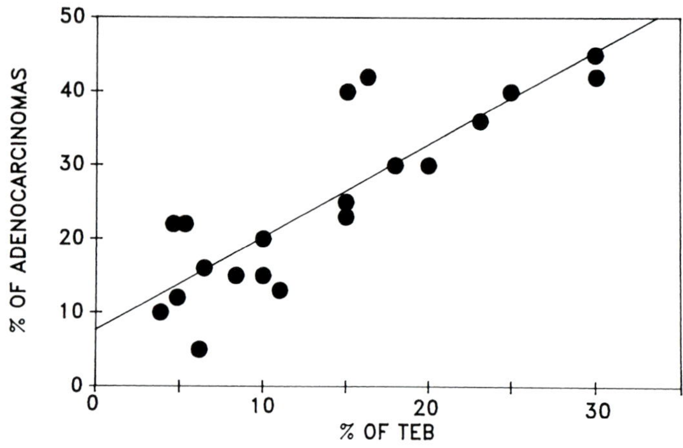

Figure 6.13

Regression curve showing the high correlation (cc 0.87 $p=$ 0.001) between percentage of adenocarcinomas and percentage of TEB

tion and early papillary projections to the widened lumen, at this stage, transformed TEBs are called intraductal proliferations (IDPs) (Fig. 6.11). Their confluence leads to the formation of microtumors that histologically are classified as adenocarcinomas, first intraductal, which progress to invasive, developing various patterns such as cribriform, comedo, or papillary types [9, 12].

Even though TEB differentiation into AB is inhibited by carcinogen treatment, not all the TEBs present in the mammary gland at the time of DMBA administration progress to IDPs. Some of them still differ-

entiate into ABs but their number is always lower than that of control animals. Occasional lobular development is observed although it is negligible. Some TEBs become smaller with an atrophic appearance being called at this stage, terminal ducts (TDs). TDs are also susceptible to neoplastic transformation and are the main target of carcinogens in older animals [4, 5]. Those TEBs that were already differentiated into ABs and early lobular structures before DMBA administration do not develop carcinomas. Most of them either remain unmodified or undergo dilatation of the lumen, giving rise to hyperplastic lesions, such as alveolar bud hyperplasia (Fig. 6.12). Others exhibit epithelial proliferation, forming tubular adenomas, give rise to cystic dilatations, or fibroadenomas (Fig. 6.12). When DMBA is inoculated to old virgin females, ranging in age from 180 to 330 days, they develop tubular adenomas that exhibit focal areas of malignant transformation, giving origin to well-differentiated adenocarcinomas with a tubular pattern. These lesions develop predominantly in the abdominal glands, in which a higher incidence of tumors is observed in older animals. The observation that mammary carcinomas arise from undifferentiated structures of the gland namely TEBs and TDs and that the number of adenocarcinomas is directly related to the number of these structure sin the mammary gland (Fig. 6.13), whereas benign lesions such as adenomas, cysts, and fibroadenomas (Fig. 6.12) arise from structures that were more differentiated at the time of carcinogen administration, indicates that the carcinogen requires and adequate structural target, and the type of lesion induced is dependent upon the area of the mammary gland that the carcinogen affects. Thus, the more differentiated the structure at the time of carcinogen administration the more benign and organized is the lesion that develops. This in turn is related to the number of cells in growth fraction, or proliferating, and the amount of binding of the carcinogen to the different structures of the mammary gland (Figs. 6.9, 6.10).

6.7.1 Cell of Origin of Rat Mammary Carcinomas

In the rat mammary gland parenchyma, three types of cells have been described, dark, intermediate and myoepithelial cells (Fig. 6.14). Whereas the morphological differences among these three cell types are clear, there are also differences in the reactivity with different ATPases. Mg++ ATPase is positive in epithelial cells and negative in myoepithelial cells, this instead presents positive reaction for Na+K+ATPase (Fig. 6.15). The three cell types are dividing cells and they incorporate ^{3}H-thymine (Fig. 6.16). The distribution of cell populations in the mammary gland during carcinogenesis varies in TEBs and TDs

(Fig. 6.17), starting as early as at 24 h post-DMBA administration, but no changes in cell composition occur in more differentiated structures such as ABs and lobules. The changes taking place in TEBs and TDs are limited to the dark-cell type, whose proportion decreases from 76 to 67% and to the intermediate cell, whose proportion increases from 11 to 19%. Myoepithelial cells are unaffected. The trend is a progressive shift of cell population distribution, with a continuous decrease in dark cells and a concomitant increase in intermediate cells (Fig. 6.17). By 14 days post-DMBA, these latter ones constitute about 40% and 50% of the proliferative compartment in TEBs and TDs, respectively. At this time the morphological manifestations of tumorigenesis have started to become apparent: increased number of epithelial cell layers, greater irregularity of the luminal border, and progressively larger intercellular spaces, which in some cases form secondary lumina are features indicative of the formation of an intraductal proliferation (IDP). The basal lamina becomes distorted, thus rendering the identification of myoepithelial cells more difficult, and the surrounding stroma becomes fibrotic and infiltrated by inflammatory cells. Between 21 and 40 days post-DMBA treatment, the descending curve of dark cells crosses over the progressively ascending curve of intermediate cells. By 40 days, the tumors display a cell distribution of greater than 65% intermediate cells with less than 35% dark cells (Fig. 6.17). The proportion of intermediate cells continues to increase with tumor age, and at 70 days they represent greater than 75% of the cells. Dark cells, at this point, have been reduced to less than 20%, whereas myoepithelial cells remain at approximately 5%. The 100-day-old tumors are dominated by intermediate cells comprising nearly 90% of the total number of cells [22]. An important change in the cell kinetic also takes place during carcinogenesis. The index of cell proliferation in itself is not increased, but the shifting occurs in the cells that proliferate. The intermediate cells are the one that increase the proliferative ratio, whereas not changes are observed in the myoepithelial or dark cells (Fig. 6.18). This agreed with the preponderance of intermediate type cells in the IDP, ductal carcinoma in situ and adenocarcinomas (Fig. 6.17).

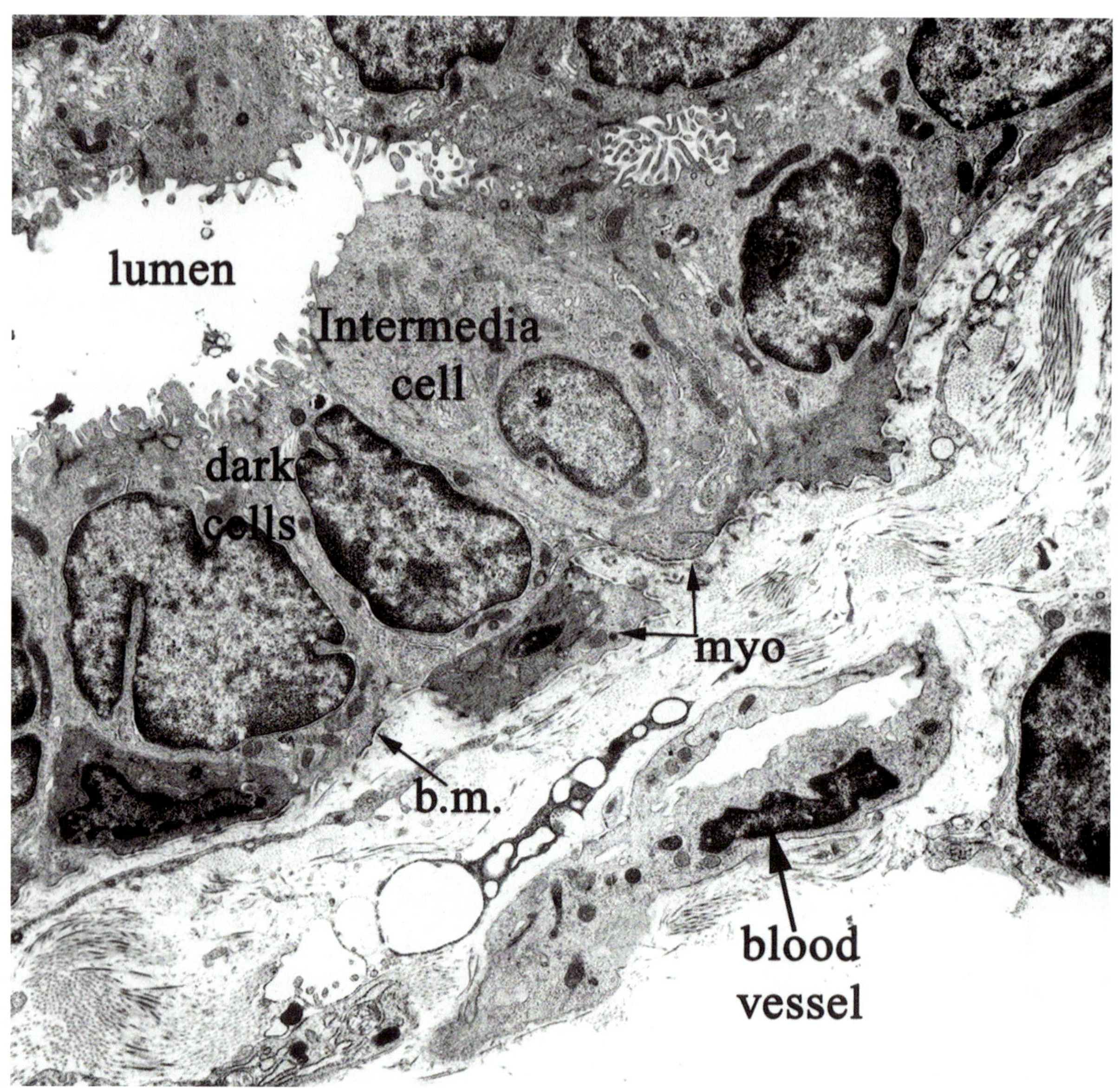

Figure 6.14

The rat mammary gland ductal system is lined by three types of cells, myoepithelial cells (*myo*); dark cells and intermediate cells. Electron micrograph of the rat mammary gland showing the three cell types. The basement membrane (*b.m.*), that separates the epithelial cells from the stroma, is opposite to the lumen. Uranyl acetate-lead citrate, × 4,000

Figure 6.15 a–c ▶

a Electron micrograph of the mammary gland showing the three cell types cytochemicaly reacted for Mg++AT-Pase. **b** Similar to **a** but reacted for Na+-K+-ATPase. Counterstained with uranyl acetate-lead citrate, × 4,000. **c** Myoepithelial cell showing positive Na+-K+-Atpase reaction in the plasma membrane, × 10,000

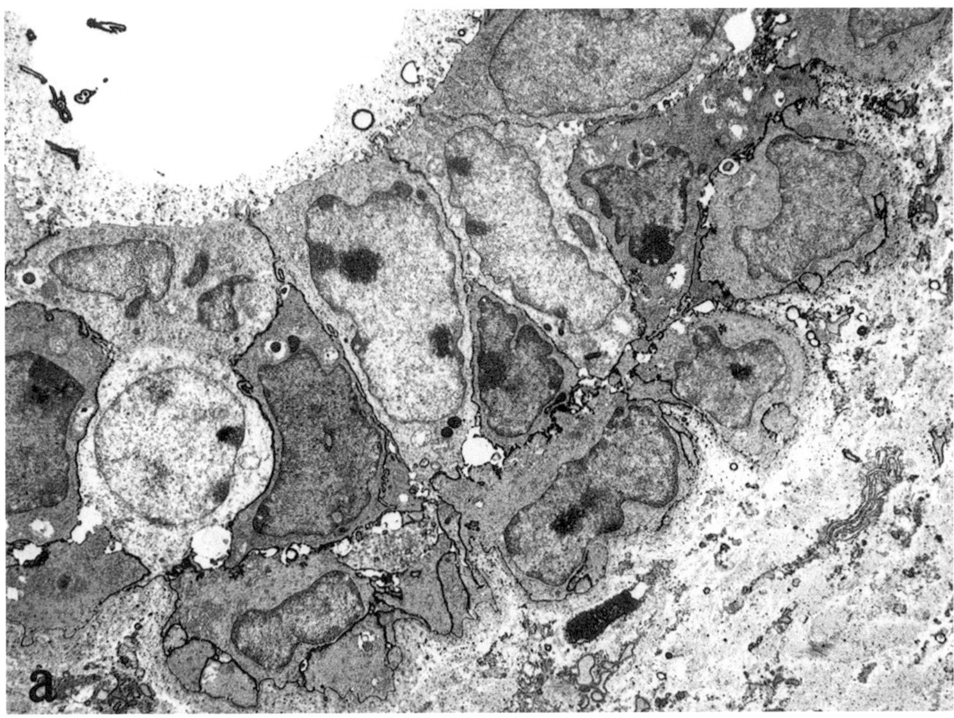

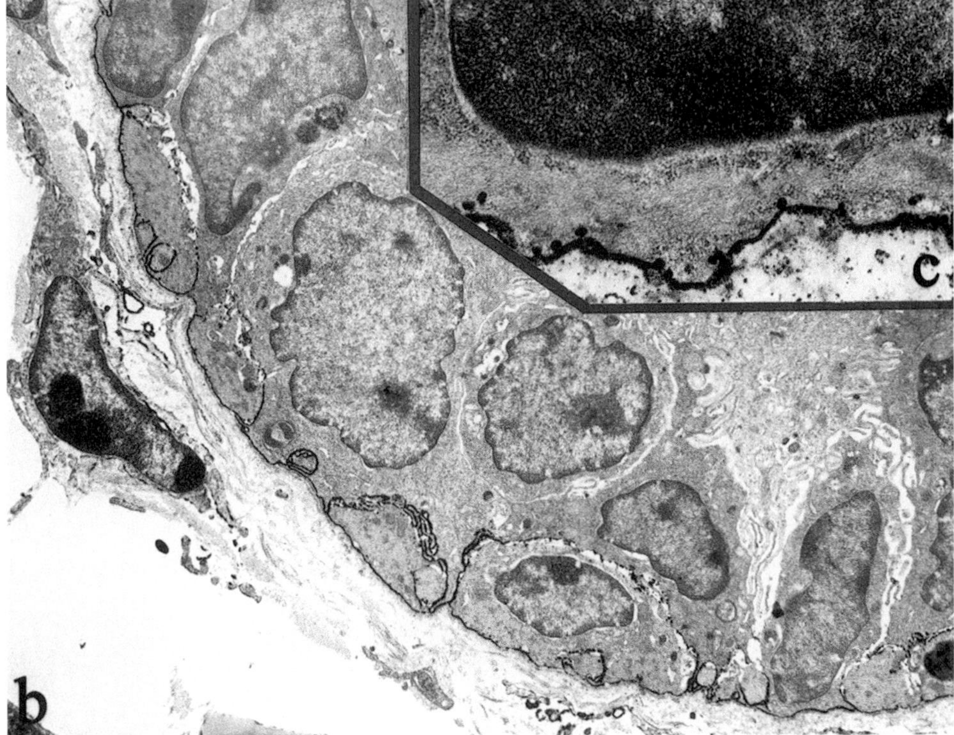

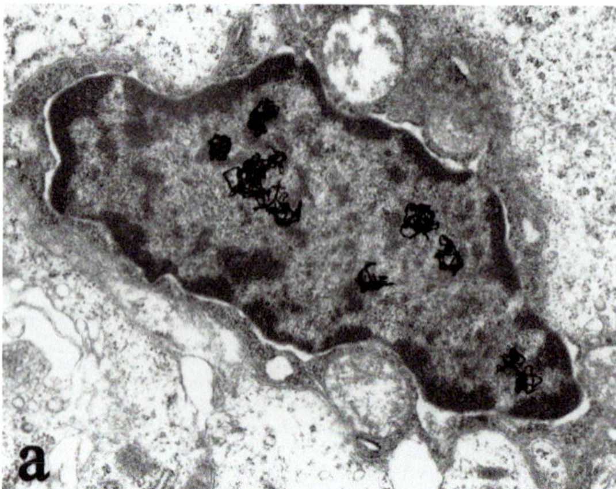

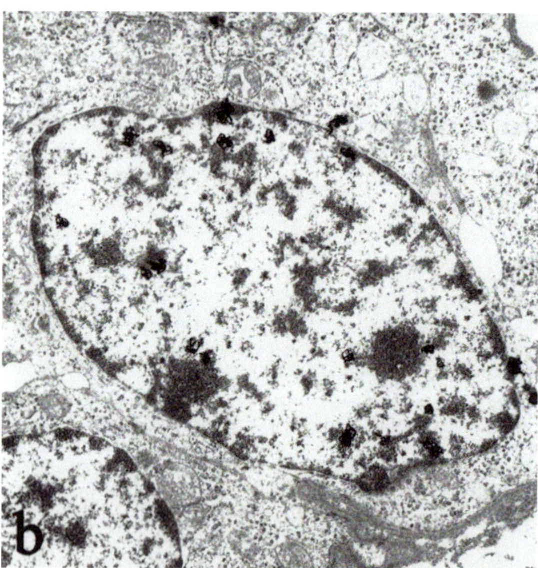

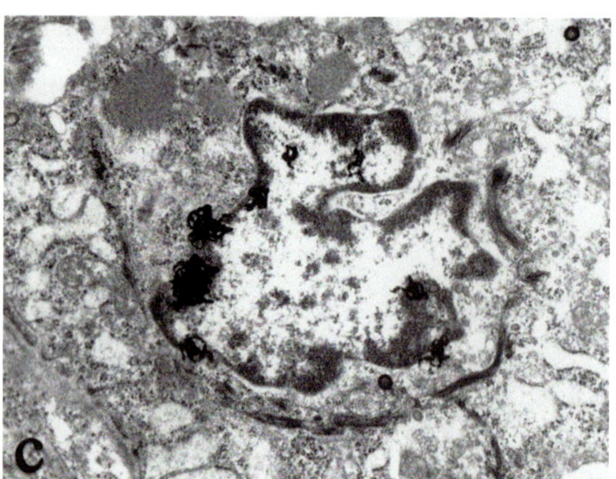

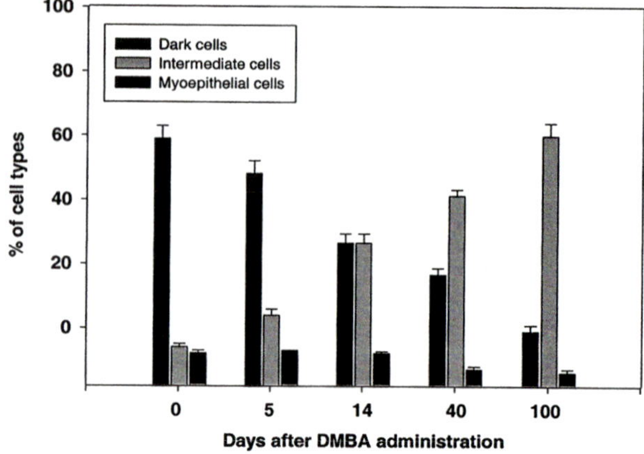

Figure 6.17

Histogram showing the relative proportion of myoepithelial, dark and intermediate cell types in the rat mammary gland of DMBA treated rats

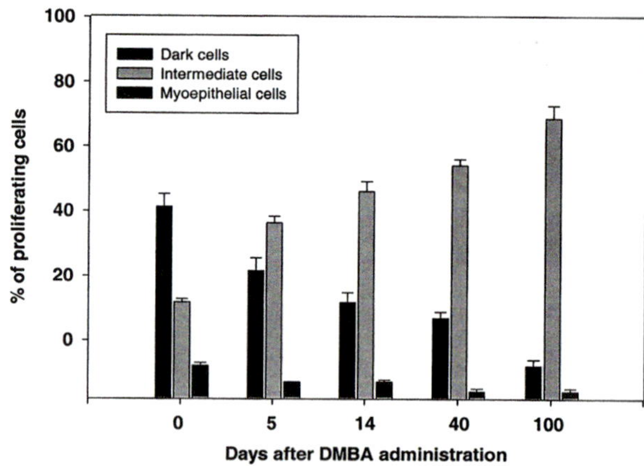

Figure 6.18

Histogram showing the percentage of proliferating cells in the different cell types in the rat mammary gland of DMBA treated rats

◀ Figure 6.16 a–c

The rat mammary gland ductal system is lined by three types of cells. Electron microscopy of autoradiograph showing **a** myoepithelial cells, **b** intermediate cells, and **c** dark cells. Counterstained with uranyl acetate-lead citrate, ×4,000

Table 6.1. Cell kinetics in mammary gland. *YV* young virgin rat, *TEB* terminal end buds, *lob* lobule

	Growth fraction	Rate of cell birth	Rate of cell loss
YV-TEB	0.55	472	44.96
YV-ducts	0.39	187	60.99
YV-lob	0.13	46	87.00
Parous-ducts	0.009	4.05	99.00
Parous-lob	0.004	0.96	98.00

The growth of the mammary gland is the result of a balance between cell birth and cell loss. The growth fraction (GF), represents the total population of cycling cells, and is determined as the rate of ^{3}H-thymidine incorporation after 5 days of continuous infusion (GF_5). It is maximal in the terminal end bud of the young virgin rat, decreasing progressively in ducts and lobules of the YV animal. Pregnancy results in a more dramatic reduction on GF in both ducts and lobules.

6.7.2 Cell Kinetics and Mammary Carcinogenesis

In every tissue, normal or abnormal, cell composition consists of a balance of three different cell populations: cycling cells, resting cells (cells in G_0), and dying cells (cell loss). In the mammary gland these three cell populations can be identified through the study of the cell cycle, and determination of the growth fraction and the rate of cell loss. The growth fraction refers to the fraction of cycling cells, while the rate of cell loss refers to the fraction of cells that die or migrate to other tissues. Both cell cycle time and the growth fraction determine the number of cells produced per unit of time, and the rate of cell loss determines the number of cells lost per unit of time. The growth of normal cells involves the net increase in cell number resulting from more cells being born than dying. In the differentiated or in the adult tissue, in which growth has ceased, the number of cells produced per unit of time is equal to the number of cells that die. The higher susceptibility of the TEB to neoplastic transformation is attributed to the fact that this structure is composed of an actively proliferating epithelium, as determined by the mitotic index (MI), DNA-labeling indices (DNA-LI), length of the cell cycle (Tc), and growth fraction (GF_5) (Figs. 6.9, 6.19–6.22; Table 6.1) [14, 15]. Both the MI and DNA-LI are very high at the tip of TEBs, decreasing progressively toward the ductal or proximal portion of the gland and even further in ABs and lobules (Figs. 6.19, 6.20). TEBs are also characterized for having the highest growth fraction, which progressively diminishes in the more differentiated ABs and lobules (Fig. 6.19, Table 6.1). By using these cell kinetic parameters we have calculated the rate of cell loss in each one of the compartments of the mammary tree. Interestingly enough, the TEB is not only the structure with the highest proliferative ratio, but also with the lowest percentage of cell loss in comparison with other parenchymal structures. The rate of cell loss is very high in the lobular structures present in the mammary gland of parous rats. This clearly indicates that the TEB of the young virgin female is the truly proliferating structure of the gland that reaches a steady state only after acquiring full differentiation. The differences in proliferative activity and growth fraction observed between TEBs and the more differentiated structures of the mammary gland are also reflected in variations in the length of Tc (Fig. 6.19). Tc in TEBs of young virgin rats has an average length of 11 h, increasing to 20.81 h and 28.18 h in TDs and ABs, respectively. Further mammary gland differentiation as a consequence of aging and pregnancy results in an even longer Tc, mainly due to a lengthening of the G_1 phase of the cell cycle (Figs. 6.20–6.23) [14]. The length of Tc also varies according to the cell type and to the specific compartment in which each given cell type is located in. The shortest Tc is observed in intermediate cells located in TEBs, whereas

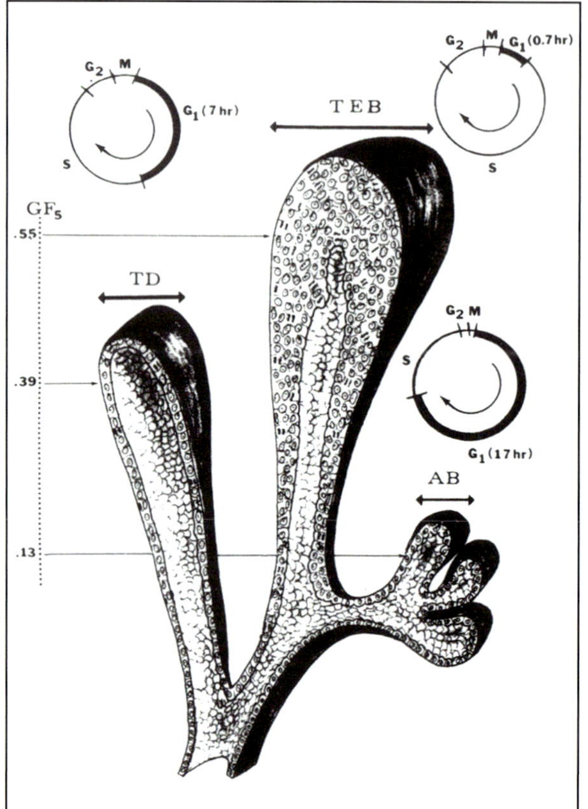

Figure 6.19

Schematic representation of terminal structures in the mammary gland of young virgin rats. The diagram of the cell cycle partitioned into its phases represents the relative length of each phase for each one of the three structures shown (reprinted with permission from: Russo, J. and Russo, I.H. Influence of differentiation and cell kinetics on the susceptibility of the rat mammary gland to carcinogenesis. Cancer Res., 40:2677–2687, 1980)

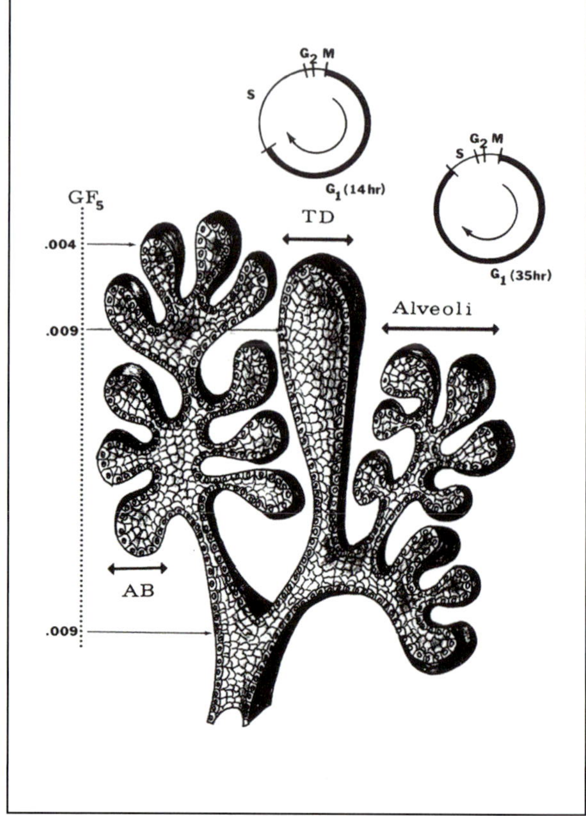

Figure 6.20

Schematic representation of terminal structures in the mammary gland of parous rats. The diagram of the cell cycle shows the relative length of the various phases of the cycle for each structure. From: Russo, J. and Russo, I.H. Influence of differentiation and cell kinetics on the susceptibility of the rat mammary gland to carcinogenesis (reprinted with permission from: Cancer Res., 40:2677–2687, 1980)

Figure 6.21 a–f ▶

a Autoradiograph of the longitudinal section of a TEB in the mammary gland of a 20-day-old rat (H&E, ×25); **b** Autoradiograph of a TEB in the mammary gland of a 30-day-old rat (H&E, ×80); **c** Autoradiograph of a TEB in the mammary gland of a 46-day-old rat (H&E, ×80); **d** Cross section at a-b level of the TEB shown in **c** (H&E, ×80); **e** Autoradiograph of a TEB in the mammary gland of a 70-day-old rat (H&E, ×80); **f** Autoradiograph of a TEB in the mammary gland of a 180-day-old rat (H&E, ×80) (reprinted with permission from: Russo, J., Wilgus, G. and Russo, I.H. Susceptibility of the mammary gland to carcinogenesis. I. Differentiation of the mammary gland as determinant of tumor incidence and type of lesion. Am. J. Pathol. 96 (3): 721–734, 1979)

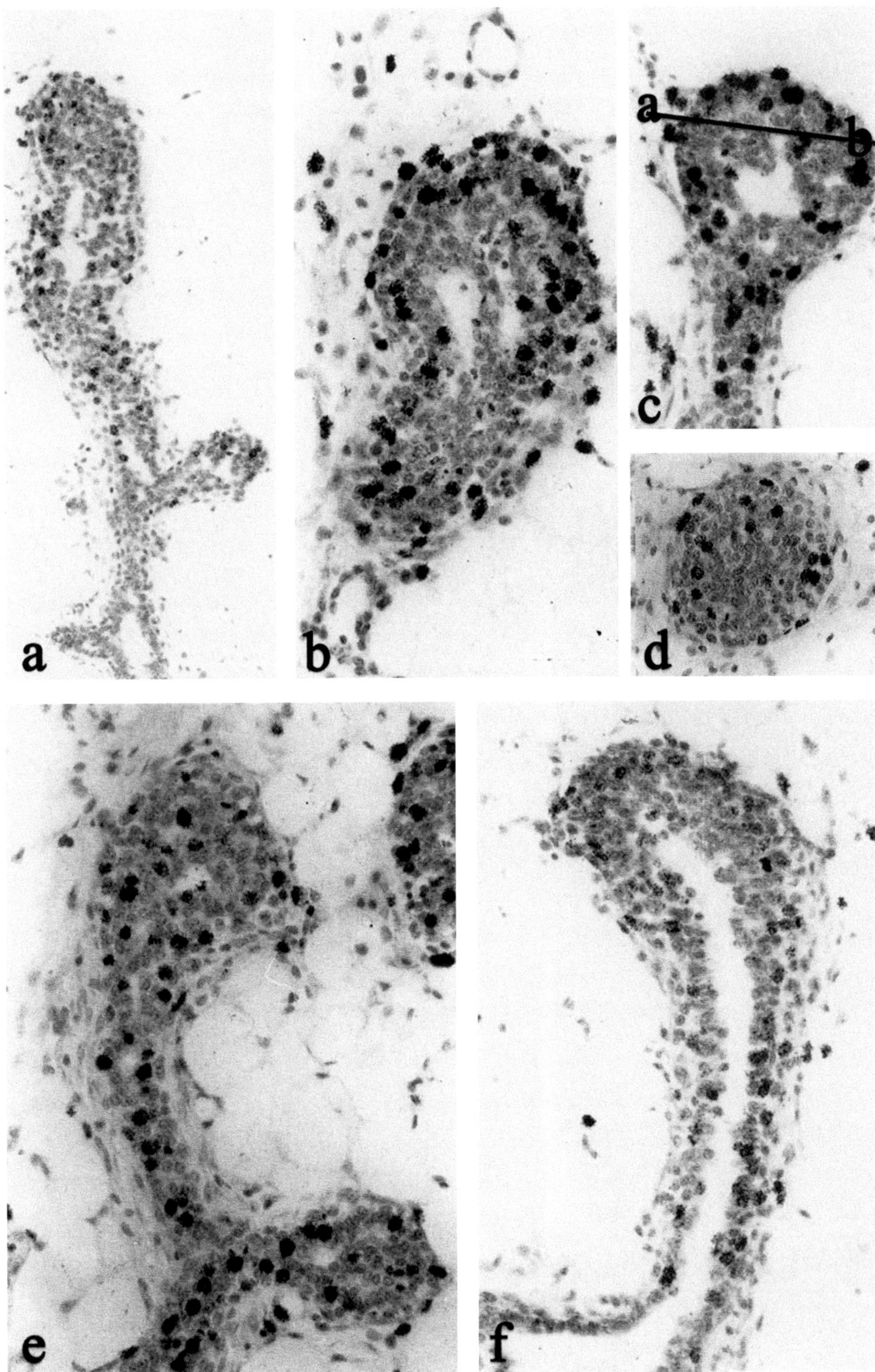
a
b
c
a
b
d
e
f

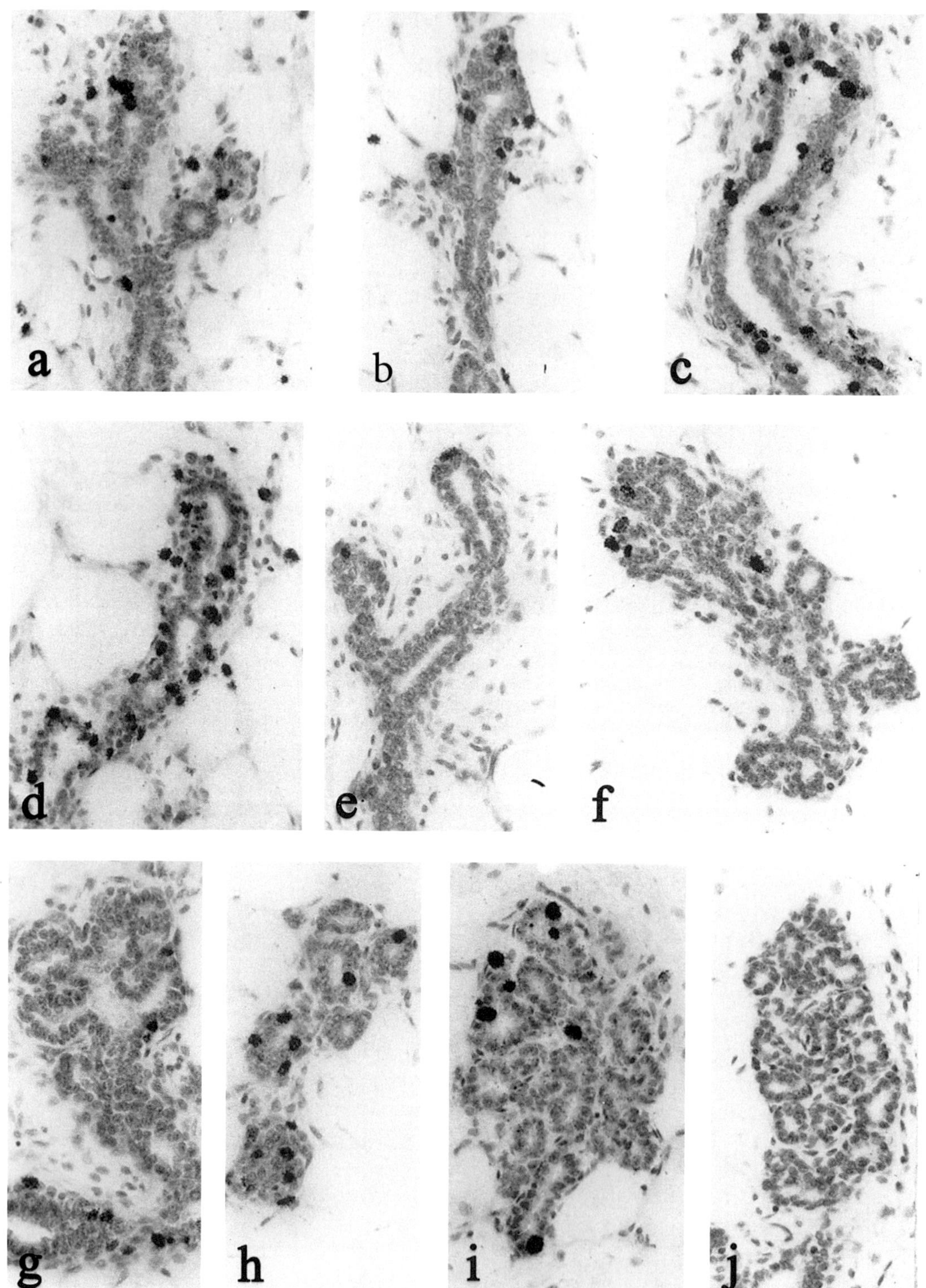

a
b
c
d
e
f
g
h
i
j

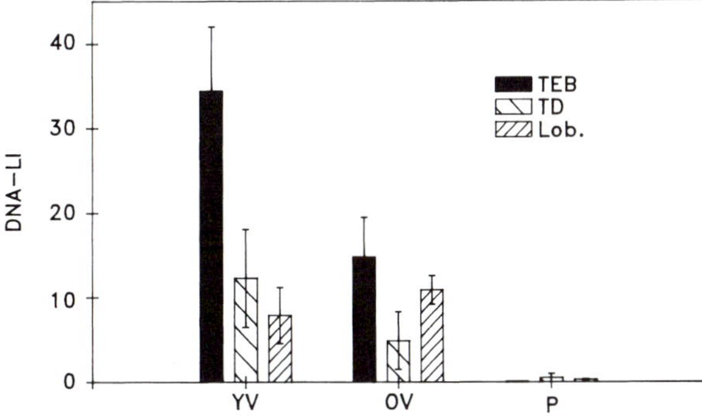

Figure 6.23

Histogram showing the percentage of proliferating cells (*DNA-LI*) in the different compartments of the rat mammary gland of young virgin rats at 50 days of age (*YV*), old virgin rats at 180 days of age (*OV*), and parous animals (*P*) at 180 days of age (reprinted with permission from: Russo, J and Russo, IH, Cancer Epidemiol Biomarkers & Prevention, 3, 353–364, 1994)

◀ **Figure 6.22 a–j**

a Autoradiograph of ducts ending in TDS, 30-day-old rat. (H&E, ×80). **b** Autoradiograph of a TD in longitudinal section, 40-day-old rat (H&E, ×80). **c–e** Autoradiographs of a TD in the mammary gland of **c** a 46-day-old rat, **d** a 55-day-old rat, and **e** a 140-day-old rat (H&E, ×80). **f–j** Autoradiographs of ABs in the mammary gland of **f** a 30-day-old rat, **g** a 40-day-old rat, **h** a 46-day-old rat, **i** a 55-day-old rat, and **j** a 180-day-old rat (H&E, ×80, all with a photographic reduction of 10%) (reprinted with permission from: Russo, J., Wilgus, G. and Russo, I.H. Susceptibility of the mammary gland to carcinogenesis. I. Differentiation of the mammary gland as determinant of tumor incidence and type of lesion. Am. J. Pathol. 96 (3): 721–734, 1979)

it lengthens when the same cell type is located in ABs or lobules. These differences in the length of Tc are due mainly to differences in the length of the G1 phase of the cell cycle, whereas all the other phases remain constant. Intermediate type cells located in TEBs have a Tc lasting 13 h. When the same cell type is located in more differentiated structures, such as ABs, exhibits a lengthened Tc, lasting 34 h. These differences in cell kinetic parameters among the differ-

ent cell types could explain the higher susceptibility of the intermediate cell of the TEBs to be affected by the carcinogen, which causes further expansion of the proliferative compartment of the intermediate cells and depression in the dark cell population after initiation of the carcinogenic stimulus [22].

Mammary epithelial cells metabolize DMBA to polar metabolites with formation of epoxides that cause DNA damage. When dissociated mammary epithelial cells of young virgin and of parous animals, that basically represent the cells of the TEBs and of the lobules, respectively, are grown in vitro, they exhibit different rates of formation of polar metabolites. TEB cells produce more polar and less phenolic metabolites than lobular cells, indicating that the former, in addition to their higher proliferative activity, are also producing more epoxides, as is manifested by a higher binding of DMBA to DNA (Fig. 6.10). Autoradiographic studies performed in vivo confirm the observation that the greatest uptake of [³H] DMBA occurs in the nucleus of epithelial cells of TEBs, and the lowest in ABs and lobules, indicating that the highest DMBA-DNA binding is associated with the structure of the gland with the highest replicative properties. The ability of the cells to remove DMBA adducts from the DNA is an indication of their capability to repair the damage. TEB cells remove adducts formed less efficiently than lobular cells. This is attributed to the shorter G_1 phase of Tc and not to a lack of reparative enzymes [1, 23, 24].

These studies support the conclusion that the differentiation of the mammary gland modifies the following parameters:

1. Glandular structure
2. Cell kinetics characteristics of the mammary epithelium, decreasing the growth fraction and lengthening the cell cycle, mainly the G_1 phase
3. Decreasing formation of polar metabolites and increasing phenolic metabolites
4. Decreasing binding of the carcinogen

All the parameters listed above affect the susceptibility of the mammary gland to carcinogenesis, and should be taken into account when assessing chemicals for cancer risk.

Table 6.2. Differential diagnosis of TEB, intraductal proliferation (*IDP*), and carcinoma in situ (*CIS*)

Tissue components	TEB	IDP	CIS
Basement membrane	Present	Present	Present
Periductal stroma	Normal	Moderate desmoplastic reaction	Marked desmoplastic reaction
Inflammatory reaction	Absent	Moderate	Marked
Luminal border	Smooth	Serrated	Irregular
Secondary luminae	Absent	Absent	Present in cribriform pattern
Micropapillae	Absent	Some	May be prominent
Epithelium	Heterogeneous three cell types	Predominance of one cell type	Predominance of one cell type
Mitoses	Numerous	Numerous	Numerous

6.7.3 Role of the Stroma in the Pathogenesis of Mammary Cancer

In the preceding sections we have shown that mammary carcinogenesis induced in Sprague-Dawley rats by administration of DMBA is the result of the interaction of the carcinogen with the TEB; when damaged, this structure further evolves to IDP and this to carcinoma (Figs. 6.11, 6.12). Intraductal proliferations are morphologically distinguishable from TEBs by their size, which is more than twice that of the TEB and by the homogenous cell composition, which consists preponderantly of intermediate cells (Table 6.2). As it is depicted in Fig. 6.24 the induction of IDPs is by no means a rare event. Within 3 weeks of DMBA administration there are between 10 and 20 IDPs per mammary gland, and this number increases with time, such that by 6 to 10 weeks after treatment there are approximately 30 lesions per gland, and around 200 per animal. Although IDPs occur in large numbers following DMBA administration, the likelihood of any one IDP of progressing to carcinoma in the intact mammary gland is lower than that, since the maximal tumorigenic response rarely goes beyond 5 to 6 adenocarcinomas per animal (Fig. 6.24). This is attributed to the fact that there are two different types of IDP. The one that we call "initiated" IDP [IDP (i)], increase in numbers steadily with a concomitant

decrease in the number of TEBS; they reach a plateau by 60 days post-DMBA (Fig. 6.24). The IDP (i) are characterized by having a diameter larger than that of the TEB, and are composed of a greater number of epithelial cells. They do not elicit a response in the surrounding stroma, and remain unchanged during the whole post carcinogen observation period. A second type of IDP, which we call "initiated and promoted" [IDP (i+p)], arises at the same time and reaches the same level as IDPs (i); by 20 to 30 days post-DMBA they are also characterized by having a larger diameter and a greater cell number than TEBS. They elicit a marked stromal reaction, consisting in collagen deposition and infiltration by mast cells and lymphocytes (Figs. 6.25, 6.26). IDPs (i+p) progress to carcinoma in situ and to invasive carcinoma. The fact that not all the IDPs progress to carcinoma indicates that although both IDPs (i) and (i+p) are preneoplastic lesions, there are factors that regulate the progression of initiated cells, which affect differently IDPs (i) and IDPs (i+p).

Figure 6.26 a, b ▶

a Whole mount of adenocarcinoma showing the mast cells surrounding the tumor, stained with toluidine blue, × 10. b Histological section of the tumor depicted in a stained with PAS-alcian blue, × 40

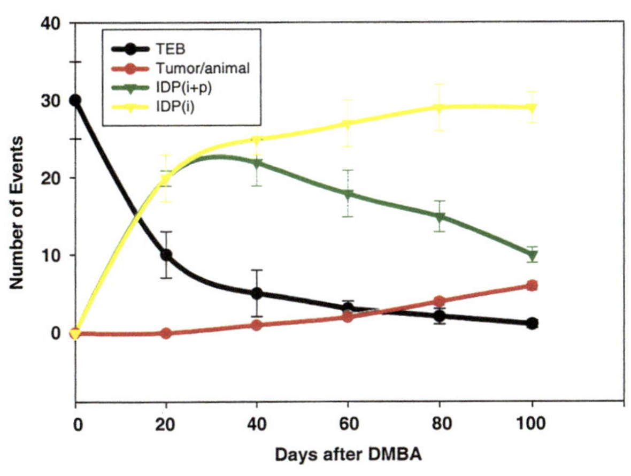

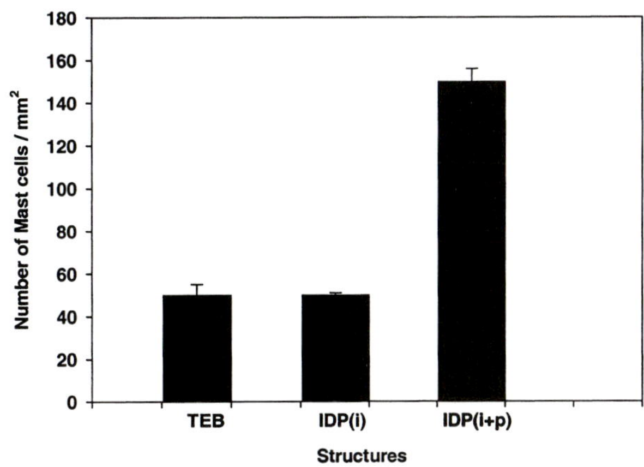

Emergence of preneoplastic lesions IDP (i); IDP (i+p) and carcinomas (*Tumor/animal*) as the number of TEB decreases with time in the mammary gland at different periods after DMBA administration

Distribution of mast cells in TEB, IDP (i); IDP (i+p)

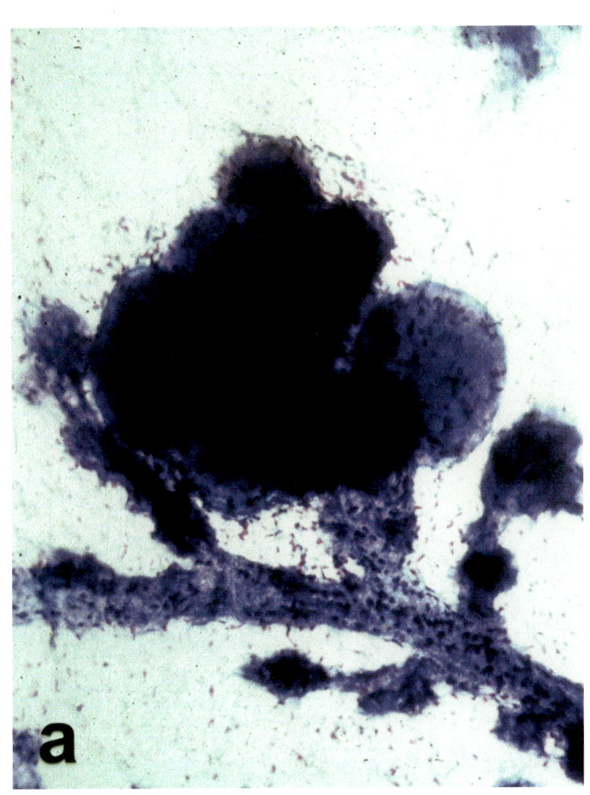

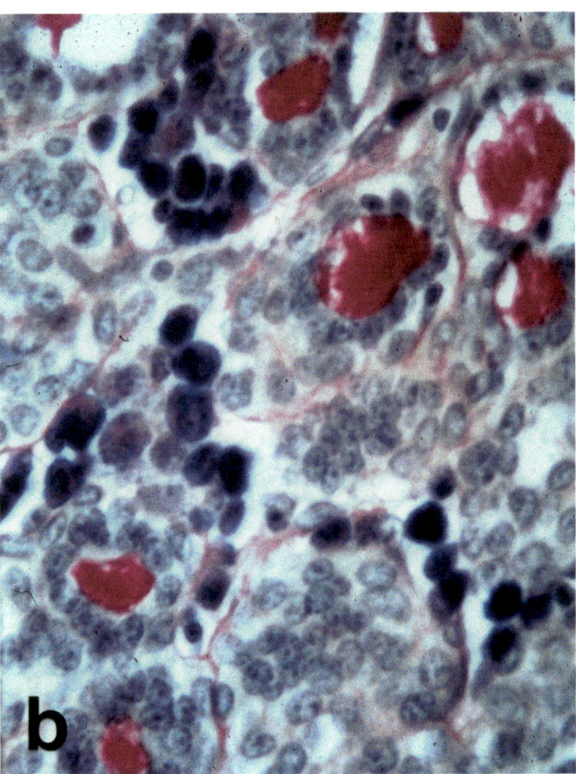

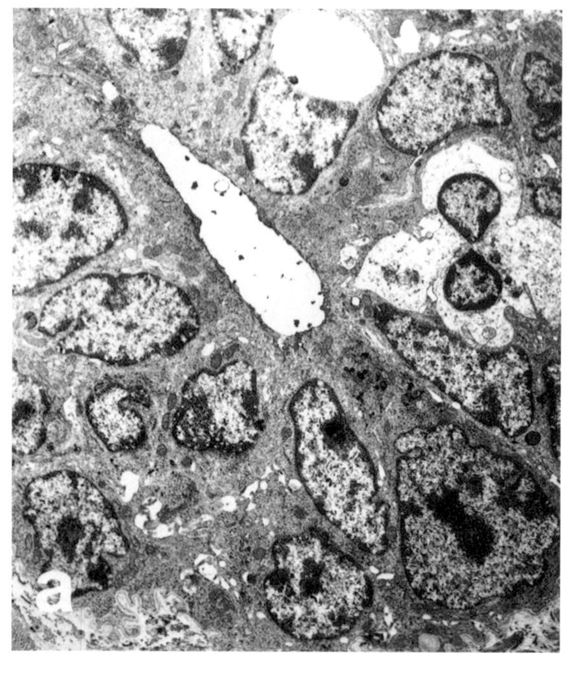

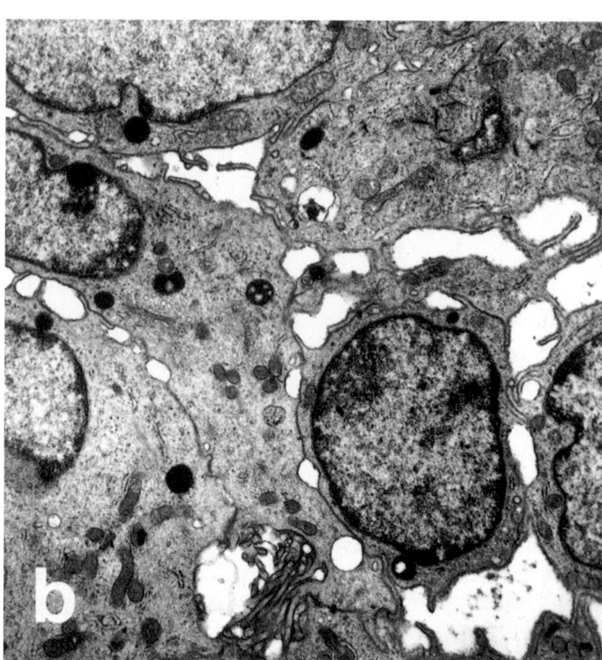

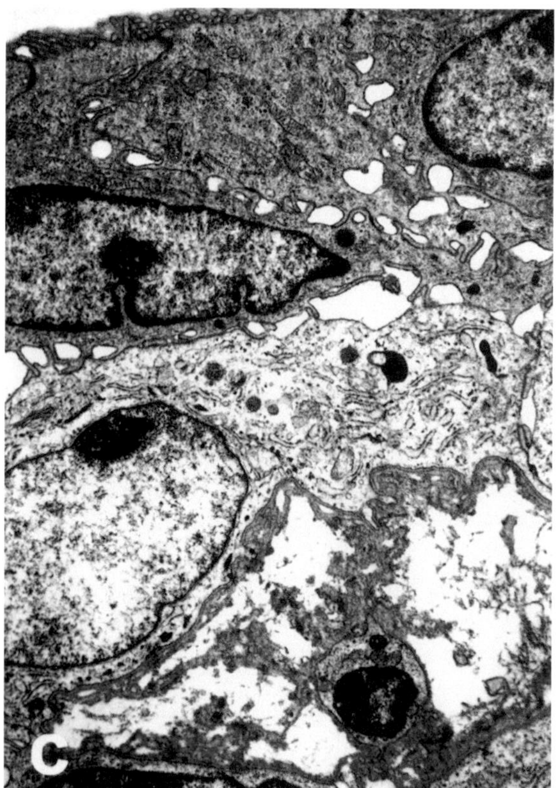

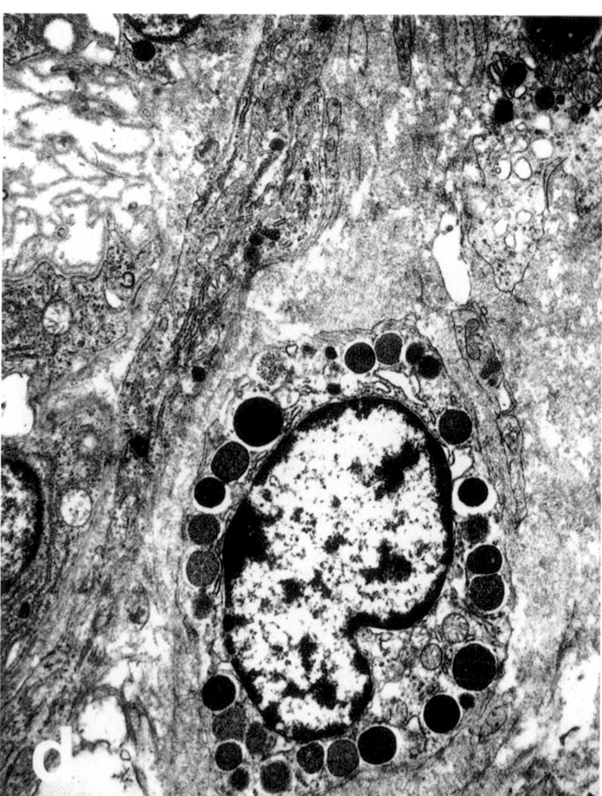

a Formation of intercellular spaces in the IDP (i+p). **b** The intercellular spaces shows electron dense material that is identified as proteoglycans. **c** Deposit of proteoglycans. **d** Deposition of proteoglycans around a carcinoma in situ, and around mast cells. Counterstained with uranyl acetate and lead citrate, × 4,000

The factors that regulate the progression of an initiated cell to preneoplasia and to neoplasia are unknown. We have been able to identify, however, a host response elicited by the initiated cells that might play a role in this mechanism. IDP (i), which does not elicit stromal reaction and fails to progress to carcinoma in situ (C.I.S.), and IDP (i+p), which is surrounded by numerous mast cells and lymphocytes and originates malignant lesions (Fig. 6.26). The number of mast cells around the IDP (i+p) is three times higher than in TEBs and IDP (i) (Fig. 6.25). This IDP (I+P) increase in mast cells is accompanied by an increase in lymphocytes, fibroblasts, collagen fibers and proteoglycans. Mast cells are found in different parts of the body, and the mammary gland is not an exception. They contain in their cytoplasm numerous granules measuring up to 0.8 μm in diameter (Fig. 6.27), which stain metachromatically with toluidine blue or alcian blue (Fig. 6.26). Mast cells have membrane receptors to IgE, which participate in the immediate and delayed type of hypersensitivity. When an antigen combines with IgE and bind the cell receptor, the cell degranulates releasing histamine and heparin. Heparin is a heparan sulfate that has been shown to stimulate cell proliferation [25]. It has been shown that transplanted tumors in the chick embryo may increase by 40-fold the number of mast cells around the tumor implant before new capillaries arise [26]. Mast cell lysates or mast cell-conditioned medium stimulate locomotion of capillary endothelial cells in vitro [27, 28], an effect that is attributed to heparin. It has been postulated that heparin or fragments of heparin on the surface of endothelial cells may selectively bind endothelial cell mitogens that are also angiogenic [25]. Interestingly enough, there are several growth factors that have great affinity for heparin [29, 30]. It has also been shown that heparin-coated tumor cells

exhibit altered transplantation and cytotoxicity reaction [31, 32], presumably due to blockage of cell surface antigens by heparin. Thus heparan sulfate proteoglycans also may be deposited in an annulus around the tumor and may modulate the immunoreactivity or accessibility of the enclosed cells. An early change observed during the process of transformation is the synthesis of a large amount of proteoglycans by IDP (i+p), which is evidenced by the deposition of an electron dense material on the cell surface of the epithelial cells, and by an increased reactivity with alcian blue pH 2.7, and PAS (Figs. 6.27, 6.28). This is accompanied by an increase in uptake of ^{3}H-fucose and ^{3}H-glucosamine (Figs. 6.28, 6.29). The number of cells taking up these precursors is almost three times the number found in TEBs and IDPs (i) (Fig. 6.29). All these data clearly indicate that the initiated cells that are progressing to malignancy are secreting proteoglycans, which accumulate in the stroma. We do not know whether these proteoglycans are influencing the response of the host by eliciting a higher mobilization of mast cells and inhibiting the cytotoxic effect of lymphocytes, or by inducing angiogenesis, desmoplasia and cell proliferation. Some of these proteoglycans, such as heparan sulfate, act as receptors for growth factors, which in turn initiate an autocrine response.

Proteoglycans occur on the plasma membranes of mammalian cells and in the extracellular matrix [33–35]. They are neutral glycoproteins, stained by PAS, which are negative with alcian blue pH 2.7 and contain fucose residues; and acid mucopolysaccharides, which react positively with alcian blue pH 2.7 and negatively with PAS. There are two types of glycosaminoglycans:

1. Glycosaminoglycans of chondroitin sulfate, containing residues of D-glucuronic acid
2. N-acetyl-D-galactosamine and glycosaminoglycans of heparan sulfate, which contain alternating residues of D-glucuronic acid or L-iduronic acid and N-acetyl-D-glucosamine

Neoplastic transformation of cells dramatically alters proteoglycan synthesis both in the tumor and in the surrounding tissues [36]. This is thought to stimulate

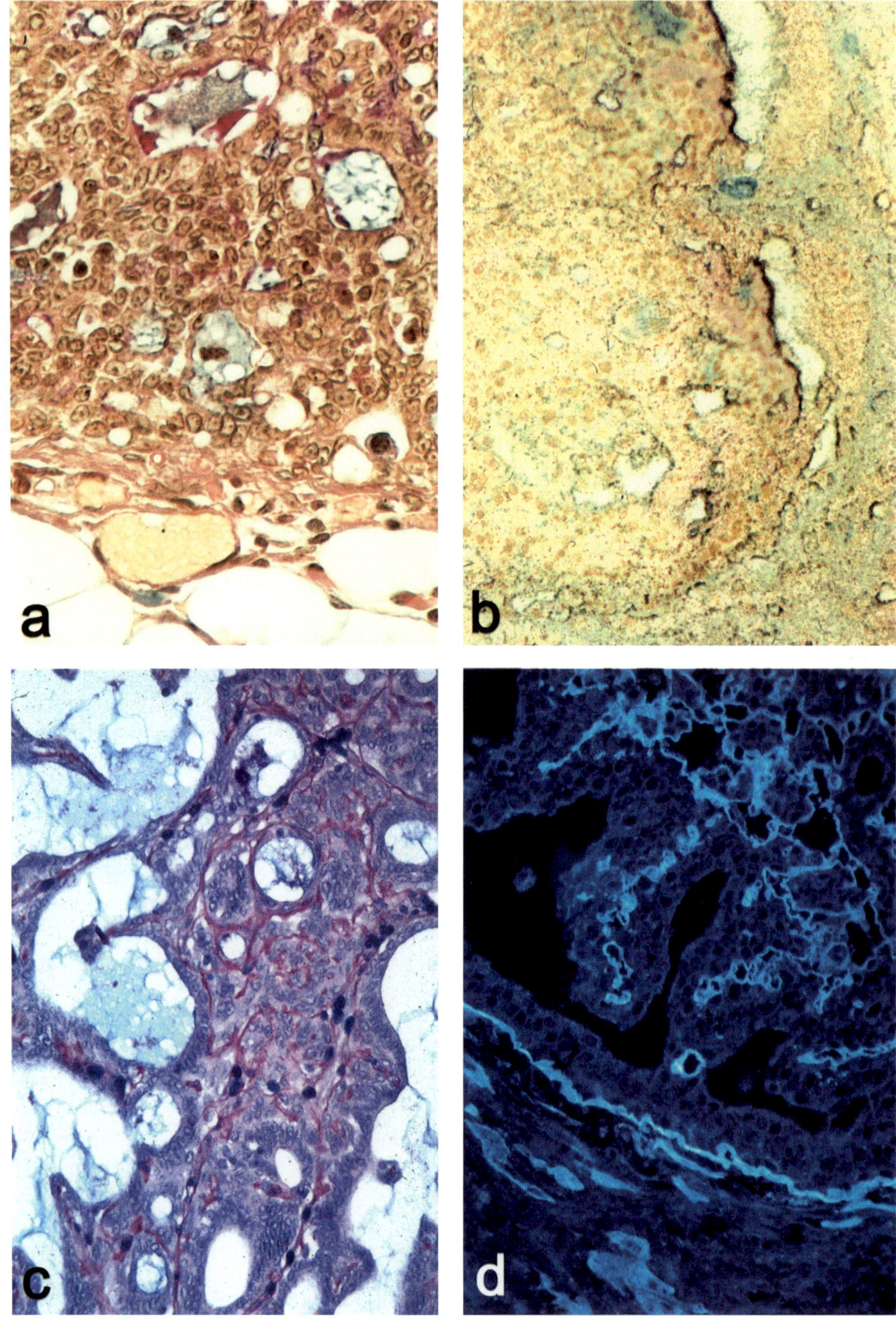

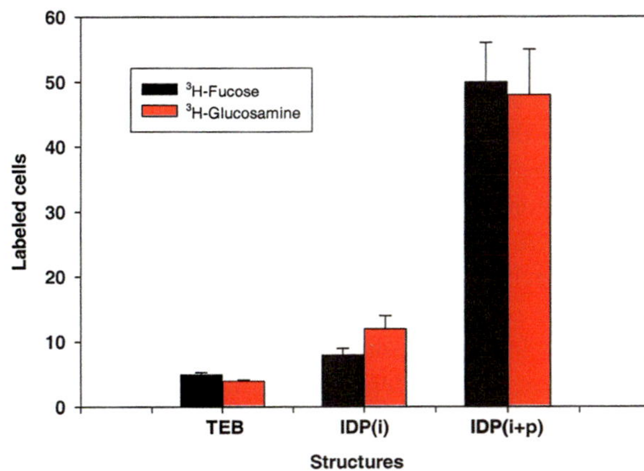

Figure 6.29

Histogram showing the percentage of cells labeled with ^{3}H-fucose and ^{3}H-glucosamine in TEB, IDP (i) and IDP (i+p)

◀ Figure 6.28 a–d

a Terminal end bud stained with alcian blue, × 40. **b** Autoradiogram of an IDP of a mammary gland of a DMBA-treated rat that received a pulse of ^{3}H fucose for 24 h and counterstained with alcian blue, × 20. **c** Cribriform adenocarcinoma stained with Alcian blue and PAS, × 40. **d** Cribriform adenocarcinoma reacted with anti basement membrane antibody and observed under fluorescence, × 40

tumorigenic growth by decreasing the adhesion of transformed cells to the extracellular matrix [36]. It is possible to speculate that the production of proteoglycans allows the IDP to progress to carcinoma in situ by stimulation of cell proliferation and by interference with an immune reaction toward the cells. Of these newly synthesized proteoglycans, both those that incorporate ^{3}H-D-glucosamine and stain with alcian blue pH 2.7 and those that uptake ^{3}H-fucose and stain with PAS may act like epiglycanin, a high molecular weight sialoglycoprotein present in mouse mammary carcinoma (Ta3) cells, which is though to mask histocompatibility antigens. These, in turn, can prevent the generation and penetration of cytolytic lymphocytes [31].

6.8 Pathological Classification of Rat Mammary Tumors

The classification presented attempts to provide a working framework for diagnosing the type of lesions found in the mammary glands of rats treated with chemical carcinogens or radiation, and to clarify criteria for establishing two basic characteristics of tumors:

1. Whether they are epithelial or stromal in origin
2. Whether they are benign or malignant

Table 6.3. Classification of rat mammary gland tumors

I. Epithelial neoplasms

A. Benign lesions
  1. Intraductal papilloma
  2. Papillary cystadenoma
  3. Adenoma
     (a) Tubular
     (b) Lactating
B. Precancerous lesions
   Intraductal proliferation (IDP)
C. Malignant lesions
  1. Noninvasive –in situ- carcinoma
     (a) Ductal papillary
     (b) Ductal solid and cribriform
     (c) Ductal comedo
  2. Invasive carcinoma
     (a) Papillary
     (b) Cribriform
     (c) Comedo
     (d) Tubular

II. Stromal neoplasms

A. Benign: fibroma
B. Malignant: fibrosarcoma

III. Epithelial-stromal neoplasms

A. Benign: Fibroadenoma
B. Malignant: Carcinosarcoma

IV. Non-neoplastic lesions

Cystic changes
  (a) Ductal
  (b) Lobular

Rat mammary tumors may be composed of a single histologic type or of combinations of several patterns. In Table 6.3 are depicted the main histological types of mammary tumors found in the rat.

6.8.1 Epithelial Neoplasms

6.8.1.1 Intraductal Papilloma

These types of lesions are well circumscribed and composed of papillary projections into the duct. A single layer of low columnar epithelial cells lines the papillae. They are separated by abundant connective tissue.

6.8.1.2 Papillary Cystadenoma

Well-circumscribed lesions that are composed of papillary projections protruding into cystic spaces are papillary cyst-adenomas. The papillae are lined by a single, double, or pseudostratified layer of low columnar epithelial cells; the lining cells may have small projections or "snouts" that give the epithelium an apocrine appearance.

6.8.1.3 Adenoma

Rat mammary gland adenomas are benign epithelial neoplasms that form glandular patterns of two types: tubular and lactating. The tubular type is characterized by proliferation of tubular or alveolar structures arranged in clusters and separated by scant connective tissue. The increased number of individual alveoli gives an appearance suggestive of a large lobule with more alveoli than usual. Individual alveoli are lined by low cuboidal epithelial cells arranged in a single layer and may have a secretion-filled lumen. Epithelial cells have small nuclei with one small, inconspicuous nucleolus. The nuclei are slightly larger than those of cells lining normal ducts and alveoli. The lumen of the alveoli composing a tubular adenoma has a round and smooth border, while in the lactating adenoma the lumina are lined by an epithe-

lium with a serrated border due to cell decapitation or supranuclear vacuolization. Lactating adenomas vary from small ones, measuring less than 1 mm in diameter, that are indistinguishable from hyperplastic lobules, to ones greater than 2 cm. The secretion-filled alveoli are lined by a single layer of low cuboidal epithelium with basal nuclei and vacuolated cytoplasm. Each individual alveolus is surrounded by a thin layer of connective tissue, whose amount progressively increases from the adenoma to the fibroadenoma. Lactating adenomas exhibit marked variation in the size of individual alveoli, some of them acquire large dimensions due to accumulation of secreted fluid, eventually forming cysts, in which the epithelium lining the lumen becomes flattened.

6.8.1.4 Precancerous Lesions: Intraductal Proliferation

The earliest change observed in the mammary parenchyma after carcinogen treatment of virgin rats is the dilation of terminal ductal structures, namely the terminal end buds (TEB). They exhibit thickening of the epithelial lining, which may be up to six layers thick (Fig. 6.30). These cells have a large, round nucleus, prominent nucleolus and coarse chromatin along the inner leaflet of the nuclear membrane. These ear-

a Whole mount of a terminal end bud (toluidine blue, × 4). **b** Histological section of a TEB (H&E, ×10). **c** High magnification of **b**, (×40). **d** Whole mount of an intraductal proliferation (IDP), in the rat mammary gland. This lesion is observed 21–41 days post-DMBA administration. The proliferation starts in the terminal end buds (TEB) and expands to the ductal structures. **e** Histological section of **d** with moderate desmoplastic reaction in the stroma (H&E, ×4). **f** Whole mount of a carcinoma in situ stained with toluidine blue, ×4. **g** Histological section of carcinoma in situ showing early papillary patterns and intense desmoplastic reaction in the stroma (H&E, ×10). **h** Whole mount of an intraductal carcinoma, cribriform pattern stained with toluidine blue, ×4. **i** Histological section of **g** showing epithelial clusters surrounded by intense desmoplastic reaction and lymphocyte infiltration (H&E, ×10)

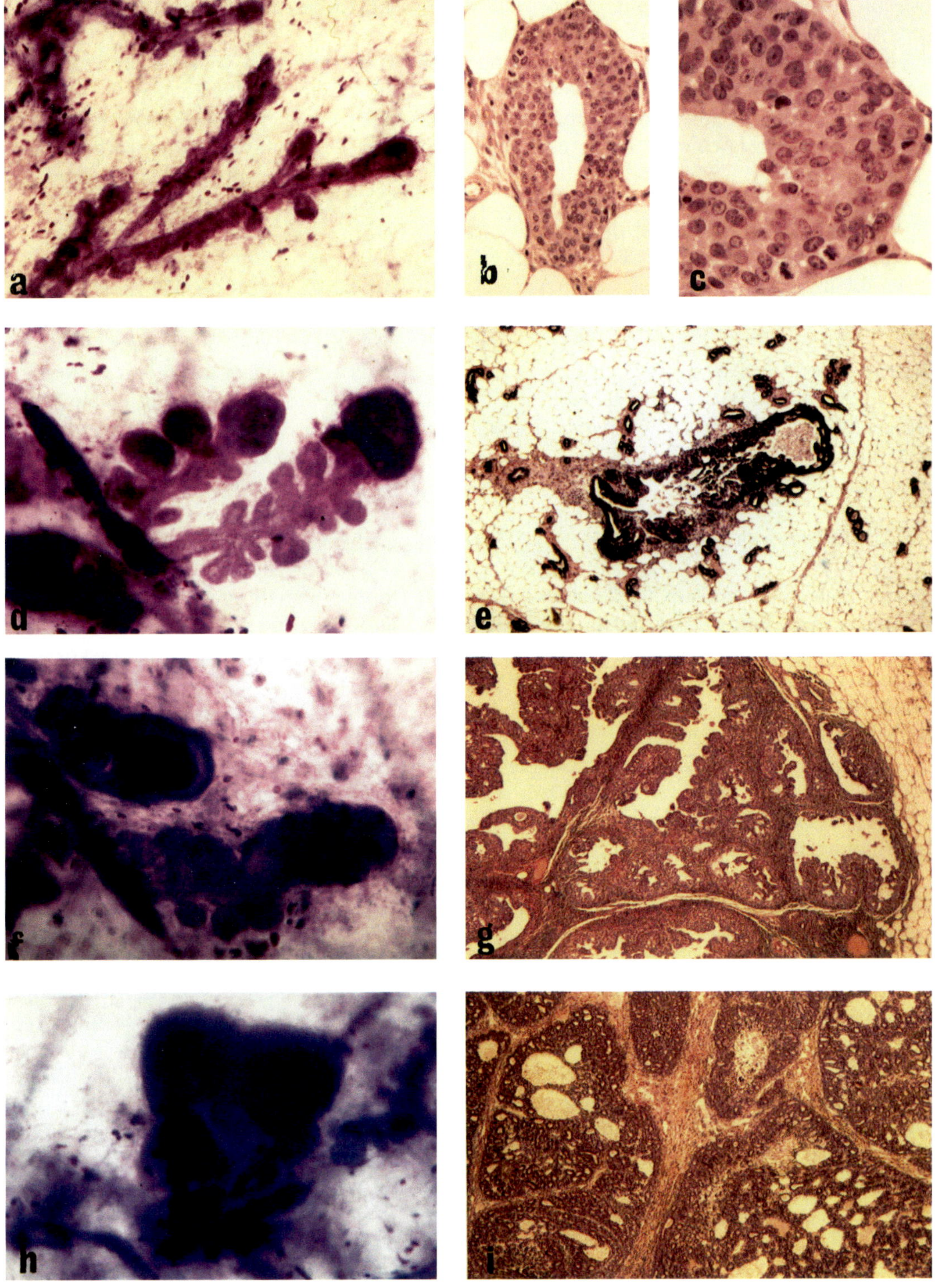

ly lesions called intraductal proliferations (IDPs) [12] represent the transition between the normal TEB [12, 13] and carcinoma in situ; the criteria for identifying these three types of structures are outlined in Table 6.2 [1, 3, 4, 12, 13]. Intraductal proliferations appear to evolve into carcinoma in situ through the development of:

1. Micropapillae, which might be the only pattern present or combined with cribriform pattern
2. Pseudolumina, forming a cribriform pattern, or
3. A comedo pattern (Table 6.2)

A progressively increasing desmoplastic reaction in the stroma surrounding the transformed ductal structures is a hallmark of neoplastic progression (Fig. 6.30).

6.8.1.5 Carcinoma In Situ

Ductal, Solid, and Papillary Carcinoma. The ductal structures are dilated, and the lining epithelium grows inward, forming epithelial papillae devoid of fibrovascular core. Most of the epithelial cell population is uniform in size and shape. Mitotic figures are often found. The stroma, which is separated from the epithelium by a well-defined basement membrane, exhibits a slight to marked desmoplastic reaction, with replacement of fat by fibroblasts, and infiltration by lymphocytes and mast cells (Fig. 6.30).

Ductal, Solid, and Cribriform Carcinoma. This type of tumor is the result of epithelial cell proliferation in a solid pattern with formation of' secondary lumina (Fig. 6.30). The tumors are cytologically similar to papillary carcinomas and like them; they elicit a stromal reaction and lymphocytic infiltration (Fig. 6.30).

Ductal Comedocarcinoma. This lesion is characterized by intraductal growth of epithelium and accumulation of necrotic cellular debris in the lumen. The surrounding stroma may exhibit a marked desmoplastic reaction. Comedo and cribriform patterns may be present simultaneously in the same tumor. Less frequently a papillary component is present as well.

6.8.1.6 Invasive Ductal Carcinomas

The diagnosis of invasive carcinomas is based upon the presence of unequivocal growth of malignant epithelial cells into the adjacent stroma. The presence of invasion can be difficult to judge because under normal conditions the mammary gland ducts grow diffusely into the fat pad, adjacent muscle, and subcutaneous tissue of the skin.

Papillary Carcinomas. The most typical and frequent of the 7,12-dimethylbenz(a)anthracene (DMBA)- and N-methyl-N-nitrosourea (NMU)-induced tumors are papillary carcinomas (Fig. 6.31) [11, 13, 20]. Most of the tumors are detectable by palpation; they efface the normal architecture of the gland, invading surrounding structures. When they invade the skin they ulcerate and undergo local necrosis. Papillary carcinomas contain delicate fibrovascular cores, often heavily infiltrated by lymphocytes and mast cells (Fig. 6.32). The fibrovascular cores are considerably thinner than those seen in intraductal papillomas. On top of the fibrovascular core grows the epithelium, which depending upon its thickness and cytologic characteristics allows one to classify these lesions into grade l or grade 2 (Table 6.4). Papillary carcinomas grade 1 are composed of 1–2 layers of epithelial cells, which in turn emit short epithelial papillae devoid of fibrovascular cores. The papillary carcinoma grade 2 is also formed by papillary projections; however, the cores of connective tissue are sparser than those observed in the papillary carcinoma grade 1, and the secondary projections (papillae) of epithelium are solid clusters of cells. The luminal borders of these cell projections are serrated, whereas those present in papillary carcinomas grade 1 are smooth (Fig. 6.32). The epithelial cells in this tumor type are slightly more pleomorphic than those of the papillary carcinoma grade 1 (Fig. 6.32). In Table 6.4 are depicted the basic histological and cytological differences between these tumor subtypes. Occasionally, in papillary carcinomas grade 2, the luminal spaces may become dilated or cystic; these lesions are called cystic papillary carcinomas. They may well represent a further evolution of a papillary or cribriform type.

Table 6.4. Differential diagnosis between papillary carcinoma grade 1 and grade 2

Components	Papillary carcinoma	
	Grade 1	Grade 2
Fibrovascular core	Prominent	Sparse
Epithelium	1–3 layer thick	5–10 layer thick
Micropapillae	Present	Present
Luminal border	Smooth	Serrated
Cytological characteristics	Moderate pleomorphism	Marked pleomorphism
Nucleolus	Inconspicuous	Prominent
Mitoses	Scarce	Numerous

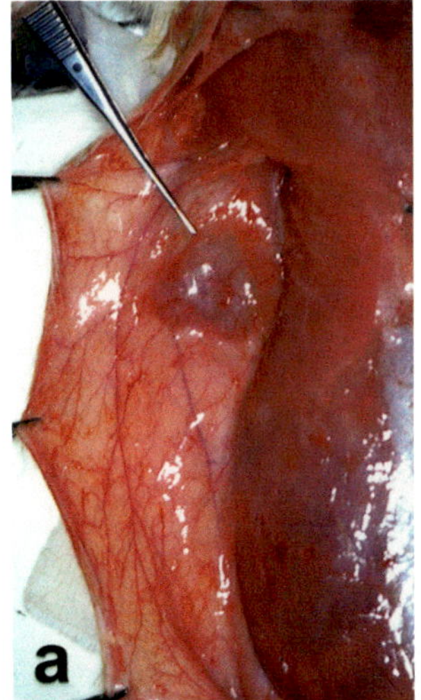
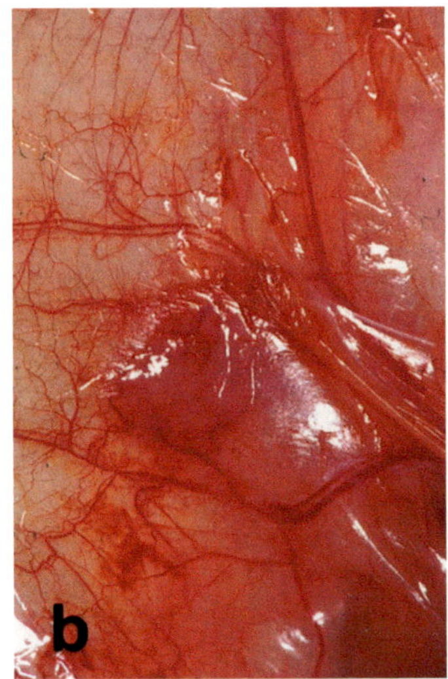
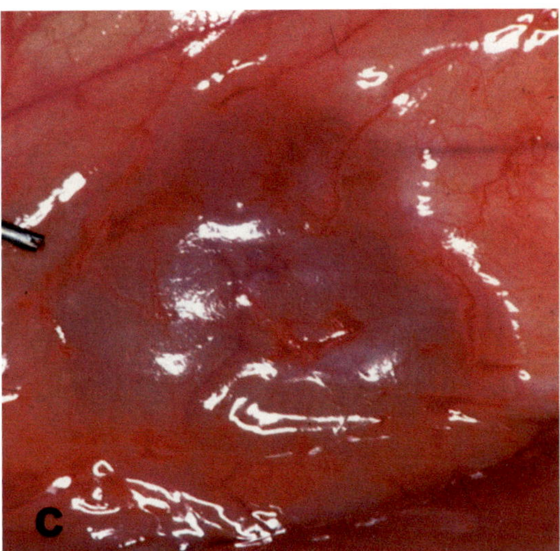

Figure 6.31 a–c

a Gross photographs of an adenocarcinoma 45 days post DMBA administration, ×1. **b** Angiogenic activity around a small adenocarcinoma 35 days after DMBA administration, ×4. **c** Close-up of **a**, ×10

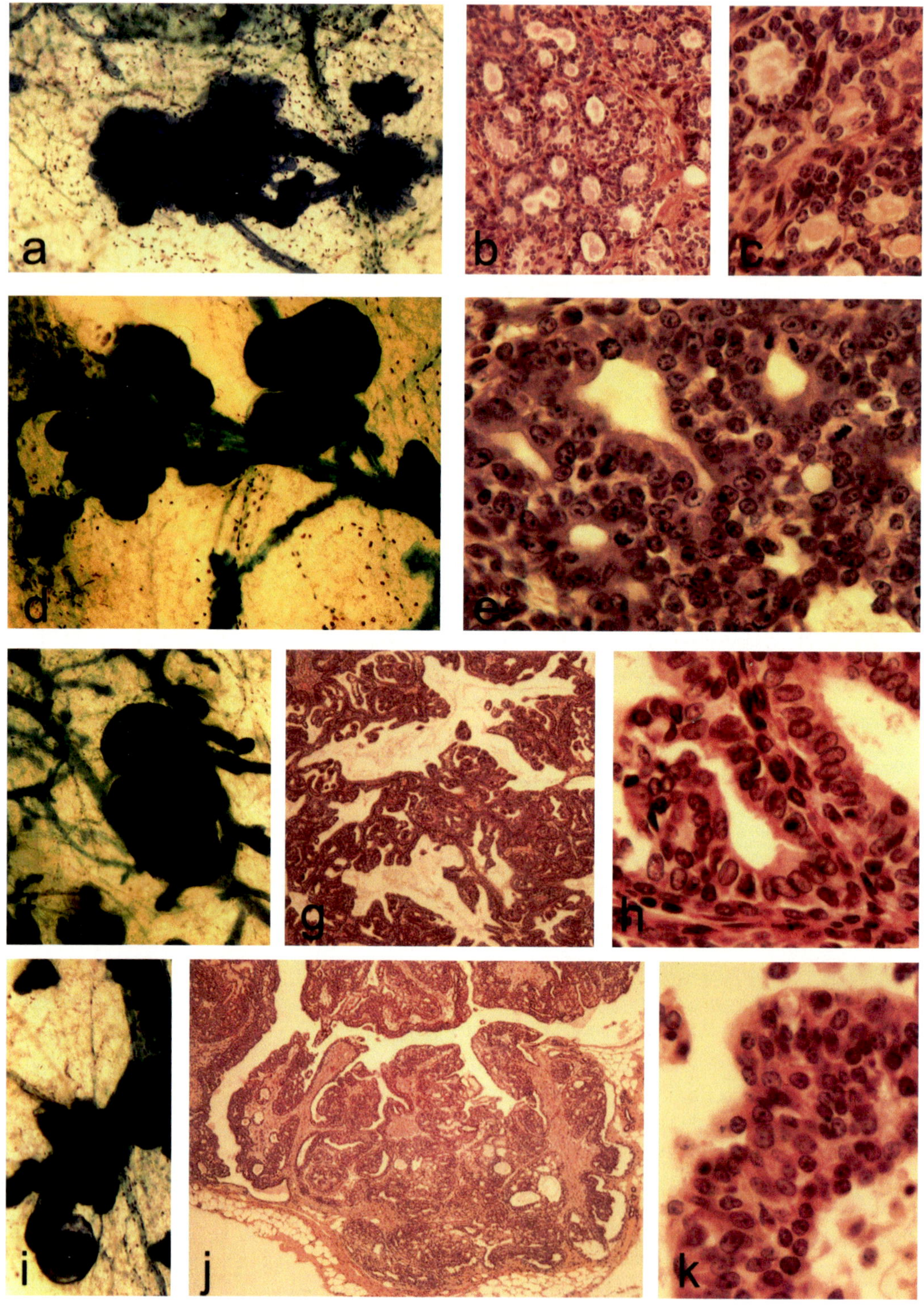

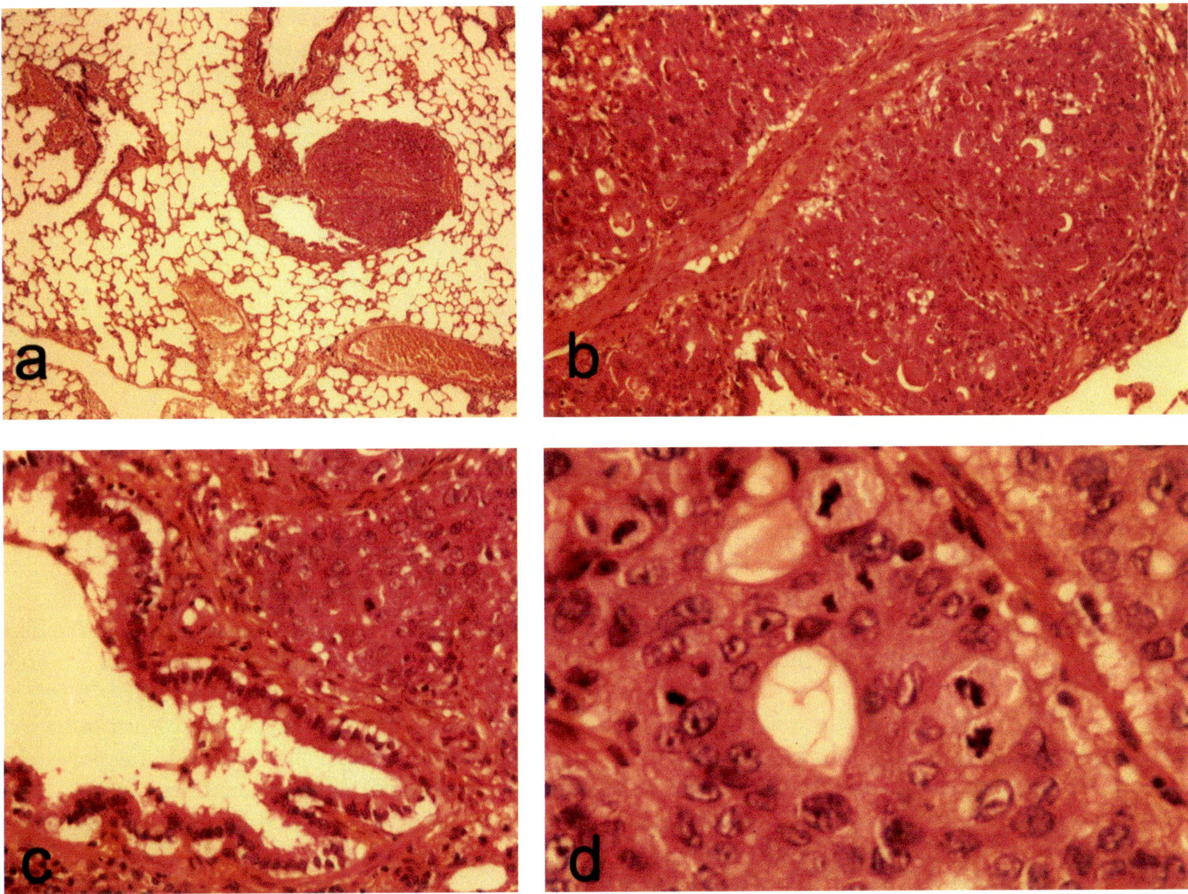

◄ **Figure 6.32 a–k**

a Tubular adenoma, stained with toluidine blue, ×4. **b** Histological section of **a** in which the tubular structures or alveoli exhibit a regular contour (H&E, ×10). **c** Individual alveoli are surrounded by a small amount of connective tissue. The lumen is circumscribed by an even and smooth glycocalyx (H&E, ×40). **d** Whole mount of a cribriform carcinoma stained with toluidine blue, ×4. **e** Adenocarcinoma with cribriform pattern (H&E, ×40). **f** Whole mount of a papillary carcinoma type 1 stained with toluidine blue, ×4. **g** Histological section of (**f**), observe the numerous papillary projections sustained by very small, thin, connective tissue cores (H&E, ×10). **h** Tall columnar cells lining the papillae of a papillary carcinoma, grade 1 (H&E, ×40). **i** Whole mount preparation of a papillary carcinoma type 2, stained with toluidine blue, ×4. **j** Papillary projection in a papillary carcinoma, grade 2 in which the number of cells per layer is higher. The luminal border has an irregular appearance (H&E, ×10). **k** Epithelium lining a papillary carcinoma, grade 2. Observe the homogeneous appearance of the cells with large nuclei and prominent nucleoli (H&E, ×40)

Figure 6.33 a–d

a Mammary carcinoma metastatic to the lung (H&E, ×4). **b–d** Higher magnification of mammary carcinoma metastatic to lung (H&E, ×40)

Cribriform Carcinoma. The invasive cribriform carcinoma exhibits the same cellular arrangement as the in situ lesions in which the solid sheets of neoplastic epithelial cells are interrupted by round or irregularly shaped secondary lumina of variable size. Invasion is characterized by penetration of haphazardly arranged, finger-like projections of epithelium into the surrounding stroma. The cribriform pattern may be maintained even in small clusters of cells infiltrating the dermis, skeletal muscle, and connective tissue, as

Table 6.5. Differential diagnosis between tubular adenomas and tubular adenocarcinomas

Components	Tubular adenoma	Tubular carcinoma
Tubular structure	Present	Present
Lumen	Prominent	Present or absent
Secretion in lumen	Present	Present; in some cases prominent
Epithelium	Three cell types	Almost always one cell type
Cell morphology	Cuboidal, polarity preserved	Pleomorphic, loss of polarity
Nuclear features	Round shape, small nucleolus	Oval, enlarged, prominent nucleolus
Stroma	Scanty, scarce	Scanty or absent

well as in metastatic lesions (Fig. 6.33). Individual neoplastic cells are moderately to markedly pleomorphic. The degree of pleomorphism varies from tumor to tumor and even in different areas of the same tumor. Interestingly enough, even in the most pleomorphic tumors the glandular pattern is still present, with secretory material within the newly formed lumina. The infiltrating neoplastic cells are in general surrounded by a connective tissue that exhibits a marked desmoplastic reaction, with heavy lymphocytic and mast cell infiltrations. The cribriform type of tumor appears in general as a uniform pattern, but it may be associated with papillary or comedo patterns in the same tumor.

Comedocarcinoma. Comedocarcinomas are more frequently found in animals that have been treated with chemical carcinogens at a young age. The lesions appear as distended ductal structures lined by a multilayered epithelium surrounding necrotic debris. Invasion occurs as an extension of duct-like structures or sheets of epithelial cells arranged in a serpiginous pattern into a stroma in which desmoplastic reaction and inflammatory cell infiltration may occur. Individual neoplastic cells are moderately pleomorphic. These tumors resemble the comedocarcinoma of the human breast [37].

Tubular Carcinoma. Under the category of tubular carcinomas are classified those tumors that are composed of well-defined tubular or alveolar structures. We postulate that this type of tumor originates from alveolar buds or from alveolar bud-derived adenomas, whereas all the other types of carcinomas described above are ductal in origin [12]. Several transitional steps between adenomas and fully manifest carcinomas are found, which in some cases makes it difficult to differentiate one from the other. Tubular carcinomas, however, differ cytologically enough from tubular adenomas to allow their identification. The epithelial cells composing the tubular carcinoma have increased nuclear size, and the nuclei contain prominent nucleoli; tubular adenomas, on the other hand, have cells with smaller nuclei, and nucleoli are absent or inconspicuous (Fig. 6.32, Table 6.5).

6.8.2 Stromal Neoplasms

6.8.2.1 Fibroma

Fibromas are well-circumscribed, non-encapsulated tumors composed of proliferating fibroblasts arranged in interlacing bundles and embedded in variable amounts of collagen fibers. In some tumors there are isolated remnants of glandular epithelium, which suggests that they originate from fibroadenomas.

6.8.2.2 Fibrosarcoma

Malignant fibroblasts exhibiting the expected anaplastic characteristics and increased number of mitoses are the essential components of fibrosarcomas.

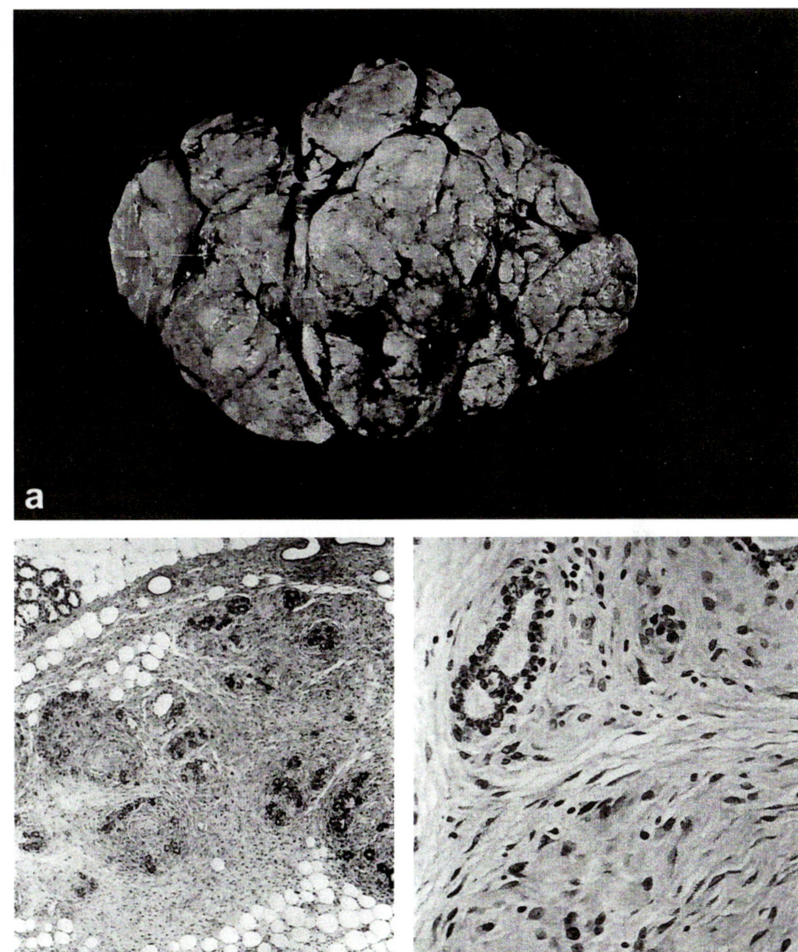

Figure 6.34 a–c

Fibroadenoma induced in DMBA parous treated rats. **a** Gross appearance of the dissected tumor. **b**, **c** Histological sections of the same tumor reveal the predominance of stromal cells with few ductules interspersed among collagenous fibers (H&E, ×4 and ×25, respectively)

6.8.3 Epithelial-Stromal Neoplasms

6.8.3.1 Fibroadenoma

Fibroadenomas are benign tumors composed of mammary epithelium and connective tissue, whose gross appearance is soft and rubbery. They are less vascularized than carcinomas. Histologically, they exhibit variations with a transition from the mainly epithelial tumors, which appear as adenomas to a more predominant proliferation of connective tissue, which determines the characteristic architecture of the pericanalicular fibroadenoma. Ductal and lobular structures are surrounded by layers of fibrous tissue (Fig. 6.34). The intracanalicular type of fibroadenoma that occurs in humans [38] is rarely found in the rat. In both types of tumors the secretory epithelium is usually one layer thick and maintains the same relation to the myoepithelium and basement membrane as does the normal mammary gland. When the fibrous tissue overgrows the epithelium to an extreme degree, ducts and alveoli become constricted, distorted, and widely separated by contracting bands of collagen.

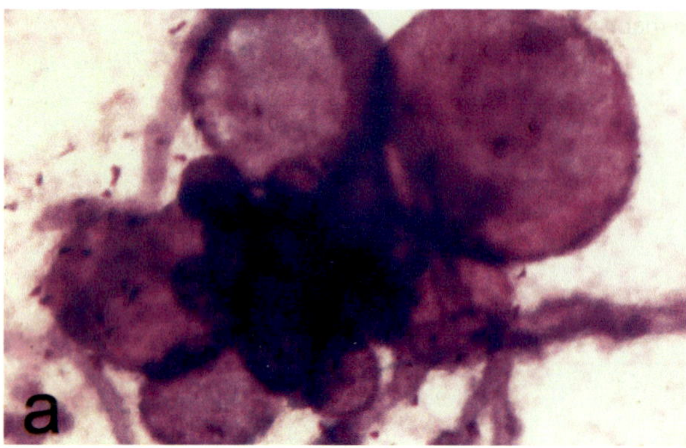

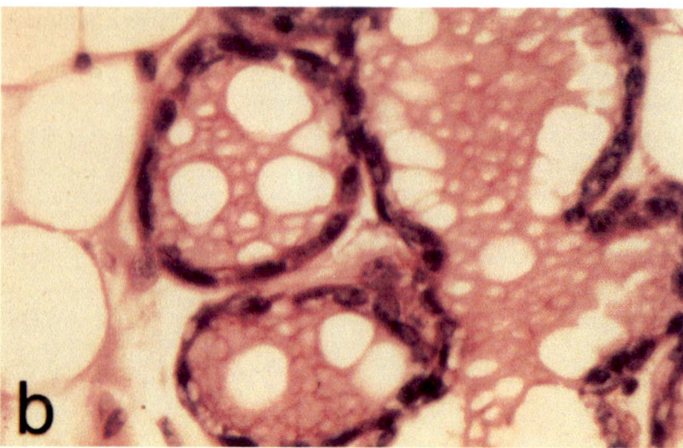

6.8.3.2 Carcinosarcoma

A rare entity, the carcinosarcoma frankly has malignant characteristics in both the epithelium and the stroma. The epithelial component varies from well-differentiated tubular structures to poorly demarcated and elongated cells, which are difficult to differentiate from neoplastic stromal cells. The specific markers keratin, myoglobin, desmin, and vimentin are useful for separating spindle-shaped epithelial cells from the stromal component. Nuclei vary in size and shape, and giant, multinucleated cells may be found. Mitoses are common in both the epithelium and the stroma.

6.8.4 Nonneoplastic Lesions

Among the nonneoplastic lesions in the mammary gland, cystic changes are the ones most frequently found. Cysts can originate from either ductal or lobular elements. Those derived from ducts exhibit a 10–100-fold increase in the normal diameter of the duct. They are lined by flat, cuboidal epithelial cells, and have myoepithelial cells, which are compressed against the basement membrane. In general, these ductal changes, that are also called duct ectasia or galactocele, are characterized by the accumulation within the lumen of eosinophilic granular material composed of lipids and protein secretion. Crystals similar to cholesterol and focal calcifications are common. Lobular cysts are characterized by a grape-

Figure 6.35 a, b

a Whole mount of cystic structures stained with toluidine blue, ×10. **b** Histological sections of cysts (H&E, ×10)

like configuration (Fig. 6.35). The small cystic dilatations can be confluent, forming one large cyst lined by low cuboidal epithelial cells, although some may contain cells with large vacuoles and decapitation of the apical portion of the cytoplasm. The nuclei are, in general, round or oval and are compressed against the basement membrane.

6.9　Differential Diagnosis of Mammary Tumors

Although a common practice for evaluating the tumorigenic response of the rat mammary gland to carcinogens is the quantitation of palpable tumors, it is important to keep in mind that palpable lesions are lumps or swellings whose nature can be determined only through histologic examination. In Table 6.6 are listed normal organs, nonneoplastic lesions, and tumors of non-mammary origin that under gross examination can be confused with mammary tumors. Whether spontaneous or carcinogen-induced rat mammary tumors are benign or malignant can be determined by criteria derived from: gross examination (macroscopic criteria), histopathologic examination, and analysis of the biological behavior of the tumor (Table 6.7).

Table 6.6. Differential diagnosis of tumoral masses developing in mammary regions

Structure or lesion	Main features
Lactating gland	Enlargement of the gland, uniformly affects all the pairs of glands
Salivary gland hyperplasia	Submandibular location; acini with serous or mucinous type epithelium
Clitoridial gland hyperplasia	Prepubic location; uniformly large cells with round, leptochromatic nuclei arranged in acini
Lymph nodes	Normal or reactive, specific locations, characteristic architecture
Abscesses	Encapsulated, tense, or fluctuant. Numerous polymorphonuclear leukocytes, macrophages, and necrotic material
Skin and adnexal tumors	Basal and squamous cell carcinomas, trichoepithelioma, tricholemmoma, sebaceous adenoma and carcinoma, fibroma, fibrosarcoma
Hibernomas	Typical architecture with numerous fat droplets of varying sizes

Table 6.7. Criteria of malignancy in mammary tumors

I. Macroscopic criteria

a) Rapid growth and skin ulceration in short period of time
b) Soft, fleshy appearance with or without areas of necrosis and hemorrhage

II. Histopathologic criteria

a) Loss of normal architecture with varying pleomorphism and layering or formation of papillae
b) One cell type, basically intermediate cells, predominate over the dark or myoepithelial cells. Varying response of the host such as fibrosis or inflammatory response
c) Increased nucleocytoplasmic ratio, round to oval nuclei with smooth contour, leptochromatic appearance, and 1 or 2 prominent nucleoli, numerous mitoses
d) Invasiveness: neoplastic cells infiltrating surrounding structures such as muscle, dermis, and fat

III. Biologic criteria

a) Metastases to lymph nodes and lungs, occasionally found in older animals, rarely found in young animals
b) Transplantability, although it may not be a reliable criterion because benign fibroadenoma may be also transplantable
c) Angiogenic response in anterior chamber of the eye, found in malignant and premalignant lesions

6.9.1 Macroscopic Criteria

The two major criteria to be taken into consideration upon gross examination of a tumor are its rate of growth and macroscopic appearance. Generally, malignant tumors tend to grow faster; however, some exceptions to this rule are observed. We have also found that tumors in the mammary glands located in the thoracic region grow faster than those arising in glands located in the abdominal region [16]. The gross appearance of carcinomas is generally soft and fleshy (Fig. 6.31). They are well vascularized and contain areas of necrosis and hemorrhage. Some tumors have cysts containing blood and necrotic material. Fibroadenomas, on the other hand, are white, with a rubbery and firm consistency, and they shell out from their capsule when they are sectioned. Carcinomas can be firm if they have elicited an intense desmoplastic response.

6.9.2 Histopathological Criteria

Among the criteria of malignancy, the most important one is the loss of the tubular-alveolar pattern of the normal mammary gland, a pattern maintained in the adenomas and fibroadenomas. Cytologically, malignant cells are larger than their normal counterparts and have an increased nucleocytoplasmic ratio. The enlarged nuclei contain coarse chromatin and more prominent nucleoli. The epithelial heterogeneity expressed by the normal gland, or even by benign lesions, in which at least myoepithelial, dark, and intermediate or clear cell types are identified, is rarely observed in malignant lesions [39]. The predominant cell in malignancy is the intermediate type, dark cells are rarely observed, and very few myoepithelial cells remain, especially in the invasive lesions. The number or mitoses is generally higher in malignant lesions than in benign ones [16]. Finally, the invasion of the stroma and neighboring tissues, such as muscle and dermis, is a hallmark of malignant tumors. The stromal response to invasion, as demonstrated by fibrosis and inflammatory infiltration, is generally more prominent in the malignant lesions than in the noninvasive or benign ones (Table 6.7).

6.9.3 Biological Criteria

The most reliable criterion of malignancy is the ability of a tumor to metastasize to distant organs, such as lymph nodes or lungs. Very few authors report the finding of metastases from either spontaneous or experimentally induced rat mammary tumors. This lack of metastasizing ability of rat tumors could be attributed to the short period of time that treated animals have been followed in most studies, since only when the study is prolonged for 2 or 3 years, essentially the whole life span of the animal, do metastases become evident. The histopathologic type of a tumor does not seem to affect its metastasizing ability, since it has been found that cribriform, comedo, or papillary carcinomas produce metastases with similar frequency [40]. Transplantability is considered another reliable criterion of malignancy in the mammary gland tumors of the rat. The ability of neoplastic lesions to elicit angiogenesis has been postulated to be a biological marker of malignancy, but it has not been extensively used [3, 40, 41].

6.10 Biological Importance of the Chemical Carcinogen-Induced Rat Mammary Tumor Model

The DMBA rat mammary model has allowed us to demonstrate that the carcinogen acts on the intermediate cell of the TEB, and that this structure is the one that evolves to IDP and carcinoma in situ. There are several factors that regulate the susceptibility of the TEB; some of them are:

1. Topographic location of the mammary gland
2. Age of the animal
3. The reproductive history

The high proliferative activity of the TEB is associated with higher binding of the carcinogen, and its short cell cycle makes them less likely to repair the DNA damaged by the carcinogen. Even though most of the TEBs are transformed to IDPS, not all of them evolve to carcinomas. The regulatory mechanism of this process is more complex due to intrinsic properties of the TEB. The fact that IDPs progress to carcinomas, secrete proteoglycans and attract lymphocytes and mast cells, emphasize the importance of the interaction of the initiated cells with the host as a mechanism in the progression of the disease. It is clear that the understanding of the mechanisms that modulate the progression of an IDP to a carcinoma will not only further our knowledge and understanding of carcinogenesis, but will also provide the tools for the prevention of the disease, as a result of the development of strategies for stopping the progression of initiated cells to fully manifested malignancy.

6.11 Genetically Engineered Mice Model

Genetic engineering of mice for mammary biology is now in its second decade. Almost 100 transgenes targeted mutations (site-directed mutations, knock outs and knock ins), combinations of transgenes and combinations of transgenes and targeted mutations have been used to study mammary cancer in mice. These mice will be referred to here under the collective term of genetically engineered mice (GEM) (summarized in Table 6.8).

6.11.1 Anatomy of the Mouse Mammary Gland

The mammary gland is anatomically divided into collecting ducts and the TDLU. The TDLU terminate in alveolar buds that share a common terminal ductule (Fig. 6.36) [42]. As will become apparent, the development of an anatomically correct classification requires knowledge of the anatomy of the mouse mammary gland. At birth the female mouse mammary gland parenchyma consists of a single primary main lactiferous duct that branches into three to five secondary ducts. From the second to the fifth weeks of life continuous branching and sprouting leads to new ducts that vary in width and length. Some of the ducts are narrow and straight, ending in club shaped terminal end buds (TEBs) (Fig. 6.36a). This period of mammary gland development is identified as the 'ductal stage'. At the beginning of ovarian function and during sexual maturity, branching continues by budding of 'lateral buds' that end in terminal ducts

(TDs). or cleavage of TEBs into two smaller buds, the 'alveolar buds' (ABs). This stage is called the 'alveolar bud stage' (Fig. 6.36a, c). The ABs, in turn, sprout new buds that are called 'ductules' at this stage. They cluster around the duct, forming a primitive lobular structure or lobule type I (Lob 1). The formation of Lob 1 signals the beginning of the 'lobular stage' that progresses from the more primitive Lob 1, composed of 6.26+4.10 ductules per cross section (Fig. 6.36a, d), to more complex lobular structures such as the lobules type 2 (Lob 2) and type 3 (Lob 3). This development takes place during pregnancy or under hormonal stimulation. Lob 2 contain 22–32 ductules per cross section (mean 26.64+5.22) (Fig. 6.36a, e). Individual ductules are small, lined by a layer of cuboidal epithelium surrounded by myoepithelial cells. The centrally located lumen is small and devoid of secretion. Lob 3 contains 53–90 ductules per cross section (mean 69.50+13.59) (Fig. 6.36f). All the ductules of the lobular structure drain into a common duct, called intralobular terminal duct. Ductules present in Lob 2 and Lob 3 accumulating secretory material within the lumen are called acini. The epithelial cells lining the lumen of the acini have vacuolated cytoplasm due to their content of lipids. During lactation, the acini become distended with milk. The distended acini become tightly packed and the boundaries between different lobules disappear. The individual lobules become very difficult to identify. At this point in the lactating gland, the term Lob 3 is no longer applicable.

The mammary lobules of mice differ from the lobules found in the human. The lobule in humans is embedded in a relatively loose connective tissue stroma that is surrounded by a denser connective tissue [42]. A clear demarcation between the intra- and interlobular spaces exists. In contrast, the lobular structures of the mouse mammary gland are surrounded mainly by fat and very small amount of connective tissue (Fig. 6.36b–f) [42]. Further, type 2 and type 3 lobules are found in the resting breasts of non-lactating, non-pregnant adult human females while the quiescent mammary gland of the mouse rarely has the more developed type I and type 2 lobules [48] (see chapter 2 for more details of the morphology of the human breast).

Table 6.8. Summary of models[a]

Models	Bitransgene/transgene	Experimental manipulation	Species	Promoters
Growth factors	FGF3 (INT2)	WNTI	Mouse	MMTV-LTR
	FGF7 (KGF)		Mouse	MMTV-LTR
	HEREGULIN (NDF)	myc	Mouse	MMTV-LTR
	HGF		Mouse	MT
	IGFII		Mouse	BGL, H19
	TGF	p53–172H, myc	Mouse	WAP, MMTV-LTR
		DMBA		MT
	TGF-β	MMTV-infected	Mouse	WAP
Receptors	TGF; DNIIR		Mouse	MMTV-LTR
	ERB-B2 (neu)	p53–172H	Mouse	MMTV-LTR
	RET-I		Mouse	MMTV-LTR
	Tpr-MET		Mouse	MMTV-LTR
Signal pathways	PyV-mT		Mouse	MMTV-LTR
	RAS		Mouse	MMTV-LTR
Cell cycle	CYCLIN DI		Mouse	MMTV-LTR
	MYC	BCL-2	Mouse	MMTV-LTR, WAP
	p53–172H, p53		Mouse	WAP, Null
	SV40TAg	BCL-2	Mouse	WAP, C(3)1
Differentiation	NOTCH4 (INT3)	TGF	Mouse	MMTV-LTR, WAP
	WNT I		Mouse	MMTV-LTR
	WNTIOb		Mouse	MMTV-LTR
	P-CADHERIN		Mouse	Null
Other transgenes	Stromelysin		Mouse	WAP
	MTSI		Mouse	MMTV-LTR
Transgenic rat models	TGF x		Rat	MMTV-LTR
	SV40Tag		Rat	C(3)1
	ERB-B2 (neu)		Rat	MMTV-LTR
Miscellaneous	DMBA treated rat		Rat	
	MNU treated rat		Rat	
	MMTV infected mouse		Mouse	
	Transplants of DMBA treated-p53 -/-mouse mammary epithelium		Mouse	

[a] Reprinted with permission, from: Cardiff, R.D., Anver, M.A., Gusterson, B.A., Green, J.E., Heninghausen, L., Jensen, R.L., Merino, M.J., Rehm, S., Russo, J., Tavassoli, F., Ward, F., and Wakefield, L. The Mammary pathology of genetically engineered mice. Oncogene 19:968–988, 2000

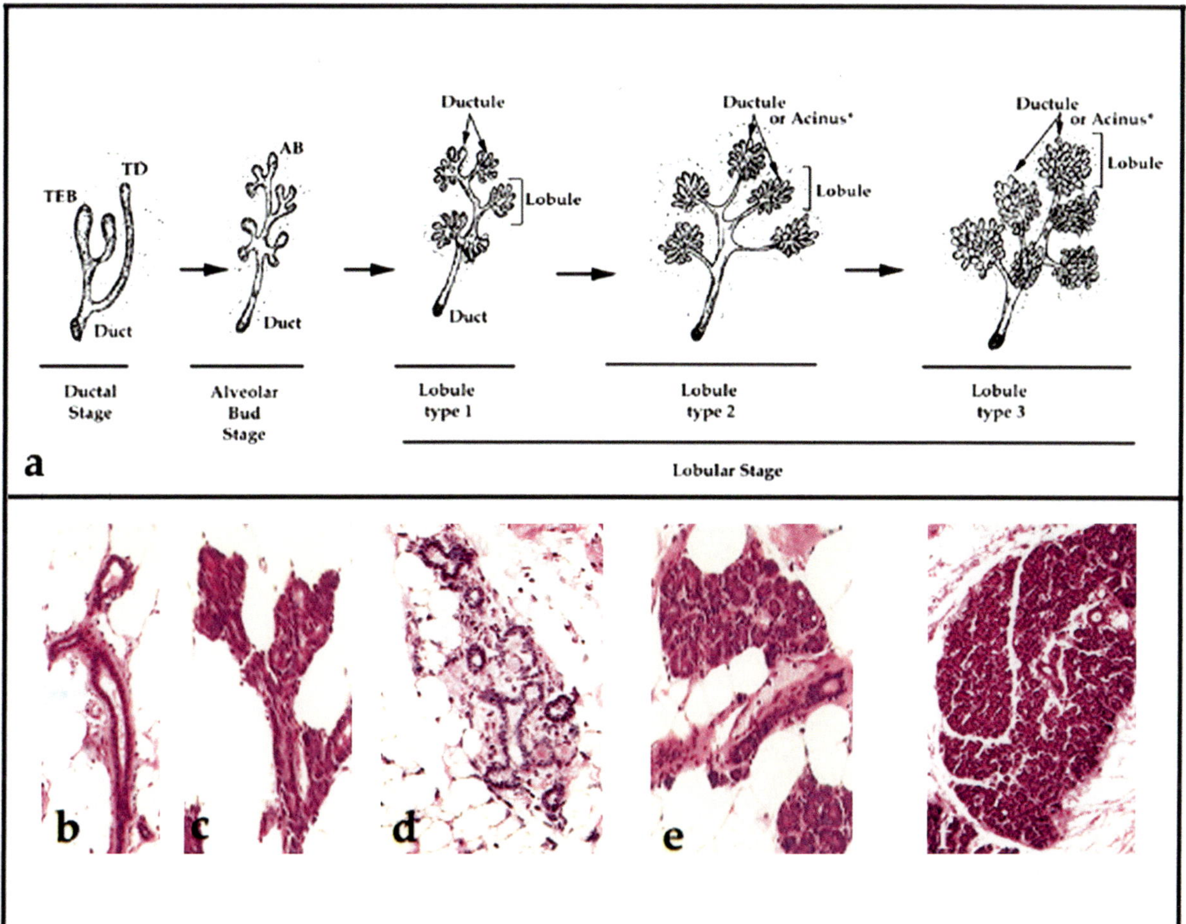

Figure 6.36 a–f

a From the 2nd to the 5th weeks of life, during the 'ductal stage,' the mammary three grows by continuous branching and sprouting of new ducts, ending in club shaped terminal end buds (TEBs). The 'alveolar bud stage' is characterized by budding of 'lateral buds' that end in terminal ducts (TDs), or cleavage of TEBs into two smaller buds, the 'alveolar buds (ABs)' (**a, c**). The ABs sprout new buds, referred to as 'ductules' that cluster around the duct, forming a primitive lobule type I (Lob 1) signaling the beginning of the 'lobular stage'. The primitive Lob I is composed of 6.26±4.10 ductules per cross section (**a, d**) and with increasing stimuli form more complex lobular structures such as the lobules type 2 (Lob 2) and type 3 (Lob 3). Lob 2 contain 22–32 ductules per cross section (mean 26.64±5.22) (**a, e**). Lob 3 contain 53–90 ductules per cross section (mean 69.50±13.59) (**f**). All the lobular ductules are associated with a duct, the intralobular terminal duct. As the ductules present in Lob 2 and Lob 3 start accumulating secretory material within the lumen they are called acini or alveoli. The mouse mammary lobular structures are surrounded mainly by fat and very small amounts of connective tissue (**b–f**). (reprinted with permission, from: Cardiff, R.D., Anver, M.A., Gusterson, B,A, Green, J.E., Heninghausen, L., Jensen, R.L., Merino, M.J., Rehm, S., Russo, J., Tavassoli, F., Ward, F., and Wakefield, L. The Mammary pathology of genetically engineered mice. Oncogene 19:968–988, 2000)

Table 6.9. Comparison of classification of mammary gland proliferative lesions[a]

Annapolis nomenclature	Alveolar or ductal origin/differentiation	Cellular origin/differentiation
Hyperplasia, functional, without atypia	Hyperplasia	Alveolar/ductal
Acinar hyperplasia, low grade, focal, non-GEM	Hyperplastic alveolar nodule (HAN)	Alveolar
Solid hyperplasia, low grade, focal, hormone-induced, non-GEM	Plaque/organoid/pregnancy-dependent 'tumor' (Type P)	Ductal
Mammary intra-epithelial neoplasia (MIN)	Preneoplasia or dysplasia	Alveolar/ductal
Adenoma/carcinoma	Adenocarcinoma	Alveolar
Glandular/acinar	Type A	Alveolar
Cribriform	Type AB/Type B/Type L	Alveolar
Papillary	Type B/Type Y	Alveolar
Solid	Type B/Type P	Alveolar/ductal
Adenosquamous	Adenoacanthoma/pale cell tumor/large cell tumor/adenosquamous carcinoma	Alveolar
Fibroadenoma	No reports	
Squamous carcinoma	Molluscoid tumor/intraductal squamous carcinoma	Ductal
Adenomyoepithelioma	Adenocarcinoma type C/carcinosarcoma/mixed tumor/adenomyoepithelioma	Alveolar and/or ductal, myoepithelial possibly with cartilage or bone

[a] Reprinted with permission, from: Cardiff, R.D., Anver, M.A., Gusterson, B.A., Green, J.E., Heninghausen, L., Jensen, R.L., Merino, M.J., Rehm, S., Russo, J., Tavassoli, F., Ward, F., and Wakefield, L. The mammary pathology of genetically engineered mice. Oncogene 19:968–988, 2000

6.11.2 Classification of Genetically Engineered Mouse Mammary Lesions

The available evidence and our experience suggest that tumors arising in many genetically engineered mice (GEM) have morphological patterns that have seldom been observed in non-GE virus-induced or carcinogen-induced mouse mammary tumors (Table 6.9). From this perspective, the histopathology of GEM mammary tumors is unique. GEM tumors have three notable phenotypes:

1. Some transgenes produce tumors closely resembling non-GEM tumors

2. Many transgenes produce tumors that have unique, transgene-specific phenotypes (signature tumors)
3. Some GEM produce tumors that mimic human breast cancer [42, 43]

6.11.3 Comparative Pathology of the Model Systems

The Annapolis consensus [42] documented that GEM produce categories of mammary tumors that are not seen in MMTV-induced or other experimentally induced mouse mammary tumors. Some of the tumors have patterns that mimic the histopathology of human breast lesions in great detail. These intriguing lesions merit much more intense study as they promise to unlock the molecular mysteries currently facing us in human breast cancer. In fact, all of the genes represented in Table 6.8 and other models merit further study because they all inform us of the normal and abnormal biology of the mammary gland. The National Cancer Institute has challenged the scientific community to develop a molecular classification of human tumors. The mouse mammary biologists have already started the marriage between pathology and molecular biology of cancer by creating animals with known genetic abnormalities that have distinctive morphological lesions. As we learn the rules of abnormal structure and function from the mouse, we should apply them to human breast cancer. One needs to be mindful that the mouse is a different species. No matter how exciting the similarities, there are differences between murine and human mammary cancer. Some of the more obvious or common similarities and differences are listed in Table 6.9 [42].

References

1. Russo, J., Tay, L.K, Russo, I.H. Differentiation of the mammary gland and susceptibility to carcinogenesis. Breast Cancer Res. Treat. 2:5–37, 1982.
2. Welsh, C.W. Rodent models to examine in vivo hormonal regulation of mammary gland tumorigenesis. In: Medina, D., Kidwell, W., Heppner, G. and Anderson, E. (eds), Cellular and molecular biology of mammary cancer. Plenum Press, New York, 1987,pp163–179.
3. Russo, J., Gusterson, B.A., Rogers, A.E., Russo, I.H., Wellings, S.R., Van Zwieten, M.J. Comparative study of human and rat mammary tumorigenesis. Lab. Invest. 62:1–32, 1990.
4. Russo, I.H., Tewari M, Russo, J. Morphology and development of rat mammary gland. In: Jones, T.C., Mohr, U., Hunt, R. D., (eds), Integument and Mammary Gland of Laboratory Animals. (Springer-Verlag, Berlin). 1989,pp. 233–252
5. Russo, I.H., Medado J., Russo, J. Endocrine Influences on mammary structure and development. In: Jones, T. C, Mohr, U., Hunt, R.D., (eds), Integument and Mammary Gland of Laboratory Animals. Springer Verlag, Berlin, 1989, pp. 252–266.
6. Russo, J., Russo, I.H. Toward a physiological approach to breast cancer prevention. Cancer Epidemiol Biomarkers & Prevention, 3:353–364, 1994.
7. Daniel, C.W., Silberstein, G.B. Postnatal development of the rodent mammary gland. In: Neville, M.C. and Daniel, C.W. (eds). The mammary gland. Development, regulation and function. Plenum Press, New York, 1987, pp 3–36.
8. Rao, G.N., Piegorsch, W.W., Haseman, J.K. Influence of body weight on the incidence of spontaneous tumors in rats and mice of long-term studies. Am. J. Clin. Nutr. 45:252–260, 1987.
9. Russo, J., Russo, I.H., van Zwieten, M.J., Rogers A.E, Gusterson, B. Classification of neoplastic and non-neoplastic lesions of the rat mammary gland. In: Jones, T. C., Mohr, U., Hunt, R. D., (eds), Integument and Mammary glands of Laboratory Animals. Springer-Verlag, Berlin, 1989, pp. 275–304.
10. Russo, J., Calaf, G., Russo, I.H. A critical approach to the malignant transformation of human breast epithelial cells. CRC Critical Reviews in Oncogenesis 4:403–417, 1993.
11. Zwieten, M. J. Normal anatomy and pathology of the rat mammary gland. In: The rat as animal model in breast, Martinus Nijhoff Publishers, Boston, 1984, pp 53–134.
12. Russo, J., Saby, J., Isenberg, W., Russo, I.H. Pathogenesis of mammary carcinoma induced in rats by 7,12-dimethylbenz(a)anthracene. J. Natl. Cancer Inst. 59:435–445, 1977.
13. Russo, J., Wilgus, G., Russo, I.H. Susceptibility of the mammary gland to carcinogenesis. I. Differentiation of the mammary gland as determinant of tumor incidence and type of lesion. Am. J. Pathol. 96:721–734, 1979.
14. Russo, J., Russo, I.H. Influence of differentiation and cell kinetics on the susceptibility of the rat mammary gland to carcinogenesis. Cancer Res. 40:2677–2687, 1980.
15. Russo, J., and Russo, I.H. Susceptibility of the mammary gland to carcinogenesis. II. Pregnancy interruption as a risk factor in tumor incidence. Am. J. Pathol. 100:497–512, 1980.
16. Russo, J., Russo, I.H. Biological and molecular bases of mammary carcinogenesis. Lab Invest. 57:112–137, 1987.
17. Isaacs, J.T. Genetic control of resistance to chemically induced mammary adeno-carcinogenesis in the rat. Cancer Res. 46:3958, 1986.
18. Russo, J. and Russo, I.H. DNA labeling index and structure of the rat mammary gland as determinant of its susceptibility to carcinogenesis. J. Natl. Cancer Inst. 61:1451–1459, 1978.
19. Huggins, C., Lorraine, C., Grand, L.C., Brillantes, F.P. Mammary cancer induced by a single feeding of polynuclear hydrocarbons and its suppression. Nature (Lond.) 1989:204–207, 1961.
20. Gullino, P.M., Pettigrew, H.M., Grantham F.H. N-nitrosomethylurea as mammary gland carcinogen in rats. J. Natl. Cancer Inst. 54:401–410, 1976.
21. Russo, I.H., Russo, J. Developmental stage of the rat mammary gland as determinant of its susceptibility to 7,12-dimethylbenz(a)anthracene. J. Natl. Cancer Inst. 61:1439–1449, 1978.

22. Russo, J., Tait, L., Russo, I.H. Susceptibility of the mammary gland to carcinogenesis III. The cell of origin of mammary carcinoma. Am. J. Pathol. 113:50–66, 1983.

23. Tay, L.K., Russo, J. Formation and removal of 7,12-dimethylbenz(a)anthracene nucleic acid adducts in rat mammary epithelial cells with different susceptibility to carcinogenesis. Carcinogenesis 2:1327–1333, 1981.

24. Tay, L.K. and Russo, J. 7,12-dimethylbenz(a)anthracene (DMBA) induced DNA binding and repair synthesis in susceptible and non-susceptible mammary epithelial cells in culture. J. Natl. Cancer Inst. 67, 155–161, 1981.

25. Folkman, J. How is blood vessel growth regulated in normal and neoplastic tissue?, Cancer Res. 46:467–473,1986.

26. Kessler, D. A., Langer, R. S., Pless, N. A., and Folkman, J. Mast cells and tumor angiogenesis. Int. J. Cancer 18:703–709, 1976.

27. Zetter, B. R. Migration of capillary endothelial cells is stimulated by tumour-derived factors. Nature 285:41–43,1980.

28. Azizkhan, R. G. Azizkhan, J. C. Zetter, B. R. and Folkman, J. Mast cell heparin stimulates migration of capillary endothelial cells in vitro. Exp. Med. 152:931–944,1980.

29. Gospardorowicz, D. Cheng, J. Lui, G. M. Baird, A. and Bohlent, P. Isolation of brain fibroblast growth factor by heparin-sepharose affinity chromatography: identify with pituitary fibroblast growth factor. Proc. Natl Acad. Sci. U.S.A. 81:6963–6967,1984.

30. Lobb R.R. and Fett, J. N. Purification of two distinct growth factors from bovine neural tissue by heparin affinity chromatography. Biochemistry 23:6295–6299,1984.

31. Lippman, M. Transplantation and cytotoxicity changes induced by acid mucopolysaccharides. Nature 219:33–36, 1968.

32. McBride W. M. and Bard, J. B. L. Hyaluronidase-sensitive halos around adherent cells, J. Exp. Med. 149:507–515,1979.

33. Ito, I. Radioactive labeling of the surface coat on enteric microvilli. Anat. Res. 151:489a, 1965.

34. Bekesi J. G. and Winzler, R. J. The metabolism of plasma glycoproteins: Studies on the incorporation of L-fucose-l-^{14}C into tissue and serum in the normai rat. J. Biol. Chem. 242:3873–3879,1967.

35. Bossmann, H. B. Hagopian, A. and Eylar, E. H. Cellular membranes: the biosynthesis of glycoprotein and glycolipids in the HeLa cell membranes. Arch. Biochem. h s. 130:573–533, 1969.

36. Esko, J. D., Rostand, S. and Weinke, J. L. Tumor formation dependent on proteoglycan biosynthesis, Science 241:1092–1096, 1988.

37. Fisher, E.R. Gregorio, R.M. Fisher, B. The pathology of invasive breast cancer. A syllabus derived from findings of the National Surgical Adjuvant Breast Project (protocol no 4). Cancer 36: 1–85, 1975.

38. Rosai, J. Ackerman's surgical pathology. Mosby, St Louis, pp 1087–1149, 1981.

39. Russo, J. Basis of cellular autonomy in susceptibility to carcinogenesis. Toxicol. Pathol. 11:149–166, 1983.

40. Brem, S.S., H.M. Jensen, H.M., Gullino, P.M. Angiogenesis as a marker of preneoplastic lesions of the human breast. Cancer 41:239–244, 1978.

41. Maiorana, A., Gullino, P.M. Acquisition of angiogenic capacity and neoplastic trans-formation in the rat mammary gland. Cancer Res. 38:4409–4414, 1978.

42. Cardiff, R.D., Anver, M.A., Gusterson, B.A., Green, J.E., Heninghausen, L., Jensen, R.L., Merino, M.J., Rehm, S., Russo, J., Tavassoli, F., Ward, F., and Wakefield, L. The Mammary pathology of genetically engineered mice. Oncogene 19:968–988,2000.

43. Cardiff, R.D., and Wellings, S.R. J. Mammary Gland Biol. Neoplasia. 4:105–122, 1999.

In Vitro Models for Human Breast Cancer

7.1 Introduction

The morphological analysis of breast cancer development indicates this to be a multi-step process that progressively evolves from ductal hyperplasia and atypical ductal hyperplasia, which represent the initial stages of neoplastic growth, to carcinoma in situ, invasive carcinoma, and ultimately metastasis, as has been documented for a number of other malignancies [1–3]. However, the possibility that normal cells give rise to ductal carcinoma in situ or invasive ductal carcinoma has not been definitively ruled out. The understanding of the cellular and molecular processes that lead a normal cell to malignancy requires the analysis of pure populations of human breast epithelial cells (HBEC) representing specific stages of neoplastic progression. Only cells in culture would provide the conditions needed for probing what effect have given etiologic agents when interacting with susceptible cells in a specific hormonal or biochemical milieu. The models that will be discussed in this chapter are:

1. The growth properties of normal human breast epithelial cells (HBEC)
2. The MCF-7 cell, a breast cancer cell line, as an in vitro model of human breast cancer
3. The growth properties of the immortal cell line MCF10F and its mechanism of cell immortalization
4. The use of primary cultures of HBEC and their susceptibility to transformation by chemical carcinogens
5. A model of transformation of human breast epithelial cells

7.2 Growth Properties of Normal Human Breast Epithelial Cells In Vitro

Like all normal diploid and differentiated somatic cells, normal HBEC have a limited capacity to divide both in vivo and in vitro. The number of doublings is higher in HBEC derived from breast tissues with a lower differentiation grade and a higher proliferation rate (Fig. 7.1) [1], indicating that the growth characteristics of HBEC in primary culture reflect the degree of lobular development and the rate of cell proliferation of the breast under in vivo conditions [1]. A characteristic of all cultured breast epithelial cells is their limited life span in vitro. The mortality of nor-

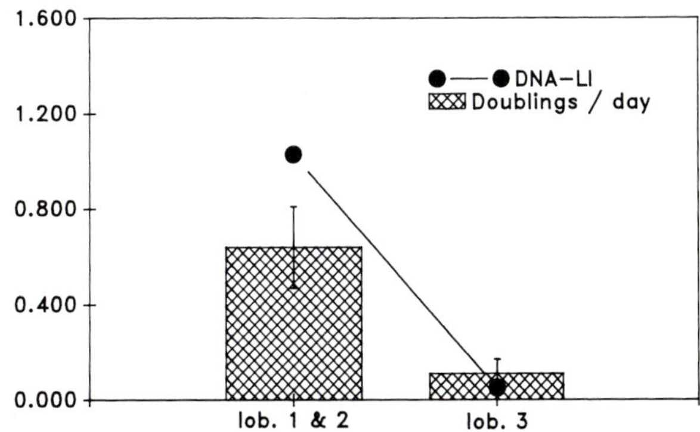

Figure 7.1

Influence of lobular development on the number of doublings/day and DNA labeling index (reprinted with permission from: Russo, J et al. Critical steps in breast carcinogenesis. The New York Academy of Sciences 698:1–20, 1993)

Table 7.1. Supplements for the growth of human mammary epithelial cells

Supplement	Serum-free-medium	Low Ca medium 0.046 mM
Insulin	5.0 µg/ml	10 µg/ml
Hydrocortisone	1.4×10^{-7} M	0.5 µg/ml
Epidermal growth factor	10 ng/ml	20 µg/ml
Cholera toxin	–	100 ng/ml
Ethanolamine	1.0×10^{-4} M	–
Phosphoethanolamine	1.0×10^{-4} M	–
Transferrin	5 µg/ml	–
Bovine pituitary extract	20–70 µg/ml	–
Serum	–	Horse serum (5 %)

Table 7.2. Comparisons of HBEC grown in two different culture conditions

	Serum-free medium	Low Ca medium
Density (cells $\times$ cm^2)	6.0×10^4	1.04×10^5
Free floating cells (cells/cm^3 media) (every 72 h)	–	$6.0–7.2 \times 10^4$
Extended growth (days)	20 passages (70–140 days)	26 passages unlimited growth
Doubling time (days)	2.3 days	1.4 days

Table 7.3. Duct formation in collagen gel

Specimen	Passage	Days in vitro	Growth in collagen	Type of growth	Days required for duct formation in gel
#73[a]	2	446	+	Ductal	24
#111[a]	2	137	+	Ductal	14
#109[a]	2	93	+	Ductal	10
#115[a]	2	66	+	Ductal	6
#118[a]	2	47	+	Ductal	7
#130[a]	36	960	+	Ductal	30
MCF-7[b]	10	291	+	Ball	–[d]
MCF-7[b]	148	1,602	+	Ball	–
Tumor #3[c]	4	102	+	Ball	–

[a] 10^4 cells from primary culture were used to initiate collagen gel culture in 2-cm^2 wells
[b] 10^4 MCF-7 cells were used to initiate gel cultures in 2-cm^2 wells
[c] 4×10^4 cells from third passage were used to initiate gel cultures in 2-cm^2 well
[d] Cultures terminated at 35 days

Figure 7.2 a–d

a Whole mount of the normal human breast showing lobules type 1. b Breast tissue disaggregated by collagenase and hyaluronidase and grown in collagen matrix reproduces the structures from which it was originated. c Normal breast tissue forming ductules in collagen matrix. d MCF-7 cells or primary tumor cells have lost the ability to form ductules in collagen matrix. Phase contrast microscopy, × 10

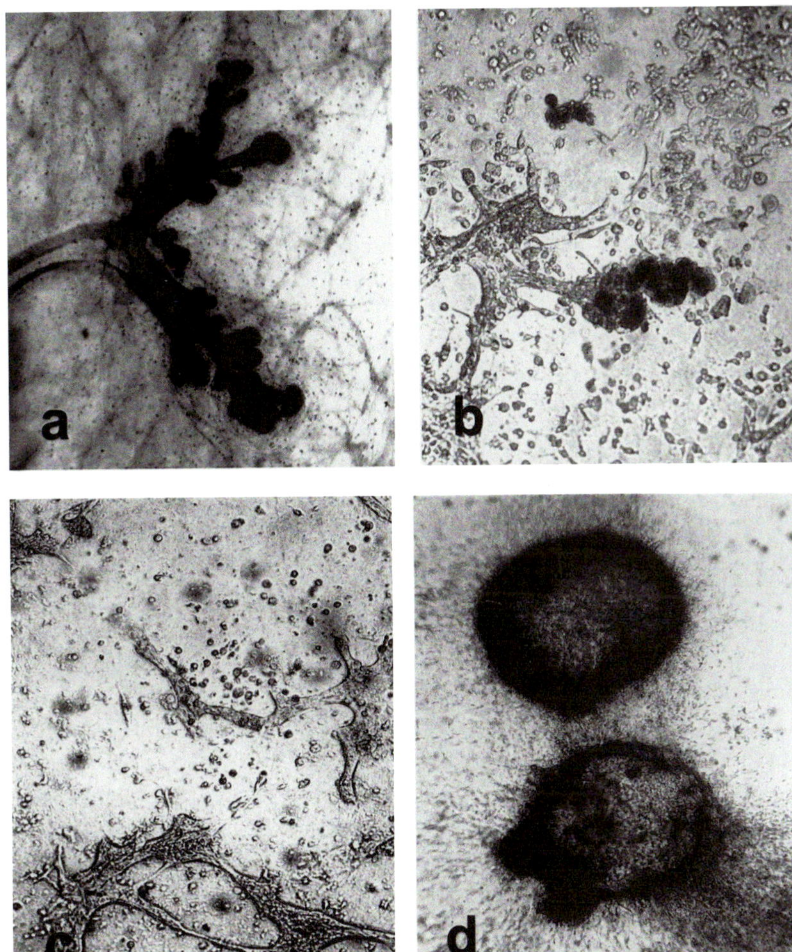

mal HBEC is characterized by a progressive cessation of cell growth in culture and senescence. HBEC cultured in standard culture medium have a life span comparable to that of adult human fibroblasts (30–40 doublings), before undergoing terminal differentiation and senescence. The survival of HBEC is profoundly affected by the concentration of calcium (Ca++) in the culture medium. Comparing two different culture conditions (Table 7.1), one with serum free medium, in which the Ca concentration is 1.05 mM, and another containing serum, but lowering Ca concentration to 0.046 mM, significantly changes the growth properties of HBEC (Table 7.2).

Extended growth without expressing terminal differentiation is observed when the Ca++ level in the culture medium is reduced from 1.05 mM to 0.046 mM (low Ca++) [4]. Under these conditions HBEC maintain their normal diploid karyotype, form domes and duct-like structures in collagen (Table 7.3) even reproducing the morphology of the structures from which the are derived from (Fig. 7.2), express specific keratin filaments and milk fat globule membrane antigen, and contain all the other structural features of breast epithelial cells [5]. When the Ca++ concentration is restored to 1.05 mM (also called high Ca++) the cells maintain the same phenotypic characteristics, but they stop their growth. This phenomenon is reversible by reducing the Ca concentration in the culture medium. The reversibility induced by the changing the Ca concentration is maintained as long as the cells maintain the normal phenotype. The response of the normal HBEC to Ca is loss during the process of cell immortalization and transformation and accompanied by the over expression of S100p [6]. Normal cells obtained from primary cultures do not form colonies in agar methocel; they instead form ductules in collagen matrix, (Table 7.3) and are unable to grow in athymic mice.

7.3 The MCF-7 Cell as a Model of Human Breast Cancer In Vitro

MCF-7 is a stable cell line derived by Soule et al. [7] from a pleural effusion from a patient with metastatic mammary carcinoma and maintained in our as well as in other laboratories around the world for more than 30 years. The abundant literature generated using this cell line is beyond the scope of this chapter and this book, but it is important to describe here some basic biology of this cell line, first in tribute to the memory of our colleague H. Soule and second to revise important experiments done in the authors laboratory that paved the further development and use of this cell line. Since its initial description [7], MCF-7 has been verified to be human both biochemically and cytologically [8]. The demonstration of human alpha-lactalbumin [9] and estrogen receptor protein [10, 11] in these cells support its origin in human breast tissue. This cell line contains receptor proteins specific for androgen, glucocorticoids and progesterone [11]. The behavior of MCF-7 cells as observed morphologically when grown in collagen coated sponges [12] and in athymic mice [13, 14] indicates the value of the cell line in understanding biological aspects of malignancy at cellular level.

7.3.1 Morphological and Growth Characteristics of MCF-7 Cells

MCF-7 was initially described by light microscopy [7] as being comprised of polyhedral epithelial cells, confirmed by scanning electron microscopy (Figs. 7.3, 7.4). In confluent cultures or in those seeded at a high cell density (Fig. 7.4a), cells tended to be compact or laterally compressed, but usually retained contact with the substratum. Cultures less than 7 days post-seeding and those not grown to confluence contained cells, which were low, cuboidal in nature. The cells maintain the epithelial pattern with separation of tissue and lumen by an interface of contiguous cell margins tightly bound together by occluded junctions (Fig. 7.4b). It has also been reported a similar degree of polarity in breast cells and tumor cultures derived from other mammals [15, 16]. The epithelial pattern in MCF-7 is also demonstrated by the presence of microvilli, which increase the luminal surface area, and by the accumulation of secretory vesicles at the free apical cell margins (Figs. 7.4c, d). Differences among individual cells are entirely consistent with the malignant origins of the cell line [12]. The combination of desmosomes, tonofilaments, and intracytoplasmic lumina, which are the markers used for identifying breast cells in culture [17], are all observed in MCF-7 cells, but seldom are all three markers present in the same cell. Desmosomes are infrequent among cells of young, growing cultures which are joined together largely by tight junctions. Microfilaments, likewise, are plentiful in most cells but are bundled into tonofilaments mostly in cells of long established cultures. Intracellular lumina were extremely rare among our samples but occurred fairly often under certain experimental conditions, as when inoculated into athymic mice [14]. Two of these characteristics, intracellular lumina and tonofilaments, have been proposed as indicators of malignancy [18], mainly since they are found in carcinoma in situ and more frequently in invasive carcinoma [18]. Derivation of the basement membrane from epithelial cells has been described in animals and in cell culture [19]. Although the presence of the basement membrane has not been fully demonstrated in normal human breast epithelium in culture, it may be significant that this

Figure 7.3 a, b

Scanning electron micrograph of MCF-7 cells growing in plastic surface, ×400

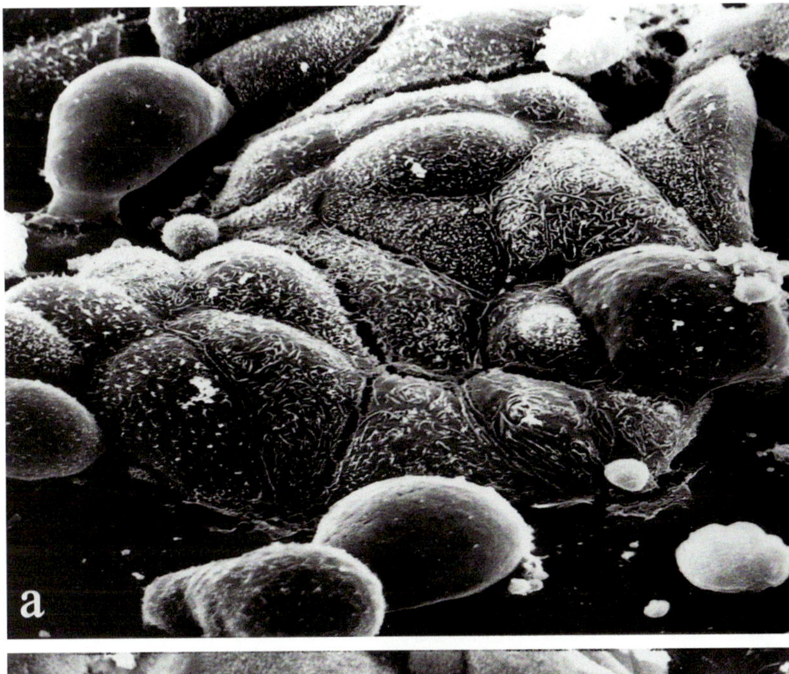

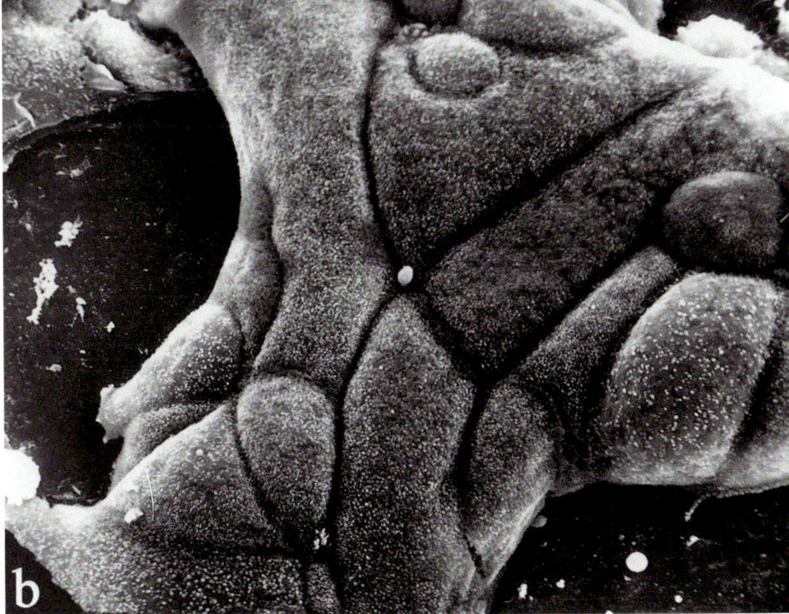

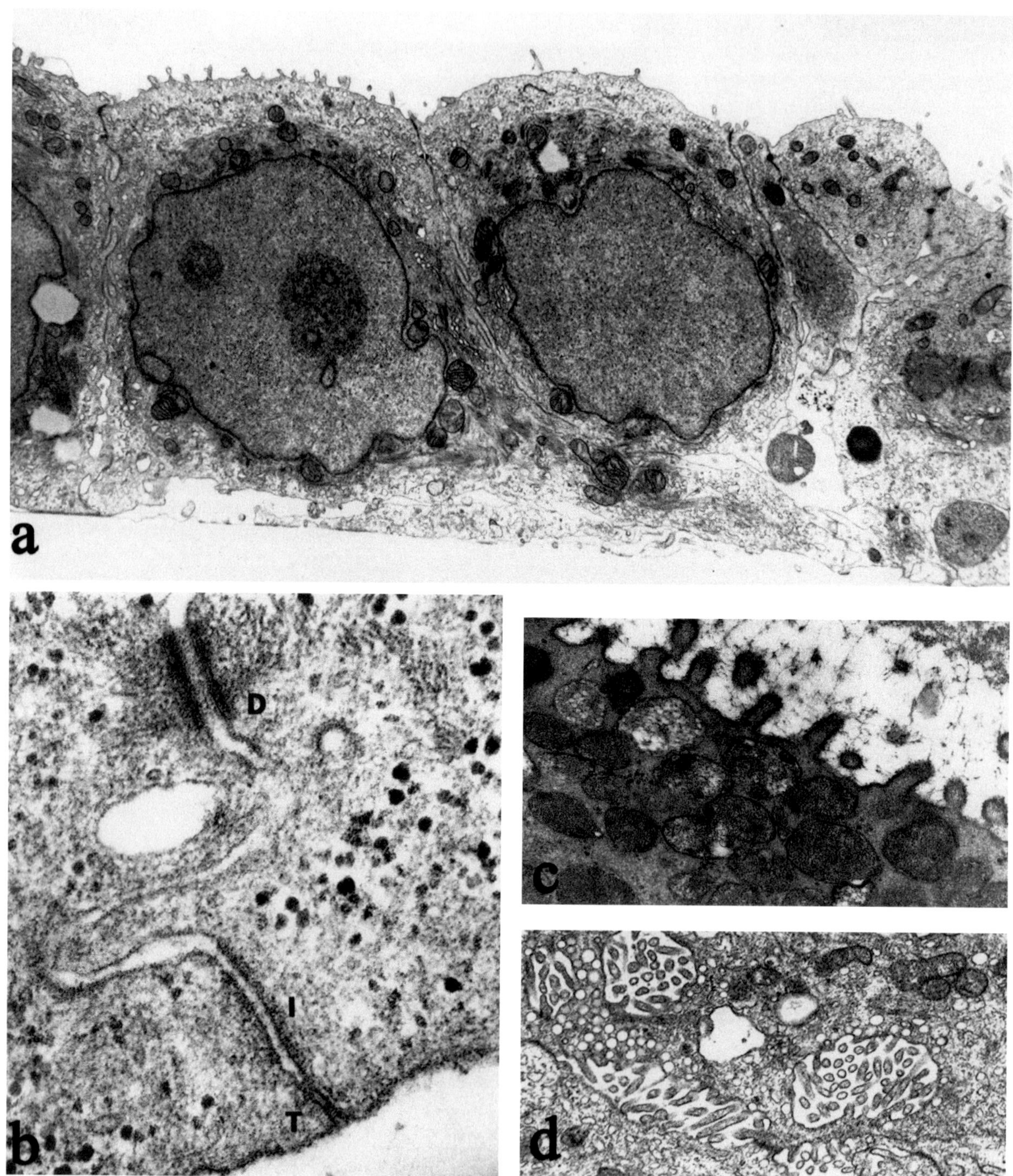
a
D
I
T
b
c
d

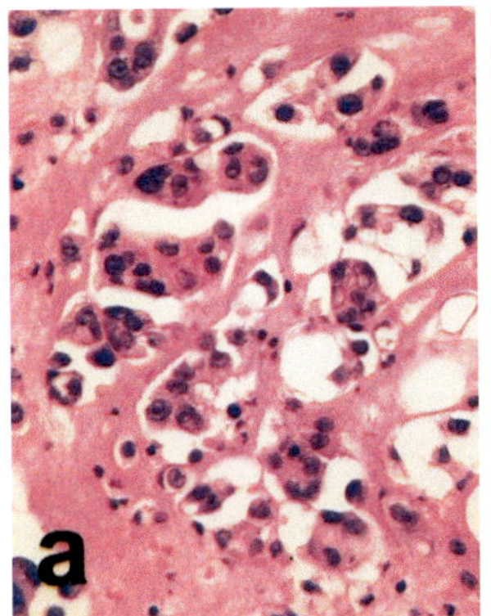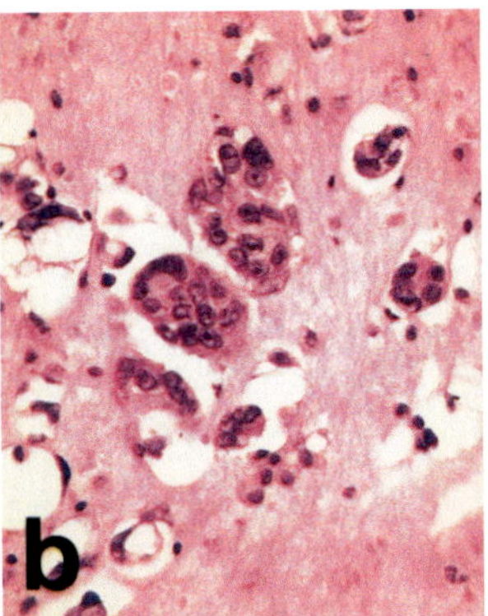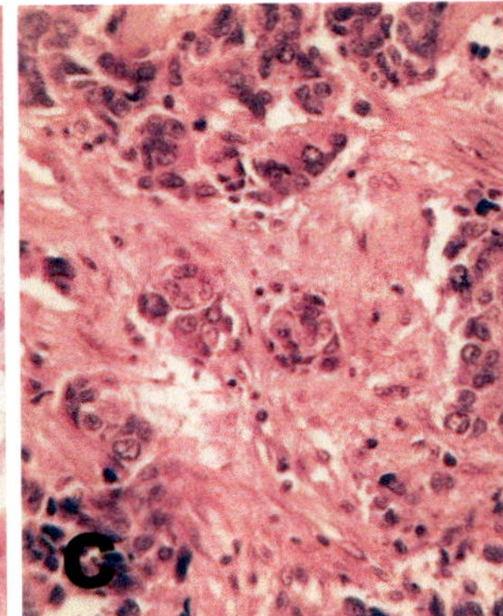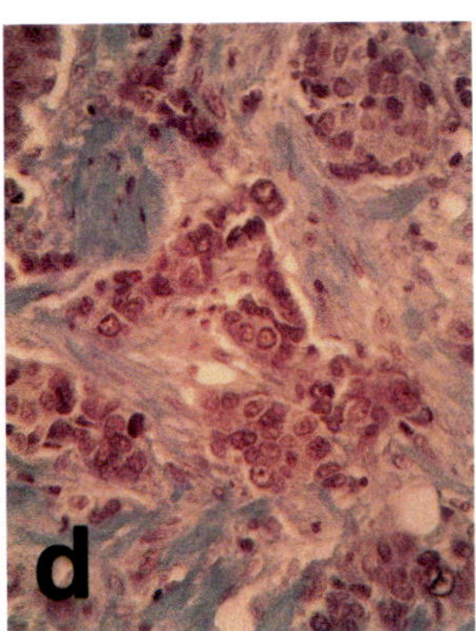

◄ Figure 7.4 a–d

a Transversal section of MCF-7 cell monolayer, ×4,000. **b** Attachment between two cells with a tight junction (*T*); intermediate junctions (*I*) and a desmosome (*D*), ×81,000. **c** Secretory vesicles clustered beneath the plasma membrane, ×60,000. **d** Microvilli on a lumen between cells, ×50,000. All sections were stained with lead citrate and uranyl acetate

Figure 7.5 a–d

a, b Histologic section of pleural effusion clot, and **c** Scirrhous carcinoma that gave rise to the pleural effusion from which MCF-7 were originated (**a, b**). Stained with H&E, ×20. **d** Same as **c** but stained with Masson's trichrome for emphasizing the stromal component, ×20

lamella is lacking in flask and collagen-coated sponge cultures of MCF-7 [20].

MCF-7 cells have a secretory potential, although it is largely inactive and unregulated. Typical indications of secretory activity are the aggregation of a few vesicles and granules just beneath the plasma membrane at the free surface and a concomitant moderate elaboration of endoplasmic reticulum and Golgi apparatus. However, a few cells bore large accumulations of membrane bound material filling the distal part of the cytoplasm, with similar structures were appearing outside the plasma membrane. Thus, in any given culture, the level of secretory activity varies from cell to cell. In this feature, MCF-7 resembles mammary malignancies and certain dysplasias previously described [18, 21] more closely than normal breast [18, 22–24]. MCF-7 is a cell line with certain ultrastructural characteristics, which allow it to be distinguished from other human breast cell cultures [17, 22, 25, 26]. It is also morphologically distinct from mammary cultures of other species [27, 28].

7.3.2 Growth of MCF-7 Cells in Tridimensional Matrix

Various in vitro methods have been used to determine and characterize the malignant potential of tumor cells [29–35]. MCF 7 cells cultured in semisolid media, like agar methocel, formed colonies and when seeded in a collagen matrix they formed ball structures or solid masses of cells (Fig. 7.2d, Table 7.3) indistinguishable of those formed by primary breast cancer cells in vitro. Another method used for testing the growth properties of breast cancer cells has been their cultivation in collagen-coated cellulose sponges, providing an excellent technique for the study of the three-dimensional expression of tumor morphology and for the investigations of its cellular interrelations. This system has been used in the study of various cells including HeLa, rodent ascites hepatoma, and explants of chick embryonic heart and liver [35]. Different tumors have been tested by the same method, including a mouse mammary carcinoma, a human cervical squamous cell carcinoma, and a human

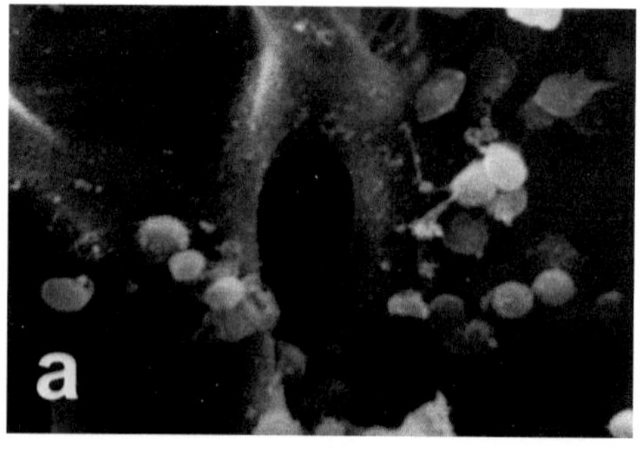

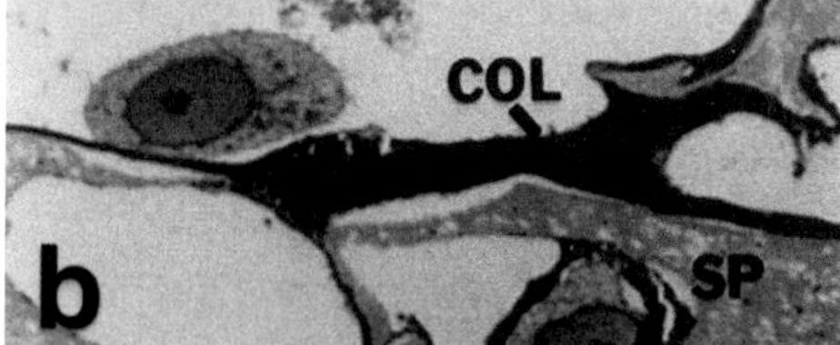
COL
SP
b

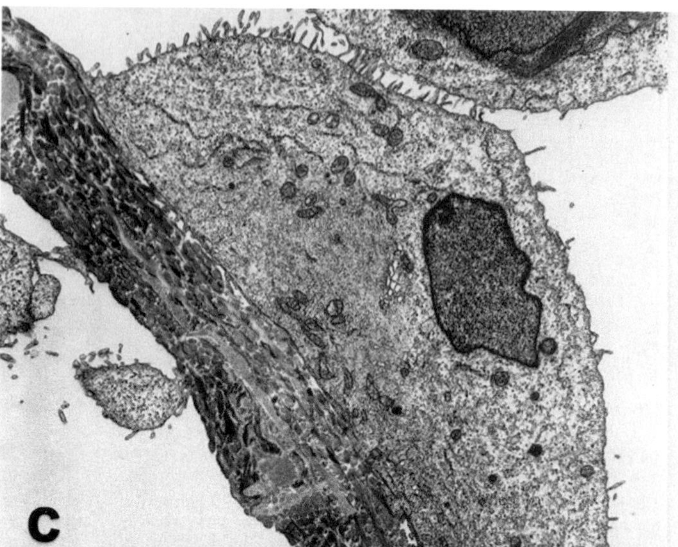
c

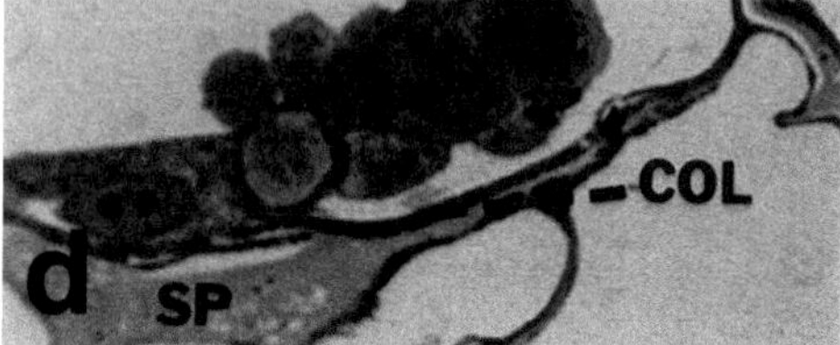
COL
SP
d

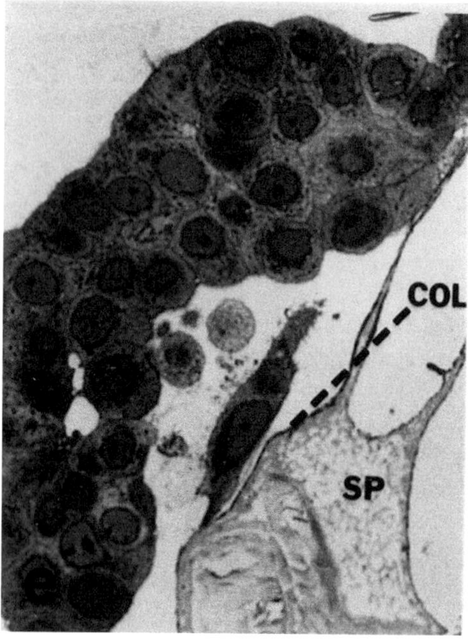
COL
SP
e

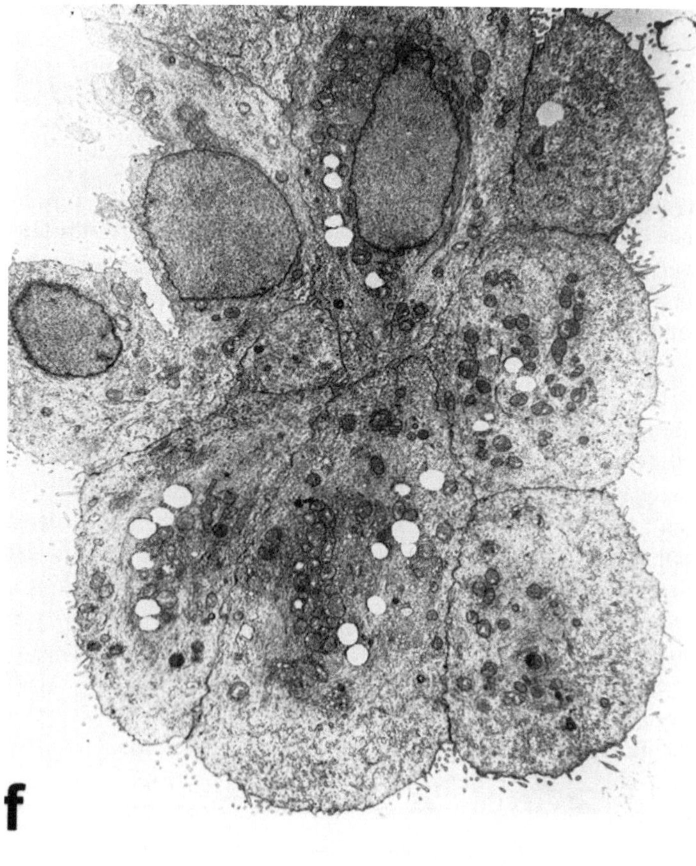
f

a Scanning electron micrograph of MCF-7 cells attached to the collagen coated sponge, ×400. **b** A single MCF-7 cell attached to the collagen (*COL*). *SP* sponge (toluidine blue, ×600). **c** A single cell attached to the collagen coated cellulose sponge, ×4,000. **d** Small cluster of MCF-7 cells partially attached to the collagen coat (*COL*). *SP* sponge (toluidine blue, ×600. **e** Large cluster of MCF-7 cells protruding intro the sponge (*SP*) cavity. The collagen (*COL*) is seen as a thin, darkly stained layer (toluidine blue, ×600). **f** A vertical section through a cluster of cells similar to that described in **e**, ×2,000 (panels **b–f** were reproduced from: Russo, J., Bradley, R.H., McGrath, C.M. and Russo, I.H. Scanning and transmission electron microscopy study of a human breast carcinoma cell line (MCF-7) cultured in collagen-coated cellulose sponge. Cancer Res. 35:2004–2014, 1977, with permission)

colon adenocarcinoma [36, 37]; in these studies, the explants grew and reproduced the organized structure of the original tumor. The morphologic pattern exhibited by the MCF-7 cells grown in the collagen-coated cellulose sponge was similar to the histologic pattern found in both the antecedent primary tumor and the pleural metastasis from which this cell line was derived (Fig. 7.5). The primary breast tumor was a scirrhous carcinoma presenting islands of atypical epithelial cells with large nuclei, prominent nucleoli, and mitoses (Fig. 7.5). In some areas, the cells were fairly close, forming clusters of 6–10 cells per level of section separated by connective tissue (Fig. 7.5b). In other areas, the clusters were larger and showed pseudolumina, which were formed by necrosis of the central cells and determined the formation of duct-like structures. Pyknotic cells and cell detritus were also observed in the interior of these formations. The metastatic cells obtained from the pleural effusion material were arranged in clusters and duct-like structures. Isolated cells were trapped in the fibrin clot, together with erythrocytes, granulocytes, and lymphocytes. The number of cells in a cluster varied from 2 to 50 per level of section. Some clusters showed a lumen-like structure (left by degenerated cells), and in some instances, nuclear pyknosis was observed (Fig. 7.5). The duct-like structure appeared

layered with cuboidal or flat, epithelial cells. The lumen contained cell debris and liquid compressing one pole of the cell. All the cells showed moderate atypia. Mitoses and pyknotic cells were frequently observed in the clusters and duct-like structures. The cells cultured in the collagen-coated sponge did not grow in monolayers, but formed clusters and acinar structures with the same pattern observed in the primary tumor and the material from the pleural effusion described above (Fig. 7.6). The cells formed large clusters with more than 100 cells per level of section (Fig. 7.6). The clusters protruded into the sponge interstices as an organoid structure that remained attached to the collagen coat by only a few cells. Like the original tumor, the clusters formed lumen-like structures via a degeneration of the central cells of the mass (Figs. 7.6, 7.7); liquid and cell detritus accumulated in the lumina. Lumen formation was at random; some large clusters did not show lumen, whereas others formed lumen eccentrically. Electron microscopic observations revealed that the cells surrounding a lumen in its early formation did not possess microvilli, but appeared in later development and were oriented toward the lumen [12, 38]. The cells grown on sponge presented the same moderate degree of atypia seen in the tumor from which they were derived, but they presented more mitotic figures and fewer pyknotic cells. Similar structure was observed in free-floating cells recovered from the culture medium (cells which apparently became detached from the collagen coating) (Figs. 7.6, 7.7). The collagen coat was easily seen when stained with Masson's trichrome or toluidine blue (Fig. 7.5). In some clusters attached to the sponge, the collagen coat was not well defined. The morphogenic memory of these cells is unaltered by long passage in vitro. This had previously been demonstrated for mouse mammary carcinoma cells [39].

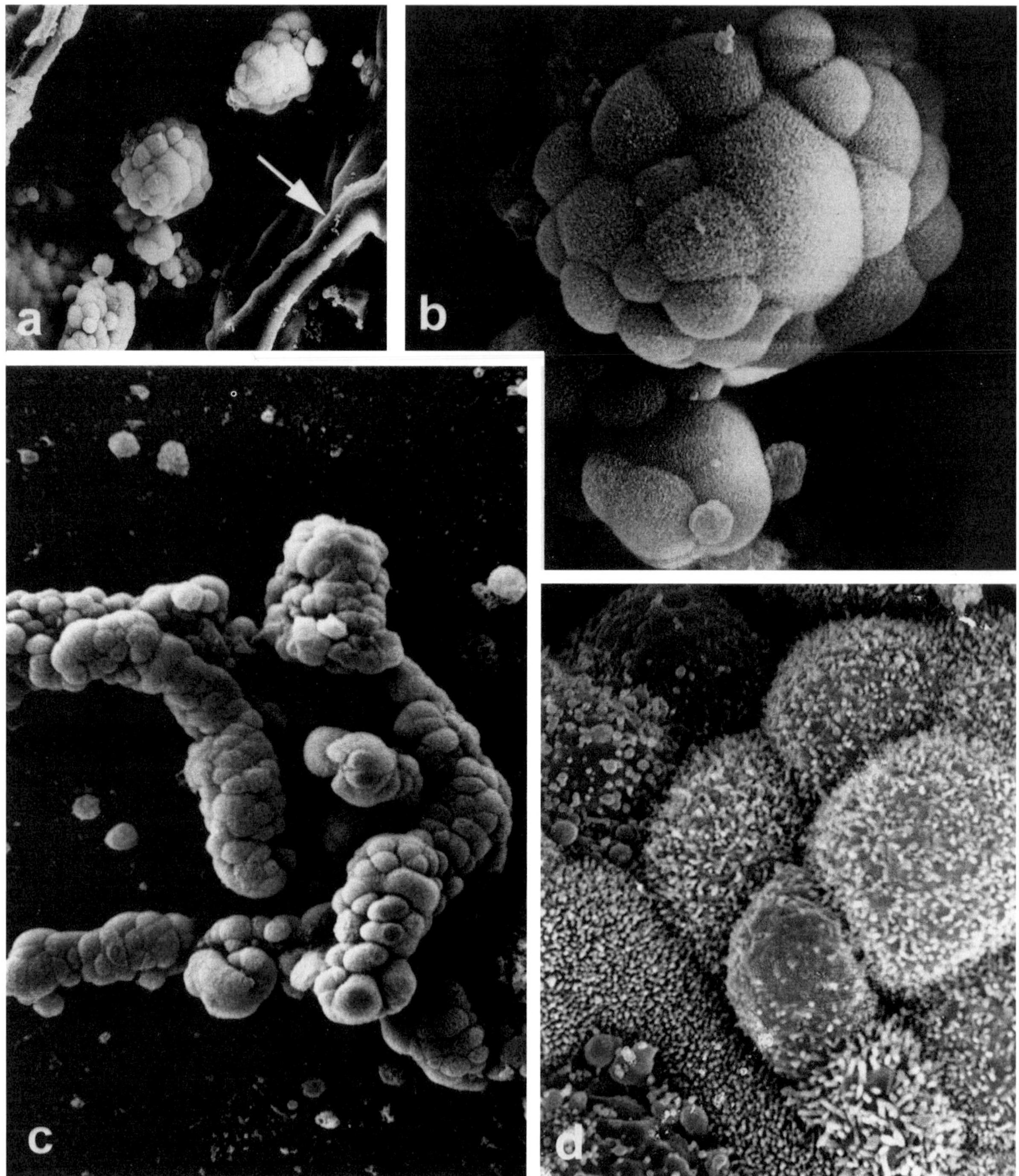

a Scanning electron microscopy of a collagen coated sponge (*arrow*) and clusters of MCF-7 cells rising above the monolayer (*left*), × 400. **b** Larger magnification of a cluster shown in **a**, × 3,500. **c** Scanning electron microscopy of cells recovered from the supernatant medium by centrifugation on a Millipore filter showing long arrays of densely packed, small round cells, with sharply defined cell limits, × 2,000. **d** Higher magnification of the surface of the cell, shown in **c**, covered by uniform type of microvilli all over the surface, but microvilli differ widely from cell to cell, × 20,000 (panels **b–d** were reproduced from: Russo, J., Bradley, R.H., McGrath, C.M. and Russo, I.H. Scanning and transmission electron microscopy study of a human breast carcinoma cell line (MCF-7) cultured in collagen-coated cellulose sponge. Cancer Res. 35:2004–2014, 1977, with permission)

7.3.3 Growth of MCF-7 Cells in Athymic Mice

An important criterion of malignancy is the ability of transformed cells to grow in an adequate heterotransplantation system [40]. Immunologically depressed athymic mice (*nu/nu*) [41–44] have the striking capability of discriminating between normal and neoplastic cells. Normal cells do not induce tumors [43], whereas malignant cells do. MCF-7 cells, cultured as previously described [12], were removed from the culture vessel by trypsinization, suspended in phosphate buffer saline (PBS) (1×10^6 cells per 0.05 ml) and transplanted in 21-day-old Balb/c (*nu/nu*) mice into the mammary gland fat pad which was cleared according to the method of DeOme [45]. The first experiment summarized in Table 7.4 demonstrated that MCF 7 cells were unable to grow neither in female nor in male athymic mice. The gross examination of the area of cell inoculation and the histological study revealed a complete absence of the inoculated cells; only disorganization of the fat and some fibrosis were observed. Only those mice that have received a transplant of pituitary glands or ovaries from syngenic mice induced the growth of MCF-7 cells (Table 7.4). Nine of the eleven (82%) inoculated female mice that received pituitary grafts developed palpable tumors within 12–18 days after inoculation. The tumors adhered to the skin and underlying muscle. No macroscopic metastatic growths were observed. Eight of the thirteen (61.5%) inoculated female mice that received ovary grafts developed palpable tumors within 12–18 days. Tumors were attached to the skin and underlying muscles; no metastatic growths were observed. The tumors were small, oblong masses of 1.5–2.5 mm at their largest diameter. They adhered to the dermis of the skin and to the muscle of the abdominal wall. The tumors were firm, of a rubbery consistency, and presented resistance to sectioning. The tumor's vascular bed was well developed. The area of the tumor was easily distinguished from the scar produced by the cauterization and the incision made during the transplant procedure. The histological pattern of the 17 tumors studied was identical. The tumors were composed of nests of cells

Table 7.4. Tumoral growth of human breast cancer cell line (MCF-7) in athymic mice

Group	Sex	Number of animals	Treatment	Number of animals with tumors/animal (%)	Latency (days)
I	Male	11	None	0/11 (0)	–
II	Female	12	None	0/12 (0)	–
III	Female	11	Pituitary isographs[a]	9/11 (82)	12–18
IV	Female	13	Ovary isographs[b]	8/13 (61.5)	12–18
V	Female	15	Estrogen pellets[c]	12/15 (80)	13–14

[a] Two pituitaries obtained from syngenic 60-day-old female mice were grafted in the perirenal fat of each animal
[b] Two ovaries obtained from syngenic 60-day-old female mice were grafted in the perirenal fat of each animal
[c] Each animal was implanted with a Silastic tube containing 5 mg of 17-β-estradiol in the interscapular region

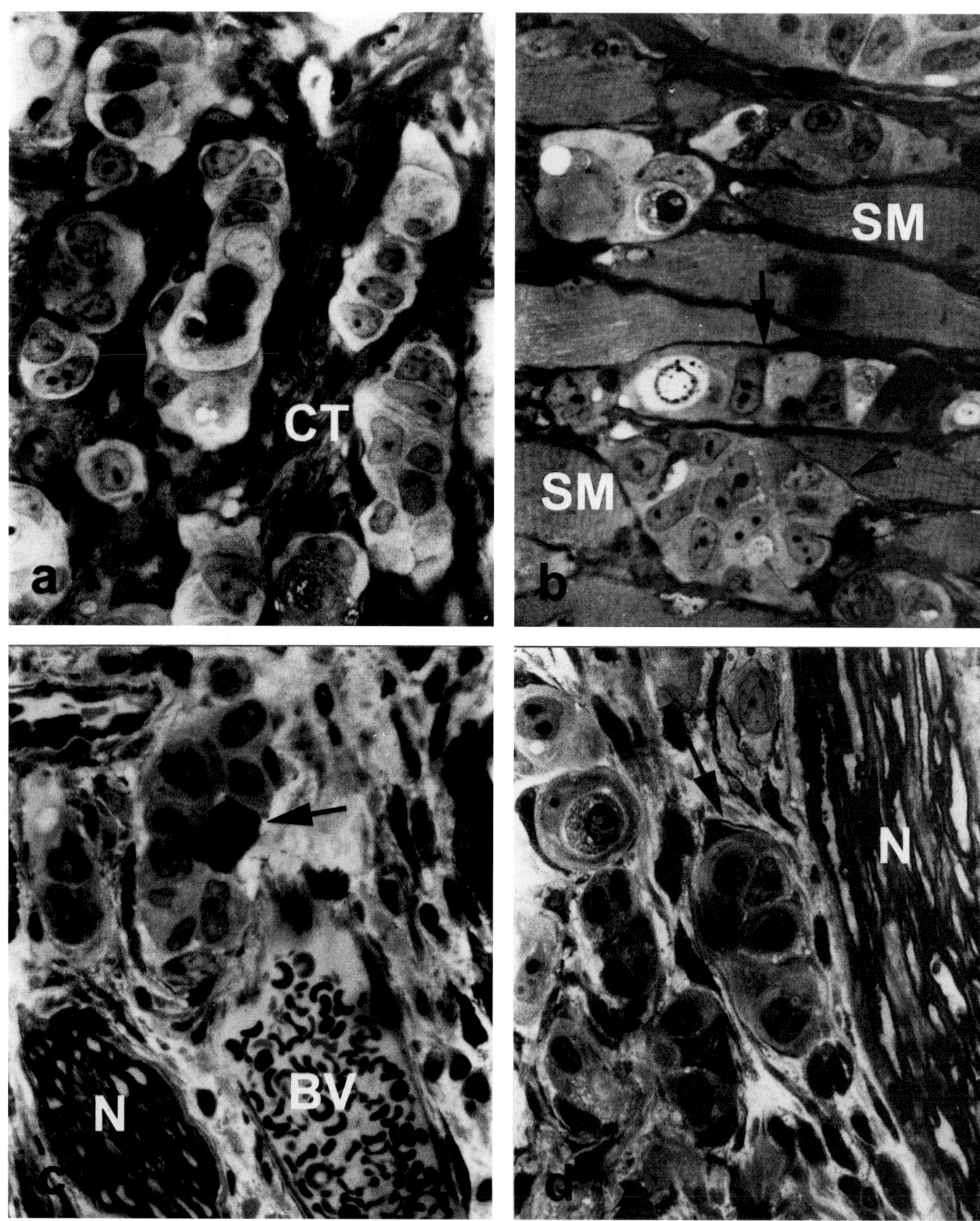
CT
SM
SM
N
BV
N
a
b
c
d

arranged in either clusters or single or double-row strands (Figs. 7.8, 7.9). The inoculated epithelial cells were surrounded by a dense stroma formed by collagen fibers and fibroblasts. Blood vessels were scarce in the central portion of the tumor and more abundant in the periphery and in areas of invasion. The cells presented a considerable degree of pleomorphism and atypia. The nucleus was oval with few indentations. The nucleoplasm was pale, and a thin layer of heterochromatin was observed on the inner side of the nuclear envelope. More than two nucleoli per nucleus were frequently observed (Figs. 7.8, 7.9). Intracellular lumina with cellular detritus within were present in some cells (Fig. 7.9). When stained with toluidine blue, the cytoplasm of most cells appeared strongly basophilic. A few cells with pale cytoplasm were also observed (Fig. 7.8). Similar epithelial cells were also observed in the dermis of the skin overlying the inoculation site and among muscular fibers of

the abdominal wall. The intense fibrous reaction observed at the inoculation site and in the dermis was not observed around cells invading skeletal muscle (Fig. 7.8). Mitoses were frequently observed in areas of invasion. No metastases were found in any of the tissues studied; however, clusters of cells attached to the adventitia of blood vessels or adjacent to the perineurium were observed in the periphery of the tumor. Invasion of blood vessels or nerves by neoplastic cells was not observed in serial sections. The tumors observed in mice isografted with pituitary glands or ovaries were indistinguishable.

The successful heterotransplantation of human tumors [44, 46] and cultured human malignant cells [41, 42] into nude mice has proven to be an excellent model for the study of neoplastic tissue and an effective diagnostic tool for differentiating malignant from benign cells [43]. The growth of MCF-7 cells as tumors in nude mice might be predicted by the malignant nature of the tumor of origin and by the demonstration of several transformation markers (Table 7.5). However, MCF-7 cells did not form tumors in all inoculated mice but only in those receiving pituitary or ovarian grafts, thus suggesting a hormone dependency for in vivo growth. The fact that more tumors were observed in mice receiving pituitary grafts (82%) than in those receiving ovarian grafts (61.5%) suggested that some pituitary hormone could be involved in the development of these tumors. The inoculation of MCF-7 cells into nude mice induces tumors morphologically similar to the

Table 7.5. Tumorigenic response of HBEC in nude mice. *NT* not tested

Specimen	Passage	Days in vitro	Growth in methocel	Chromosome pattern	Site of implantation[a]	Number of animals inoculated	Number of animals with tumors
MCF-7	185–189	1,650	+	Aneuploid 60–80	Fat pad	16	12
HBEC-#130	33–45	1,030	–	46	Fat pad	10	0
Primary breast cancer cells (tumor #5)	2–3	44	NT	46	Fat pad	6	3

[a] 1×10^7 cells in 0.2 ml of PBS were inoculated in the mammary fat pad of castrated nude male mice supplemented with Silastic implant containing 5 mg of 17-β-estradiol

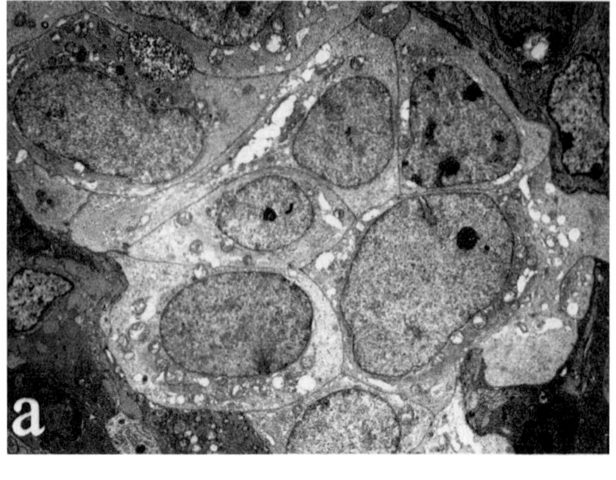
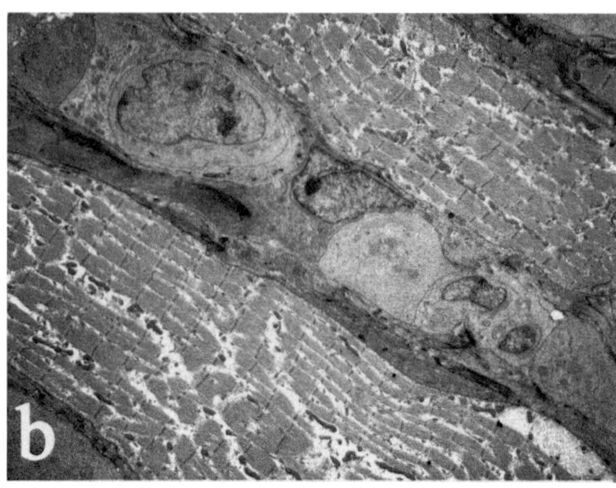
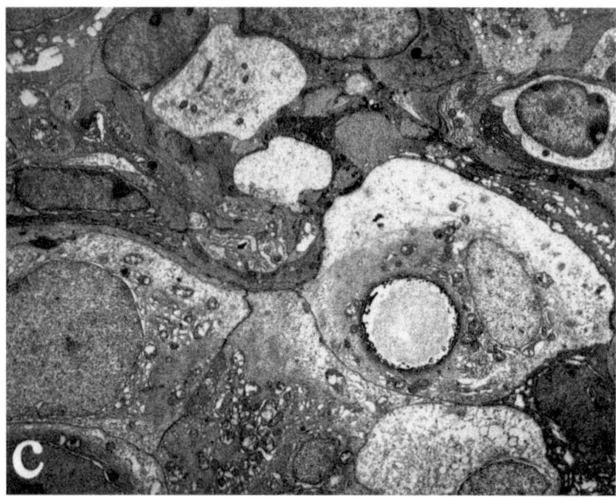
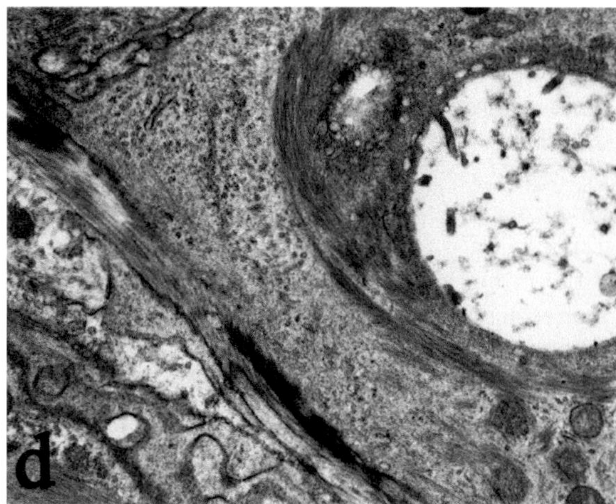
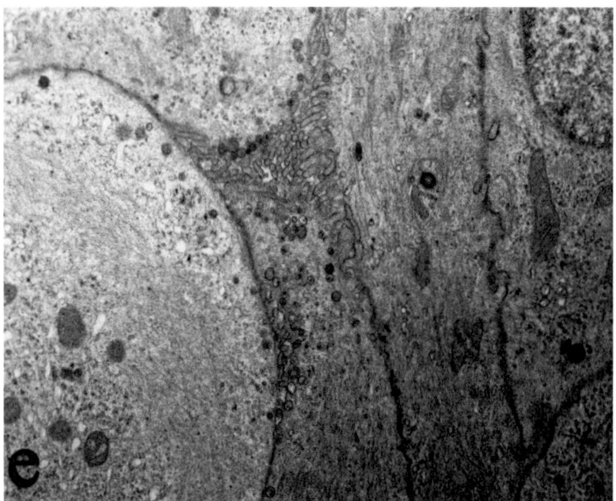
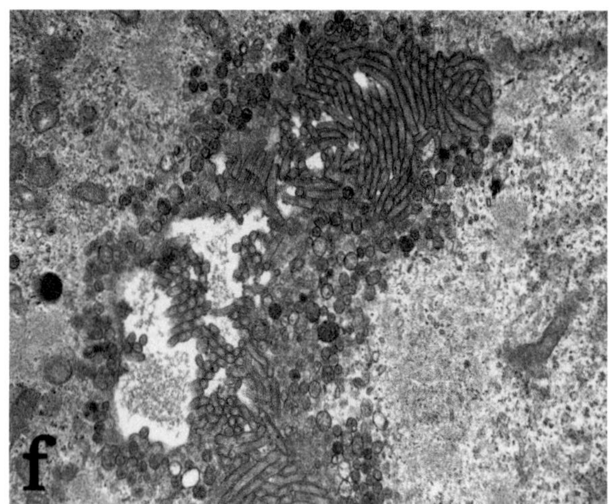

Figure 7.9 a–f

Electron micrographs of a tumor induced by heterotransplantation of MCF-7 cells in athymic mice. **a** Cluster of MCF-cells, ×2,000. **b** Strands and clusters of MCF-7 cells among muscle fibers, ×2,000. **c** Cluster of MCF 7 cells showing the formation if intracellular lumen surrounded by short microvilli, ×2,000. **d** Intracellular lumen surrounded by numerous tonofilaments, ×4,000. **e** Intercellular spaces forming small lumina surrounded by numerous microvilli, ×2,000. **f** Detail of an intercellular spaces and microvilli surrounding the lumen, ×4,000

tumor of origin. This property of malignant cells has been described for other cell lines maintained for almost 100 passages in vitro [43] and transplanted into nude mice, and for human tumors transplanted into the anterior chamber of the guinea pig eye [47]. MCF-7 cells develop a histological pattern in the nude mice similar to that observed in the tumor of origin. The tumor of origin was an infiltrative ductal carcinoma with productive fibrosis (commonly called scirrhous carcinoma). This same pattern of epithelial cells surrounded by a dense stroma is observed in the mouse, suggesting that it is the neoplastic epithelial cell that elicits a stromal response in the host. This observation was also supported by results obtained in an experimental model developed for the study of scirrhous carcinoma [48].

The absence of tumors in untreated animals could be explained by an inadequate hormonal milieu for the growth of MCF-7 cells. The fact that the original tumor from which MCF-7 cells were derived was responsive to hormones and that MCF-7 cells still retain specific high-affinity estradiol and progesterone receptors after more than 160 passages in culture, supports this explanation. The utilization of hormonal supplementation in the growth of MCF-7 cells in 1976 [14], suggested the replacing the isografts by hormone pellets [49]. We found out that the use of castrated male, estrogen supplemented, was also suitable for the growth of MCF 7 cells (Table 7.4). The removal of the uterus and supplementation with estradiol either as pellets or Silastic tube containing 5 mg of 17-β-estradiol in female mice is also a standard

procedure (Table 7.5). The removal of the uterus avoids the swelling and accumulation of fluid in this organ due to the estrogenic stimulation.

7.4 Growth Properties of Immortal Human Breast Epithelial Cells In Vitro

Induction of immortality or immortalization involves abrogation of cellular programs for limiting the rate and the number of cell replications and is generally perceived as the key event of an oncogenic process. The spontaneous immortalization of HBEC is a rarely occurring event. Numerous investigators have tried to induce immortalization of HBEC using various physical, chemical, and biological approaches, such as radiation, benzo(a)pyrene, viruses, and gene transfer, respectively. The most consistent approach has been the biological one. Human papilloma virus 16 (HPV-16), the oncogenes E6 and/or E7 [50, 51], and the simian virus 40 (SV40) [52] have successfully induced immortalization of HBEC. Interestingly, HBEC immortalized with viral oncogenes often express phenotypes indicative of neoplastic transformation, such as increase in anchorage-independent growth and tumorigenesis in nude mice, even though these viruses have not been linked with the origin of human breast cancer. Therefore a normal HBEC without expressing any transformed phenotypes is essential to any studies on experimentally induced transformation. We have reported that a mortal human breast cell, Sample #130, derived from a subcutaneous mastectomy specimen of a 36-year-old woman with no family history of breast cancer acquired the immortal phenotype in vitro [5, 53]. The breast was composed of lobule type 2 [54] and was free of neoplasia, exhibiting only stromal fibrosis, cystic changes and ductal hyperplasia without atypia. Original explants of the tissue, maintained for over a year, exhibited a normal diploid chromosomal pattern [53]. MCF-10F cells, which exhibited immortality after extended cultivation in low calcium medium [5, 53], retained the characteristics of the normal breast epithelium, such as lack of tumorigenicity in nude mice, three-dimensional growth in collagen, hormone and growth factor dependency for in vitro

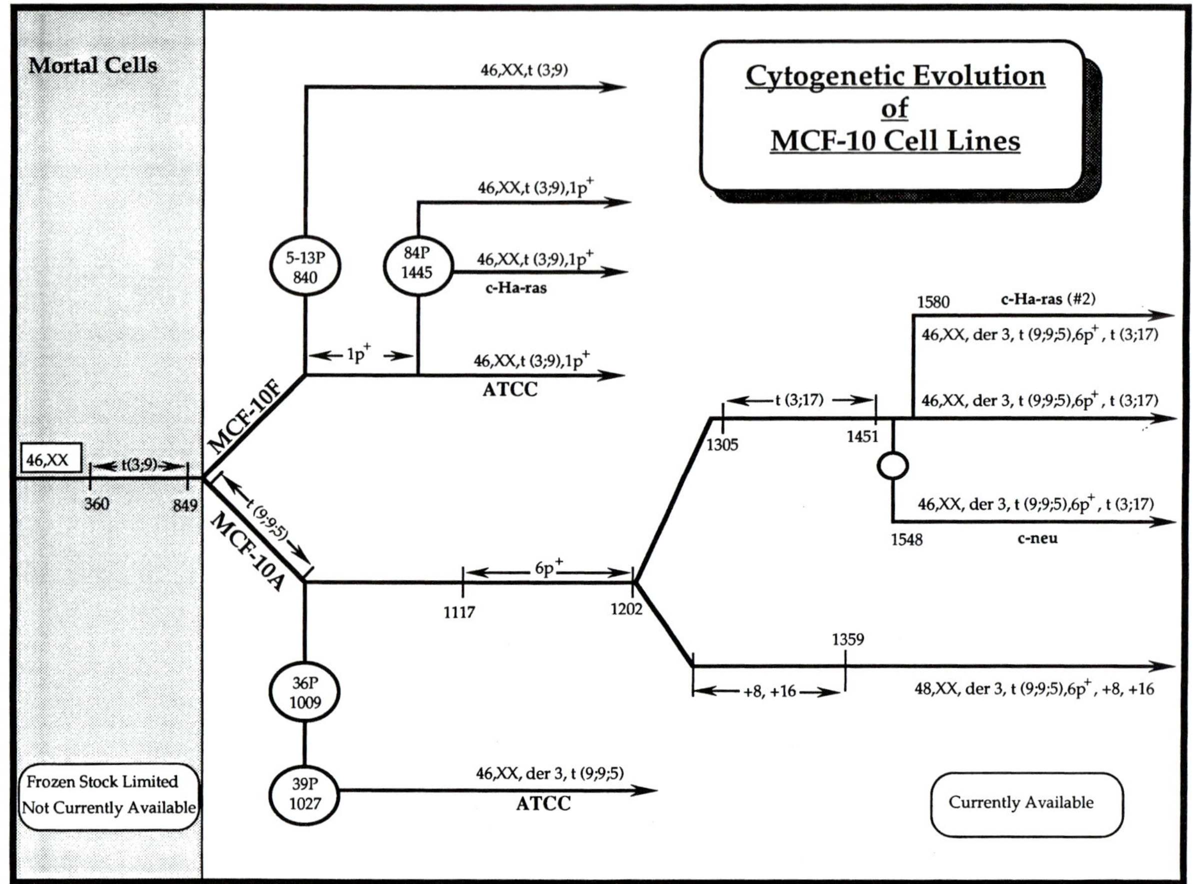

Figure 7.10

Cytogenetic evolution of MCF-10 cells. Diagram drawn by James Elliott and Jose Russo

growth, lack of anchorage-independent growth and dome formation in confluent cultures (Fig. 7.10) [5, 21]. Immortalization of these cells was characterized by their continuous growth in culture medium containing either low Ca++ or the conventional level of Ca++ (1.05 mM) without entering senescence, and without expressing phenotypes indicative of neoplastic transformation, such as colony formation in agar or in agar-methocel. MCF-10F cells are bona fide normal HBEC in nature, expressing genetic, cytogenetic, ultrastructural and phenotypic characteristics of normal human breast epithelium, representing the cell line closest to a normal HBEC available. The phenotype of MCF-10F cells has been maintained stable for more than 118 passages in vitro (Fig. 7.10). Several mechanisms are considered to play a role in cell immortalization. Among them are the activation of telomerase, abrogation of cell cycle control, and activation of specific genes.

Table 7.6. Comparison of the sequence of p53 exon 7 in MCF-10 M and MCF-10F cells (reprinted with permission from: Barnabas, N.; Moraes, R., Calaf, G., Estrada, S. and Russo, J. Role of p53 in MCF-10F cell immortalization and chemically induced neoplastic transformation. Int. J. of Oncology 7:1289–1296, 1995)

Codon number	253	254	255	256	257	258	259	260	261	262	263
MCF-10M[a]											
– Antisense	TGG	TAG	TAG	TGT	GAC	CTT	CTG	AGG	TCC	agt	cct
– Sense	ACC	ATG	ATG	ACA	CTG	GAA	GAC	TCC	AGG	tca	gga
– Amino acid	Thr	Ileu	Ileu	Thr	Leu	Glu	Asp	Ser	Ser		
MCF-10F[b]											
– Antisense	TGG	TTA	GTA	GTG	TGA	CCT	TCT	GAG	GTC	CAG	TCC
– Sense	ACC	AAT	CAT	CAC	ACT	GGA	AGA	CTC	CAG	GTC	AGG
– Amino acid	Thr	Asn	His	His	Thr	Gly	Arg	Leu	Gln	Val	Arg

[a] MCF-10M cells exhibit the wild-type sequence as reported by Buchman et al (Gene 70:245,1988)
[b] MCF-10F cells show a frame shift mutation by the insertion of a base at codon 254

7.4.1 Telomerase Activation

There is evidence that the repetitive TTAGGG sequences located at the ends of human chromosomes (i.e., telomeres) may act as a molecular mitotic clock [55]. It is generally believed that each successive genomic replication is accompanied by gradual shortening of 50–200 bp due to incomplete replication of the 3' ends and cellular senescence occurs when telomeres reach a critically-short length that replication of the genome can not be maintained [56]. The stabilization of the telomeric sequences at the ends of chromosomes, which is required for the continuous proliferation of immortal cells, involves the activation of the enzyme telomerase, which adds TTAGGG repeats to the 3' ends of chromosomes [57, 58]. The genetic nature of cellular senescence implicates activation of telomerase as a key element of cell immortalization [58, 59]. Elevated levels of telomerase activities have been detected in a number of immortal cell lines and human tumor tissues [60, 61]. We have observed telomerase activity in immortal MCF-10F, but not in the mortal MCF-10 M cells [62] (see Chapter 8), suggesting that telomerase activation may play a role in the spontaneous immortalization of MCF-10F cells.

7.4.2 Abrogation of Cell Cycle Control

Cell fusion studies indicate that the phenotype of cellular senescence is dominant and immortality results from recessive changes in normal regulatory genes. Conceivably, inactivation of the genes that restrict cell cycle progression is essential to cell immortalization. Cyclin-dependent kinase (CDK) complexes and their inhibitors are essential components of the cell cycle machinery, controlling cell cycle arrest in the G_1 phase of the cycle. Since p53 acts to regulate cell cycle progression through transcriptional activation of p21$^{\text{WAF-1}}$, an inhibitor of all G_1 CDKs, abrogation of p53 function has been implicated in the immortalization of HBEC. Insertional mutation in exon 7 of the p53 gene has been implicated in the spontaneous immortalization of MCF-10F cells (Table 7.6) [63], a postulate supported by the observation of the spontaneous immortalization of breast cells from a Li-Fraumeni patient that carried a point mutation in the p53 gene [64]. However, the immortalized MCF-10F cells are still able to produce the wild-type p53 protein [65] and maintain wild-type p53-mediated functional responses, such as expression of p21$^{\text{WAF-1}}$ and mdm2 [66]. Furthermore, the introduction of a single-amino acid deletion mutant (del239) of p53 gene abrogates wild-type p53-mediated cellular responses and induces immortalization of HBEC. A recent study indicates that alterations in p53 appear to be

Table 7.7. Phenotypic profile of normal, immortalized and neoplastic HBEC in vitro

Cell type number/ chromosome pattern	Passage	Days in vitro	Growth in agar	Growth in collagen	Tumorigenesis in SCID mice
MCF-10M/diploid	22–29	1,030	(–)	(+) (ductal)	0/10
MCF-10F/diploid t(3:9)	130	>2,000	(–)	(+) (ductal)	0/10
MCF-7/aneuploid (60–80)	>89	>1,650	(++)	(+) (ball)	12/16

important in overcoming the M1 blockade [66]. However, the introduction of seven missense mutants of p53 genes failed to induce immortalization in the same cell line, even though all of these p53 mutants have been shown to abrogate p53-mediated transactivation in other cell types [67]. Therefore, the role of p53 in immortalization of HBEC needs further evaluation.

The CDK-4 inhibitor (CDKN2), commonly referred to as p16, is also an inhibitor of the cell cycle and has been localized to 9p21–22. Homozygous deletion of this chromosomal subregion has been observed in the immortalized MCF-10F cells, which contain a balanced reciprocal translocation, t(3;9) (3p13;9p22) [53]. Similarly, loss of the 9p21 subregion has been correlated with the acquisition of an immortal phenotype of neoplastic human head and neck keratinocyte cell lines.

It is currently accepted that transition between different cell cycle states are regulated at checkpoints; cell cycle checkpoints are regulated by a highly conserved family of protein kinases, the cyclin-dependent kinases (cdks), and their activating partners, the cyclins. The D-type cyclins bind to several different cdks, one of their main partners being cdk4 [68], and drive the cells into mid/late GI-phase; an almost immediate consequence is the activation of cyclin E: cdk2 complexes, which carry the cell forward to the end of the GI-phase. Cyclin A: cdk2 activity increases in concert with entrance into S-phase and likely triggers the GI/S transition; as the cells move through S-phase, cyclin A switches partners and affiliates increasingly with CDC2 [69]. The connections between the D-type cyclins and tumorigenesis are strengthened by the evidence that these cyclins are essential

for cell cycle regulation of the retinoblastoma tumor suppressor protein (Rb). It has been proposed that the exclusive role of cyclin DI is to inactivate Rb so that cells can enter S-phase and replicate their DNA [70]. E-type cyclins, on the other hand, are thought to act after D-type cyclins at the GI/S transition and in the initiation of DNA replication; cyclin E deregulation might also contribute to transformation [71]. Although a mutant cyclin A, lacking the cyclin destruction box, was one of the first cyclins to be implicated in transformation [72], the mechanism of this event is not yet known. Most studies on the control of animal cell proliferation have been performed in model systems in vitro, in which cell proliferation can be modulated in a controlled fashion. In studying the process of cell immortalization we have compared critical components of the ell cycle regulatory proteins in the mortal cells derived from Sample #130 (MCF10 M) (Table 7.3), that originates the MCF10F cell line (Fig. 7.10) with the tumor cell line MCF-7. The phenotypic profile of the mortal MCF-10 M cells, the immortal non-tumorigenic MCF-I0F cell line, and the breast cancer cell line MCF-7 is shown in Table 7.7. MCF-7 cells were aneuploid and formed colonies in semi-solid medium, while MCF-10 M and MCF-10F cells were both diploid and did not form colonies. MCF-10 M and MCF-10F cells grew in a similar fashion when plated in collagen gel. They formed three-dimensional tubular structures 3 weeks post-plating. MCF-7 cells, on the other hand, did not show evidence of organization, remaining as isolated cells or forming balls. The differences observed in the in vitro growth characteristics correlated with the in vivo properties of the three HBEC lines analyzed. The tumorigenic assay was negative for MCF-10 M and

Figure 7.11 ▶

The *left panels* show the quantitation of the Western blot shown in the *right panels* for each of the protein studied. Modified from: Salicioni, A.M., Russo, I.H. and Russo, J. Correlation between cell cycle regulators and the immortalization and transformation of human breast epithelial cell lines. Int. J. of Oncology, 13:65–71, 1998, with permission

MCF-IOF cells, while MCF-7 cells induced mammary tumors in 75 % of the SCID mice injected. The protein expression of HBECs cell cycle regulators in vitro correlates with their tumorigenic properties in vivo (Table 7.7). The tumorigenic potential of HBECs can be related to the level of cell cycle regulators as well as protein expression of the early-genes (Fig. 7.11). The presence and differential expression of cyclin E- and cyclin A-related proteins and their putative relevance in the tumorigenic properties of HBECs. A direct connection between cell cycle and cancer has been evident for some time. There is very high level of cyclin D1 protein expression in the breast carcinoma cell line MCF-7 in comparison with the normal or immortal non-tumorigenic HBECs studied; this increase was correlated with the loss of ductulogenic capabilities of HBEC in semisolid media, forming ball-like structures in vitro, and the tumorigenicity in SCID mice in vivo (Fig. 7.11). Cyclin D1 is encoded by the *CCDNI gene* on chromosome llql3, which has been identified as the PRADI proto-oncogene. Overexpression of cyclin D1 in MCF-7 cells correlate with the reported overexpression of cyclin D1 in breast, gastric and esophageal carcinoma specimens [73] as a result of amplification of the 11q13 region, and in one breast carcinoma cell line due to stabilization of its mRNA [74]. Interestingly, cyclin D3 differences seen in the three cell lines were not parallel to those observed in cyclin D1 (Fig. 7.11), supporting further the possibility that D-type cyclins may not be functionally redundant and may have different roles during G1/S-phase according to the cell type [75]. The fact that cdk4 levels were markedly higher in MCF-7 breast carcinoma cells than in the mortal and the immortal HBEC (Fig. 7.11), in association with overex-

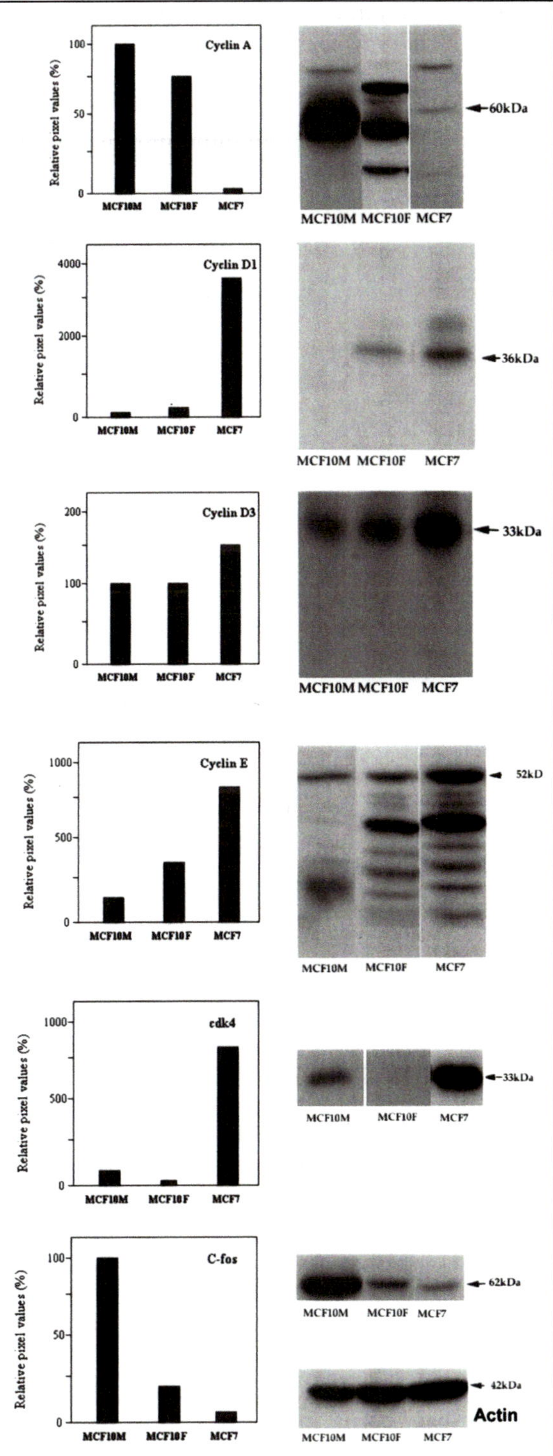

Table 7.8. Cyclin E protein expression in mortal, immortal and neoplastic HBECs in vitro. OD optical density (reprinted with permission from: Salicioni, A.M., Russo, I.H. and Russo, J. Correlation between cell cycle regulators and the immortalization and transformation of human breast epithelial cell lines. Int. J. of Oncology, 13: 65–71, 1998)

Cell type	Cyclin E (50–52 kDa)		Cyclin E (52 kDa)		Cyclin E (~50 kDa)	
	OD	Fold difference[a]	OD	Fold difference[a]	OD	Fold difference[a]
MCF-10M	346	1.0	282	1.0	82	1.0
MCF-10F	1,132	3.3	369	1.3	693	8.4
MCF-7	3,197	8.8	1,087	3.9	1,741	21.2

[a] The protein expression of cyclin E obtained by Western blotting after densitometric analysis. Bands detected at either 50 or 52 kDa were quantified separately; all bands from 50 to 52 kDa were also analyzed. Results are expressed in terms of optical density (OD) in pixels; a fold-difference was calculated relative to OD values obtained in MCF-10 M cells

Table 7.9. Cyclin A protein expression in mortal, immortal and neoplastic HBECs in vitro (reprinted with permission from: Salicioni, A.M., Russo, I.H. and Russo, J. Correlation between cell cycle regulators and the immortalization and transformation of human breast epithelial cell lines. Int. J. of Oncology, 13: 65–71, 1998)

Cell type	Cyclin A (45–70 kDa)		Cyclin A (>60 kDa)	Cyclin A (~60 kDa)		Cyclin A (–45 kDa)
	OD	Fold difference[a]	OD	OD	Fold difference[a]	OD
MCF-10 M	8,179	1.0	(+) (~70 kDa)	7,691	1.0	(–)
MCF-10F	6,194	0.76	2,218 (~65 kDa)	4,698	0.61	139.3
MCF-7	214	0.03	(+) (~70 kDa)	134	0.02	(+)

[a] The protein expression of cyclin A obtained by Western blotting after densitometric analysis. Bands were quantified either together (45–70 kDa), or separately, observed at either >60 kDa, ~60 or ~45 kDa. Results are expressed in terms of OD (optical density) in pixels; a fold-difference was calculated relative to OD values obtained in MCF-10M cells

pression of cyclin D1, may explain the remarkable tumorigenicity of these cells observed in vivo. Both cyclin D1 and estrogens have an essential role in regulating proliferation of breast epithelial cells. There is a clear evidence [76] on the cyclin D1 dependent potentiation of estrogen receptor regulated genes in T47D cancer cells in a cdk-independent fashion. Cyclin D1 was able to activate ER-mediated transcription in the absence of estrogen, due to a direct physical binding to the hormone-binding domain of the ER. Expression of type β of ER has recently been reported in association with the process of immortalization of MCF-10F cells [77]. These observations may explain the high proliferative rate of MCF-10F cells in the absence of ER protein observed in HBEC in vitro [78]. Deregulation of cyclin DI is associated with an ER negative status and high cyclin E [79]. In this context, MCF-10F cells may provide a good predictive in vitro model since the presence of ER type β could be an alternative way that the HBECs utilize for abnormal proliferation.

D-type and E-type of cyclin-cdk complexes appear to regulate different aspects of the G1-phase of the cell cycle. Cyclin E revealed a major band at 52 kDa, which was present in the three HBEC lines; the polyclonal anti-cyclin E antibody also recognized another band –50 kDa, as well as other minor bands (Fig. 7.11). Quantification of all bands together (from 50 to 52 kDa) showed that the level of expression of cyclin E protein was 3-times higher in MCF-10F than in MCF-10 M cells, and showed a 9-fold or 3-fold increase in MCF-7 cells when compared to MCF-10 M or MCF-10F cells, respectively (Fig. 7.11). As seen in Table 7.8, the two major cyclin E-like proteins detected by Western blotting displayed a different degree of expression in the three cells lines analyzed: the significant differences in cyclin E protein expression among the three HBEC lines observed in Fig. 7.11 were mainly due to higher levels of the 50 kDa protein. The breast carcinoma cells MCF-7 showed significantly higher levels of both 52 kDa and 50 kDa cyclin E proteins than MCF-10 M or MCF-10F cells. The involvement of cyclin E in breast cancer has been demonstrated [71, 80], although the nature of this phenomenon is not presently known. There is a clear correlation between increased levels of cyclin E protein expression in the neoplastic HBEC line MCF-7 and its tumorigenicity observed in vivo (Fig. 7.11). Furthermore, these data raise the possibility of alternative splicing variants of cyclin E being involved in the immortalization and transformation of HBECs in agreement with previous observations [81]. The expression of cyclin A, on the other hand, was maximal in MCF-10 M cell line and significantly lower in MCF-10F than in its mortal counterpart MCF-10 M cells; MCF-7 cells showed almost undetectable levels ofcyclin A (Fig. 7.11). Table 7.9 shows cyclin A protein expression when the three major bands detected by Western blotting were quantified together (45–70 kDa) or independently. A major cyclin A-related protein of –60 kDa was detected in the three HBEC lines, whose expression was maximal in MCF-10 M cells and very low in neoplastic cells. In addition to the –60 kDa cyclin A, MCF-10F cells also displayed two cyclin A-related proteins of –65 and 45 kDa, whose expression was significantly higher than in the other HBEC analyzed. MCF-10 M cells showed a minor cyclin A form of –70 kDa, also detected in MCF-7 cells; quantification of these bands was difficult due to its low optical density. As seen in Fig. 7.14, a 45 kDa cyclin A-related protein was also detected in the neoplastic cells; this signal was absent in the mortal HBEC. The existence of novel cyclin A-related proteins in the MCF-10F cell line suggests a possible involvement in the process of immortalization of HBECS. Interestingly, a 56-kDa cyclin A has been de-

scribed in a mouse mammary epithelial cell line after retrovirus-induced overexpression of cyclin DI [82]. In MCF-10F cells, however, the presence of these cyclin A-like proteins was associated with low endogenous levels of cyclin D1 protein. Further studies are required to better understand the biological relevance of cyclin A-related proteins in cell cycle regulation during transformation of HBECS. There is a progressive reduction in cyclin A protein as cyclin A were parallel to increasing levels of cyclin E with the progression from a normal to a neoplastic HBEC phenotype and could be related to the differential regulation of ER-dependent transcription of genes required for the S-phase by these two cyclins [83]. It is also possible that a gradual decrease in the capability of undergoing cyclin A-dependent apoptosis [84] occurs, as HBECs become neoplastic.

An abnormal expression in early-response genes such as *c-fos*, involved in AP-1 transcription factor activity, could be related to the increase in growth advantage seen in HBECs from the normal to a tumorigenic phenotype. Our results show a progressive decrease in c-fos proto-oncoprotein as these HBECs become immortal, and with a further decrease in the malignant MCF-7 cells. In agreement with these observations in vitro, Smith et al. [85] have recently reported that breast cancer cells display a lower AP-1 activity than do normal HBEC. Moreover, we demonstrate here that a low AP-1 activity observed in vitro can be correlated with an increased in vivo tumorigenic ability of HBECs.

Another inhibitor of the cell cycle, prohibitin [86], has been implicated in the process of cell immortalization. Prohibitin gene is localized to chromosome 17q21 where mutations have been reported in certain forms of breast cancer, suggesting that it may be a tumor suppressor gene.

7.4.3 Genes Preferentially Expressed During Cell Immortalization

In furthering the efforts to determine whether specific genes were involved in the process of immortalization, subtractive hybridization and differential display analysis between the immortal MCF-10F cell line and its parental mortal #130 cells using a 10F(+)/130(−) subtractive cDNA library has been performed. Among the 15 clones isolated one contained sequence identical to H-ferritin and another one to a calcium binding protein [87, 88]. The amplification of H-ferritin gene and overexpression of H-ferritin protein have been associated with the progression of human breast cancer. It has been postulated that the up-regulation of H-ferritin may be a source of iron necessary for growth and clonal expansion [87]. Ferritin iron, once released, may increase the level of reactive iron, leading to an increase in oxygen free radical generation, oxidative DNA damage and mutation. The observed increase in the expression of the calcium binding protein S100p [88] in the immortalized cells acquired importance to the light that immortal cells maintained a level of intracellular Ca++ lower than mortal cells [89], suggesting that this protein and/or Ca++ had played an important role in the spontaneous immortalization of MCF-10F cells [4]. This was further demonstrated by showing that S100p is expressed differently in normal, immortal, and neoplastic cells. Interestingly whereas mortal and immortalized cell lines did not form colonies in agar methocel plates, but mammary carcinoma cell lines did form colonies (Fig. 7.12), mortal and immortalized cell lines formed branching ductules, and mammary carcinoma cell lines, formed solid masses characteristic of transformed cells. An important difference between the mortal and the immortal phenotypes was the expression of S100p, which was significantly increased in the immortalized and mammary carcinoma cell lines over that of mortal cell lines. Mortal cell lines showed little to no S100p expression, while immortalized and mammary carcinoma cell lines showed varied expression of S100p (Fig. 7.13). Both agar methocel and collagen matrix assays and measurement of S100p expression via Northern blotting are, together, valuable techniques in assessing cell normality, immortalization, and malignancy. Agar methocel and collagen matrix assays are consistent markers of malignancy. They can distinguish between normal and neoplastic cells, however they cannot differentiate between mortal and immortal cells instead S100p is consistently expressed during spontaneous and induced cell immor-

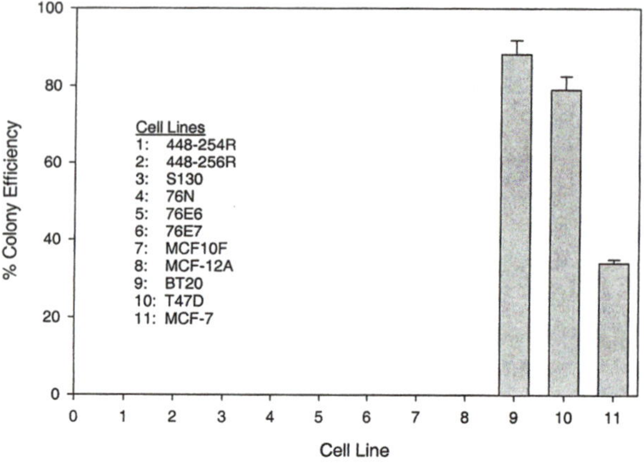

Figure 7.12

Colony efficiencies for cells in agar methocel at 21 days post-plating. Primary, normal, and immortal cell lines do not form colonies in agar methocel whereas neoplastic cell lines do. The data depicted in this figure were presented as an abstract by: Slater, C.M., Lareef, M.H., Russo, I.H., Tomaz, J., Band, V., and Russo, J. S100p is a marker of cell immortalization, preceding phenotypic expression of neoplastic transformation in human breast epithelial cells. Proc. Am. Assoc. Cancer Res. 42:4784a, 2001

Figure 7.13 a, b ▶

S100p and beta-actin Northern blots. a S100p Northern blot. Primary and mortal cell lines showed no S100p expression. Immortal cell lines, 76E6, 76E7, MCF12A, and MCF10F showed 1-, 11-, 50-, and 33-fold increases in S100p expression compared to beta-actin primary cells. Neoplastic cell lines BT20, MCF-7, and T47D showed 16-, 11-, and 0.3-fold increases. b Beta-actin Northern blot used as control. The data depicted in this figure were presented as an abstract by: Slater, C.M., Lareef, M.H., Russo, I.H., Tomaz, J., Band, V., and Russo, J. S100p is a marker of cell immortalization, preceding phenotypic expression of neoplastic transformation in human breast epithelial cells. Proc. Am. Assoc. Cancer Res. 42:4784a, 2001

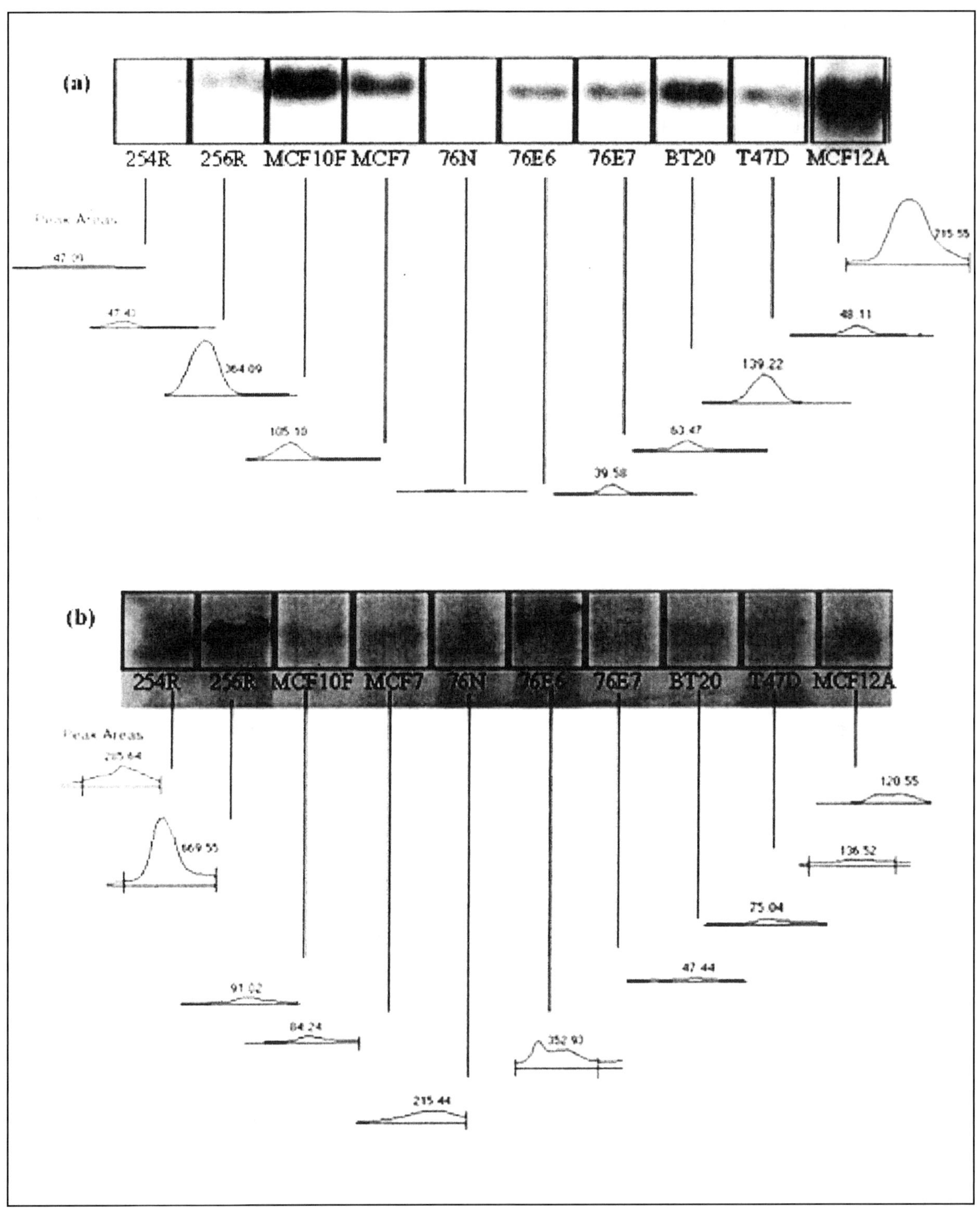
(a)
254R 256R MCF10F MCF7 76N 76E6 76E7 BT20 T47D MCF12A
Peak Areas
47.09
47.40
364.09
105.10
39.58
63.47
139.22
48.11
715.55
(b)
254R 256R MCF10F MCF7 76N 76E6 76E7 BT20 T47D MCF12A
Peak Areas
287.64
669.55
91.02
84.24
215.44
352.93
47.44
75.04
136.52
120.55

talization, but cannot distinguish between immortal and neoplastic cells.

It is conceivable that an increase in the expression of the Ca++-binding protein may facilitate the process of cell immortalization by mobilizing intracellular Ca++ to the medium, thus maintaining a low intracellular concentration that might facilitate cell proliferation. It is plausible that the overexpression of H-ferritin, which might have contributed to the formation of free radicals that are known to be mutagenic, and the overexpression of S100p, that might result in higher cell proliferation, have acted in combination for inducing genomic changes, such as the observed translocation between chromosomes 3 and 9 [53], mutation of the tumor suppressor gene *p53* [65], and microsatellite instability (MSI) of chromosomes 11p13, and 17p [90]. The role played by telomerase activation and its association with the above mentioned changes still needs to be clarified. Nevertheless, those changes described above suggest that more than one event is involved in the induction and maintenance of the immortalized status. Additional studies are needed in order to definitively clarify what is the driving force in the immortalization of epithelial cells in the female breast.

7.5 Transformation of Primary Cultures of Human Breast Epithelial Cells with Chemical Carcinogens

Chemical carcinogens are mutagens in nature, and play a major and probably an etiological role in the initiation of human cancer [2]. Based upon their in vitro transforming potential in rodent cells, a number of environmental agents have been identified as human carcinogens [91, 92]. However, extrapolation of data from experimental carcinogenesis to the human situation has been challenging due to inherent differences between human and experimental animals in susceptibility to chemically-induced neoplastic transformation, resulting in frequent failure in attempts to demonstrate transformation by carcinogenic agents with human cells as targets [93]. Only in a few cases have environmental chemical carcinogens, such as polycyclic hydrocarbons and aromatic

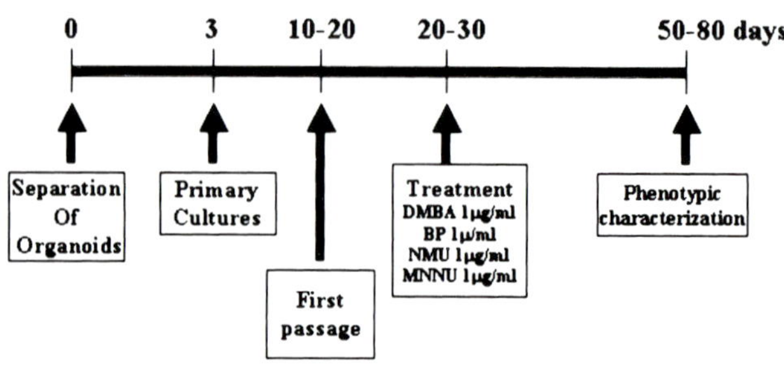

Figure 7.14

Protocol for transformation of human breast epithelial cells with chemical carcinogens

amines, been shown to experimentally induce transformation of human breast epithelial cells (HBEC) in vitro [94–97]. Full induction of malignant phenotypes by chemical carcinogens occurs only in the HBEC that have undergone immortalization [4], a process associated with multiple genetic alterations [4, 98]. As a result, none of the chemical carcinogens has been considered as a serious risk factor for human breast cancer. To date, there is little information concerning the interactions of various risk factors and environmental chemical carcinogens. It remains essentially unknown whether, for example, genetic predisposition influences the response of HBEC to chemical carcinogens. Understanding of the causative agents of breast cancer and mechanisms responsible for carcinogenic progression necessitates establishment of a reliable system to transform human breast epithelial cells in vitro. Primary cultures of HBEC established from women without and with familial history of breast cancer, as evidenced by linkage analysis have been utilized to determine their response to environmental chemical carcinogens [99]. Basically the experimental schedule that has been utilized is depicted in Fig. 7.14. The breast tissue samples have been obtained from reduction mammoplasties from women that when to surgery either by cosmetic reasons or prophylactic mastectomies. The primary cultures were established from outgrowths of organoids following the procedures described previously [96, 97] and treated for 24 h [99] with either

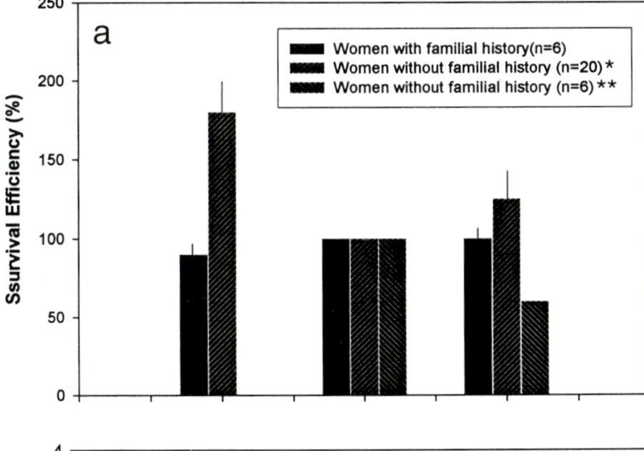

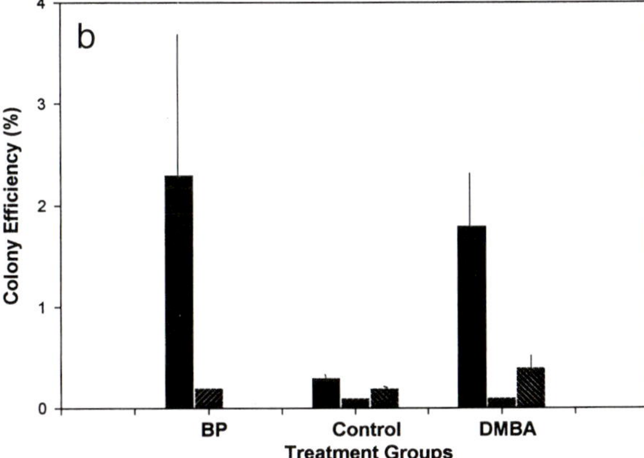

Figure 7.15 a, b

a Survival efficiency and **b** colony efficiency in soft agar of chemical carcinogen-treated HBEC from women with and without familial history of breast cancer (mean ± SD). Survival efficiencies were calculated as percentage of the values of controls for each sample to minimize derivations in responses among samples and to compare with the values of our previous results on carcinogen-treated HBEC from women with no familial history of breast cancer (* from reference [1]; ** from reference [96]); (reprinted with permission from: Hu, Y.F., Russo, I.H., Zalipsky, U., Lynch, H.T and Russo, J. Environmental chemical carcinogens induce transformation of breast epithelial cells from women with familial history of breast cancer. In vitro Cell. Dev. Biol. Volume 33, number 7, pages 495–498, 1997)

0.1 µg/ml benzo(a)pyrene (BP) or 0.1 µg/ml 7,12-dimethylbenz(a)anthracene (DMBA). The effect of carcinogens was evaluated by measuring anchorage-independent growth (i.e., survival efficiency and colony efficiency) in agar methocel. As compared to the DMSO-treated controls, BP and DMBA did not affect the survival efficiency, but significantly increased colony efficiency of the treated cells (Fig. 7.15). Colonies formed from the treated cells showed considerable anchorage-independent growth during the 21-day assay period. However, when individual colonies were isolated, they failed to expanded grow. Since formation of colonies in agar is generally construed as indicating anchorage-independent growth, a hallmark of neoplastic cells, our results clearly showed that HBEC from women with familial history of breast cancer manifested phenotypic changes indicative of initial stages of neoplastic transformation in response to the carcinogen treatment. In contrast, carcinogen treatments of HBEC from women without familial history of breast cancer induced only phenotypic alterations indicative of partial transformation, such as increased survival efficiency in agar methocel [96, 97], which is perceived to precede the acquisition of anchorage independence [100, 101]. Therefore, genetic predisposition in women with familial history of breast cancer confers inherited susceptibility to environmental chemical carcinogens. Conceivably, neoplastic transformation occurs as a consequence of cumulative genetic alterations in regulatory mechanisms influencing cellular proliferation and/or programmed cell death or apoptosis.

Two molecular mechanisms responsible for cell transformation have been associated with the expression of bcl-2, an apoptosis inhibitor that is highly expressed in breast carcinomas with a low apoptotic index [102, 103], and cyclin D1, a proliferation-associated gene which is frequently amplified or overexpressed in all forms of breast carcinoma [104–108]. The levels of bcl-2 and cyclin D1 expression were unaffected by chemical carcinogen treatments during the initial phases of cellular transformation in vitro. Therefore, the role of bcl-2 and cyclin D1 in the etiology of human breast cancer, if any, appears to be subsequent to the initial stage of neoplastic transformation. In this regard, even though bcl-2 has been implicated as an early event in epithelial malignancies of skin [109–112], endometrium, and gastrointestinal tracts, overexpression of bcl-2 failed to immortalize normal human keratinocytes, or to transform SV40 immortalized human mammary epithelial cells [113] in vitro, or to increase the incidence of epithelial malignancies in vivo in transgenic mice [114]. Similarly, overexpression of cyclin D1 prolonged the s-phase of the cell cycle and inhibited growth of human breast epithelial cells [115], yet shortened G1 phase and promoted the completion of the cell cycle in G1-arrested human breast cancer cells [116], in spite of the fact that cyclin D1, an important component driving cells through the restriction point START to complete the cell cycle [117], has been shown to complement a defective adenovirus E1A oncogene to immortalize cells [118]. In addition, expression of cyclin D1 has been associated with malignant progression, defining a major transition from a benign state to commitment to carcinoma in human breast neoplasia [108].

Human breast epithelial cells from women with familial history of breast cancer manifest phenotypic changes indicative of initial stages of neoplastic transformation in response to treatments with environmental chemical carcinogens. Since carcinogen treatments of HBEC from women without familial history of breast cancer induced only phenotypic alterations indicative of partial transformation, such as increased survival efficiency in agar methocel [4], it is reasonable to conclude that genetic predisposition in women with familial history of breast cancer confers inherited susceptibility to environmental chemical carcinogens. In addition, utilization of HBEC from women with different genetic background provides a novel system to transform human breast epithelial cells in vitro, thus allowing one to identify the causative agents of breast cancer and mechanisms responsible for carcinogenic progression. Finally, in agreement with previous clinical and experimental observations, the role of bcl-2 and cyclin D1 in the etiology of human breast cancer, if any, appears to be subsequent to the initial stage of neoplastic transformation. Therefore, the molecular mechanisms responsible for the transformation of normal human breast epithelium remain to be elucidated.

7.6 In Vitro System of Cell Transformation

We have developed an in vitro experimental system for the transformation of HBEC with chemical carcinogens [1]. Our studies led us to conclude that in order to induce full neoplastic transformation, i.e., expression of advantageous growth, anchorage independence, enhanced chemo-invasiveness, absence of ductulogenesis, and tumorigenesis in a heterologous host [1], the cells need to be immortalized prior to carcinogen exposure [1]. Our in vitro model of cell transformation was developed utilizing the immortalized HBEC MCF-10A transfected with *c-Ha-ras* oncogene and MCF-10F treated with the carcinogen benzo(a)pyrene (BP).

7.6.1 Transformation of Human Breast Epithelial Cells with c-Ha-ras Oncogene

A significant event in cancer research has been the identification and the subsequent characterization of oncogenes in both human and experimental animal tumors [119–122]. In particular, activation of the ras gene family has been found in human tumors [123] as well as in animal tumor model systems [120, 121, 124]. The role of activated *c-Ha-ras* in the initiation of human breast cancer is not clear yet, although approximately 60–70% of primary human breast carcinomas exhibit overexpression of *c-Ha-ras* mRNA and p2 l ras protein [125–127]. Nevertheless, there is evidence in experimental systems that a point-mutated *c-Ha-ras* proto-oncogene may be involved in the development of mouse and rat mammary tumors induced by treatment with chemical carcinogens [128, 129]. In addition, introduction of the *v-Ha-ras* oncogene into transgenic mice leads to the development of mammary tumors [130], and overexpression of a point mutated *c-Ha-ras* proto-oncogene or of a *v-Ha-ras* oncogene in rodent mammary epithelial cell lines leads to their in vitro transformation and in vivo tumorigenicity [131–133]. HBEC previously immortalized with benzo(a)pyrene have been transfected with *v-Ha-ras* oncogene using a retrovirus vector, but the expression of the fully malignant phenotype in those cells required the cooperation of two oncogenes, *v-Ha-ras* and large T antigen [134]. It has been reported [53] that, in contrast to other human breast tumor and cell lines [135–137], immortalized MCF-10A and MCF-10F cells lacked amplification, rearrangement, or mutational activation of cellular proto-oncogenes such as *c-erbB-2/HER2/neu*, *c-erbA-1*, *int-2*, and *c-Ha-ras-1* [53]. It has also been reported that restriction fragment length polymorphism analysis and DNA sequencing did not detect activating missense mutations in the common activation sites of *Ha-ras* oncogenes.

MCF-10A [53], which was derived without viral or chemical intervention from mortal diploid HBEC with extended life span (Fig. 7.10), has allowed to test whether the insertion of an activated Ha-ras oncogene alone is capable of inducing malignant transformation in breast epithelium. MCF-10A cells were transfected with the *c-Ha-ras* oncogene contained in the plasmid pHo6-Tras [138]. Their growth pattern in plastic, tridimensional growth in collagen, expression of anchorage-independent growth, independence from hormones and growth factors for growth, and tumorigenicity in nude mice were then tested and compared with those of MCF-10A parent cells or cells transfected with the neomycin-resistant gene alone or with the proto-oncogene (pHo6neo).

c-Ha-ras gene transfected into MCF-10A cells was inserted in the DNA of the cells (Figs. 7.16, 7.17) and expressed itself by the production of the mutated p21 protein (Fig. 7.18). This insertion did not result in activation, rearrangement, or amplification of other oncogenes known to be associated with breast carcinoma, such as *c-erbB-2/HER-21neu* and *int-2* [135, 139–141]. The insertion of the *c-Ha-ras* has been mainly localized in chromosome 11 using in situ hybridization (Fig. 7.19), however, autoradiographic silver grains were also detected in chromosomes 1, 2, 3, 5, 9, 12, and 16 (Fig. 7.19). Indicating the possibility that the insertion of the mutated *c-Ha-ras* oncogene either activated or rearranged other unknown oncogenes that might have acted jointly with the *c-Ha-ras* oncogene to produce the malignant phenotype, or that it is the strength of the enhancer flanking the activated *c-Ha-ras* oncogene that cooperated in producing the malignant phenotypes [138, 142].

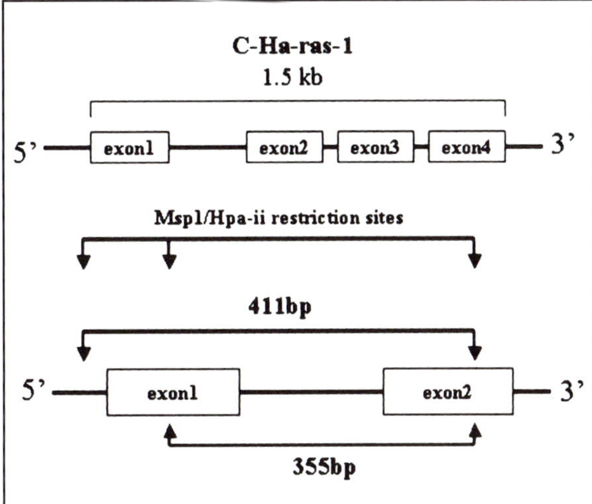

Figure 7.16

Restriction sites for c-Ha ras oncogene

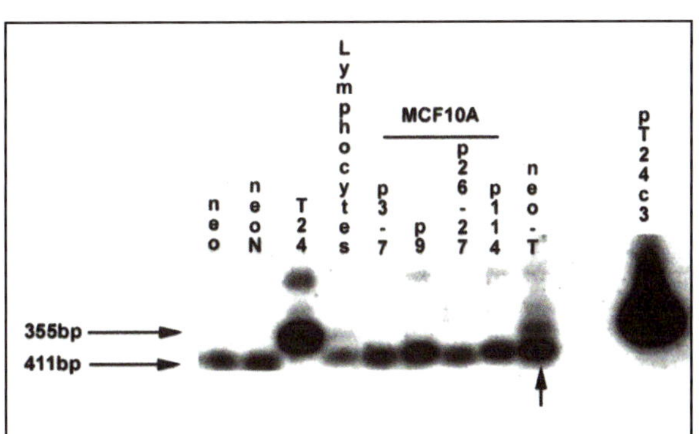

Figure 7.17

MCF-10AneoT and T24 cells contained a 411-bp *MspI–HpaII* fragment, indicating the presence of a mutated *ras* gene

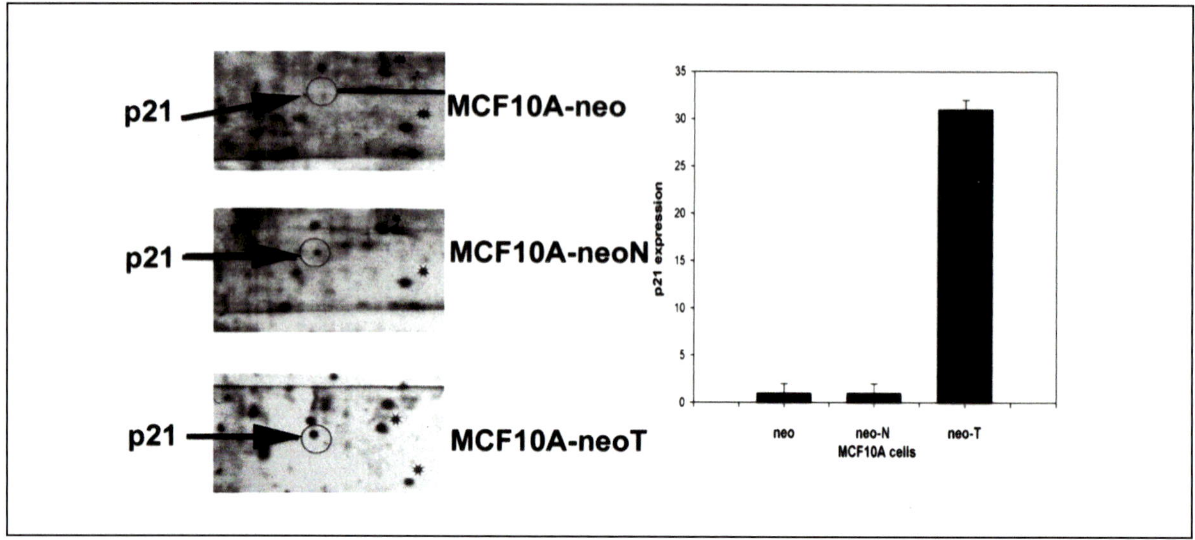

Figure 7.18

Two-dimensional gel Western blot profiles of *ras* gene products in MCF-10Aneo, MCF-10AneoNras and MCF-10Aneo-Tras. The panreactive antibody against mutated (activated) p2 I (pan-p2I, *left panels*) is recognized only in MCF-10AneoT. The non-mutated (*arrows, in circle*) is also over-expressed in the transformed cells. Modified from: Basolo, F., Elliott, J., Tait, L., Chen, X.Q., Maloney, T., Russo, I.H., Pauley, R., Momiki, S., Caamano, J., Klein-Szanto, A.J.P., Koszalka, M. and Russo, J. Transformation of Human Breast Epithelial Cells by *c-Ha-ras* oncogene. Molecular Carcinogenesis, 4:25–35, 1991, with permission

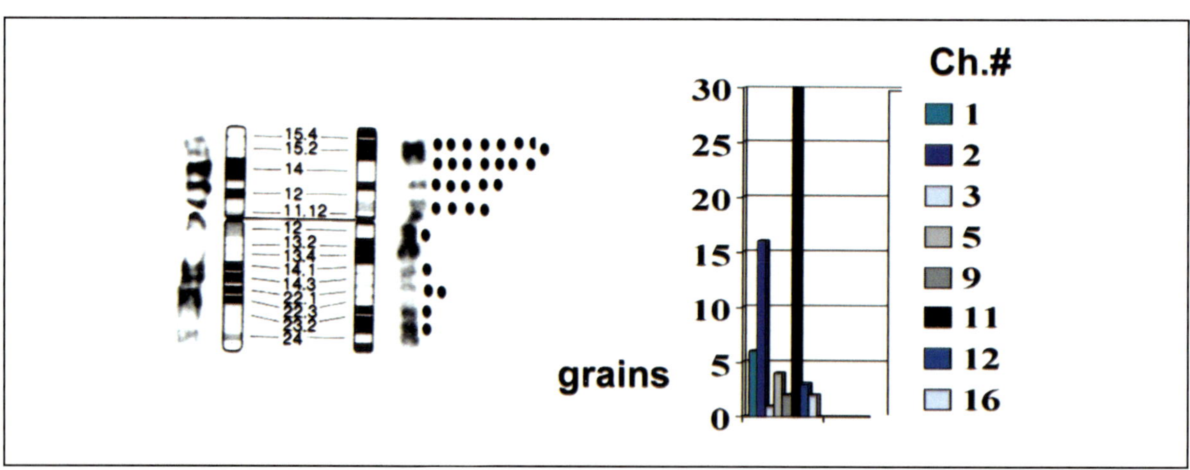

Figure 7.19

Autoradiographic data on the number of silver grains detected in chromosome 11 when hybridized with the cDNA probe for c-Has ras oncogene. The histogram in the *right panel* shows the other chromosomes that have hybridized with the probe

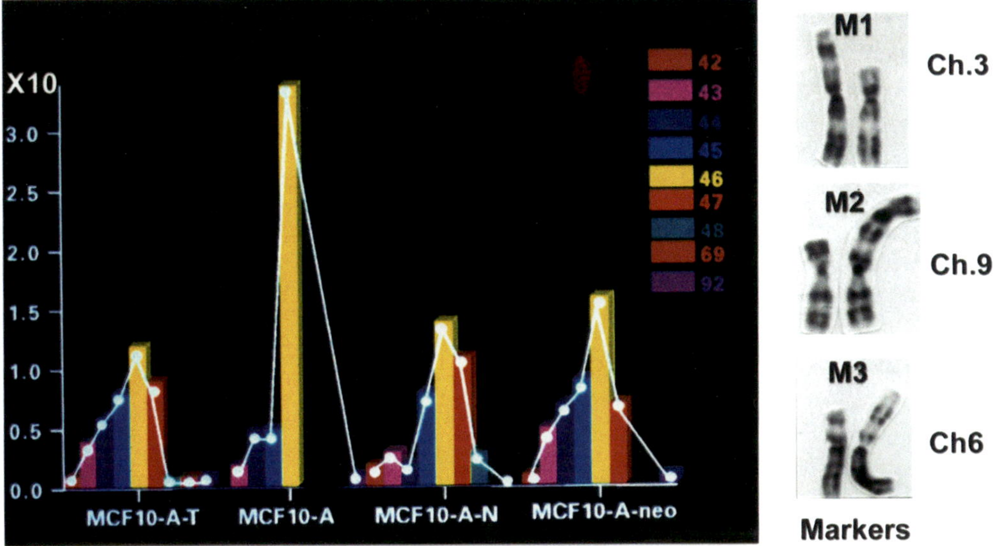

Figure 7.20

Modal distribution of the chromosomes in the *c-Ha-ras* transformed and non-transformed cells. The *right panels* show the chromosome markers for MCF-10A

The karyotype of transfected cells remained pseudodiploid, with a mode of 46 chromosomes, practically identical to that of parent cells (Fig. 7.20). Similar results have been reported for early passages of *c-Ha-ras*-transformed rat embryo fibroblasts that remained diploid even after becoming metastatic in nude mice [143, 144]. Even though transfection resulted in chromosomal losses and additions, these changes were not restricted to cells transfected with activated *c-Ha-ras*; they were also found in cells transfected with pHo6 and normal *c-Ha-ras*, an observation that supports the concept that the expression of *c-Ha-ras* oncogene does not lead to gross chromosomal abnormalities.

The malignant phenotypes expressed by transfected MCF-10A cells were anchorage-independent growth (Figs. 7.21–7.23), hormone and growth factor independence (Figs. 7.24, 7.25), alterations in the tridimensional pattern of growth in collagen matrix

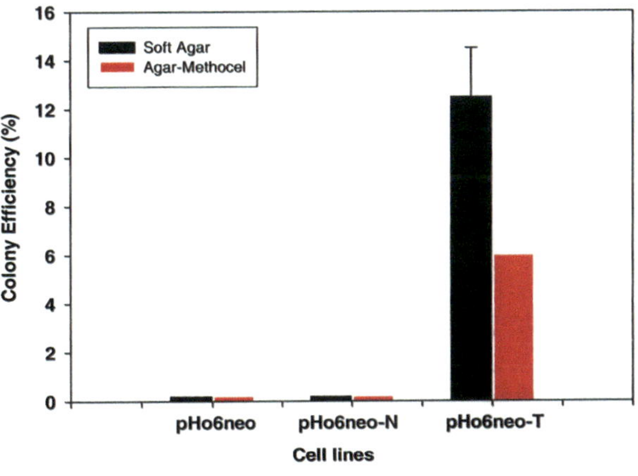

Figure 7.21

Histogram depicting the colony efficiency of *c-Ha-ras* transformed MCF-10A cells

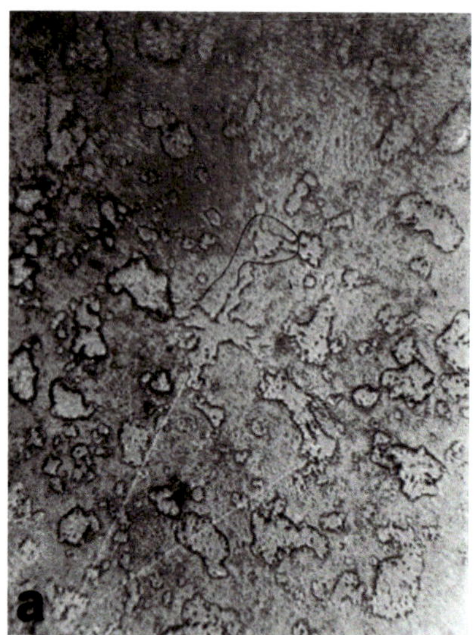
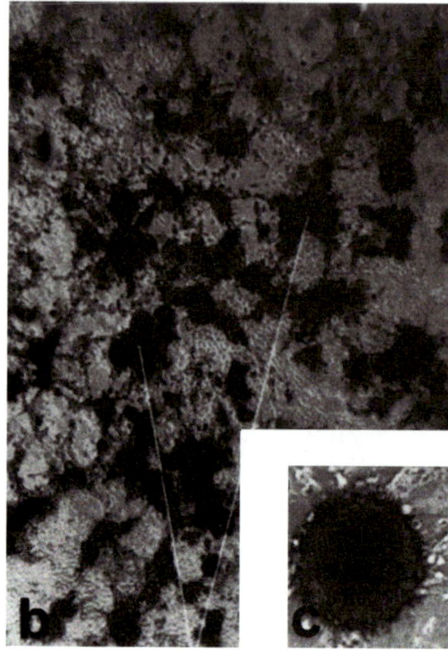

Figure 7.22 a–c

a Morphology of post-confluent MCF-10A cells, ×40. **b** Morphology of post-confluent MCF-10A-neoT cells showing loss of contact inhibition; growing cells overlap forming foci, ×40. **c** Enlargement of an individual focus from panel **b**, ×100. All the photographs were taken under phase contrast microscopy

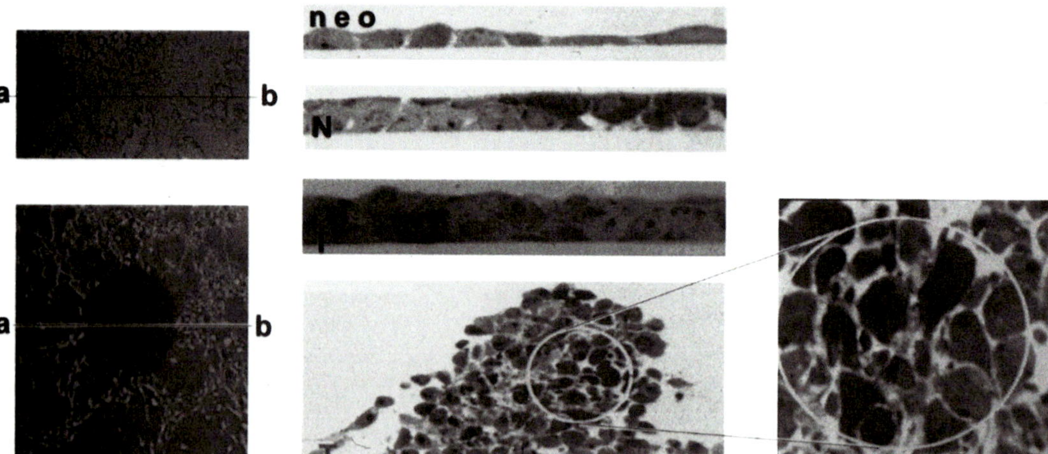

Figure 7.23

Composite showing monolayers of MCF-10A*neo* cells transfected with plasmid containing the neomycin resistant gene, *MCF-10AneoN*, transfected with the normal ras sequence, and *MCF-10AneoT*, transfected with mutated ras sequence. The *upper left corner* is a monolayer of MCF-10Aneo showing the *a–b* levels at which the histological section was performed shown in *neo*, the *upper middle panel*. The *lower left corner* shows the MCF-10AneoT focus and the line *a–b* at which the histological section was taken and shown in the *lower middle panel*. The *right panel* shows the cluster of epithelial cells transformed by *c-Ha-ras* transfection at higher magnification. *Middle panel N* monolayer of MCF-10AneoN, *middle panel T* monolayer of MCF-10AneoT

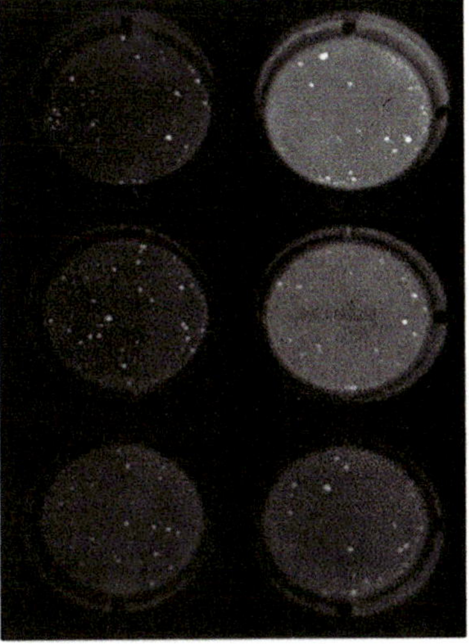
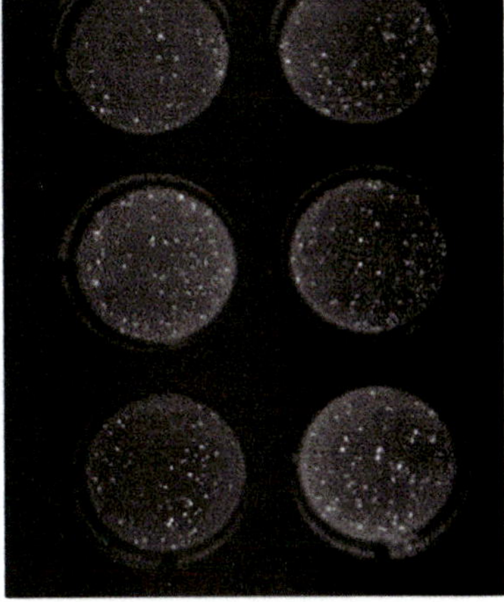

(Fig. 7.26), increased invasiveness (Fig. 7.27) and collagenolytic activity (Fig. 7.28), and tumorigenesis in nude mice, all properties observed in transformed cells [97, 134, 145–147].

Among the phenotypic markers indicative of in vitro cell transformation, the ability of cells to grow in an anchorage-independent manner is a reliable criterion (Figs. 7.21, 7.24) [146], especially when accompanied by tumorigenicity, since many normal cells are able to grow in methocel or agar but are unable to produce tumors [148–150]. In rodent cells, anchorage-independent growth is usually expressed as a relatively late marker [98]. In MCF-10-neoT cells, however, this property was detected early, after the third passage post transfection, and was associated with tumorigenicity in nude mice, a phenomenon also expressed by breast tumor cell lines such as MDA-MB-231, BT-20, and MCF-7 [49, 151].

The exact mechanism by which *c-Ha-ras* is involved in the tumorigenic process is not clear, although it has been postulated that *c-Ha-ras* activation affects the ductulogenic process, a phenomenon observed in transfected MCF-10A cells and also reported in the rodent system [134, 152]. *C-Ha-ras*-transfected MCF-10A cells formed large spherical masses lined by an epithelium two to three layers

Figure 7.24

Colony formation in agar methocel by MCF-10AneoT is growth factor and hormone independent. *H* horse serum, *CT* cortisol, *EGF* epidermal growth factor

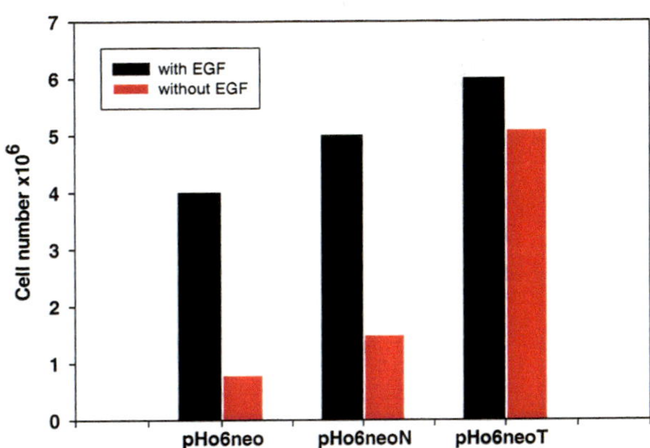

Figure 7.25

Histogram depicting cell growth in the presence or absence of EGF

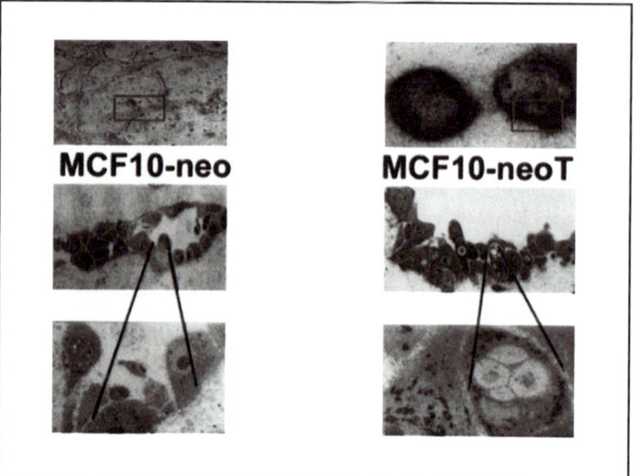

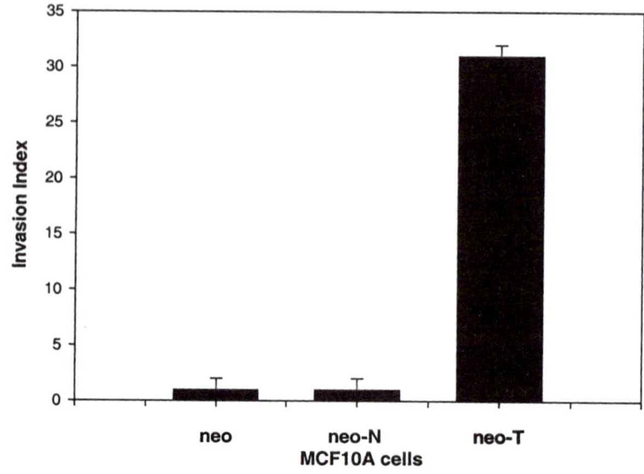

Figure 7.26

The *left panel* shows the MCF-10Aneo cells growing forming ductules in a collagen matrix forming well developed ductules (×40) lined by cuboidal epithelial cells (×250), that is confirmed by electron microscopy (×2,000). The *right panel* shows the MCF10-AneoT cells that lack the ability to form ductules and formed hollow masses (×40), lined by a multilayer of atypical cells (×250), some of them with intracellular lumen (×2,000)

thick exhibiting an altered morphologic appearance; individual cells were two-fold larger than non transfected cells and had an increased nuclear:cytoplasmic ratio (Fig. 7.23). The ultrastructural appearance of these cells was significantly different from that of normal cells, showing formation of numerous intracellular lumens with secretory like material (Fig. 7.26), such as those described in many breast cancer cell lines and human primary breast cancers [18, 153]. The cell surface is significantly changed in the transformed cells by increasing the number, length and thickness of the microvilli (Fig. 7.29). The expression of breast epithelial markers like cytokeratin, milk fat globule membrane antigens were more similar to those expressed by MCF-7 cells than those transfected by the vector alone (neo) or the non-mutated ras (pHo6neoN) (Fig. 7.30). Immunoblots with specific cytokeratin AE1 and AE3 antibodies showed identical molecular weight species of cytokeratins in MCF-10A, MCF-10neo, MCF-10FneoN and MCF-10FneoT

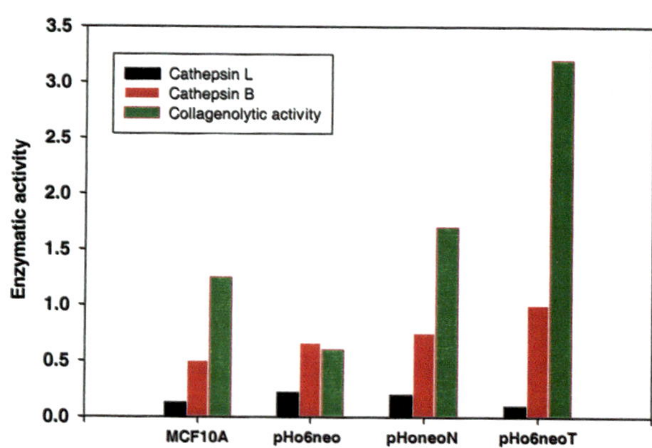

Figure 7.27

Histogram depicting the invasion index

Figure 7.28

The enzymatic profile of the c-Has ras transformed cells (pHo6neoT) is significantly different from the parental cell (MCF-10A), the transfected cells by the plasmid alone (pHo6neo), or the one transfected by the non-mutated ras (pHo6neoN)

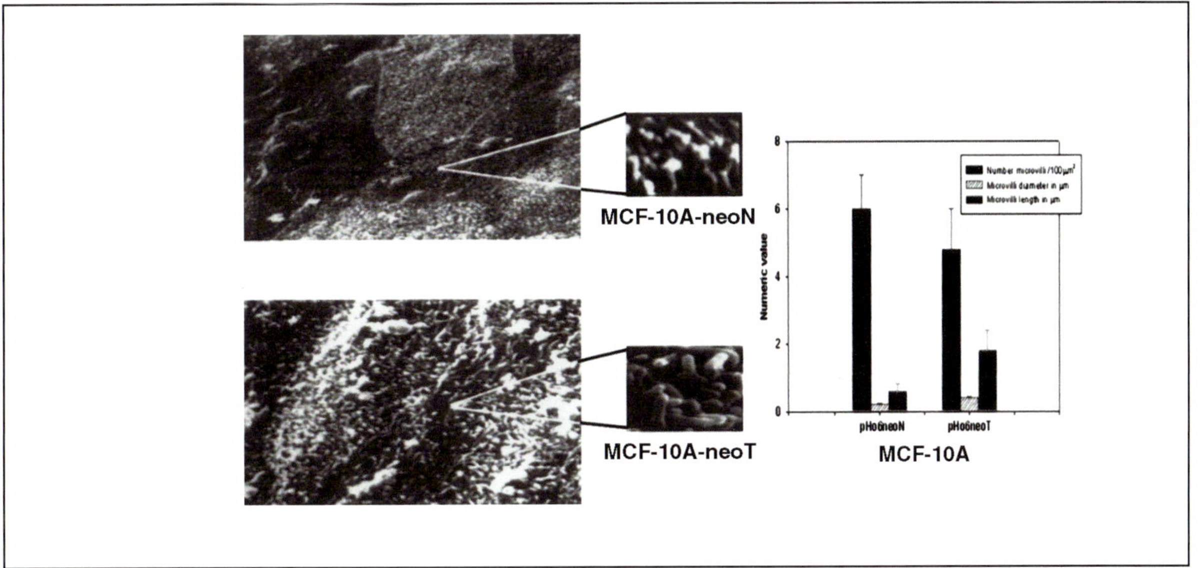

The mutated c-Ha ras oncogene induces significant changes in the cell surface by increasing the number of microvilli by unit area, the length and the thickness of the microvilli

cells (Fig. 7.31); however in MCF-10FneoT cells the intensity of immunostaining and the number of immunoreacted phosphorylated polypeptides keratin 7, 8, 15, and 16 was decreased. This altered morphology in vitro could explain the undifferentiated pattern of tumors developed in vivo (Fig. 7.39c). In addition to alterations in the morphogenetic properties of the mammary epithelium, *c-Ha-ras*-transfected cells had a reduced requirement for epidermal growth factor (EGF) (Figs. 7.24, 7.25), as has been reported in other systems. In the rodent model, transfected cells synthesize and secrete their own transforming growth factor (TGF-α), which binds the EGF receptor [154, 155]; this mechanism also appears to operate in transfected MCF-10A cells [156], in which transfection induces an increase in TGF-α-mRNA expression and TGF-α protein secretion [157]. This increase in TGF-α production may partly account for the enhanced growth rate of these cells in hydrocortisone-

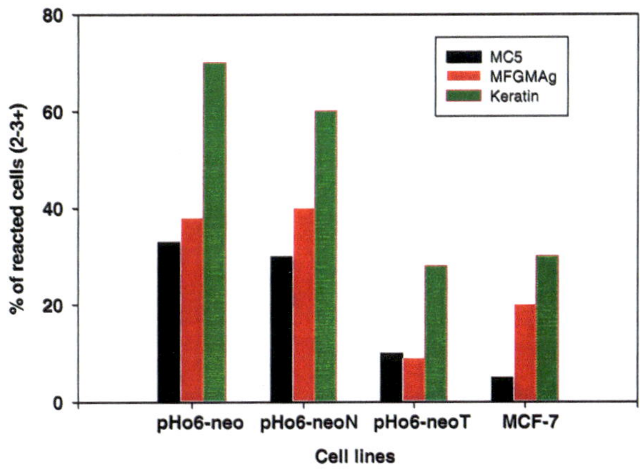

Histogram depicting the changes in the phenotype of the cells transfected by the mutated *c-Ha-ras*. There is a significant difference in the expression of keratin, and milk fat globule membrane antigen (MC5 and MFGMA)

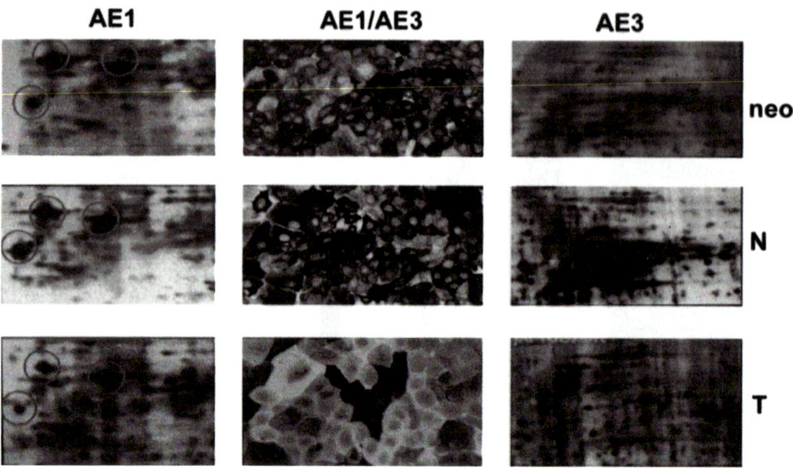

Figure 7.31

Identification of cytokeratins in 2-D gel Western blots of MCF-10Aneo, MCF-10AneoN and MCF-10AneoT. 100 µg of total cellular protein were separated on 2-D gels and transferred to nitrocellulose. Polypeptide profiles were visualized with gold stain, then appropriate areas of the blot were cut out and immunoreacted with anti-cytokeratins antibody. Antibody AE1 detected acidic keratins 15 and 16 (*circled*). Antibody AE3 detected keratins 7 and 8. The immunocytochemical profile shown in the *middle panel* shows less number of reacting cells in the MCF-10AneoT. Modified from: Maloney, T., Geronimo, I., Fontanini, G., Basolo, F., Elliott, J.W. and Russo, J. Transfection of a normal human breast epithelial cell line with *c-Ha-ras* oncogene alters the expression of p21 and cytokeratins. Am. J. Pathol. 140:1483–1488, 1992, with permission

and cholera toxin-deprived medium or in serum-free medium and for their ability to grow in soft agar [157]. Results on *ras* transformation and TGF-α production in MCF-10A cells contrast with those recently reported in another human mammary epithelial cell line [158] in which no significant change in the levels of TGF-α production could be detected in v-Haras-infected cells or in cells transformed by a combination of *v-Ha-ras* and SV40T oncogenes as compared with their parental cells [158]. In separate experiments published elsewhere [156, 157], MCF-10AneoT cells expressed a 5- to 1 0-fold increase in the level of 1.4-kb *c-Ha-ras* RNA transcripts in comparison with the parental cell line and the other transfectants. In addition, there was a corresponding increase in p2 l ras protein expression and in TGF-α production. These data could explain the biological differences in anchorage-independent growth in the absence of EGF and may be functionally relevant in the process of ductulogenesis. Transfection of MCF-10A cells with the activated *c-Ha-ras* oncogene induces the expression of invasive characteristics similar to those of tumorigenic or transformed cells of intermediate malignancy (Table 7.9) [159, 160] or of NIH 3T3 and 10T1/2 ras oncogene-transformed cells [161–168]. In an in vitro chemoinvasive assay, MCF-10AneoT cells were more invasive than MCF-10A cells transfected with the neomycin-resistant gene alone or with the proto-oncogene (Table 7.9), but less invasive than metastatic melanoma cells [169] or ras-transfected NIH 3T3 cells. Like NIH 3T3 cells [164, 165] and human bronchial epithelial cells (147), MCF-10AneoT cells also produced more type IV collagenase than non transfected cells, an important property in the process of invasion and metastasis (Fig. 7.28).

MCF-l0AneoT cells exhibited greater chemotaxis than cells transfected with the neomycin-resistant gene alone or the ras proto-oncogene, although chemotactic activity was not significantly different from that of MCF-10A parent cells, a phenomenon also observed in immortalized human bronchial epithelial cells (Table 7.9) [147]. Ras transfection of immortalized HBEC MCF-10A cells can also be involved in early steps of tumor progression in vitro. This observation agrees with a study reporting that activation of the *ras* oncogene preceded the onset of mammary neoplasia [170], although in that case the presence of the activated oncogene alone did not suffice to induce the expression of malignancy, since it was first necessary that active cell proliferation be induced by estrogenic hormones for the neoplastic phenotype to be manifested [170]. MCF-10A cells, which are immortal and actively proliferating, express the fully malignant phenotype upon insertion of the activated oncogene. This is an excellent model for understanding the mechanisms whereby the *c-Ha-ras* oncogene induces malignant phenotypes. Collectively, all of these data support the concept that *c-Ha-ras* oncogene could be involved in both early and late stages of mammary carcinogenesis.

7.6.2 Transformation of Human Breast Epithelial Cells with Chemical Carcinogens

Polycyclic hydrocarbons and aromatic amines induce mammary carcinomas both in vivo [171–174] and in vitro [47]. The susceptibility of the mammary epithelium to prototype carcinogens has been demonstrated in vivo [1, 171–173], and in vitro using mammary explants [1, 175, 176], or cell cultures [174, 177, 178, 179]. These studies have provided important leads to the identification of several molecular, metabolic and cellular events that are required for the initiation of mammary cancer [174, 179, 180]. An important requirement for cell transformation is proliferation in the presence of carcinogens; the proliferating mammary epithelium is thus able to metabolize and bind the carcinogens, and to replicate damaged DNA, which carries carcinogen-induced alterations to the subsequent cell population [174, 179, 180]. Under ideal conditions, the evaluation of the carcinogenic potential of a substance requires that the target cells have not been previously affected by viral or chemical agents either in vivo or in vitro, in order to ensure that the effect measured is truly that of the carcino-

gen tested. For these reasons, studies have been performed in MCF-10F using two carcinogenic compounds that require metabolic activation, DMBA and B(a)P, and two direct-acting carcinogens, NMU and MNNG, were used (Figs. 7.32–7.36) [1, 179, 181].

Although long-lived HBEC lines have been obtained by treatment with SV40 virus [98] and immortalization has been achieved by treatment with B(a)P [95], there are few reports of spontaneously arising, long-lived cell lines [18, 53, 151, 152]. HMT-3522 is a breast cell line derived from breast tissue with fibrocystic disease, which exhibits extensive chromosomal aberrations [151]. MCF-10F cells, in addition of expressing the normal phenotype of HBEC, are pseudodiploid and express minimal chromosomal alterations [46xx,lp+,t(3;9)(pl3:p22)] [53]. MCF-10F cells in that sense are unique because even though they are long lived, they have retained the features of normal differentiation that allow one to test small deviations after they are treated with chemical carcinogens in vitro. Although definitive phenotypic markers of human breast epithelial cell transformation have not been determined yet [95, 98, 152], indicators of cell transformation have been shown to be common for human and rodent mammary and other epithelial cells [47]. MCF-10 M, the cells that gave origin to the immortal MCF-10F and MCF-10A cells, exhibited increased survival efficiency in agar methocel after treatment with chemical carcinogens in vitro [182]. However, neither these cells nor other breast primary cultures exhibited a progression in the expression of phenotypes associated with neoplastic transformation (Fig. 7.32) [182]. Since in vitro treatment of HBEC primary cultures with chemical carcinogens did not succeed in inducing the full expression of transformation phenotypes, it was decided to use the protocol developed for primary cultures of breast epithelial cells (Fig. 7.16) for testing the response of the spontaneously immortalized cells MCF-10F to the same carcinogens, in order to elucidate whether immortalization is required for the expression of the fully transformed phenotype [96, 183]. Similar data have been reported for other cell types [184–186] in which the survival in agar preceded the acquisition of anchorage independence [186]. MCF-10F cells treated with carcinogens in vitro (Figs. 7.33–7.36) express

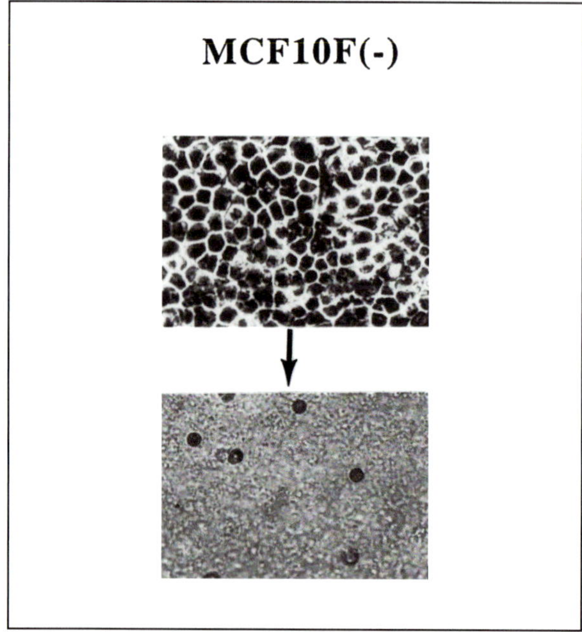

Figure 7.32

MCF-10F control cells, phase contrast. *Upper panel:* In plastic Petri dish, ×40. *Lower panel:* In agar methocel, 21 days after seeding, ×16 (reprinted with permission from: Calaf, G., and Russo, J. Transformation of human breast epithelial cells by chemical carcinogens. Carcinogenesis 14:483–492, 1993)

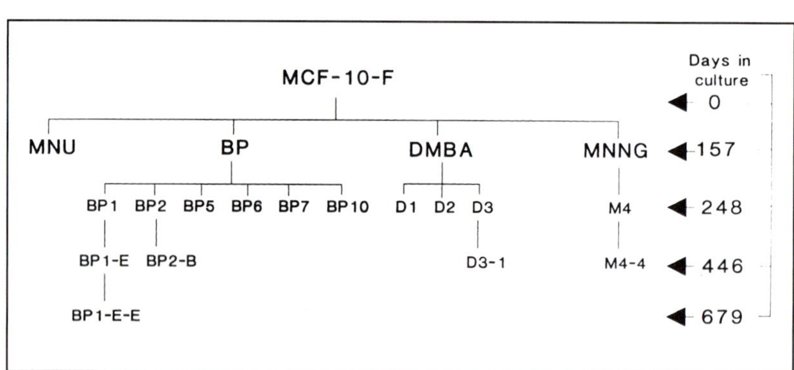

Figure 7.33

Flow chart showing the evolution of MCF-10F cells after treatment with the carcinogens NMU, B(a)P, DMBA, or MNNG. Days in culture indicate the number of days in vitro that it took each cell line to emerge (reprinted with permission from: Calaf, G., and Russo, J. Transformation of human breast epithelial cells by chemical carcinogens. Carcinogenesis 14:483–492, 1993)

Table 7.10. Cell kinetic changes induced by chemical carcinogens during the transformation of MCF-10F cells. *TPS* total passages, *TD* total doublings, *DT* doubling times

	Days in vitro	TPS	TD	DT (h)
MCF-10F	141	8	33.9	100
DMBA	119	8	40.5	71
D1	277	14	64.8	69
D2	277	13	56.9	78
D3	292	20	101.2	47
MNNG	119	10	43.0	66
M4	292	14	54.4	88
NMU	171	20	ND	ND
BP	141	8	43.8	77
BP1	292	18	86.9	55
BP2	292	16	60.1	79
BP5	292	18	77.0	63
BP6	292	16	58.0	83
BP7	292	17	70.4	60
BP10	292	16	70.4	61

phenotypes indicative of neoplastic transformation, such as increased total number of doublings and decreased DT, expression of anchorage-independent growth, in vitro invasive capability, altered cell growth patterns in collagen matrix and tumor formation in SCID mice. MCF-10F cells treated with either DMBA, MNNG, NMU or B(a)P express an early increase in growth and changes in the rate of cell proliferation, as indicated by a shorter DT, which becomes progressively shorter with the number of passages (Table 7.10). This phenomenon suggests that in each passage there is a selection of highly proliferating cells that booster cell growth advantage, thus each passage resulted in the selection of more aggressive phenotypes. There are clear morphological changes observed either by light microscopy as well as by ultrastructural means (Fig. 7.37). The progressive and stepwise process of selection of more aggressive phenotypes supports the hypothesis of a multistep process in the progression of carcinogenesis, as has been suggested in other systems [18, 187].

Evidence exists that tumor development in vivo is a complex process involving multiple steps through qualitative different stages [18, 187, 188]. We have presented evidence that neoplastic transformation in vitro, like neoplastic development in vivo, is a progressive process. In the case of MCF-10F cells treated with chemical carcinogens, alterations in the ductulogenic pattern in collagen gel preceded morphological changes observed in monolayers. These morphologically transformed cells were able to grow in agar methocel, and this latter phenotype was expressed with more intensity in later passages (Figs. 7.33–7.36). A similar phenomenon has been observed in Syrian hamster cells [189], and in human fibroblasts [190]. In the case of MCF-10F cells, the acquisition of anchorage independence was manifested at 157 days in culture, and the efficiency varied from carcinogen to carcinogen, being the highest for DMBA and B(a)P. NMU was the least efficient in inducing colony formation and did not originate clones; MNNG originated four colonies from which only one clone, M4,

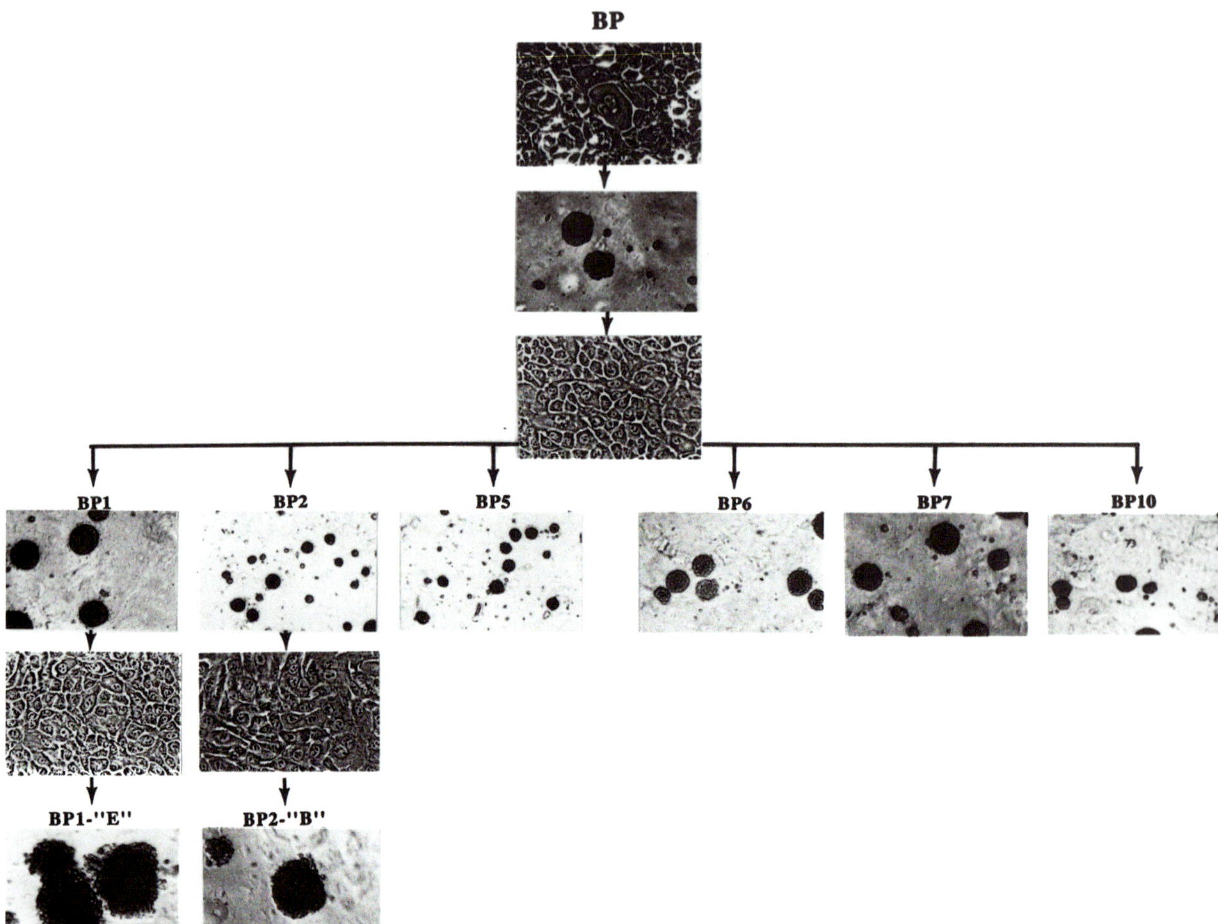

Figure 7.34

BP-treated MCF-10F cells (phase contrast) form colonies that isolated and expanded were reseeded in agar methocel originating the cell lines, BP1, BP2, BP5, BP6, BP7, and BP10. From BP1 and BP2 originates the clones BP1-E and BP2B. BP1-E is the clone that will induce tumors in heterologous host (reprinted with permission from: Calaf, G., and Russo, J. Transformation of human breast epithelial cells by chemical carcinogens. Carcinogenesis 14:483–492, 1993)

emerged at 248 days post-treatment. M4 exhibited greater CE than the parental cells, and generated other subclones that emerged by 446 days in culture (Fig. 7.33, Table 7.11). We observed that the apparent refractory nature of human breast epithelial cells to express the phenotypes of neoplastic transformation upon treatment with carcinogens in vitro [47, 95, 147, 152] could be overcome by isolating and reseeding the colonies formed in agar methocel, which are further selected by reseeding in semisolid medium. Whereas this selective pressure in vitro may not represent the same forces that are operational in vivo, our observations indicate that the emergence of neoplastic phenotypes is a continuum expressed only in those cells that exhibit further growth advantage.

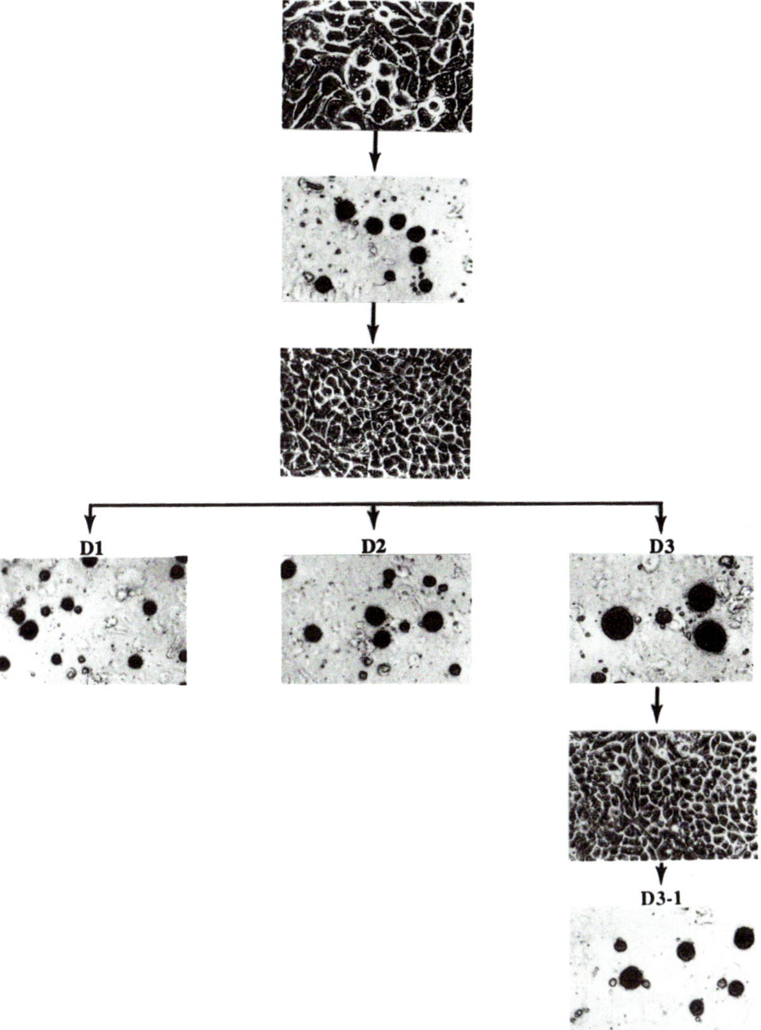

Figure 7.35

DMBA-treated MCF-10F cells (phase contrast) form colonies that isolated and expanded were reseeded in agar methocel originating the cell lines, D1, D2 and D3. D3 originates the clone D3-1 (reprinted with permission from: Calaf, G., and Russo, J. Transformation of human breast epithelial cells by chemical carcinogens. Carcinogenesis 14:483–492, 1993)

It has been shown that chemoinvasion, or the ability of cells to cross basement membranes in vitro, as well as chemotaxis, or the ability of the cells to respond to a chemoattractant, are cell properties that are enhanced in transformed cells and correlate with malignant characteristics in vivo [191–196]. The chemoinvasive and chemotactic capabilities of the different cell lines tested by their ability to traverse a reconstituted basement membrane utilizing published methods [191, 197] is depicted in Table 7.12. The

Table 7.11. Anchorage independent growth of MCF-10F and carcinogen-treated cells. *CN* colony number, *CE* colony efficiency, *CS* colony size

	Days in vitro	Passage	CN	CE (%)	CS (µm)
MCF-10F	141	8	0	0	0
DMBA	119	8	52	9.7	111
D1	277	14	26	0.8	59
D2	277	13	165	4.7	45
D3	292	20	829	90.0	157
D3-1	163	10	2,200	83.6	476
MNNG	119	10	15	1.5	127
M4	292	14	30	3.6	30
NMU	171	20	5	0.2	96
BP	141	8	43	3.2	165
BP1	246	13	76	4.5	20
BP1	292	18	554	45.0	167
BP1-E	206	14	1,700	88.0	687
BP2	292	16	21	0.5	60
BP2-B	156	6	595	23.0	418
BP5	292	18	115	17.5	18
BP6	292	16	37	3.2	13
BP7	292	17	26	6.2	57
BP10	292	16	145	30.2	32

Table 7.12. Chemoinvasion and chemotaxis of MCF-10F and carcinogen-treated cells

	Days in vitro	Number of passages after treatment	Chemotactic index	Invasive index
MCF-10F	395	34	56	93
T24	NA	NA	677	1,124
D3	290	21	112	182
D3-1	155	8	438	523
BP-1	344	20	970	457
BP-1-E	171	10	682	820
BP-5	280	12	122	329
BP-7	409	22	258	281
BP-10	169	8	102	121

Table 7.13. Tumorigenic assay

	Passage number	Number of animals with tumors	Size (mm³)	Latency (days)
MCF-10-F	32-37	0/3, 0/2	–	–
T24	NA	3/3	5.3	10
MCF-7	142	2/2	20.0	28
D3	20-21-26	0/3, 0/3, 0/3	–	–
D3-1	6-8-13	0/3, 0/3, 0/4	–	–
M4	14-20	0/3, 0/3	–	–
NMU	27	0/3	–	–
BP 1	21-32	0/4, 0/4	–	–
BP 1-E	5	3/3	9.5	101–124
BP5	19-22-25	0/3, 0/3, 0/2	–	–
BP6	21	0/3	–	–
BP7	25	0/3	–	–

Figure 7.36 ▶

MNNG-treated MCF-10F cells (phase contrast) form colonies that isolated and expanded were reseeded in agar methocel originating the cell line M4 (reprinted with permission from: Calaf, G., and Russo, J. Transformation of human breast epithelial cells by chemical carcinogens. Carcinogenesis 14:483–492, 1993)

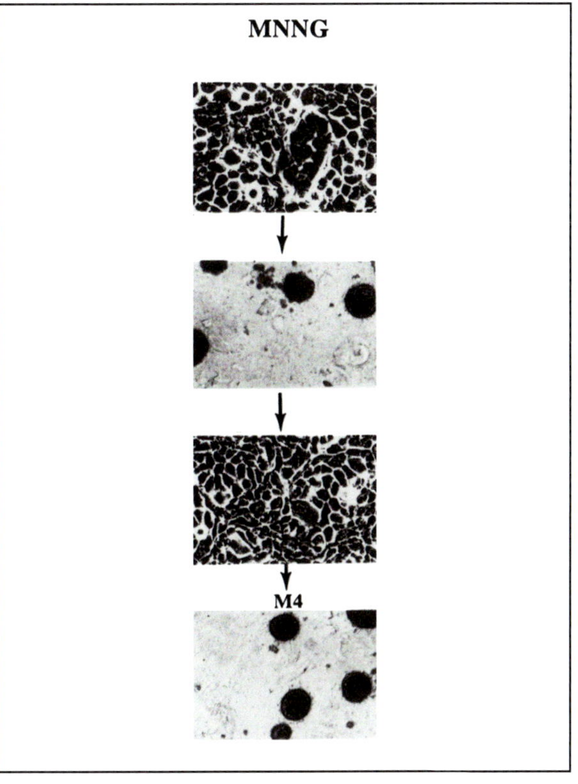

clones derived from DMBA- and B(a)P-treated cells, i. e., D3-1 and BPI-E respectively, exhibited greater invasive and chemotactic capabilities than MCF-10F control cells, and both parameters were similar to those of the tumorigenic T24 cells. The clones BP5, BP7 and BP10 presented greater values for invasion and chemotaxis than MCF-10F control cells, but less than BPI-E, D3-1 and T24 cells. The higher chemoinvasive and chemotactic capacity of BP1-E and D3-1 cells was observed in late passages and correlated with their higher CE in agar methocel. Similar results in transformed cells have been reported by other authors [193].

In the experimental system of HBEC transformed with chemical carcinogens (Table 7.13) the SCID

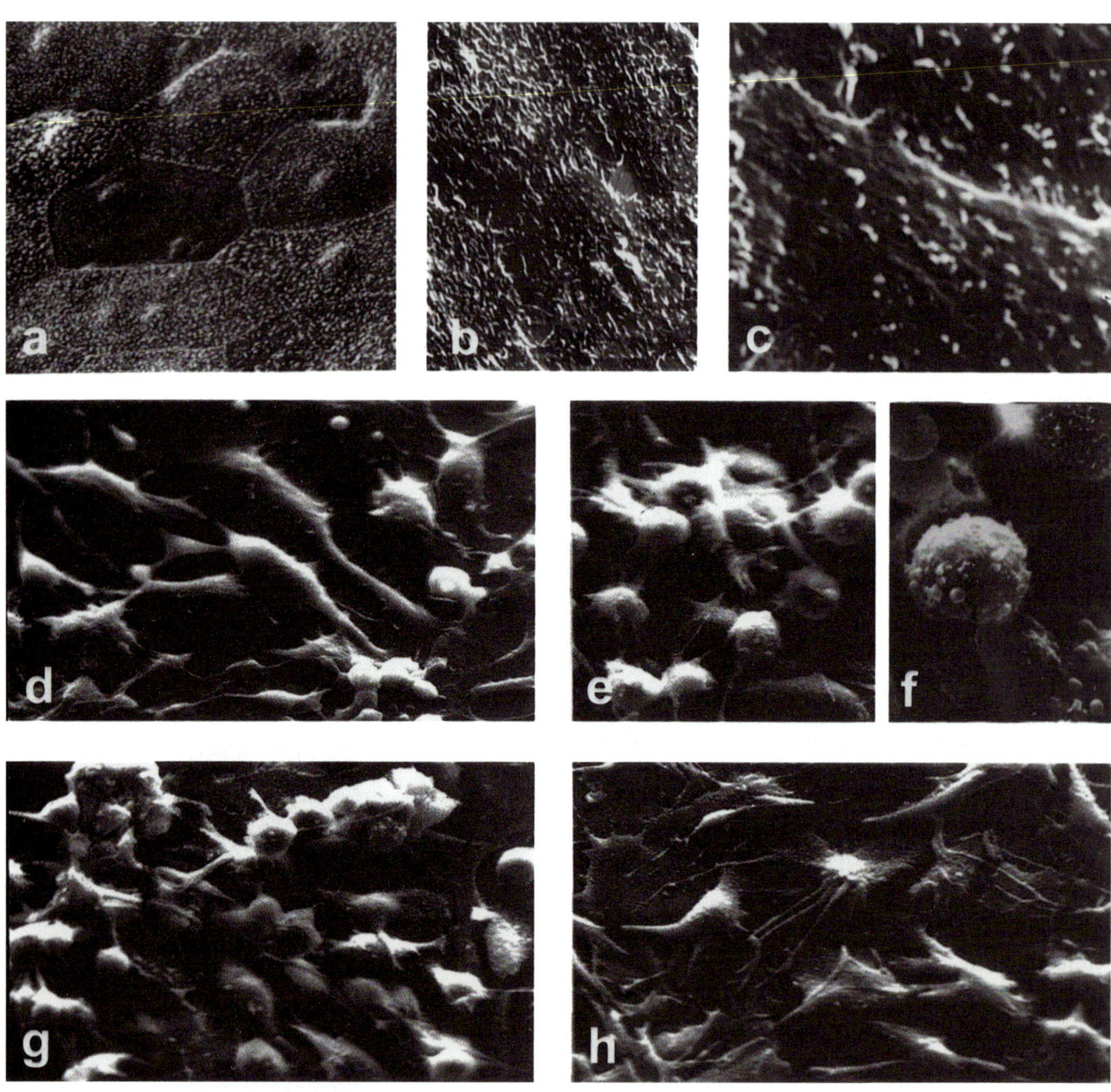

Figure 7.37 a–h

Scanning electron micrographs of MCF-10F and the transformed clones. **a** MCF-10F cells, ×400. **b** Cell surface of MCF-10F cells ×4,000. **c** Microvilli of MCF-10F cells, ×10,000. **d** DMBA-treated cells, ×400. **e** BP1 cells transfected with *c-Ha-ras*, ×400. **f** Higher magnification of **e**, ×2,000. **g** BP transformed cells, ×400. **h** MMNG-treated cells, ×400

mice as heterologous hosts for testing tumorigenicity has been used. SCID mice have an autosomal dominant recessive defect that impairs the rearrangement of antigen receptor genes in both T and B lymphocyte progenitors. SCID mice also lack functional T and B cells, which make these animals a suitable host for heterotransplantation. Tumorigenesis in heterologous hosts is considered to be the final reliable criterion for assessing complete transformation of human cells [47, 147], even though the validity of this model has been questioned, since many human malignancies or cell lines derived from them are not tumorigenic in the nude mouse [197]. The adequacy of SCID mice for testing tumorigenicity has been validated by the observations that 100% of the mice inoculated with either T24 or MCF-7 cells developed tumors with a short latency period. SCID mice proved to be more adequate as a host for MCF-7 cells than nude mice, since in our model they did not require estrogen supplementation [14]. The tumors developed in inoculated SCID mice were proven to be of human origin by determination of Alu sequences [198], which showed that they were derived from the cells inoculated and not a host reaction. T24 and BPI-E, the two cell lines expressing tumorigenesis in SCID mice (Table 7.13), also exhibited the highest in agar-methocel in MNNG-treated cells. BP1-E cells also exhibited a higher CE, larger CS and higher CN than the other non-tumorigenic clones, which indicated that these phenotypes need to be sequentially expressed prior to the manifestation of the tumorigenic phenotype. Although anchorage independent growth is considered to be a predictor of tumorigenesis in other cell systems [47, 152], in the experimental model neither anchorage independence nor any of the other parameters served, when considered individually, as an indicator of the tumorigenic potential of a cell. These observations are supported by results on human breast epithelial cells obtained from milk, which have been reported to acquire anchorage independent growth and immortalization after SV40 infection, but do not elicit tumorigenesis in nude mice [18, 47, 53, 152] and by the observation that the extended lifespan induced in human breast epithelial cells treated with B(a)P in vitro was not accompanied by the expression of anchorage independence or tumorigenicity [95]. The ultimate mechanism that determines the expression of the tumorigenic phenotype by cells derived from chemically treated human breast epithelial cells is not known, but other studies have allowed us to conclude that tumorigenesis in a heterologous host emerges in chemically treated immortal cells as a consequence of clonal expansion, in which phenotypes indicative of neoplastic transfor-

mation are cumulatively expressed through successive processes of selection over long periods of time. During the process of neoplastic transformation no chromosomal changes were detected. The molecular events that are operational in each phase of the transformation process indicate that each carcinogen induces different degrees of point mutations in codons 12 and 61 of the *c-Ha-ras* oncogene [199] as an event detectable by the 10th passage post-carcinogen treatment. Other genes such as p53, Rb and erbB2 were differently expressed by the various clones derived from carcinogen-treated cells [200, 201].

7.6.3 Ha-ras Enhances the Transformation of Human Breast Epithelial Cells with Chemical Carcinogens

The levels and localization of ras expression in normal and malignant breast tissues have been examined and quantitated by analyzing breast tissue samples for the expression of ras related mRNA and p2 1 ras protein which has been found to be expressed in biopsies of both normal and malignant breast tissues [202]. However, whether the ras oncogene is a causative agent of human breast cancer have not been proved as yet. Therefore, one way to evaluate the contribution of ras genes in the development of the tumorigenic phenotype is to introduce this gene into suitable acceptor cells. Transfection of the non tumorigenic cell lines, clones D3-1 and BP1, derived from the carcinogen-treated MCF-10F cell lines, and the MCF-10F cell line with the cHa-ras oncogene not only enhanced colony formation in agar-methocel and invasiveness but induced tumorigenicity with a short latency period in SCID mice (Tables 7.14, 7.15).

The MCF-10F cells, DMBA or BP-treated cells and the clones D3-1 and BPI did not exhibit tumorigenicity in SCID mice. We have already shown that the subclone BP1-E derived from BP1, expressed the tumorigenic phenotype after 101 days of inoculation (Table 7.15) whereas the MCF-10F-Tras had lower tumorigenicity because it took 99 days to induce tumors in 3/14 animals, the clones D3-1-Tras and BPI-Tras were highly tumorigenic and the tumors appeared between 47 and 60 days post-inoculation, in 4 out of 4

Table 7.14. Anchorage independency and invasion assay (reprinted with permission from: Calaf, G., Zhang, P.L., Alvarado, M.V., Estrada, S. and Russo, J. *C-Ha-ras* enhances the neoplastic transformation of human breast epithelial cells treated with chemical carcinogens. Int. J. Oncol. 6: 5–11, 1995)

Cell lines (cells/filter)	Days in vitro	Number of passages	Colony[g] number (CN)	Colony[h] efficiency (%) mean ± SE	Chemotactic[i] Index (cells/filter) mean ± SE	Chemoinvasive[j] index mean ± SE
MCF-10F	308	31–37[a]	0±0	0.0±0	53±6	121±12
MCF-10F-Tras	160	128–131[b]	1,850±100	52.6±1	260.2±26	180.0±45
T24 cell line	NA	NA	1,990±100	50.0±1	677.0±136	1,124±489
MCF-7 cell line	NA	NA	2,050±200	52.0±1	215.0±58	93±48
DMBA	119	8[c]	52±2	9.7±1	138.0±42	170±90
Clone D3	292	20–21[d]	829±139	90.3±2	112.0±10	182±3
Subclone D3-1	455	8–10[e]	2,200±180	83.6±9	438.0±11	523±137
Clone D3-1-Tras	455	5[b]	2,850±300	94.0±4	540.0±50	1,680±300
BP	141	8[f]	43±2	3.2±1	ND	ND
Clone BPI	292	18–20,32,42[d]	554±77	45.0±12	970±79	457±43
Subclone BPI-Eh	498	10–20[e]	1,700±100	88.0±10	682±230	820±180
Clone BPI-Tras	480	131[b]	4,400±100	97.0±10	2,376.0±548	2,421±792

[a] Number of passages after DMSO (control) treatment
[b] Number of passages after insertion of *c-Ha-ras* oncogene in the control MCF-10F, D3-1 and BPI cell lines, respectively
[c] Number of passages after DMBA treatment
[d] Number of passages after colony emergence in agar methocel from DMBA and BP-treated cells
[e] Number of passages of D3-1 and BPI-E after removal of the colonies derived from D3, and BPI generation
[f] Number of passages after BP treatment
[g] CN numbers of colonies per well formed in the agar methocel
[h] Colony efficiency (%), mean ± SE of three experiments, standard error of the mean (SE)
[i] Number of cells attached to the lower surface of the filter in the Boyden-type chamber mean ± SE of three experiments
[j] Number of cells that crossed a reconstituted basement membrane; mean ± SE of three experiments. Student's *t*-test for the differences in the chemotactic and chemoinvasive indices were significant ($p < 0.001$) between MCF-10F cells and all the other cell lines tested

animals and 11 out of 14 animals, respectively (Table 7.15). All the tumors derived from D3-1-Tras and BP1-Tras cells were poorly differentiated adenocarcinomas (Figs. 7.38, 7.39; Table 7.15). They were immunocytochemically positive for keratin (Fig. 7.39e) whereas the human milk fat globule membrane antigen (HMFGMA) was frankly expressed only in tumors induced by BP1-E cells; tumors derived from *c-Ha-ras* transfected cells showed either a notably reduced expression of this antigen, as observed in D3-1-Tras induced tumors, in which only 10% of the tumor cells were positive (Fig. 7.39f), or complete abolishment of HMFGMA reactivity, as in the BP1-Tras induced tumor cells. Tumor cell lines derived from the tumors thus originated have been an important resource for understanding the molecular basis of mammary carcinogenesis (Fig. 7.40) (see Chapter 8).

Altogether the data presented in this chapter summarize an in vitro model of breast cancer in which

Table 7.15. Tumorigenic assay and immunohistochemical studies (reprinted with permission from: Calaf, G., Zhang, P.L., Alvarado, M.V., Estrada, S. and Russo, J. *C-Ha-ras* enhances the neoplastic transformation of human breast epithelial cells treated with chemical carcinogens. Int. J. Oncol. 6: 5–11, 1995)

Cell lines	Number of cells injected ($\times 10^6$)	Number of animals with tumors/total animals[a]	Tumor size (mm^3)	Latency[b] (days)	Keratin[c] (immunochemical reaction)	HMFGMA[d] (immunochemical reaction)
MCF-0F	7–30	0/5	–	–	+	+
MCF-10F-Tras	17	1/14	4.8	99	+	+
T24 cell line	10	3/3	5.3	10	+	–
MCF-7 cell line	9	2/2	20.0	28	+	+
Clone D3	37	0/9	–	–	+	+
Subclone D3-1	16	0/10	–	–	+	+
Clone D3-1-Tras	10	4/4	6.1	47	+	+
Clone D3-1-Tras tumor	–	–	–	–	+	+ (10%)
Clone BP1	20	0/8	–	–	+	+
Subclone BPI-E	10	3/11	9.5	101–124	+	+
Clone BPI-Tras	13	11/14	6.8	60	+	+
Clone BPI-Tras tumor	–	–	–	–	+	–

[a] Number of animals with tumors per total number of animals injected
[b] Number of days between the day of cell injection and the day the first tumor appeared
[c] and [d] keratin and HMFGMA expression detected by immunochemical reactions

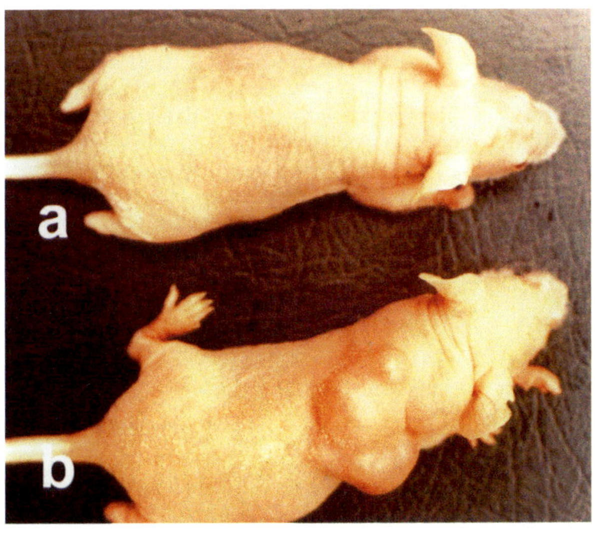
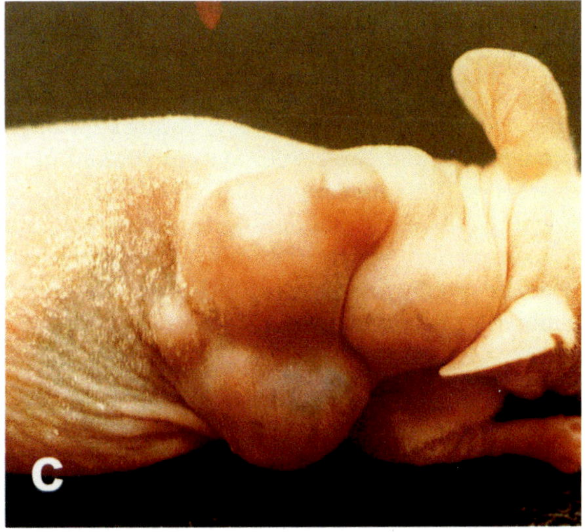

Figure 7.38 a–c

a Nude mice inoculated with MCF10F cells. **b** Nude mice inoculated with BP1-T-ras cells. **c** Detail of tumors induced in nude mice by the inoculum of BP1-Tras cells

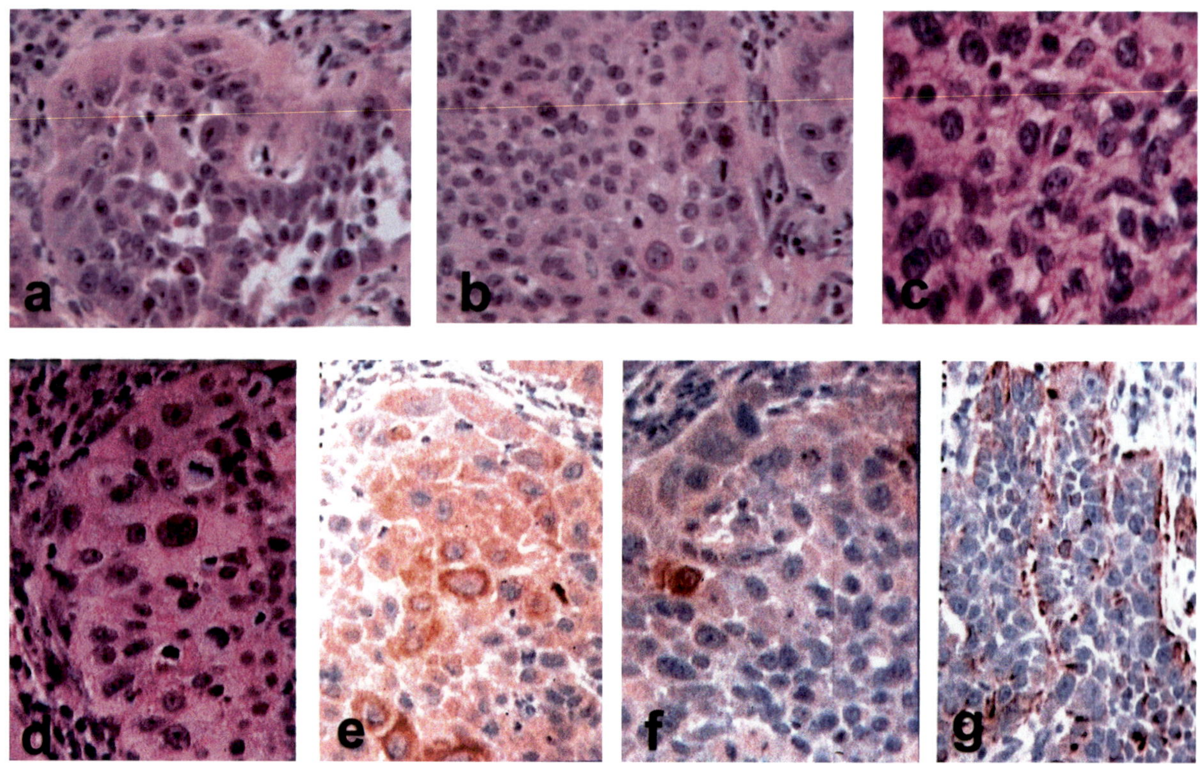

the final malignant phenotype of tumorigenesis can be induced in HBEC by carcinogen treatment alone or in combination with *ras* oncogene, provided that the treated cells are previously immortalized and enough time and clone selection are allowed for its expression. This model provided clones of cells expressing different stages of progression to malignant transformation, which are useful for determining whether specific phenotypes are the result of specific genotypic alterations.

Figure 7.39.a–g

Histological sections of tumors induced in heterologous hosts. **a, b** Sections stained with H&E of tumors induced by BP1-E cells, ×40. **c, d** Poorly differentiated adenocarcinomas induced by c-Has ras transformed cells, ×40. **e** Immunocytochemical reaction against keratin AE1 and AE3 in tumors induced by BP1-Tras, ×40. **f** Same tumor as shown in **e** immunoreacted against milk fat globule membrane antigen, ×40. **g** Same tumor as shown in **e** immunoreacted against vimentin, ×40

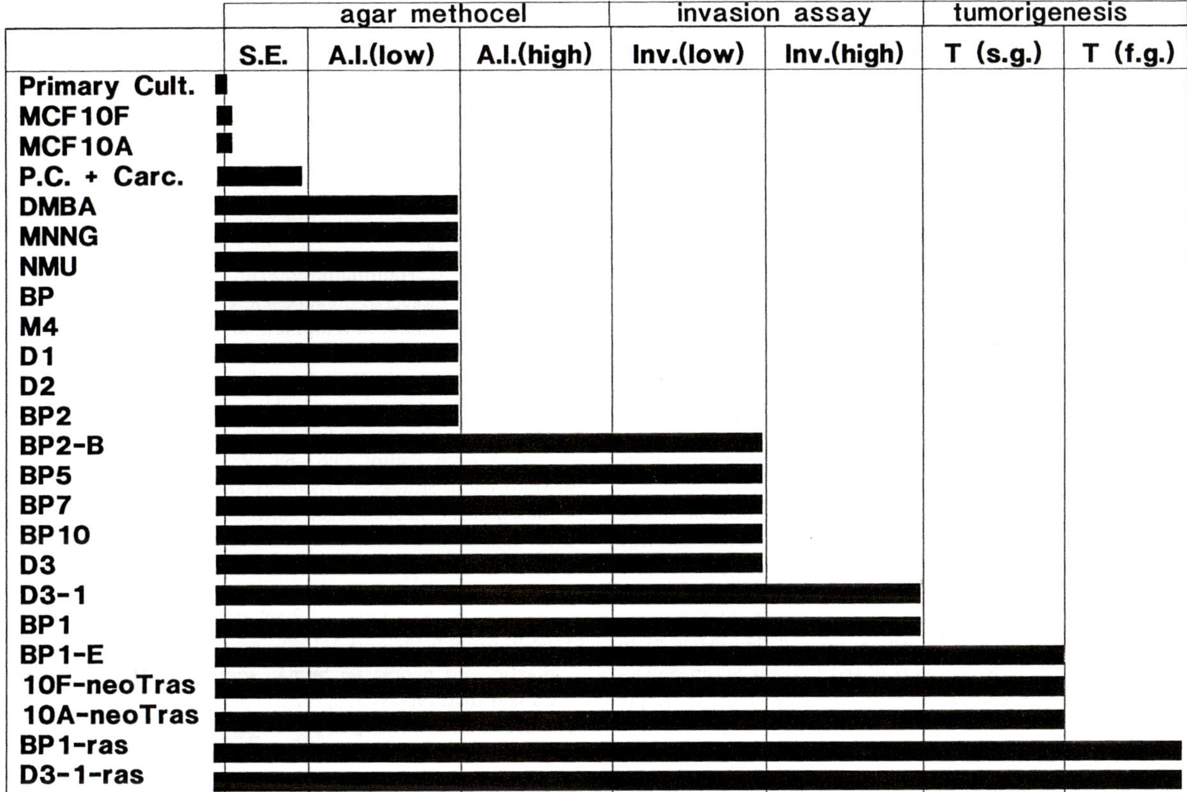

Figure 7.40

Expression of malignant phenotypes. Comparison of HBEC primary cultures, MCF-10A and MCF-10F, carcinogen-treated cells, derived clones, and c-ras transfected cells respectively. *S.E.* survival efficiency, *A.I.* anchorage independent growth, *Inv.* invasiveness, *T* tumorigenesis, *s.g.* slow growth, *f.g.* fast growth (reprinted with permission from: Russo, J et al. Critical steps in breast carcinogenesis. The New York Academy of Sciences 698: 1–20, 1993)

References

1. Russo, J., Calaf, G., and Russo, I.H. A critical approach to the malignant transformation of human breast epithelial cells with chemical carcinogens. Crit. Rev. Oncogenesis 44:403–417, 1993.
2. Farber, E. The multistep nature of cancer development. Cancer Res. 44:4217–4223, 1984.
3. Page, D.J. and Dupont, W.D. Anatomic markers of human premalignancy and risk breast cancer. Cancer 66:1326–1335, 1990.
4. Russo, J., Calaf, G., Sohi, N., Tahin, N.Q., Zhang, P.L., Alvarado, M.E., Estrada, S., and Russo, I.H. Critical steps in breast carcinogenesis. Ann. NY Acad. Sci. USA 698:1–20, 1993.
5. Tait, L., Soule, H.D. and Russo, J. Ultrastructural and immunocytochemical characterization of an immortalized human breast epithelial cell line, MCF-10. Cancer Res. 50: 6087–6094, 1990.
6. Slater, C.M., Lareef, M.H., Russo, I.H., Tomaz, J., Band, V., and Russo, J. S100p is a marker of cell immortalization, preceding phenotypic expression of neoplastic transformation in human breast epithelial cells. Proc. Am. Assoc. Cancer Res. 42:4784a, 2001.

7. Soule, H.D., Vazquez J., Long A., Albert S., Brennan, M. A human cell line from a pleural effusion derived from a breast carcinoma. J Natl. Cancer Inst. 51: 1409–1416, 1973

8. McGrath, C., Grant, P.M, Soule, H.D., Glancy, T., Rich, M.A. Replication of oncornavirus-like particle in human breast carcinoma cell line, MCF-7. Nature 252: 247–250, 1974

9. Rose HN, McGrath C. α-Lactalbumin production in human mammary carcinoma. Science 190: 673–675, 1975.

10. Brooks, S.C., Locke, E.R., Soule, H.D. Estrogen receptor in a human cell line (MCF-7) from breast carcinoma. J. Biol. Chem. 248: 6251–6253, 1973.

11. Horwitz, K.B., Costlow, M.E., McGuire, W.L. MCF-7: A human breast cancer cell line with estrogen, androgen, progesterone and glucocorticoid receptors. Steroids 26: 785–795, 1975.

12. Russo, J., Soule, H.D., McGrath, C., Rich, M.A. Re-expression of the original tumor pattern by a human breast. carcinoma cell line (MCF-7) in sponge cultures J. Natl. Cancer Inst. 56: 279–282, 1976.

13. Russo, J., Brennan, M.J., Rich, M.A. Induction of tumor growth by inoculation of a human breast cancer cell line MCF-7 into ovary or pituitary grafted nude mice. Proc. Amer. Cancer Soc.17: 116a, 1976.

14. Russo, J., McGrath, C.M., Russo, I.H. and Rich, M.A. Tumoral growth of a human breast cancer cell line (MCF-7) in athymic mice. In: Nieburgs H.E.. (ed.), III Int. Symp. on Detection and Prevention of Cancer, New York, 1976, pp. 617–626.

15. Arnold, W.J., Soule, H.D., Russo, J. Fine structure of a human mammary carcinoma cell line, MCF-7. In Vitro 10: 356, 1975.

16. Pickett, P.B., Pitelka, D.R., Hamamoto, S.T., Misfeldt, D.S. Occluding junctions and cell behavior in primary clusters of normal and neoplastic mammary gland cells. J. Cell Biol. 66: 316–332, 1975.

17. Buehring, G.C., Hackett, A.J. Human breast tumor cell lines: Identity evaluation by ultrastructure. J. Natl. Cancer Inst. 53: 621–629, 1974.

18. Ozzello, L., Ultrastructure of the human mammary gland. In: Summers SC. (ed), Pathology Annual. Appleton-Century-Crofts, New York. 1971. pp 1–59.

19. Pierce, G.B., Nakane, P.K. Basement membranes: Synthesis and deposition in response to cellular injury. Lab Inv 21: 27–41, 1969.

20. Russo, J., Bradley, R., Soule, H.D. Ultrastructural study of human mammary carcinoma cells (MCF-7) grown in collagen-coated sponge. Proc. Electron Microsc. Soc. Amer. 1975, p 392–393.

21. Murad, T.M. Ultrastructure of ductular carcinoma of the breast (in situ and infiltrating lobular carcinoma). Cancer 27: 18–28, 1971.

22. Russo, J., Furmanski, P., Bradley, R., Wells, P., Rich, M. Differentiation of normal mammary epithelial cells in culture: An ultrastructural study. Amer. J. Anat. 145: 57–78, 1976.

23. Tannenbaum M, Weiss M, Marx AJ: Ultrastructure of the human mammary ductule. Cancer 23: 958–978, 1969.

24. Fanger, H., Ree, H.J. Cyclic changes of human mammary gland epithelium in relation to the menstrual cycle–An ultrastructural study. Cancer 14: 574–585, 1974.

25. Young, R.K., Cailleau, R., Mackay, B., Reeves, W.J. Establishment of epithelial cell line MDA-IIB-157 from metastatic pleural effusion of human breast carcinoma. In Vitro 9: 239–245, 1974.

26. Cailleau, R., Young, R., Olive, M., Reeves, W.J. Breast tumor cell lines from pleural effusions. J Natl. Cancer Inst. 53: 661–674, 1974.

27. Pitelka, D.R., Hammamoto, S.T., Duafala, J.G., Nemanic, M.K. Cell contacts in the mouse mammary gland. I Normal gland in postnatal development and the secretory cycle. J. Cell Biol. 56: 797–818, 1973.

28. Arnold, W.J., Soule, H.D., Russo, J.: Fine structure of a murine mammary carcinoma cell line. In Vitro 12: 57–64, 1976.

29. Archer, F.L. Normal and neoplastic human tissue in organ culture. Arch. Pathol. 85:62–69, 1968.

30. Matoska, J., Siracky, J. Histology and ultrastructure of human breast cancer in organ culture. Neoplasma 21:685–696, 1974.

31. Tchao, R., Easty, G.C., Ambrose, E.J., et al. Effect of chemotherapeutic agents and hormones on organ culture of human tumors. Eur. J. Cancer 4:39–45, 1968.

32. Wellings, S.R., Jentoff, V.L. Organ culture of normal, dysplastic, and neoplastic human mammary tissues. J. Natl. Cancer Inst. 49:329–338, 1972.

33. Mareel, L.M., Varaet, L., De Ridder, L.A. Possibility of distinction between normal and neoplastic cells through transplantation into chick blastoderms. J. Natl. Cancer Inst. 51:809–815, 1973.

34. Mareel, L.M., Varaet, L., De Ridder, L. A., et al: Possibility of distinction between malignant and nonmalignant cells by transplantation into chick blastoderms: Further evidence from animal and human biopsy specimens. J. Natl. Cancer Inst 53:1351–1358, 1974.

35. Leighton, J., Justh, G., Esper, M., et al. Collagen-coated cellulose sponge: Three dimensional matrix for tissue culture of Walker tumor 256. Science 155:1259–1261, 1967.

36. Leighton, J., Mark, R., Justh, G. Patterns of three-dimensional growth in vitro in collagen coated cellulose sponge: Carcinomas and embryonic tissues. Cancer Res. 28:286–296, 1968.

37. Leighton, J. Collagen-coated cellulose sponge. In Tissue Culture-Methods and Applications (Kruse PF, Patterson MK, eds.). New York, Academic Press, 1973, pp 367–371.

38. Russo, J., Soule, H.D., McGrath, C., Rich, M.A. Reexpression of the original tumor pattern by a human breast carcinoma cell line (MCF-7) in sponge culture. J. Natl. Cancer Inst.56: 279–282,1976.

39. Sandford, K.K., Dunn, T.B., Westfall, B.B., et al. Sarcomatous change and maintenance of differentiation in long-term cultures of mouse mammary carcinoma. J Natl. Cancer Inst 26:1139–1183, 1961.

40. Sanford, K.K. Biologic Manifestation of Oncogenesis In Vitro: A critique. J. Natl. Cancer Inst., 53: 1481–1485, 1974.

41. Giovanella, B.C., Stehlin, J.S., and Williams, L.J. Jr. Development of Invasive Tumors in the "Nude" Mouse after Injection of Cultured Human Melanoma Cells. J. Natl. Cancer Inst., 48: 1531–1533, 1972.

42. Giovanella, B.C., Stehlin, J.S. Heterotransplantation of Human Malignant Tumors in "Nude" Thymusless Mice. I. Breeding and Maintenance of "Nude" Mice. J. Natl. Cancer Inst., 51: 615–619, 1973.

43. Giovanella, B.C., Stehlin, J.S., and Williams, L.J. Jr. Heterotransplantation of Human Malignant Tumors in "Nude" Thymusless Mice. II. Malignant Tumors Induced by Injection of Cell Cultures Derived from Human Solid Tumors. J. Natl. Cancer Inst., 52: 921–930, 1974.

44. Povlsen, C.O., Fialkow, P.J., Klein, E. Growth and Antigenic Properties of a Biopsy-Derived Burkitt's Lymphoma in Thymusless (Nude) Mice. Intl. J. Cancer, 11: 30–39, 1973.

45. DeOme, K.B., Faulkin, J.1 t. Jr., Bern, H.A., and Blair, P.B. Development of Mammary Tumors from Hyperplastic Alveolar Nodules Transplanted into Gland-Free Mammary Fat Pads of Female C3H Mice. Cancer Res., 19: 350–359, 1959.

46. Rygaard, J., Povlsen, C.O. Heterotransplantation of a Human Malignant Tumor to "Nude" Mice. Acta Pathol. Microbiol. Scand.,77: 758–760, 1969.

47. Greene, H.S.N. The Significance of the Heterologous Transplantability of Human Cancer. Cancer, 5: 24–44, 1952.

48. Russo, J., and McGrath, C.M. Scirrhous Carcinoma in the Mouse: A Model for Human Mammary Carcinoma. Excerpta Medica, Amsterdam, 488, 1975.

49. Shafie, S.M., Giartham, F.H., Role of hormones in the growth and regression of human breast cancer cells (MCF-7) transplanted into athymic mice. J. Natl. Cancer Inst. 67:51–56, 1981.

50. Band, V., Zagetowski, D., Kulesa V., and Sager, R. Human papilloma virus DNAs immortalize normal human mammary epithelial cells and reduce their growth factor requirements. Proc. Natl. Acad. Sci. USA 87:463–467 1990.

51. Band, V., Dalal, S., Delmolino, L., and Androphy, E.L. Enhanced degradation of p53 protein in IIPV-6 and BPV-1 E6-immortalized human mammary epithelial cells. EMBO J. 12:1847–1852, 1993.

52. Yilmaz, A., Gaide, A.C., Sordat, B., Borbeny, Z., Lahm, H., Imam, A., Shreyer, M., and Odartehenko, L. Malignant progression of SV40-immortalized human milk epithelial cells. Br. J. Cancer 68:868–873, 1993.

53. Soule, H.D., Maloney, T.M., Wolman, S.R., Peterson, W.D., Brenz, R., McGrath, Ch.M., Russo, J., Pauley, R.J., Jones, R.F. and Brooks, S.C. Isolation and characterization of a spontaneously immortalized human breast epithelial cell line, MCF-10. Cancer Res., 50, 6075–6086, 1990.

54. Russo, J. and Russo, I.H. (1987) Development of the human mammary gland. In Neville, M.C. and Daniel, C. (eds), The Mammary Gland Development, Regulation and Function. Plenum, New York, Chap. 3, p. 67.

55. Harley, C.B. Telomere loss: mitotic clock or genetic time bomb? Mutat. Res. 256:271–282, 1991.

56. Hopfer, U., Jacobberger, J.W., Gruenert, D.C., Eckert, R.L., Jat, P.S., Whitsett, J.A. Immortalization of epithelial cells. Am. J. Physiol. 270:C1-C11, 1996.

57. Blackburn, E.H. Structure and function of telomeres. Nature 350:569–573, 1991.

58. Shay, J.W., Wright, W.E., Werbin, H. Loss of telomeric DNA during aging may predispose cells to cancer. Int. J. Oncol. 3:559–563, 1993.

59. Shay, J.W., Wright, W.E., Werbin, H. Defining the molecular mechanisms of human cell immortalization. Biochem. Biophys. Acta. 1072:1–7, 1991.

60. Bacchetti, S., Counter, C.M. Telomeres and telomerase in human cancer. Int. J. Oncol. 7:423–432, 1995.

61. Avilion, A.A., Piatyszek, M.A., Gupta, J., Shay, J.W., Bacchetti, S., Greider, C.W. Human telomerase RNA and telomerase activity in immortal cell lines and tumor tissues. Cancer Res. 56:645–650, 1996.

62. Higgy, N.A., Russo, J., Mgbonyebi, P., Salicioni, A.M., Russo, I.H. Human chorionic gonadotropin inhibits telomerase activity in human breast epithelial cells in vitro. Proc. Am. Assoc. Cancer Res. 39:541, 1998.

63. Barnabas, N., Moraes, R., Calaf, G., Estrada, S., and Russo, J. Role of p53 in MCF-10F cell immortalization and chemically-induced neoplastic transformation. Int. J. Oncol. 7:1289–1296, 1995.

64. Shay, J.W., Wright, W.E., and Werbin, H. Toward a molecular understanding of human breast Cancer – A hypothesis. Breast Cancer Res. Treat. 25:83–94 1993.

65. Russo, J., Barnabas, N., Higgy, N., Salicioni, A.M., Wu, Y.L. and Russo, I.H. Molecular basis of human breast epithelial cell transformation. In: Breast Cancer. Advances in biology and Therapeutics. (F. Calvo, M. Crepin and H. Magdelenat, Eds) John Libbey, Eurotext, 1996. pp. 33–43.

66. Gollahon, L.S. and Shay, J.W. Immortalization of human mammary epithelial cells transfected with mutant p53 (273[his]). Oncogene 12:715–725, 1996.

67. Gao, Q., Hauser, S.H., Liu, X.L., Wazer, D.E., Madoc-Jones, H. and Band, V. Mutant p53-induced immortalization of primary human mammary epithelial cells. Cancer Res. 56:3129–3133, 1996.

68. Matsushime, H., Ewen, M.E., Strom, D.K., Kato, J.Y., Hanks, S.K., Roussel, M.F. and Sherr, C.J. Identification and properties of an atypical catalytic subunit (p34PSKJIIcII4) for mammalian D type G1 cyclins. Cell 71: 323–334, 1992.

69. Hunter, T., and Pines, J. Cyclins and cancer. Cell 66: 1071–1074, 1991.

70. Lukas, J., Pagano, M., Staskova, Z., Draetta, G. and Bartek, J. Cyclin D1 protein oscillates and is essential for cell cycle progression in human tumor cell lines. Oncogene 9: 707–718, 1994.

71. Keyomarsi, K., O'Leary, N., Molnar, G., Lees, E., Fingert, H.J. and Pardee, A. Cyclin E, a potential prognostic marker for breast cancer. Cancer Res. 54: 3 80–3 85, 1994.

72. Wang, J., Zindy, F., Chenivesse, X., Lamas, E., Henglein, B., and Brechot, C. Modification of cyclin A expression by hep-

atitis B virus DNA integration in a hepatocellular carcinoma. Oncogene 7:1653–1656, 1992.

73. Lammie, G.A., Fantl, V., Smith, R., Schuuring, E., Brookes, S., Michalides, R., Dickson, C., Arnold, A. and Peters, G. D11S128, a putative oncogene on chromosome 11q13 is amplified and expressed in squamous cell and mammary carcinomas and lined BCL-1. Oncogene 6: 439–444, 1991.

74. Lebwohl, D.E., Muise-Helmericks, R., Sepp-Lorenzino, L., Serve, S., Timaul, M., Bol, R., Borgen, P. and Rosen, N. A truncated cyclin D1 gene encodes a stable MRNA in a human breast cancer cell line. Oncogene 9: 1925–1929, 1994.

75. Sherr, C.J. Mammalian G1 cyclins. Cell 73: 1059–1065, 1993.

76. Zwijsen, R.M., Wientjens, E., Klompmaker, R., van der Sman, J., Bemards, R., and Michalides, R.J.A.M. CDK-independent activation of estrogen receptor by cyclin D1. Cell 88: 405–415, 1997.

77. Hu, Y.F., Lau, K.M., Ho, S.M. and Russo, J. Increased expression of estrogen receptor β in chemically transformed human breast epithelial cells. Int. J. Oncol. 12: 1225–1228, 1998.

78. Zajchowski, D.A. and Sager, R. Induction of estrogen-regulated genes differs in immortal and tumorigenic human mammary epithelial cells expressing a recombinant estrogen receptor. Mol, Endocrinol, 5: 1613–1623, 1991.

79. Nielsen, N.H., Emdin, S.O., Cajander, J,. and Landberg, G. Deregulation of cyclin E and D1 in breast cancer is associated with inactivation of the retinoblastoma protein. Oncogene 14: 295–304, 1997.

80. Buckley, M.F., Sweeney, K.J., Hamilton, J.A., Sini, R.L., Manning, D.L., Nicholson, R.I., De Fazio, A., Watts, C.K., Musgrove, E.A. and Sutherland, R.L. Expression and amplification of cyclin genes in human breast cancer. Oncogene 8: 2127–2133, 1993.

81. Sewing, A,. Ronicke, V., Burger, C., Funk, M. and Muller, R. Alternative splicing of human cyclin E. J. Cell Sci. 107: 581–588, 1994.

82. Han, E.K.H., Begemann, M., Sgambato, A., Soh, J.W., Doki, Y., Xing, W.Q., Liu. W., and Weinstein, I.B. Increased expression of cyclin D1 in a murine mammary epithelial cell line induces p27 ^{kipl}, inhibits growth, and enhances apoptosis. Cell Growth Differ. 7: 699–710, 1996.

83. Dynlacht, B.D., Flores, 0., Lees, J.A. and Harlow, E. Differential regulation of E2F trans-activation by cyclin/cdk2 complexes. Genes Dev. 8: 1772–1786, 1994.

84. Meikrantz, W., Gisselbrecht, S., Tam, S.W. and Schlegel, R. Activation of cyclin A-dependent protein kinases during apoptosis. Proc. Natl. Acad. Sci. USA 91: 3754–3758, 1994.

85. Smith, L.M., Birrer, M.J., Stampfer, M.R. and Brown, P.H. Breast cancer cells have lower activating protein I transcription factor activity than normal mammary epithelial cells. Cancer Res. 57: 3046–3054, 1997.

86. Jupe, F.R., Liu, X.T., Kielbauch, J.L., McClung, J.K. and Dell'Orco, R.T. Prohibitin antiproliferative activity and lack of heterozygosity in immortalized cell lines. Exp. Cell Res. 218:877–880, 1995.

87. Higgy, N.A., Salicioni, A.M., Russo, I.H., Zhang, P.L. and Russo, J. Differential expression of human ferritin H chain gene in immortal human breast epithelial cells MCF-10F. Mol. Carcinog. 20:332–339, 1997.

88. Silva, D.C.G., Hu, Y-F., Russo, I.H., Ao, X., Salicioni, A.M., Yang, X., and Russo, J. S100P CA^{+2} –binding Protein Overexpression is Associated with Immortalization and Neoplastic Transformation of Human Breast Epithelial Cells in vitro and Tumor Progression in vivo. Int. J. Oncol. 16:231–240, 2000.

89. Ochieng, J., Tahin, Q.S., Booth, C.C. and Russo, J. Buffering of intracellular calcium in response to increased extracellular levels in mortal, immortal and transformed human breast epithelial cells. Journal of Cellular Biochemistry 46:1–5, 1991.

90. Huang, Y., Bove, B., Wu, Y., Russo, I.H., Tahin, Q., Yang, X., Zekri, A., Russo, J. Microsatellite Instability During the Immortalization and Transformation of Human Breast Epithelial Cells In vitro. Mol. Carcinog. 24:118–127 1999.

91. Montesano, R. and Tomatis, L. Legislation concerning chemical carcinogens in several industrialized countries. Cancer Res., 37:310–316, 1977.

92. Doll, R. An epidemiological perspective of the biology of cancer. Cancer Res., 38:3573–3583, 1978.

93. DiPaolo, J.A. Relative difficulties in transforming human and animal cells in vitro. J. Natl. Cancer Inst., 70:3–8, 1983.

94. Chang, S.E. In vitro transformation of human epithelial cells. Biochim. Biophys. Acta, 823:161–194, 1986.

95. Stampfer, M.R. and Bartley, J.C. Induction of transformation and continuous cell lines from normal human mammary epithelial cells after exposure to benzo[a]pyrene. Proc. Natl Acad. Sci. U.S.A., 82:2394–2398, 1984.

96. Russo, J., Reina, D., Frederick, J. and Russo, I.H. Expression of phenotypical changes by human breast epithelial cells treated with carcinogens in vitro. Cancer Res., 48:2837–2857, 1988.

97. Calaf, G. and Russo, J. Transformation of human breast epithelial cells by chemical carcinogens Carcinogenesis, 14:483–492, 1993.

98. Russo, J., Barnabas, N., Zhang, P.L. and Adesina, K. Molecular basis of breast cell transformation. Radiat. Oncol. Invest., 3:424–429, 1996.

99. Hu, Y.F., Russo, I.H., Zalipsky, U., Lynch, H.T and Russo, J. Environmental chemical carcinogens induce transformation of breast epithelial cells from women with familial history of breast cancer. *In vitro* Cell. Dev. Biol. 33: 495–498, 1997.

100. Traul, K.A., Takayama, K., Kachevsky, V., Hink, R.J. and Wolff, J.S. A rapid in vitro assay for carcinogenicity of chemical substances in mammalian cells utilizing an attachment independence endpoint-2-assay validations. J. Appl. Toxicol. 1:190, 1981.

101. Putnam, D.L., Park, D.K., Rhim, J.S., Stever, A.F. and Ting, R.C.. Correlation of cellular aggregation of transformed

cells and their growth in soft agar and tumorigenic potential. Proc. Soc. Exp. Biol. Med., 155:487–494, 1977.

102. Chan, W.K., Poulsom, R., Lu, Q.L., Patel, K., Gregory, W., Fisher, C.J. and Hanby, A.M. Bcl-2 expression in invasive mammary carcinoma: correlation with apoptosis, hormone receptors and p53 expression. J. Pathol., 169:153A, 1993.

103. Gee, J.M., Robertson, J.F., Ellis, I.O., Willsher, P., McClelland, R.A., Hoyle, H.B., Kyme, S.R., Finlay, P., Blamey, R.W. and Nicholson, R.I. Immunocytochemical localization of BCL-2 protein in human breast cancers and its relationship to a series of prognostic markers and response to endocrine therapy. Int. J. Cancer, 59:619–628, 1994.

104. Buckley, M.F., Sweeney, K.J.E., Hamilton, J.A., Sini, R.L., Manning, D.L., Nicholson, R.I., deFazio, A., Watts, C.K.W., Musgrove, E.A. and Sutherland, R.L. Expression and amplification of cyclin genes in human breast cancer. Oncogene, 8:2127–2133, 1993.

105. Bartkova, J., Lukas, J., Müller, H., Lützhoft, D., Strauss, M. and Bartek, J. Cyclin D1 protein expression and function in human breast cancer. Int. J. Cancer, 57:353–361, 1994.

106. Gillet, C., Fantl, V., Smith, R., Fisher, C., Bartek, J., Dickson, C., Barnes, D. and Peters, G. Amplification and overexpression of cyclin D1 in breast cancer detected by immunohistochemical staining. Cancer Res., 54:1812–1817, 1994.

107. Zhang, S.Y., Camano, J., Cooper, F., Guo, X. and Klein-Szanto, A. Immunohistochemistry of cyclin D1 in human breast cancer. Am. J. Clin. Path., 102:695–698, 1994.

108. Weistat-Saslow, D., Merino, M.J., Richard, E.M., Lawrence, J.A., Bluth, R.F., Wittenbel, K.D., Simpson, J.F., Page, D.L. and Steeg, P.A. Overexpression of cyclin D mRNA distinguish invasive and in situ breast carcinomas from non-malignant lesions. Nature Med., 1:1257–1260, 1995.

109. Nakagawa, K., Yamamura, K., Maeda, S. and Ichihashi, M. bcl-2 expression in epidermal keratinocytic diseases. Cancer, 74:1720–1724, 1994.

110. Sabourin, J.C., Martin, A., Baruch, J., Truce, J.B., Gompel, A. and Poitout, P. bcl-2 expression in normal breast tissue during the menstrual cycle. Int. J. Cancer, 59:1–6, 1994.

111. Lauwers, G.Y., Scott, G.V., Hendricks, J. Immunohistochemical evidence of aberrant bcl-2 protein expression in gastric epithelial dysplasia. Cancer, 73:2900–2904, 1994.

112. Bronner, M.P., Culin, C., Reed, J.C. and Furth, E.E. The bcl-2 proto-oncogene and the gastrointestinal epithelial tumor progression model. Am. J. Pathol., 146:20–26, 1995.

113. Lu, P.J., Lu, Q.L., Rughetti, A. and Taylor-Papadimitriou, J. bcl-2 overexpression inhibits cell death and promotes the morphogenesis, but not tumorigenesis of human mammary epithelial cells. J. Cell Biol., 129:1363–1378, 1995.

114. McDonnell, T.J. and Korsmeyer, S.J. Progression from lymphoid hyperplasia to high-grade malignant lymphoma in mice transgenic for the 4(14:18). Nature, 349:254–256, 1991.

115. Han, E.K., et al., Stable overexpression of cyclin D1 in a human mammary epithelial cell line prolongs the S-phase and inhibits growth. Oncogene, 10:953–961, 1995.

116. Musgrove, E.A., Lee, C.S., Buckley, M.F. and Sutherland, R.L. Cyclin D1 induction in breast cancer cells shortens G1 and is sufficient for cells arrested in G1 to complete the cell cycle. Proc. Natl Acad. Sci., U.S.A., 91:8022–8026, 1994.

117. Sherr, C.J., G1 phase progression: cycling on cue. Cell, 79:551–555, 1994.

118. Hinds, P.W., Dowdy, S.F., Eaton, E.N., Arnold, A. and Weinberg, R.A. Proc. Natl. Acad. Sci. U.S.A., 91:709–713, 1994.

119. Bishop, J.M. The molecular genetics of cancer. Science 235:305, 1987.

120. Zarbl, H., Sukumar, S., Arthur, A.V., Martin-Zanca, D., Barbacid, M. Direct mutagenesis of Ha-ras-1 oncogenes by N-nitroso-N-methylurea during initiation of mammary carcinogenesis in rats. Nature 315:382–385, 1985.

121. Balmain, A., Pragnell, I.B. Mouse skin carcinoma induced in vivo by chemical carcinogens have a transforming Harvey-ras oncogene. Nature 303:72–74, 1983.

122. Barbacid, M. Ras genes. Annu. Rev. Biochem. 56:779–827, 1987.

123. Bos, J.L. The *ras* gene family and human carcinogenesis. Mutat. Res. 195:255–271, 1988.

124. Sukumar, S. Ras oncogenes in chemical carcinogenesis. In: Current Topics in Microbiology and Immunology, Vol. 148. Springer Verlag, Berlin, 1989, pp. 93–114.

125. Thor, A., Qhuchi, N., Hand, P.N., et al. *Ras* gene alterations enhanced levels of *ras* p2i expression in a spectrum of benign and malignant human mammary tissues. Lab. Invest. 55:603–615, 1986.

126. DeBortoli, M.E., Abou-Issa, H., Haley, B.E., Cho-Chung, Y.S. Amplified expression of p2 1 *ras* protein in hormone-dependent mammary carcinomas of humans and rodents. Biochem. Biophys. Res. Commun. 127:699–706, 1985.

127. Clair, T., Miller, W.R., Cho-Chung, Y.S. Prognostic significance of the expression of a *ras* protein with a molecular weight of 21,000 by human breast cancer. Cancer Res. 47:5290–5293, 1987.

128. Sukumar, S., Notario, V., Martin-Zanca, D., Barbacid, M. Induction of mammary carcinomas in rats by nitrosomethylurea involves malignant activation of *H-ras-1* locus by single point mutations. Nature 306:658–661, 1983.

129. Dandekar, S., Sukumar, S., Zarbl, H., Young, U.T., Cardiff, R.D. Specific activation of the cellular Harvey-ras oncogene in dimethylbenzanthracene-induced mouse mammary tumors. Mol. Cell Biol. 6:4104–4108, 1986.

130. Sinn, E., Muller, W., Pattengale, P., Tepler, I., Wallace, R., Leder, P. Coexpression of MMTV/*v-Ha-ras* and MMTV/c-myc genes in transgenic mice: Synergistic action of oncogenes in vivo. Cell 49:465–475, 1987.

131. Redmond, S.M.S., Reichmann, E., Muller, R.G., Friis, R.R., Groner, B., Hynes, N.E. The transformation of primary and established mouse mammary epithelial cells by p2 1 *ras* is concentration dependent. Oncogene 2:259–265, 1988.

132. Hynes, N.E., Jaggi, R., Kozman, S.C., et al. New acceptor cell for transfected genomic DNA: Oncogene transfer into a

mouse mammary epithelial cell line. Mol Cell Biol 5:268–272, 1985.

133. Gunzburg, W.H., Salmons, B., Schlaeffti, A., et al. Expression of oncogenes *mil* and *ras* abolishes the in vivo differentiation of mammary epithelial cells. Carcinogenesis 9:1849–1856, 1988.

134. Clark, R., Stampfer, M.R., Milley, R., et al. Transformation of human mammary epithelial cells by oncogenic retroviruses. Cancer Res. 48:4689–4694,1988.

135. Liderau, R., Callahan, R., Dickson, C., Peters, G., Escot, C, Ali, I.U. Amplification of the *int-2* gene in primary human breast tumors. Oncogene Res. 2:285–291, 1988.

136. Kraus, M.H., Uyasa, Y, Aaronson, S.A. A position 12-activated H-ras oncogene in all HS578T mammary carcinosarcoma cells but not normal mammary cells of the same patient. Proc. Natl. Acad. Sci, USA 81:5384–5388, 1984.

137. Sukumar, S., Carney, W.P., Barbacid, M. Independent molecular pathways in initiation and loss of hormone responsiveness of breast carcinomas. Science 240:524–526, 1988.

138. Spandidos, D.A., Wilkie, N.M. Malignant transformation of early passage rodent cells by a single mutated human oncogene. Nature 310:469–475, 1984

139. Slamon, D., Godolphin, W., Jones, L.A., et al. Studies of *HER-2/neu* proto-oncogene in human breast and ovarian cancer. Science 24:707–712, 1989.

140. Yamamoto, T., Ikawa, S., Akiyama, T., et al. Similarity of protein encoded by the human c-erbB-2 gene to epidermal growth factor receptor. Nature 319:230–234, 1986.

141. Casey, G., Smith, R., McGillivray, D., Peters, G., Dickson, C. Characterization and chromosome assignment of the human homolog of *int-2*, a potential proto-oncogene. Mol Cell Biol 6:502–510,1986.

142. Spandidos, D.A., Anderson, M.L. A study of mechanisms of carcinogenesis by gene transfer of oncogenes into mammalian cells. Mutat. Res. 185:271–291, 1987.

143. Wolman, S.R., Smith, H.S., Stampfer, M., Hackett, A.J. Growth of diploid cells from breast cancer. Cancer Genet. Cytogenet. 16:49–64, 1985.

144. Muschel, R.J., Nakahara, K., Chu, E., Pozzatti, R., Liotta, A.L. Karyotypic analysis of diploid or near diploid metastatic *Ha-ras*-transf6rmed rat embryo fibroblasts. Cancer Res 46:4104–4108, 1986.

145. Chang, S.E., Ken, J., Lane, E.B., Taylor-Papadimitriou, J. Establishment and characterization of SV40-transformed human breast epithelial cell lines. J. Cancer Res. 42:2040–2053, 1982.

146. Yoakum, G.H., Lechner, J.F., Gabrielson, E.W., et al. Transformation of human bronchial epithelial cells transfected by Harvey-ras oncogene. Science 227:1174–1179, 1985.

147. Ura, H., Bonfil, R.D., Reich, R., et al. Expression of type IV collagenase and procollagen genes and its correlation with the tumorigenic, invasive and metastatic abilities of oncogene-transformed human bronchial epithelial cells. Cancer Res 49:4615–4621, 1989.

148. Soule, H.D., Maloney, T., McGrath, C.M. Phenotypic variance among cells isolated from spontaneous mouse mammary tumors in primary suspension culture. Cancer Res. 41:11 54–1167, 1981.

149. Sporn, M.B., Roberts, A.B. Autocrine growth factors and cancer. Nature 31 3:745–747, 1985.

150. Lang, W.E., Tokes, Z.A., Benedict, W.F., Sargente, N. Anchorage independent growth and plasminogen activator production by bovine endothelial cells. J. Cell Biol. 84:281–293, 1980.

151. Soule, H.D., McGrath, C.M. Estrogen-responsive proliferation of clonal human breast carcinoma cells in athymic mice. Cancer Letter 10:177–189, 1980.

152. Strange, R., Aguilar-Cordova, E., Young, U.T., Billey, H.T., Dandekar, S., Cardiff, R. Harvey-ras mediated neoplastic development in the mouse mammary gland. Oncogene 4:309–315,1989.

153. Russo, J., Tay, L., Russo, I.H. Tumor Diagnosis by Electron Microscopy. Field, Rich &Assoc., New York, 1986, pp. 15–126.

154. Salomon, D.S, Perroteau, I., Kidwell, W.R., Tam, J., Derynck, R. Loss of growth responsiveness to epidermal growth factor and enhanced production of alpha-transforming growth factors in ras-transformed mouse mammary epithelial cells. J. Cell Physiol. 130:397–409,1987.

155. Derynck, R. Transforming growth factor-alpha. Cell 54:593–595, 1988.

156. Saeki, T., Ciardello, F., McGeady, M. Transformation of a human mammary epithelial cell line following overexpression of a human transforming growth factor-alpha (TGF-alpha) gene. Proc. Am. Assoc. Cancer Res. 31:228a, 1990.

157. Ciardiello, F., McGeady, M.L., Kim, N. TGF-alpha expression is enhanced in human mammary epithelial cells transformed by an activated *c-Ha-ras* proto-oncogene but not by the *c-neu* protooncogene, and overexpression of the TGF-alpha cDNA leads to transformation. Growth and Differentiation, 1:407–420, 1990.

158. Valverius, E.M., Bates, S.E., Stampfer, M.R. Transforming growth factor-alpha production and epidermal growth factor receptor expression in normal and oncogene transformed human mammary epithelial cells. Mol. Endocrinol. 3:203–214, 1989.

159. Koszlowsky, J.M., McEvan, R., Keer, H. Prostate cancer and the invasive phenotype: Application of new in vivo and in vitro approaches. In: Fidler, I.J., Nicholson, G. (eds.) Tumor Progression and Metastasis. Alan R. Liss, Inc., New York, 1988, pp. 189–231.

160. Albini, A., Iwamoto, Y., Kleinman, H.K. A rapid in vitro assay for quantitating the invasive potential of tumor cells. Cancer Res. 47: 3239–3245, 1987.

161. Egan, S.E., McClarty, G.A., Jarolim, L., et al. Expression of H-ras correlates with metastatic potential: Evidence for direct regulation of the metastatic phenotype in 10T1/2 and NIH/3T3 cells. Mol. Cell Biol. 7:830–837, 1987.

162. Varani, J., Fliegel, S.E.G., Wilson, B. Motility of ras-H oncogene transformed NIH/3T3 cells. Invasion Metastasis 6:335–346, 1986.

163. Bolscher, J.G.M., van der Bijl, M.M.W., Neefjes, J.J., Hall, A., Smets, L.A., Ploegh, H.L. Ras (proto) oncogene induces N-linked carbohydrate modification: Temporal relationship with induction of invasive potential. EMBO J. 7:3361–3368, 1988.

164. Bondy, G.P., Wilson, S., Chambers, A.F. Experimental metastatic ability of *H-ras* transformed NIH/3T3 cells. Cancer Res. 45:6005–6009, 1985.

165. Thorgeirrson, U.P. Turpeenniemi-Hujanen, T., Williams, J.E., et al. NIH/3T3 cells transfected with human tumor DNA containing activated *ras* oncogene express the metastatic phenotype in nude mice. Mol. Cell Biol. 5:259–262, 1985.

166. Greig, R.G., Koestler, T.P., Trainer, L., et al. Tumorigenic and metastatic properties of "normal" and ras-transfected NIH/3T3 cells. Proc. Natl. Acad. Sci. USA 82:3698–3701, 1985.

167. Collard, J.G., Schijven, J.F., Roos, E. Invasive and metastatic potential induced by ras-transfection into mouse BW5147 T-lymphoma cells. Cancer Res. 47:754–759, 1987.

168. Egan, S.E., Broere, J.J., Jarolim, L, Wright, J.A., Greenberg, A.H. Coregulation of metastatic and transforming activity of normal mutant *ras* genes. Int. J. Cancer 43:443–448, 1989.

169. Albini, A., Ankerman, S.L., Noonan, D.M. The in vivo invasiveness and interactions with laminin of K-1735 melanoma cells. Clin. Exper. Metastasis 7:436–451, 1989.

170. Kumar, R., Sukumar, S., Barbacid, M. Activation of *ras* oncogene preceding the onset of neoplasia. Science 248:1101–1104,1990.

171. Huggins, C., Grand, L.C. and Brillantes, F.P. Critical significance of breast structure in the induction of mammary cancer in the rat. Proc. Natl. Acad. Sci. USA, 45, 1294–1300, 1959.

172. Russo, I.H. and Russo, J. Developmental stage of the rat mammary gland as determinant of its susceptibility to 7,12-dimethylbenz(a)anthracene. J. Natl. Cancer Inst., 61: 1439 – 1442,1978.

173. Dao, T.L., Bock, F.G. and Greiner, M. Mammary carcinogenesis by 3-methylcholantrene. Inhibitory effect of pregnancy and lactation on tumor induction. J. Natl. Cancer Inst., 25: 991–1003, 1960.

174. Russo, J. and Russo, I.H. Biological and molecular basis of mammary carcinogenesis. Lab. Invest. 57: 112–137, 1987.

175. Telang, N.T., Bannerjee, M.R., Lyer, A.P. and Kundu, A.B. Neoplastic transformation of epithelial cells in whole mammary gland in vitro. Proc. Natl. Acad. Sci. USA, 76: 5886–5890, 1979.

176. Guzman, R.C., Osbom, R.C., Bardey, J.C., Imagawa, W., Asch, B.B. and Nandi, S. In vitro transformation of mouse mammary epithelial cells grown serum free inside collagen gels. Cancer Res., 47: 275–280, 1987.

177. Miyamoto, S., Guzrnan, R.C., Osbome, R.C. and Nandi, S. Neoplastic transformation of mouse mammary epithelial cells by in vitro exposure to N-nitrosourea. Proc. Natl. Acad. Sci. USA, 85: 477–481, 1988.

178. Moore, C.J., Eldrich, S.R., Tricomi, W.R. and Gould, M.N. Quantitation of benzo(a)pyrene and 7,12-dimetylbenz(a)-anthracene binding to nuclear macromolecules in human and rat mammary epithelial cells. Cancer Res., 47: 2609–2613, 1987.

179. Russo, J., Tay, L.K. and Russo, I.H. Differentiation of the mammary gland and susceptibility to carcinogenesis. Breast Cancer Res. Treat. 2: 5–73, 1982.

180. Russo, J. and Russo, I.H. Influence of differentiation and cell kinetics on the susceptibility of the rat mammary gland to carcinogenesis. Cancer Res. 40: 2677–2687, 1980.

181. Gullino, P.M., Pettigrew, H.M. and Grantham, F.H. N-Nitrosomethylurea as mammary gland carcinogen in rats. J. Natl. Cancer Inst. 45: 401–404,1975.

182. Russo, J., Gusterson, B.A., Rogers, A.E., Russo, I.H., Wellings, S.R. and Van Zwieten, M.J. Comparative study of human and rat mammary tumorigenesis. Lab. Invest. 62: 244–278, 1990.

183. Russo, J. and Russo, I.H. Role of differentiation on transformation of human breast epithelial cells. In Medina, D. and Kidwell, W. (eds) Cellular and molecular biology of mammary cancer. Plenum Press, NY, 1987, pp. 399.

184. Stever, A.F., Rhim, J.S., Hentosh, P.M. and Ting, R.C. Survival of human cells in the aggregate form: potential index of in vitro transformation. J. Natl. Cancer Inst. 58: 917–921, 1978.

185. Putnam, D.L., Park, D.K., Rhim, J.S., Stever, A.F. and Ting, R.C. Correlation of cellular aggregation of transformed cells with their growth in soft agar and tumorigenic potential. Proc. Soc. Exp. Biol. Med. 155: 487–494, 1977.

186. Traul, K.A., Takayama, K., Kachevsky, V., Hink, R.J. and Wolff, J.S. A rapid in vitro assay for carcinogenicity of chemical substances in cells utilizing an attachment independence endpoint-2-assay validations. J. Appl. Toxicol. 1: 190–195, 1981.

187. McCormick, J.J. and Maher, V.M. Toward an understanding of malignant transformation of diploid human fibroblasts. Mutat. Res. 199: 273 –291, 1988.

188. Salomon, D.S., Ciardiello, F., Valverius, E., Sacki, T. and Kim, N. Transforming factors in human breast cancer. Biomed. Pharmacother. 43: 661–667, 1989.

189. Barrett, J.C. and Ts' O.P.0.P. Relationship between somatic mutation and neoplastic transformation. Proc. Natl. Acad. Sci. USA, 75: 3297–3301, 1978.

190. Kakunuoka, T. Neoplastic transformation of human diploid fibroblast cells by chemical carcinogen. Proc. Natl. Acad. Sci. USA, 75: 1334–1388, 1978.

191. Ochieng, J., Basolo, F., Albini, A., Melchiore, A., Watanabe, H., Elliott, J., Raz, A., Paredi, S. and Russo, J. Increased invasive chemotactic and locomotive abilities of *c-Ha-ras-*

transformed human breast epithelial cells. Invasion Metastases, 11: 38–47, 1991.

192. Liotta, L.A. Tumor invasion and metastases: the role of basement membrane. Am. J. Pathol. 117: 339–348, 1984.

193. Bonfil, R.D., Reddel, R., Ura, H., Reich, R., Fridman, R., Harris, C.C. and Klein-Szanto, A.J.P. Invasive and metastatic potential of a *v-Ha-ras* transformed human bronchial epithelial cell line. J. Natl. Cancer Inst. 81: 587–594, 1989.

194. Zimmermann, A. and Keller, H.V. Locomotion of tumor cells as an element of invasion and metastasis. Biomed. Pharmacother. 41: 337 – 344, 1987.

195. Mensing, H., Albini, A. and Kreig, T. Enhanced chemotaxis of tumor derived and virus transformed cells to fibronectin and fibroblasts conditional medium. Int. J. Cancer. 33:43–48, 1984.

196. MacCarthy, J.B., Basara, M.I., Palon, D.F. and Funcht, L.T. The role of cell adhesion proteins, laminum and fibronectin in the movement of malignant and metastatic cells. Cancer Metastases Rev. 4: 12–152, 1988.

197. Smith, H.S., Wolman, S.R. and Hackett, A.J. The biology of breast cancer at the cellular level. Biochim. Biophys. Acta. 738: 103–123, 1984.

198. Cooper, C.S., Blair, D.G., Oskarsson, M.K., Tainsky, M.A., Eader, L.A. and Vande Woude, G.F. Characterization of human transforming genes from chemically transformed teratocarcinoma, and pancreatic carcinoma cell lines. Cancer Res. 44, 1–10, 1984.

199. Zhang, P.L., Calaf, G. and Russo, J. Point mutation in codons 12 and 61 of the *c-Ha-ras* gene in carcinogen-treated human breast epithelial cells (HBEC). Proc. Am. Assoc. Cancer Res. 33: 669a, 1992.

200. Abarca-Quinones, J., Calaf, G., Estrada, S., Barnabas-Sohi, N., Zhang, P.L., Garcia, M. and Russo, J. Phenotypic progression of human breast epithelial cells HBEC transformed with chemical carcinogen. Proc. Am. Assoc. Cancer Res. 33: 670a, 1992.

201. Calaf, G. and Russo, J. Emergence of progressive neoplastic phenotypes of human breast epithelial (HBEC) treated with chemical carcinogens in vitro. Proc. Am. Assoc. Cancer Res. 33: 1141a, 1992.

202. Rochlitz, C.F, Scott, G.K., Dodson, J.M., Liu, E., Dollbaum, C.H., Smith, H.S., Benz, C.H. Incidence of activating ras oncogene mutations associated with primary and metastatic human breast cancer. Cancer Res. 49: 357–360, 1989.

Genomic Basis of Breast Cancer

8.1 Introduction

The Human Genome Project (HGP) is having a significant impact on the way that we are studying the biology and pathology of breast cancer and in turn it will have a significant impact in the way that medicine will be practiced in this century. The final objective of the HGP is to identify the genes and their function as a physical unit of heredity that passes from parents to offspring. These pieces of DNA contain information for making specific protein that is the following challenge in our understanding of the biologic process under discussion. To find a gene, and its function it was first needed to define the DNA sequence that determines the gene and how many genes make up the human genome. Whereas approximately 3 billion DNA base pairs have been sequenced, only 3% of the human genome DNA is used to make proteins. Therefore, 97% of the human genome is in excess of DNA accumulated from viral infections, erroneous duplications, and other events. At the present time, it is not clear how many genes are contained in the 3 billion DNA bases. It is estimated between 33,630 to 134,000 possible genes. The challenge is to identify which is or are the genes relevant for understanding the biology of the human breast and how those genes are modified in order to turn a normal breast cell into a cancer cell [1–3].

In the present chapter we apply the knowledge and technology gained through the HGP to understand the emergence of the immortalization and transformation of human breast epithelial cells, and outline strategies for manipulating the genes involved in this process for reverting the malignant phenotype. The knowledge outlined in the biology of the immortalization and transformation process in HBEC discussed in the previous chapter is pivotal to understand the biology behind the molecules.

8.2 Genomic Changes Observed in Breast Cancer

Genetic alterations such as microsatellite instability (MSI) and loss of heterozygosity (LOH) may contribute to the initiation and progression of human breast cancer [4–7]. MSI has been found in breast carcinomas on 1q, 3p, 6p, 6q, 7p, 11p, 16q, 17p, 17q, 18q, 19q, and Xq [8–11]. The emergence of MSI may involve defects in DNA replication or mismatch repair (MMR) mechanisms [12–17], which are considered to be a driving force in the multistage process of carcinogenesis [18–20]. LOH has been observed in both in situ and invasive breast carcinomas on multiple chromosomal arms, including 1p, 1q, 3p, 6q, 7q, 11p, 11q, 13q, 16q, 17p, 17q, and 18q [21–26]. This type of genetic alteration may indicate deletion of the remaining normal allele of a tumor suppressor gene (or genes), which is a generally accepted mechanism of carcinogenesis initially hypothesized by Knudson [27] in his two-hit theory. The multiplicity of these genetic alterations in various tumor stages has provided evidence that primary and secondary events accumulate and hence contribute to stepwise neoplastic progression. The alterations are complex making difficult to precisely identify the early events that have contributed to initiation and/or progression of breast cancer.

An in vitro model consisting of mortal, immortalized, and transformed human breast epithelial cells (HBECS) established in our laboratory (Fig. 8.1)

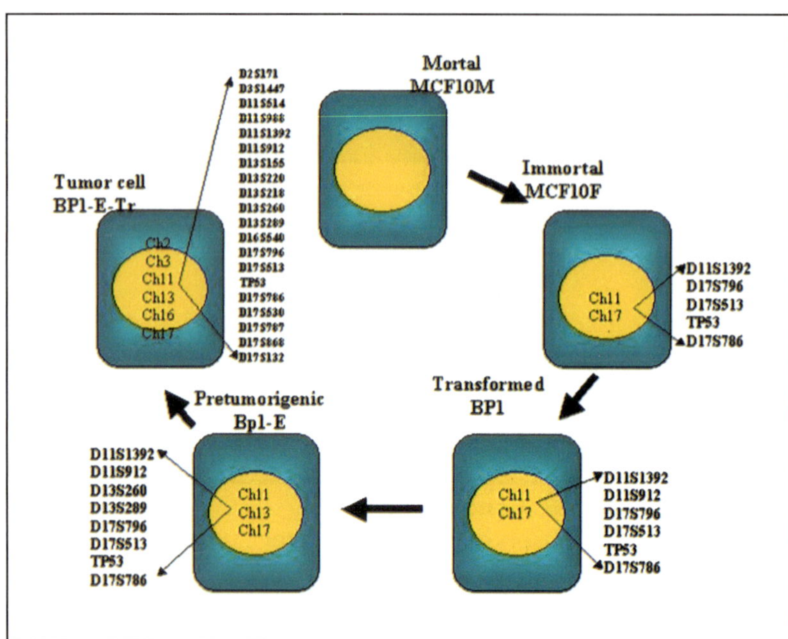

Figure 8.1

Schematic drawing of the evolution of the mortal cells MCF10 M to the tumor cell line BP1E-Tr. The chromosome markers and loci depict the changes observed during the process of immortalization, transformation, and tumorigenesis

[28–31], and described in Chapter 7, has been a useful tool for studying phenotypic changes and their relationship to the genomic changes that develop during the initiation and progression of chemically induced carcinogenesis. By using this system, a frameshift mutation in *p53* at exon 7 was demonstrated to be associated with the immortalization of MCF-10F cells [32], supporting the notion that inactivation of p53 is an early event in breast carcinogenesis [33]. HBECs treated with the carcinogens benzo(a)pyrene (BP) and 7,12-dimethylbenz(a)anthracene (DMBA) express phenotypes indicative of neoplastic transformation after clonal selection, such as increased colony formation in agar-methocel and chemo-invasion [29, 30]. These phenotypic changes are associated with the loss of the normal allele and point mutations at codons 12 and 61 of the *c-Ha-ras* oncogene [34] as well as amplification of several other oncogenes such as *c-erbB2*, *int-2* and *mdm2* [30, 35]. These findings indicate that activation of oncogenes and inactivation of tumor suppressor genes are involved in the initiation and progression of breast carcinogenesis. In addition MSI was detected in several chromosomes (see next section 8.3) during the process of cell

immortalization and transformation, indicating that it is an underlying mechanism pointing toward a defect in DNA replication and mismatch repair (MMR) in the initiation of breast cancer.

Figure 8.2 ▶

Ideographic presentation of microsatellite markers used in the analysis of the immortalized and transformed human breast epithelial cells. *Vertical bars* along the chromosomes indicate the region(s) to which each marker was mapped (reprinted with permission from: Huang. Y., Bove, B., Wu, Y.L., Russo, IH., Yang, X., Zekri, A., and Russo, J. Microsatellite instability during immortalization and transformation of human breast epithelial cells in vitro. Molecular Carcinogenesis, 24:118–127, 1999)

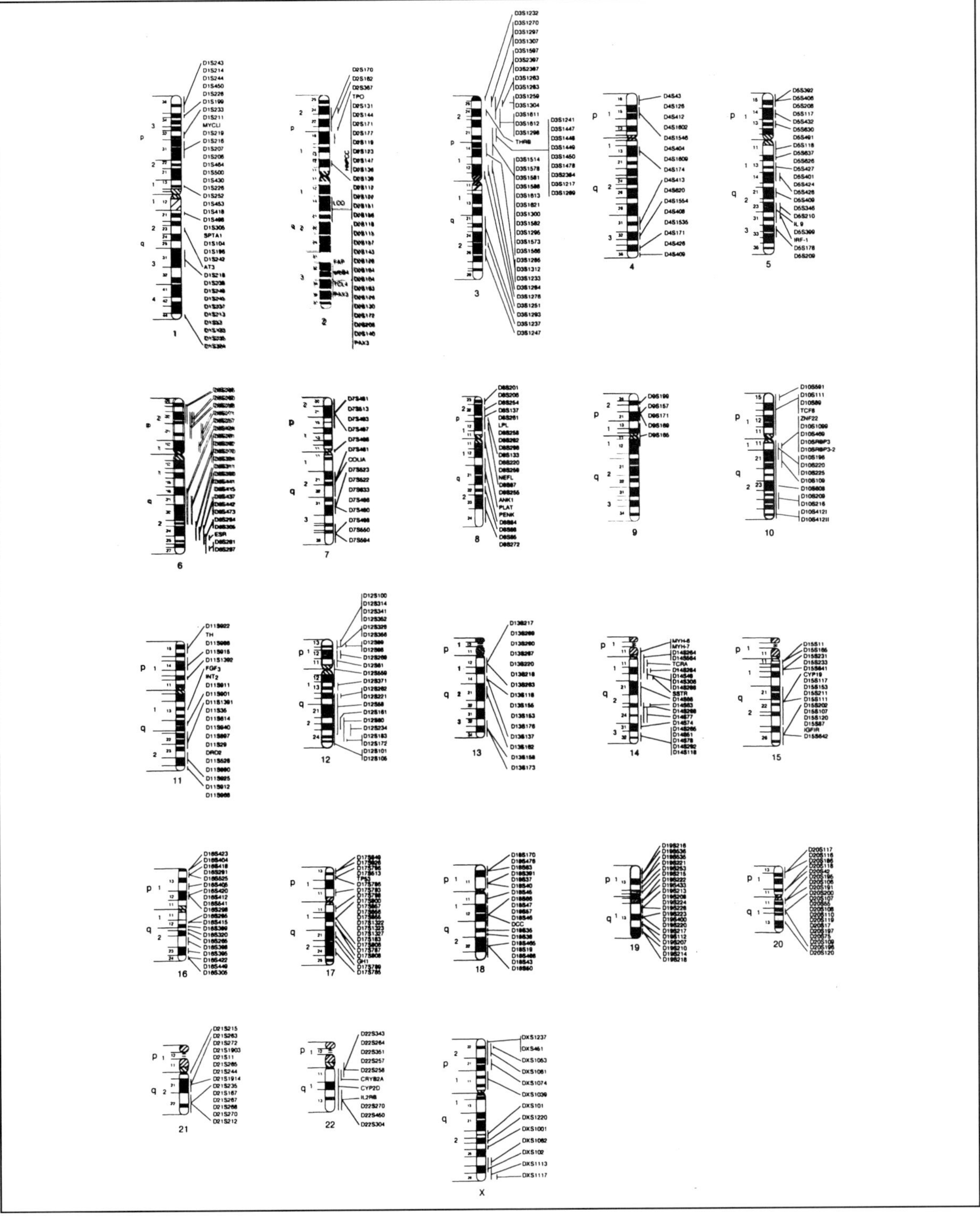

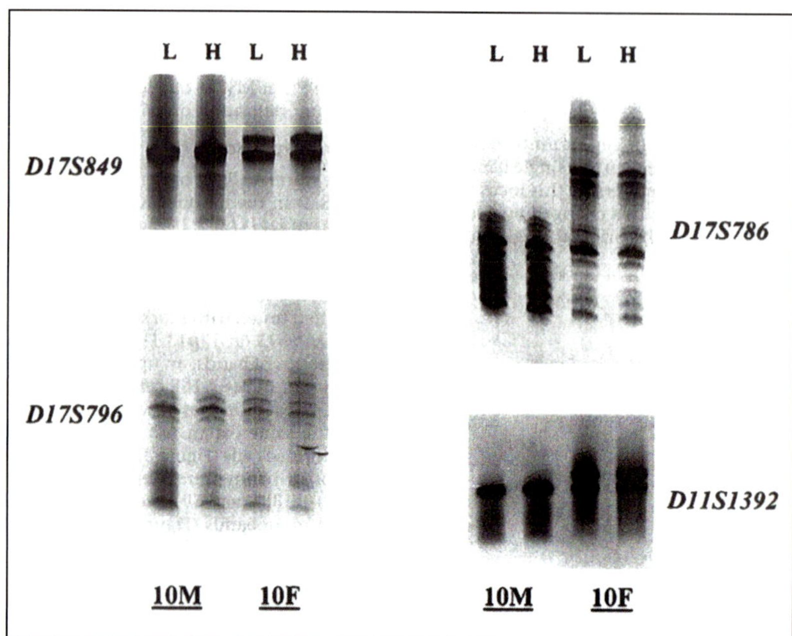

Figure 8.3

Determination of microsatellite patterns on chromosome 11 and 17 in MCF-10 M (10 M) and MCF-10F (10F) cells cultured in low (*L*) and high (*H*) calcium concentrations (reprinted with permission from: Huang. Y., Bove, B., Wu, Y.L., Russo, IH., Yang, X., Zekri, A., and Russo, J. Microsatellite instability during immortalization and transformation of human breast epithelial cells in vitro. Molecular Carcinogenesis, 24: 118–127, 1999)

8.3 Microsatellite Instability as an Early Genomic Event in Breast Cancer Initiation

Microsatellite instability (MSI) is a unique type of genomic alteration that may reflect the presence of defective DNA replication and/or DNA MMR mechanisms during the processes of immortalization and transformation of HBECs [14, 15, 36]. We have used 466 markers to perform a genome-wide microsatellite analysis to map representative regions of the 22 human autosomes and the X chromosome, to determine the targets of MSI in the processes of HBEC immortalization and carcinogen-induced transformation using the basic experimental model outlined in Fig. 8.1 (see Chapter 7 for more details). The markers included chromosomal regions and genes frequently implicated in human malignancies involved in mechanisms such as cell-growth control, cell-cycle regulation, and DNA repair (Fig. 8.2) [37]. Analysis of genomic DNA of MCF-10F cells and of the BP-transformed cells BP1 and BP1E revealed the presence of MSI in several loci on chromosomes 11 and 17 in

MCF-10F cells and MSI in additional loci on chromosomes 11 and 13 in BP1 and BP1E (Figs. 8.1, 8.3–8.6). MSI was also found on chromosomes 13 and 16 in the DMBA-transformed lines D3 and D3-1 (Figs. 8.5, 8.6) [38]. LOH, which has been shown to be involved in multiple regions on at least eight individual chromosomes in spontaneous breast cancers [21, 23, 25], was not found in any of the cell lines tested with the markers used. These findings could indicate that in the immortalized and the transformed HBECs, LOH, an indicator of deletion or inactivation of tumor suppressor genes, may not be a dominant mechanism in the early stages of cell transformation.

Allelic imbalances on chromosomes 11p and 17p have been implicated in the development of invasive cancer of the urinary bladder [39]. Chromosome 11p also shows abnormal methylation at the CpG island locus in spontaneously immortalized and transformed human bronchial epithelial BEAS-2B sublines sequentially induced by simian virus 40 T-antigen and various oncogenes [40]. The same phenomenon has also been observed on chromosome 17p in the immortalized BEAS-2B cells [40]. We have previously reported that a mutation in exon 7 in the well-

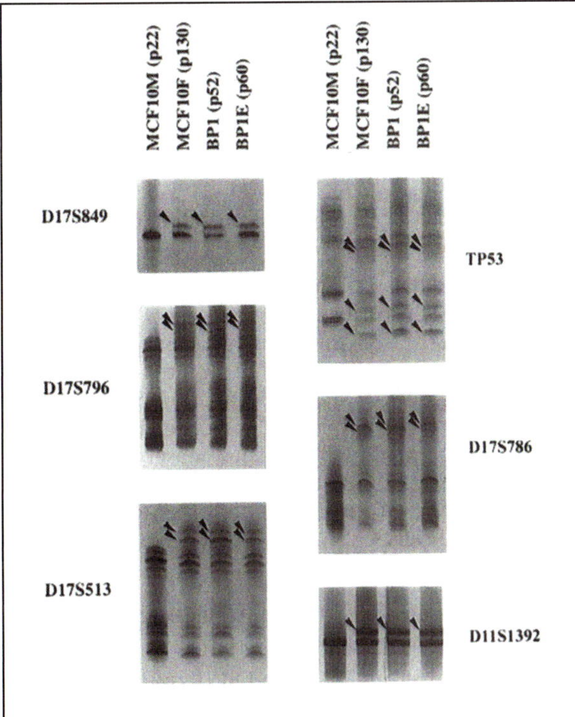

Figure 8.4

Microsatellite instability (MSI) on chromosome 11p and 17p in immortalized HBEC MCF10F and derived transformed cell lines. The markers used were *D17S849* (at 17p13.3), *D17S796* (at 17p13), *D17S513* (at 17p13.1), *D17S786* (at 17p13.1) *D11S1392* (at 11p13) and TP53. The *arrowheads* indicate abnormal bands (reprinted with permission from: Huang. Y., Bove, B., Wu, Y.L., Russo, IH., Yang, X., Zekri, A., and Russo, J. Microsatellite instability during immortalization and transformation of human breast epithelial cells in vitro. Molecular Carcinogenesis, 24:118–127, 1999)

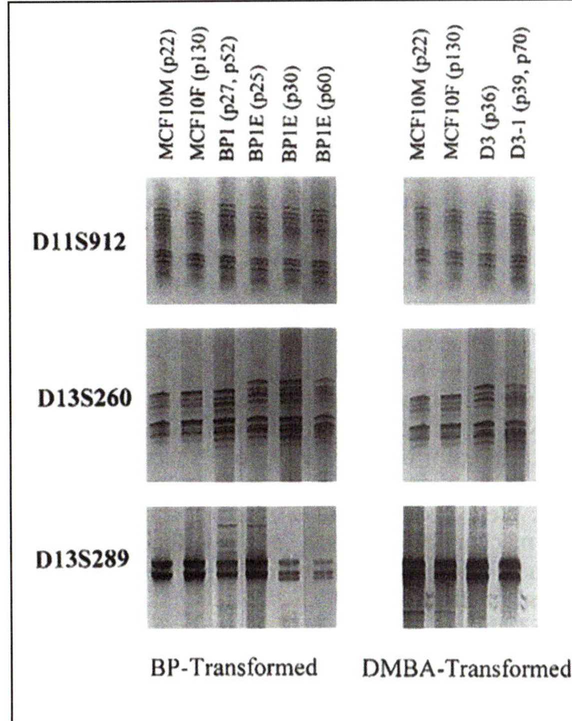

Figure 8.5

MSI detected in BP1 and BP1E cells with markers *D11S912* (at 11q25), *D13S260* (at 13q12–13), and *D13S289* (at 13q12–13) and in D3 and D3-1 cells with marker *D13S260* (at 13q12-13) (reprinted with permission from: Huang. Y., Bove, B., Wu, Y.L., Russo, IH., Yang, X., Zekri, A., and Russo, J. Microsatellite instability during immortalization and transformation of human breast epithelial cells in vitro. Molecular Carcinogenesis, 24:118–127, 1999)

known tumor suppressor gene TP53, which is at 17p13.1, occurred in association with the immortalization of MCF-10F cells [32]. There are indications that additional tumor suppressor genes may map to the short arm of chromosome 17 at p13.3 [41–46].

Among the MSI-positive loci in the BP-transformed HBECS, *D11S912* (at 11q25) has been shown to be affected in ovarian cancers [47] and in breast tissues exhibiting ductal hyperplasia (Table 8.1) [48].

Two other loci, *D13S260* and *D13S267* (both of which flank the BRCA2 locus at 13q12–13), have been shown to manifest instability in sporadic breast cancer [49, 50] and in early-onset familial breast cancer [51–54]. These two loci have been found to exhibit MSI correlated with the progression of human breast cancers from carcinoma in situ to invasive carcinoma (Table 8.2) [55].

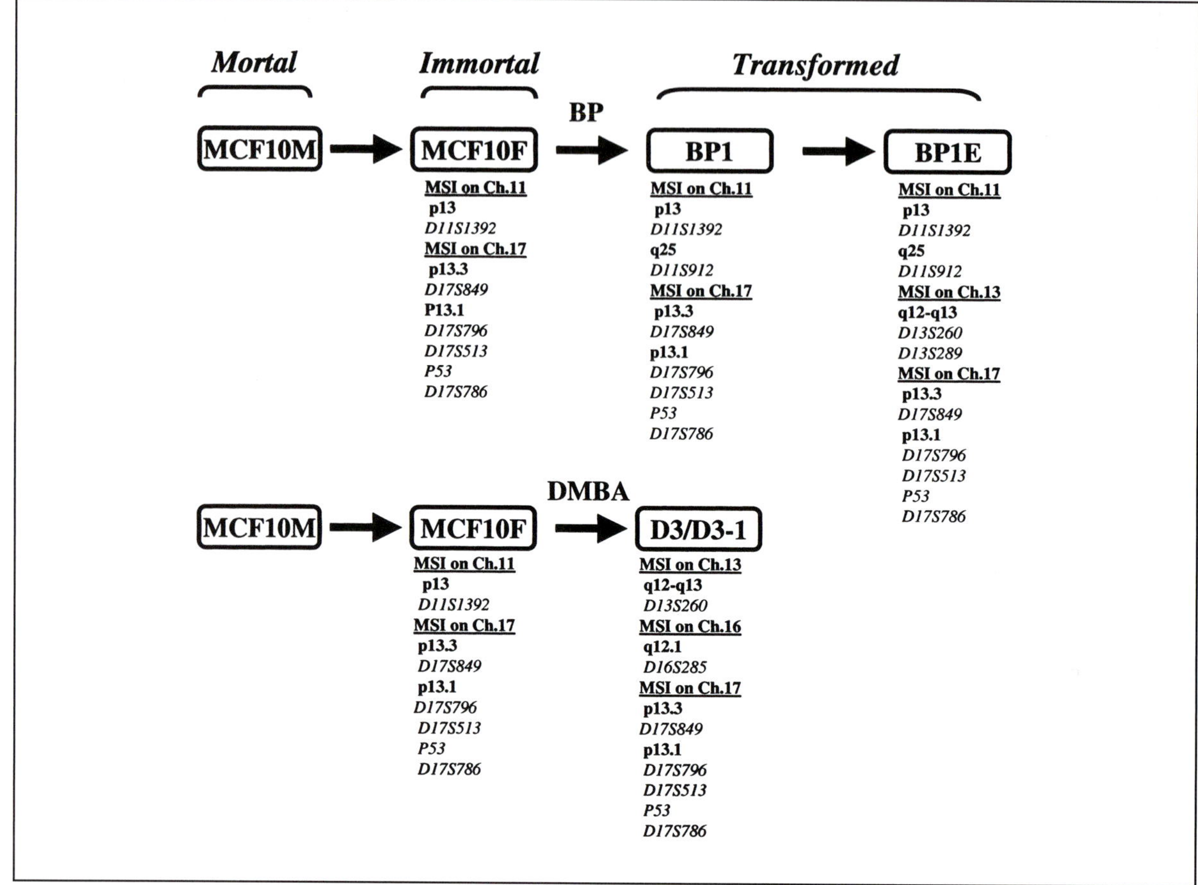

Microsatellite instability first appeared during the process of immortalization, emerging on chromosomes 11pl3 (at *D11S1392*) and 17p (at *D17S849*, *D17S796*, *D17S513*, *TP53*, and *D17S786*) in the immortalized MCF-10F cells (Figs. 8.1, 8.3). In chemically transformed HBECs, MSI was found involving one locus on 11q25 (*D11S912*) in BP1 cells and in two additional loci (*D13S260* and *D13S289*) on chromosome 13ql2–13 in the phenotypically more transformed BP1E cells. Huang et al. [56], found MSI in the DMBA-transformed D3 and D3-1 cells at marker *D13S260*, and Wu et al. [38] reported the same phenomenon in *D16S285* (Fig. 8.5). Therefore, these findings further strengthen the notion that MSI is correlated with the initiation and the progression of neoplastic transformation of human breast epithelial cells.

Figure 8.6

MSI on chromosomes 11p, 17p, 11q, 13q and 16q correlated with the immortalization of MCF10 M cells and the expression of transformation phenotypes in BP- and DMBA-treated cells (reprinted with permission from: Huang. Y., Bove, B., Wu, Y.L., Russo, I.H., Yang, X., Zekri, A., and Russo, J. Microsatellite instability during immortalization and transformation of human breast epithelial cells in vitro. Molecular Carcinogenesis, 24: 118–127, 1999)

Table 8.1. Microsatellite instability (*MSI*) and loss of heterozygosity (*LOH*) in ductal hyperplasia (*DHP*), carcinoma in situ (*CIS*), and invasive carcinoma (*INV*)

Markers	Location	Histopathological type of breast lesions					
		DHP		CIS		INV	
		MSI	LOH	MSI	LOH	MSI	LOH
Int2	11q13.3	2/24 (8.3)[a]	0/24 (0)	4/35 (11.4)	2/35 (5.7)	2/14 (14.3)	0/14 (0)
D11S614	11q21–23.3	2/33 (6.1)	0/30 (0)	3/38 (7.9)	0/38 (0)	2/16 (12.5)	0/16 (0)
D11S912	11q25	3/37 (5.4)	1/33 (3.03)[c]	15/54 (27.8)[b]	5/54 (9.2)[c]	3/22 (13.6)[b]	8/22 (36.4)[c]
D11S940	11q21–23.3	1/27 (3.7)	0/37 (0)	2/39 (5.1)	1/39 (2.6)	2/16 (12.5)	0/16 (0)
D13S260	13q12–13	0/14 (0)	0/14 (0)	3/23 (13)	3/23 (13)	2/13 (15)	4/13 (31)
D13S267	13q12–13	0/11 (0)	0/11 (0)	3/21 (14)	7/21 (33)	1/12 (8)	2/12 (17)
D13S289	13q12–13	0/7 (0)	0/7 (0)	3/11 (27)	2/11 (18)	1/5 (20)	3/5 (60)

[a] Number of lesions affected/number of informative cases (%) – applies to MSI and LOH in all cases.
[b] Fisher's exact test $p<0.05$
[c] Fisher's exact test $p<0.01$

Table 8.2. MSI and LOH in ductal carcinoma in situ of the breast

Markers	Map	Total cases[a]	MSI (%)	LOH (%)	MSI and LOH (%)
D13S260	13q12–13	35	5 (14)	4 (11)	9 (26)
D13S267	13q12–13	33	3 (9)	8 (24)	11 (30)
D13S289	13q12–13	23	5 (22)	2 (9)	7 (30)

[a] Including both informative and uninformative cases

Consistent with the hypothesis [18, 19] that a "mutator phenotype" arises early as a driving force in the initiation and progression of carcinogenesis, MSI has been found to be positively correlated with the histopathologic progression of human breast carcinoma in situ to invasive carcinoma [10, 57–60]. Importantly, MSI is associated with the acquisition of the immortalized phenotype and the progressive expression of transformation phenotypes induced in HBECs by chemical carcinogens in vitro.

MSI not only indicates defective DNA replication, MMR, and/or transcription-coupled DNA repair [14, 15, 17, 36] but also induces hypermutability or alters the expression and/or functions of genes in which the affected microsatellites reside [17, 61–64]. Because MSI was detected [56] in the transformed HBECs in the markers *D13S289* and *D13S260*, which flank the breast cancer susceptibility gene *BRCA2*, PCR-SSCP analysis was performed in the 26 exons of this gene. No mutations were found, suggesting that this gene was not involved in the immortalization and/ or transformation of HBECs.

Altogether these data clearly indicate that MSI is an early event in the immortalization and transformation of HBEC. In section 8.6 of this chapter we will discuss the studies on MMR genes that are affected during the early stages of neoplastic transformation.

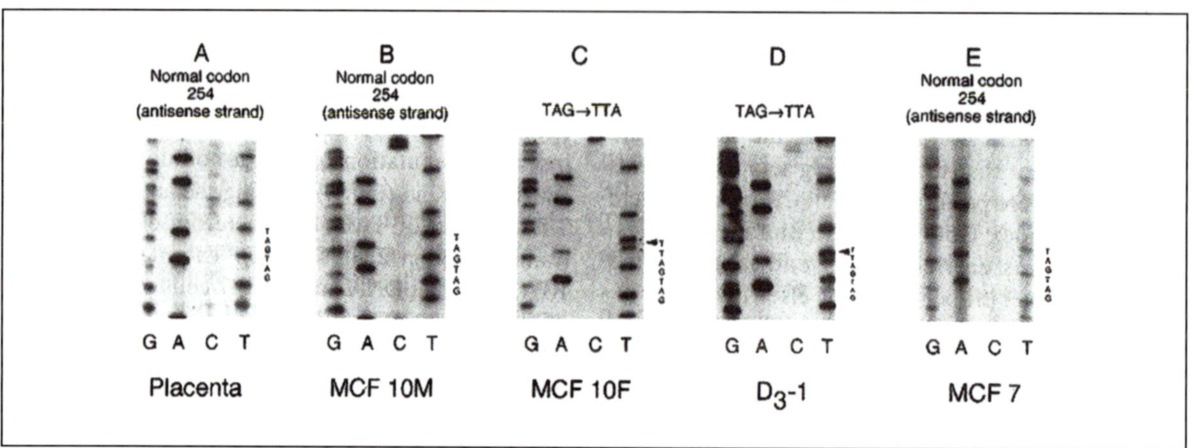

8.4 Other Genomic Changes Associated with Immortalization, Transformation, and Tumorigenesis

8.4.1 Tumor Suppressor Gene p53

Cell immortalization, such as that induced by either HPV16-E6 or by gamma radiation, has been associated with loss of p53 [65]. The involvement of p53 in cell immortalization has been confirmed by the observation that breast epithelial cells derived from women carrying germline p53 mutations, such as in Li Fraumeni syndrome families; undergo spontaneous immortalization [66]. The p53 gene has been identified as an important tumor suppressor gene in normal cells. Loss of normal p53 function is associated with genomic instability, in vitro cell transformation and in vivo tumor development [67]. This gene, located in the short arm of the human chromosome 17 at position p13.1, has a product of a 393-amino-acid nuclear phosphoprotein that exhibits antiproliferative activity, regulating the transition from the G_1 to the S phase of the cell cycle, and determining cell death through apoptosis. It functions as a genomic guardian, monitoring the integrity of the genome. By blocking the cell cycle it protects the genome against damaging agents, suppresses cell proliferation and inhibits malignant transformation. In order to determine whether p53 was involved in the immortaliza-

Figure 8.7

Direct DNA sequencing of the PCR amplified products generated from exon 7 of the p53 gene of placenta, MCF-10 M, MCF-10F, D3-1 and MCF-7 cells. The mortal cells line MCF-10 M, placental DNA and MCF-7 cells showed the wild type p53 sequence. An insertional mutation of a T at codon position 254 in the antisense strand in MCF-10F and D3-1 cells, causing the antisense strand to read TTA instead of TAG, changing the reading at codon 254

tion of MCF-10F cells, we compared these cells with the mortal MCF-10 M utilizing Northern and Southern blots, polymerase chain reaction (PCR) amplification and sequencing of the p53 gene, and single strand conformation polymorphism (SSCP), which is a rapid and sensitive method for the detection of mutations and/or deletions. Southern and Northern blot analyses did not reveal any changes, whereas SSCP analysis of exons 5–9 of the p53 gene showed a conformational shift in exon 7 in the MCF-10F cell line that was not present in the mortal cells MCF-10 M [32]. Sequence analysis using asymmetric PCR-amplified products of exon 7 and an antisense primer revealed an insertional mutation of thymine at codon 254 in MCF-10F, but not in MCF-10 M cells (Fig. 8.7). In order to determine whether p53 mutations were the driving force in the immortalization of MCF-10F cells, we transfected these cells with the wild p53 using the pC53-SN3 vector containing *neo* as selectable marker; this transfection did not restitute the mortal phenotype, indicating that the mutation of p53 is not the only factor responsible of the immortalization. It is possible, however, that the p53 mutation detected in the immortal MCF-10Fcells had resulted in genetic instability, such as the MSI reported above, that facilitated the emergence of other associated genes leading to immortalization (see section 8.6).

8.4.2 Oncogenes

8.4.2.1 c-Ha-ras

There is evidence that the c-Ha-ras oncogene plays a role in the development and the progression of human and animal malignancies [68]. Approximately 60–70 % primary human breast carcinomas exhibit overexpression, and 27 % LOH of this gene [69, 70]. Approximately 10 % of all human neoplasms carry a mutated ras gene, although mutations in human breast cancer are rarely found at any stage [34]. The exact mechanism of action of the *c-Ha-ras* gene is not clear; it has been suggested that the mutation may inactivate this locus on chromosome 11, thus leading to cell transformation. Supporting this contention is the finding that clones D1 and D3, derived from DMBA treated MCF-10F cells exhibited mutations in codons 12 and 61 of the *c-Ha-ras* gene. The clones BP1 and BP1E, derived from BP treated cells exhibited mutations in codon 61, but not in codon 12 [34]. The observations that there was an increase in colony efficiency after a mutation was detected, whereas cells which exhibited a more invasive or the tumorigenic phenotype did not differ in number of mutations from cells exhibiting a less aggressive phenotype, indicate that mutations of *c-Ha-ras* oncogene are associated with the early event of cell transformation. LOH in the locus of the c-Ha-Ras oncogene, on the other hand, has been observed in the BP1E tumor and tumor derived cell lines [71].

8.4.2.2 c-neu, int-2, and c-myc Oncogenes

Genetic alterations of the *c-neu*, *int-2*, and *c-myc* oncogenes have been reported in human breast cancer at different stages of progression of the disease [71]. Amplification of the *c-neu* oncogene is a frequent event in primary breast cancers, occurring in 18–33 % of the cases, and a high percentage of tumors show overexpression of the c-neu protein, indicating that deregulation of the gene might be involved in the neoplastic process. In our in vitro system, c-neu gene transcript was detected as a 4.5-kb band in the MCF-10F cell line, and the intensity of the signal was increased 8.0-fold in both BP1 and BP1E cell lines [35]. Southern blot data also showed gene amplification in the same cell lines [35].

The *int-2* gene was first described as a cellular gene activated by insertional mutagenesis using the MMTV provirus in mouse mammary tumors; *int-2* is amplified in 10–20 % of human breast cancers. Although the physiological role of this gene has not been clearly established, its homology with the fibroblast growth factor gene family suggests that it might play a role in several biological processes, such as differentiation and development. The *int-2* oncogene produces a 4.6-kb mRNA transcript that was present in the MCF-10F cell line. The intensity of the signal was increased 1.5-, 1.8-, 1.3- and 2.0-fold above the values found in MCF-10F control cells in BP1, BP1E, D3 and D3-1 cell lines, respectively [34]. The analysis showed that both, gene amplification and gene rearrangement were associated with increased mRNA levels in BP1, BP1E and D3-1 cell lines. Genomic DNA changes may affect the level of transcription during the process of cell transformation, which, in turn, may facilitate the evolution of BP1 to BP1E cells.

The importance of *c-myc* in breast tumorigenesis has been demonstrated in transgenic mice in which overexpression of *c-myc* results in mammary cancer development. Over-expression of the *c-myc* gene as the result of translocation, mutation, or amplification has been implicated in the genesis and progression of a variety of human tumors, including breast cancer [72]. Amplification of the *c-myc* gene is present in 17–33 % of primary human breast tumors. Northern blot analysis allowed the characterization of the c-myc gene transcript as a single band of 2.3 kb in MCF-10F cells. The intensity of the signal was increased 1.5-fold only in D3-1 cells, but none of the other cell lines studied exhibited any changes [34].

8.4.3　mdm2 Gene

mdm2 expression may be regulated by wild type *p53* [32]. Since the ability to regulate *mdm2* expression is lost in *p53* mutants, and MCF-10F and transformed cells have a demonstrable *p53* mutation, we hypothesized that *mdm2* expression might be altered in these cells. The Southern blot analysis of the Eco RI digested genomic DNA of immortal MCF-10F and transformed cells did not reveal any demonstrable amplification of the *mdm2* gene in any of the cell lines studied (Fig. 8.8). Northern analysis of total cellular RNA using *mdm2* specific cDNA, on the other hand, iden-

tified a 5.5 Kb transcript in all the cell lines (Fig. 8.8). An interesting observation was the 2.5-fold increased expression of the *mdm2* RNA transcript in the BP-IE cell line, which was absent in the precursor cell line BP1 (Fig. 8.8) [32]. This observation is consistent with the progression of the BP-treated cell lines from BP1 to the tumorigenic and more aggressive clone BP1E (Fig. 8.1). Since p53 protein was detectable in all the cell lines, including the parental cell lines, without increased *mdm2* expression, it is reasonable to suggest that up-regulation of *mdm2* expression in BP-1E cells may have played a distinct role in the expression of the tumorigenic phenotype by BP-1E cells, apart from its *p53* binding effect. This finding is supported by the reported amplification and overexpression of *mdm2* and *p53* mutation in human soft tissue sarcomas as alternative/exclusive regulatory mechanisms to inactivate the pathway to cell growth suppression.

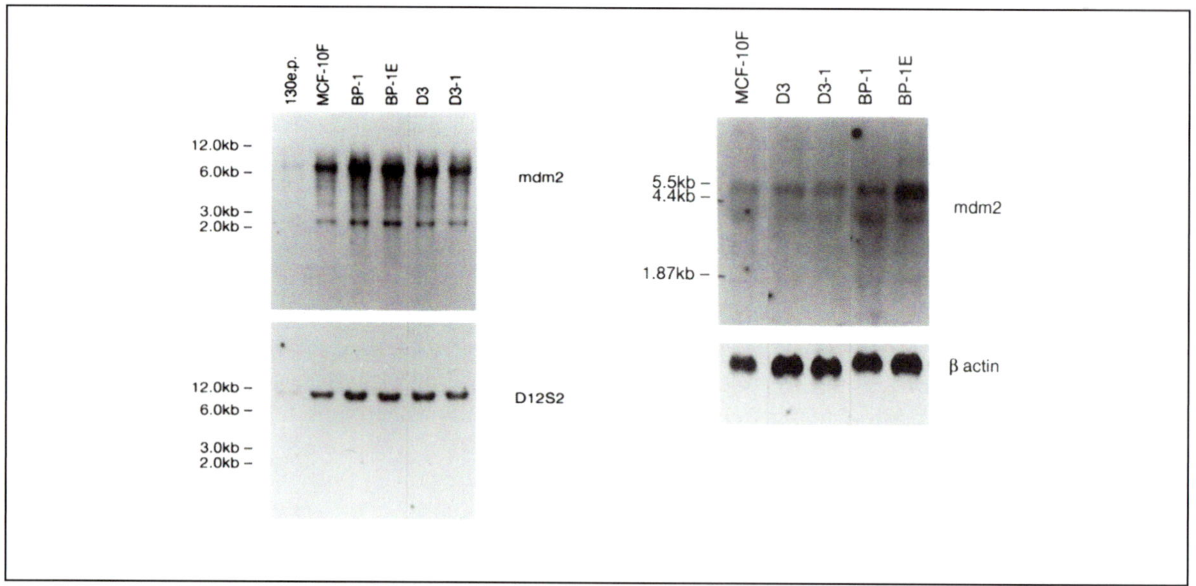

Figure 8.8

Left panel, Southern blot analysis of *Eco*R1-digested genomic DNA of HBEC hybridized with cDNA fragment of *mdm2.* Correction for differential loading and chromosome 12 polysomy (DS282) showed no amplification of the *mdm2* gene. Molecular size markers are shown on the left. *Right panel,* Northern blot analysis of total RNA of HBEC hybridized with *mdm2* cDNA probe, showing a 2.5-fold increased expression of *mdm2* in BP1E cells, in comparison with BP-1. Hybridization with β actin was done to normalize RNA loading

8.4.4 Loss of Heterozygosity and Fluorescence In Situ Hybridization Analysis of Chromosome 17p

The fact that the frequency of allele loss in breast cancer has been reported in chromosome 17p [73–75] suggests that genes located in that chromosome arm might be likely targets for this event. A gene located in the telomeric portion of chromosome 17p, on 17p13.3, distal to *p53*, has been observed to be host in primary breast cancer [76]. LOH of this region, using the probe p144D6, has been found in 75 % of primary breast cancers and in cells that are progesterone receptor negative. LOH of 17p has been associated with high cell proliferation in primary breast tumors, and with a shorter doubling time in the tumorigenic cell line BP1E. A number of breast tumors have been reported to lose the tip of 17p without affecting the *p53* gene, suggesting that a second gene, distinct from *p53*, may be involved in breast cancer. With this concept in mind we performed DNA analysis for allelic loss on chromosome 17p 13.3 using probes pYNZ22 and p144D6 for detecting variable number of tandem repeats (VNTR) (Fig. 8.9). The Southern blots showed that the cell lines MCF-10 M and MCF-10F are heterozygous for probe pYNZ22 (Fig. 8.9). Clones D3, D3-1, BP1 and BP1E, derived from DMBA and BP treated cells, respectively, showed the same heterozygous restriction length polymorphism pattern (RFLP). RFLP analysis with probe pl44D6 revealed a heterozygous pattern in MCF-10 M, MCF-10F cells and in clones D3, D3-1 and BP1. Only the cell line BP1E exhibited LOH, which probed with p144D6 (Fig. 8.9). This phenomenon was also demonstrated by fluorescence in situ hybridization (FISH) analysis (Fig. 8.10) [77]. Conventional banding analysis did not reveal any alterations of 17p in either MCF-10F or BP1E cells. FISH analysis showed that both pl44D6 and the chromosome 17 centromeric probe hybridized to both copies of chromosome 17 in MCF-10F cells (Fig. 8.10). In these cells, the hybridization signals were in parallel in both chromatids of both homologues (Fig. 8.10a, b). In transformed BP1E cells, the 17 centromeric probe was positive, but the p144D6 probe did not hybridize both chromatids in the two homologues, but only two chromatids of one

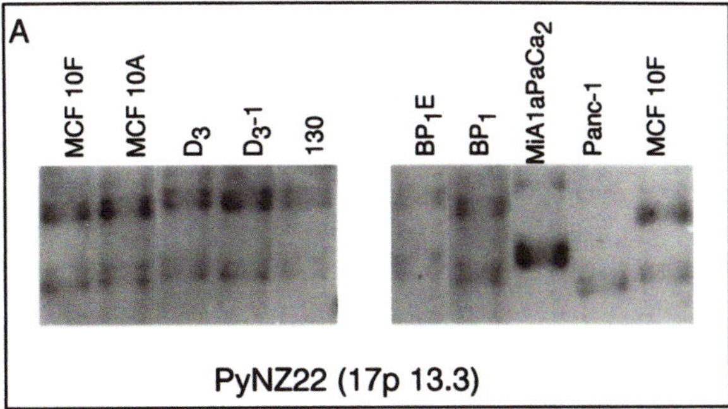

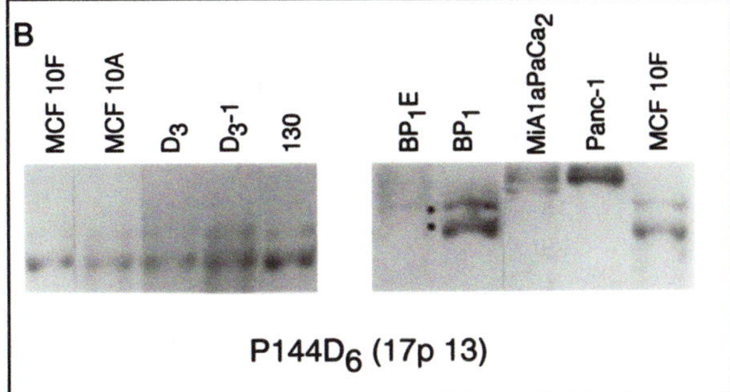

Figure 8.9 a, b

Southern blot analysis of chromosome 17p using the VNTR probes **a** pYNZ22.1 and **b** p144D6. Loss of heterozygosity (LOH) was observed in BP1E cells with the probe p144D6. An *asterisk* indicates the loss of an allelic band. MiA1a-PaCA2–139 and Panc-1–15, two human pancreatic carcinoma cell lines, used as positive controls at passages 139 and 15, respectively, showed the expected LOH and homozygosity

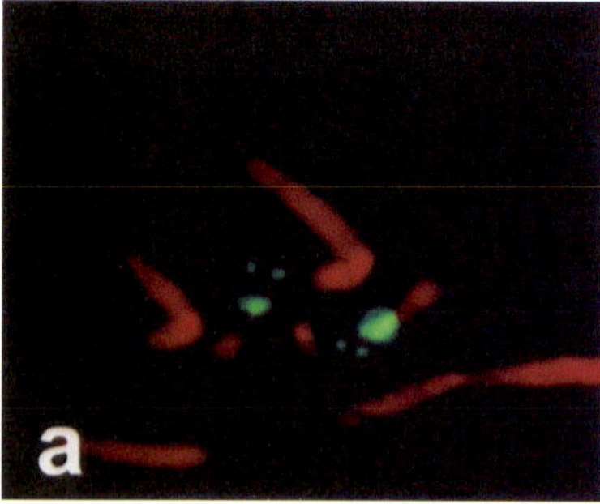
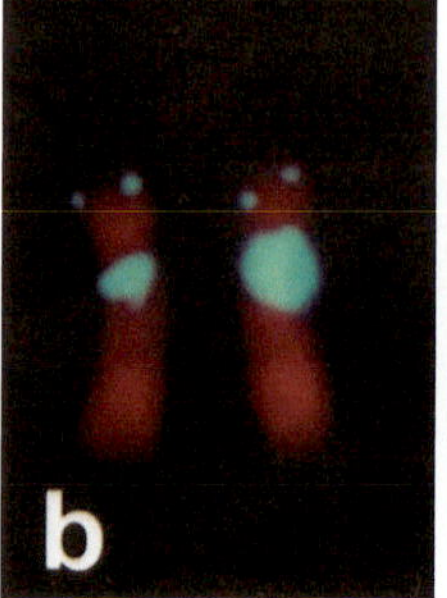
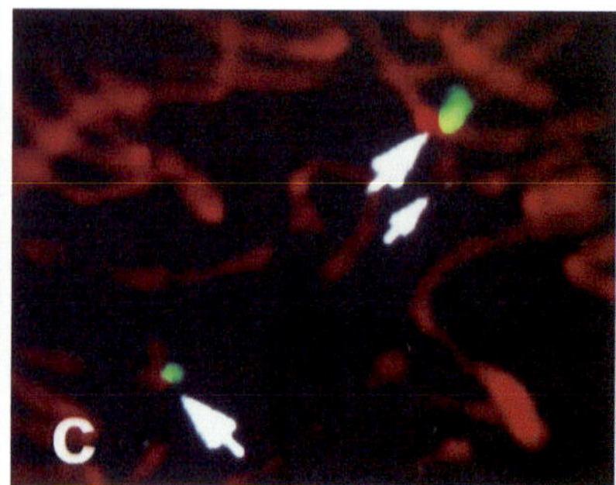
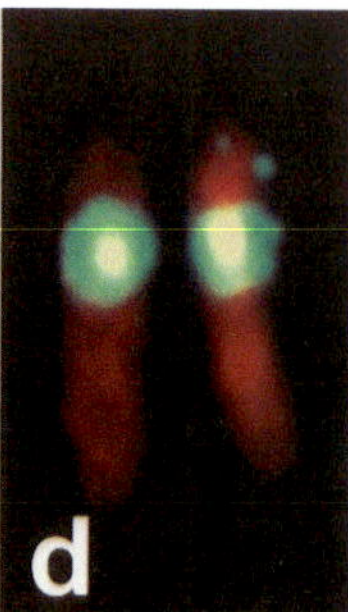

Figure 8.10 a–d

a Fluorescence in situ hybridization (FISH) analysis showed that both pl44D6 and the chromosome 17 centromeric probe hybridized to both copies of chromosome 17 in MCF-10F cells. **b** Details in which the chromosome 17 shows the hybridization signals in parallel in both chromatids of both homologues. **c** In transformed BP1E cells, the 17 centromeric probe was positive, but the p144D6 probe did not hybridize both chromatids in the two homologues (*arrows*). **d** Two chromatids of one homologue were positive, indicating that LOH in the telomeric position of chromosome 17p

homologue were positive (Fig. 8.10 c,d), indicating that LOH in the telomeric position of chromosome 17p was observed only in the cell line expressing the pretumorigenic phenotype [77], that resulted in a pretumorigenic cell line that evolved to a tumorigenic one.

8.5 Search for Specific Functional Relevance of the Genomic Changes

8.5.1 Reversion of the Immortalization Phenotype

To investigate the functional role of genomic changes during the process of cell immortalization and transformation described in the previous sections, we have chosen chromosomes 11, 13 and 17, that were detected to be affected in the immortalized and transformed cells. Single normal human fibroblast A9-derived chromosome 11, 13, or 17, tagged with a

neomycin resistant gene, was transferred into 6×10^6 transformed BP1E cells (Fig. 8.11). Surviving cells or clones of microcell hybrids from chromosome 11 or 17 were designated BP1E-11*neo* or BP1E-17*neo* cells. A total of 16 colonies were isolated from BP1E-11*neo* and BP1E-17*neo* cells each. The transfer efficiency in BP1E cells was approximately 2.6×10^{-6} cells. During a selection period of up to 6 months BP1E-17*neo* cells, and to a lesser degree BP1E-11*neo* cells, exhibited altered cellular morphology and growth pattern, such as contact inhibition and cellular senescence [29, 30]. In addition to the acquired ability to survive in the G-418 selection medium that indicates the active function of the neomycin resistance gene tagged on the donor chromosome 11 or 17 (Fig. 8.12), the physical presence of these chromosomes was further confirmed by dual color-fluorescence in situ hybridization (FISH) analysis (Fig. 8.13). The parent BP1E cells contained two cytogenetically normal chromosomes 17 (Fig. 8.13 a,b); the microcell hybrid BP1E-17*neo*#100 cells acquired an additional chromosome 17, showing a positive signal of pSV2*neo*, further confirming its identity as the donor copy from the A9–17*neo* cells (Figs. 8.13 c,d). With chromosome 11 and pSV2*neo* probes, BP1E cells showed to contain two chromosomes 11 (Fig. 8.13 e,f), while PB1E-11*neo* #145 cell metaphases showed an extra chromosome 11 with positive pSV2*neo* signal (Figs. 8.13 g,h). In addition, DAPI-banded images showed that the donor chromosome 11 had lost the majority of its p-arm (p11-pter) and distal q-arm (q24-qter) (Fig. 8.13 g,h).

Whereas MCF-10F cells grew forming a monolayer of polyhedral cells without overlapping (Fig. 8.14),

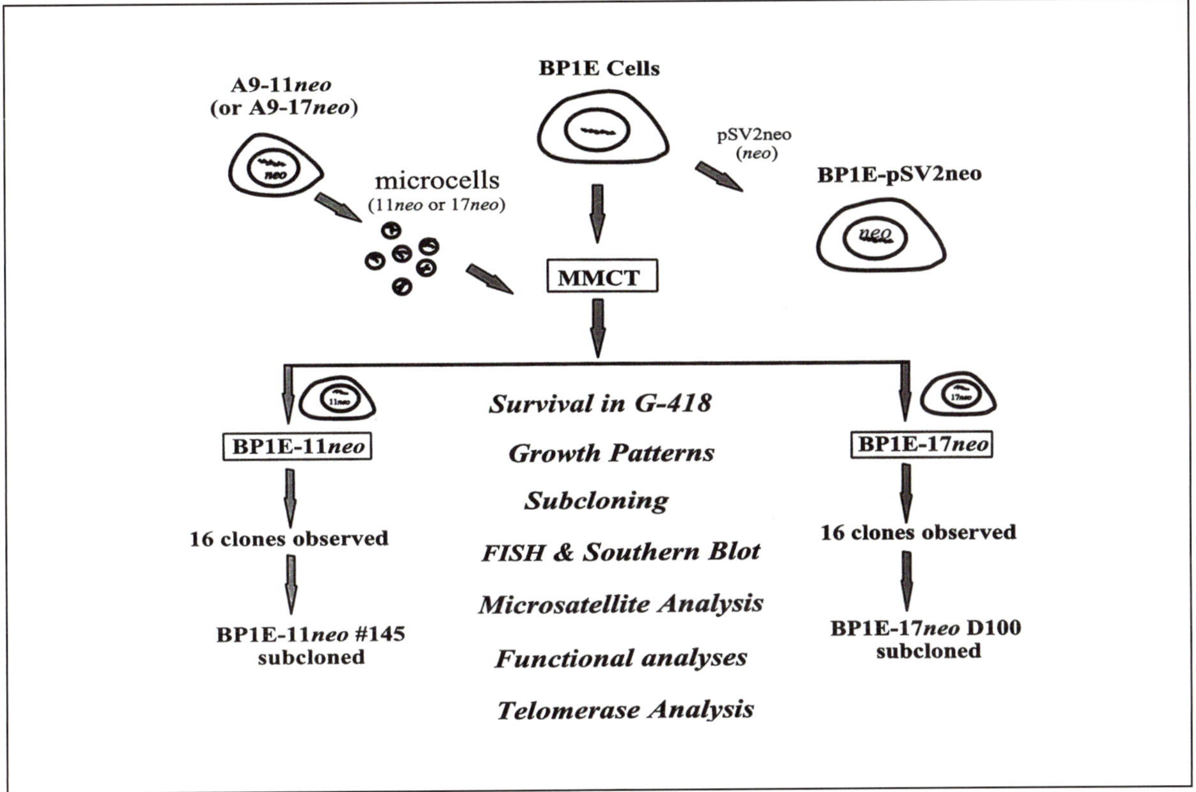

Figure 8.11

Transfer of chromosome 11 and 17 in BP1E cells by microcell mediated chromosome transfer (MMCT). Human chromosome donor cells A9-11*neo* or A9-17*neo* were utilized for generating microcell hybrids BP1E-11*neo* and BP1E-17*neo* cells respectively. Colonies surviving in G-418 were examined for growth pattern, and when possible sub cloned. Expandable clones BP1E-11*neo* #145 and BP1E-17*neo* D100 were subjected to FISH, Southern blot, microsatellite polymorphism, functional and telomerase analyses. PSV2neo plasmid was used to transfect BP1E cells to produce vector transfectant BP1E-pSV2neo as vector control (reprinted with permission from: Yang, X., Huang, Y., Russo, I.H., Balsara, N.R., Barrett, C. and Russo, J. Functional roles of chromosomes 11 and 17 in the transformation of human breast epithelial cells in vitro. Int. J. Onc. 15:629–638, 1999)

as previously described [28], BP1E cells exhibited a growth pattern similar to that of MCF-10F cells, although the cells showed a tendency to overlap. Individual cell morphology varied; some cells appeared smaller in size and slightly spindly in morphology (Fig. 8.14) [29]. *BP1E-pSV2neo* cells were both morphologically and in growth pattern identical to BP1E cells. Clone BP1E-11*neo* #145 was the only expandable one from the 16 colonies originally isolated (Figs. 8.11, 8.14). These cells were able to continue growing for many passages and could be retrieved from frozen stocks for further growth. Their growth pattern retained features of the parental cells. This clone has been passaged for more than 10 times without significant morphological variations from early passages, and without evidence of cellular senescence. From the 16 clones originally isolated from chromosome 17 hybrids only BP1E-11*neo* D100 cells were subcloned. BP1E-17*neo* D100 cells were able to

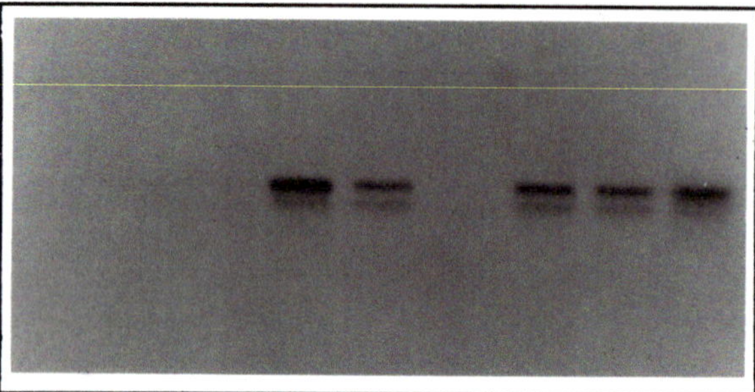

pSV2neo

Figure 8.12

Southern blot analysis of pSV2*neo* plasmid. A fragment of 444 bp pSV2*neo* plasmid was amplified from genomic DNA using PCR. Lane 1, no template control; lane 2, MCF-10F cells; lane 3, A9 cells; lane 4, A9–11*neo*; lane 5, A9–17*neo* cells; lane 6, BP1E cells; lane 7, BP1E-pSV*neo*; lane 8, BP1E-11*neo* #145; lane 9, BP1E-17*neo*D100 (reprinted with permission from: Yang, X., Huang, Y., Russo, I.H., Balsara, N.R., Barrett, C. and Russo, J. Functional roles of chromosomes 11 and 17 in the transformation of human breast epithelial cells in vitro. Int. J. Onc. 15:629–638, 1999)

Figure 8.13 a–h ▶

Dual-color FISH analysis of chromosomes 11 and 17. **a, c, e, g** DAPI stained metaphases showing gross morphology of chromosomes; **b, d, f, h** Specifically labeled chromosome 11 or 17 (*red*) with or without positive pSV2*neo* signal (*green*). **a, b** BP1E cells hybridized with chromosome 17 and pSV2*neo* probes containing two normal chromosomes 17; **c, d** BP1E-17*neo* D100 cells hybridized with chromosome 17 showing an inserted chromosome 17 tagged with the neomycin gene detected with the pSV2*neo* probe; **e, f** BP1E cells hybridized with chromosome 11 and pSV2*neo* probes; **g** and **h** BP1E-11*neo* #145 cells hybridized with chromosome 11 and pSV2*neo* probes; **h** shows the inserted chromosome 11 tagged with the neomycin gene, and detected with the pSV2*neo* probe (reprinted with permission from: Yang, X., Huang, Y., Russo, I.H., Balsara, N.R., Barrett, C. and Russo, J. Functional roles of chromosomes 11 and 17 in the transformation of human breast epithelial cells in vitro. Int. J. Onc. 15:629–638, 1999)

divide only for a limited period of time (approximately 16–20 doublings), as senescence became apparent as early as at passage two. Further loss of growth ability and failure to reach full confluence occurred by passage four (Fig. 8.14). The other 15 colonies of microcell hybrids BP1E-11*neo* and BP1E-17*neo* cells, on the other hand, manifested a significant extent of growth arrest and cellular senescence during a selection growth period of over six months. BP1E-11*neo* colonies could not reach full confluence, and individual cells were enlarged or flattened with irregular cellular shape, and condensed or vacuolated nuclei. BP1E-17*neo* hybrids did not divide, and underwent progressive cellular senescence.

BP1E cells grew slowly for the first 60 h of plating, starting then a fast logarithmic phase of growth that continued up to 196 h in culture without ever reaching a plateau (Fig. 8.15). BP1E-pSV2*neo* cells showed almost identical growth curve to that of BP1E cells. The growth of BP1E-11*neo* #145 cells showed a rate of growth significantly slower than that of the parental BP1E cells; although the cells entered in the logarithmic phase of growth at 60 h post-plating, a slower rate of growth became apparent by 100 h, and the cells

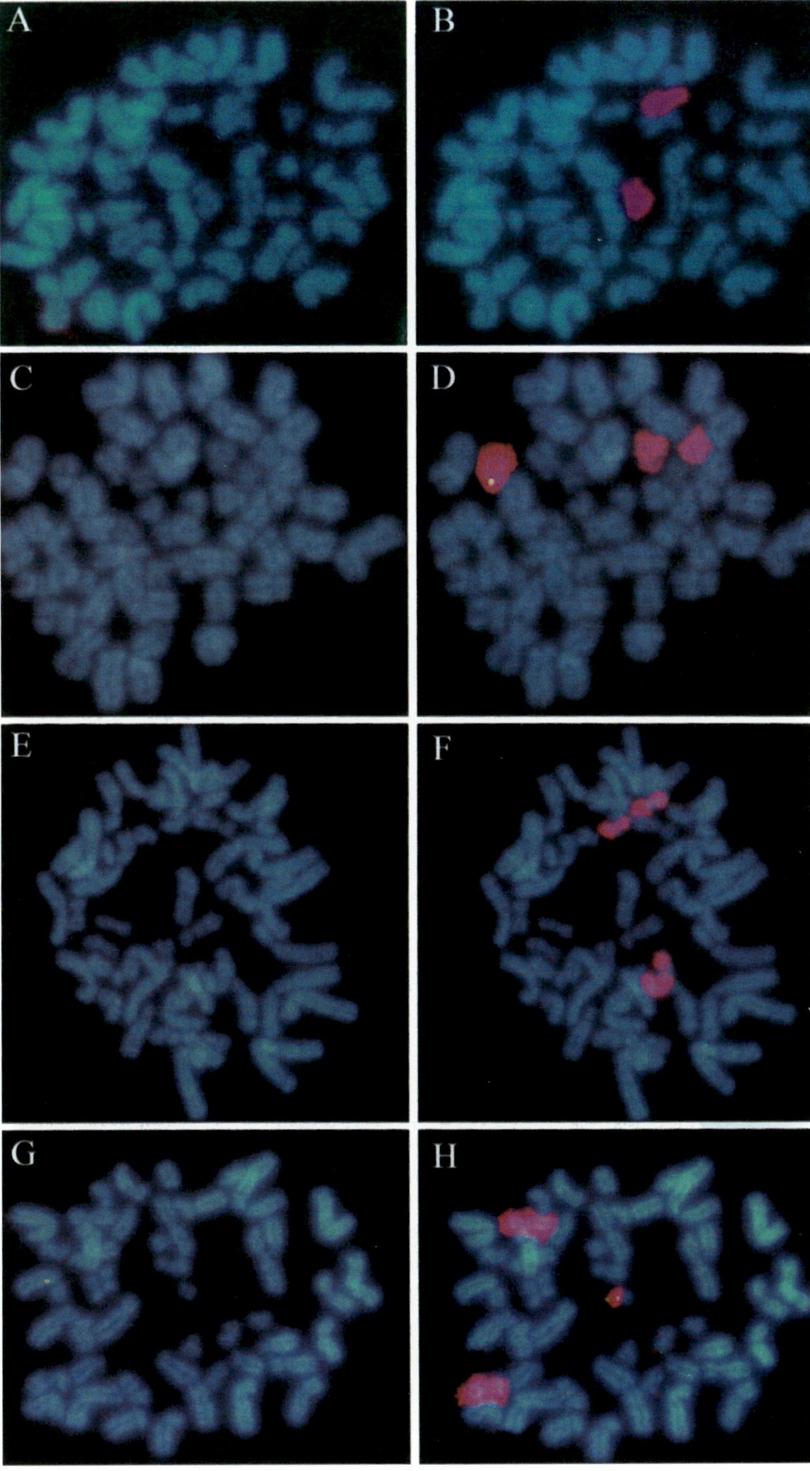

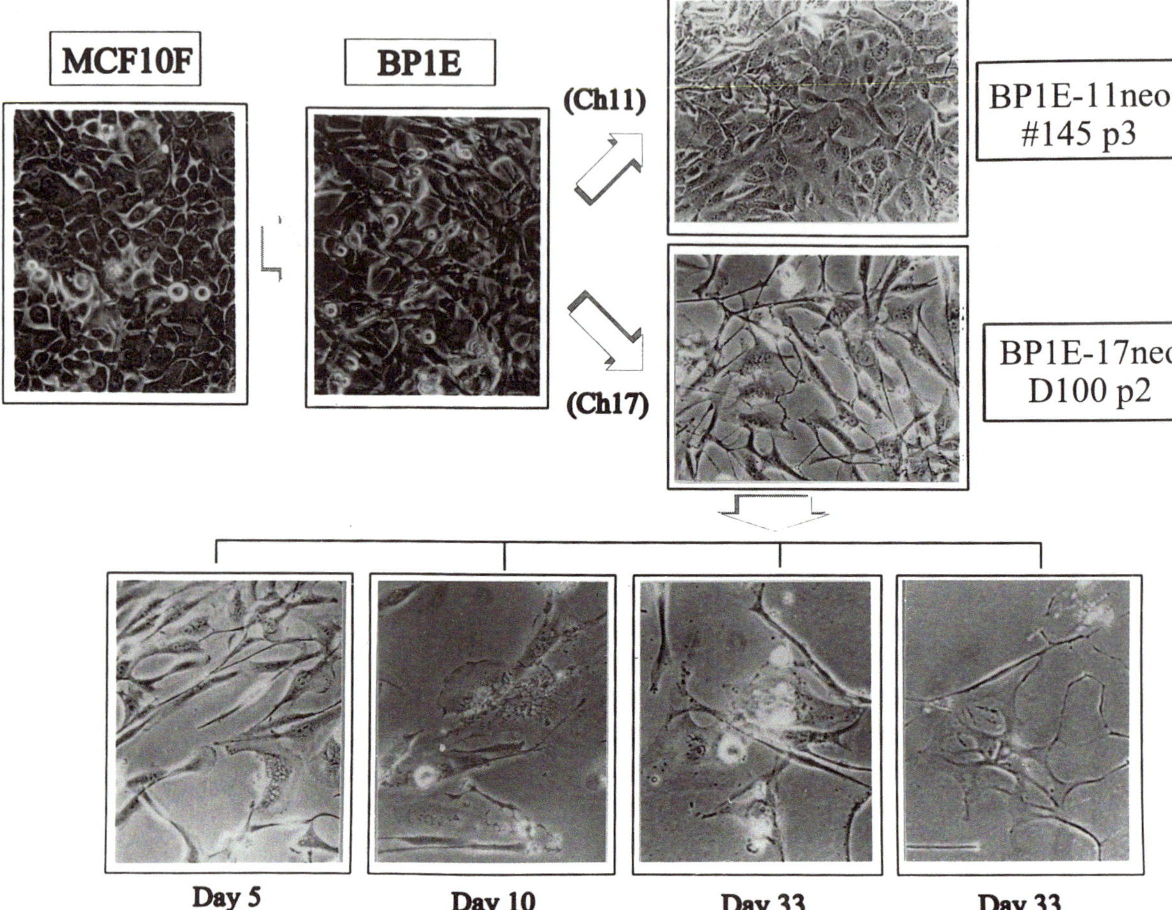

Figure 8.14

Cultures of MCF-I0F and BP1E cells showing characteristic morphologies. Chromosome 11 (*Ch11*) and chromosome 17 (*Ch17*) generated BP1E-11*neo* #145 and BP1E-17*neo* D100 cells

Figure 8.16 ▶

Comparison of anchorage independent growth and colony formation efficiency among MCF-10F, BP1E, BP1E-pSV2*neo*, BP1E-11*neo* #145, and BP1E-17*neo*D100 cells in agar-methocel. Relative colony formation efficiency is plotted in the *upper graph*. Appearance of the corresponding cultures in agar methocel is shown in the *lower panels* photographed in phase contrast (×100) (reprinted with permission from: Yang, X., Huang, Y., Russo, I.H., Balsara, N.R., Barrett, C. and Russo, J. Functional roles of chromosomes 11 and 17 in the transformation of human breast epithelial cells in vitro. Int. J. Onc. 15:629–638, 1999)

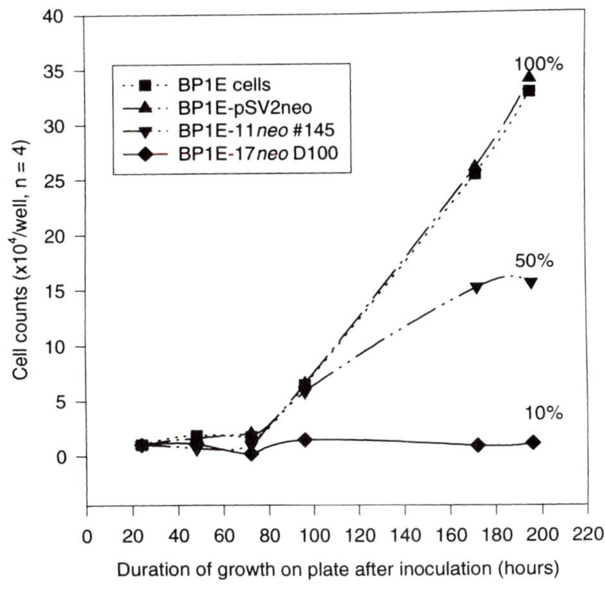

Figure 8.15

Comparison of growth rates among BP1E, BP1E-pSV2*neo*, BP1E-11*neo* #145 and BP1E-17*neo* D100 cells. Cells were plated in quadruplicates in 24-well chambers at a density of 10^4 cells per well. Cell counts were plotted against time (abscissa) and expressed as the mean of four wells per time point (ordinate). Cell numbers were also expressed as the percentage of cells in relation to the number of BP1E cells at the 196th hour in culture, which was arbitrarily set as 100% (reprinted with permission from: Yang, X., Huang, Y., Russo, I.H., Balsara, N.R., Barrett, C. and Russo, J. Functional roles of chromosomes 11 and 17 in the transformation of human breast epithelial cells in vitro. Int. J. Onc. 15:629–638, 1999)

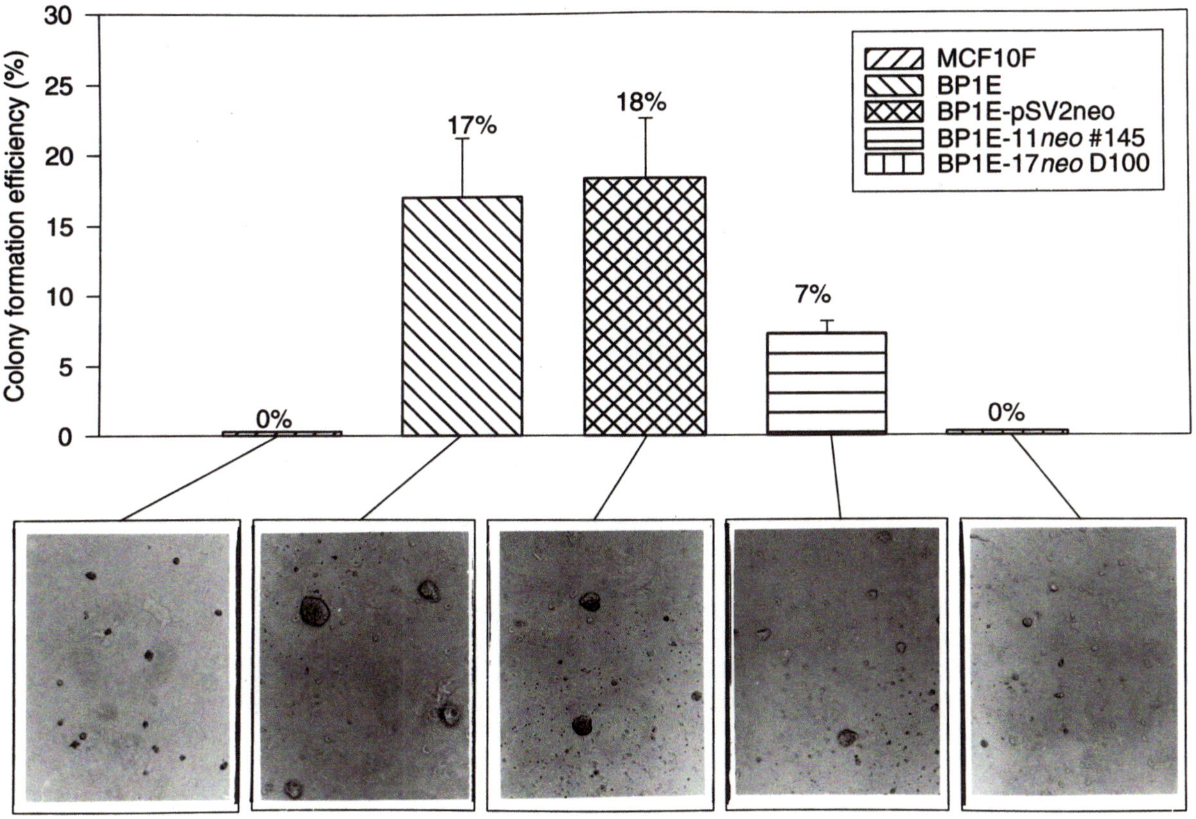

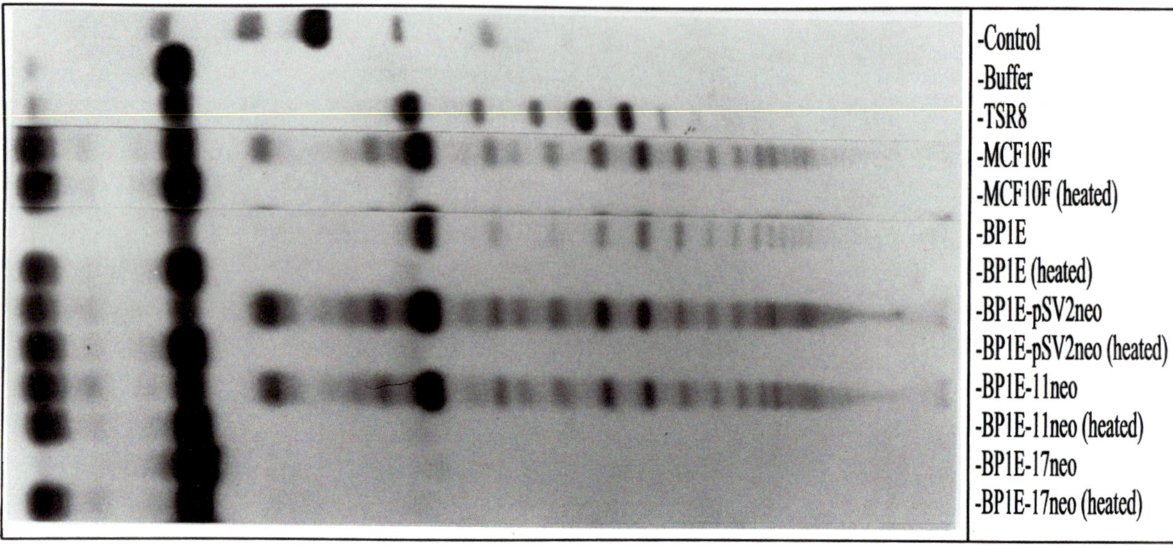

Figure 8.17

Analysis of telomerase activity in control, TSR8, MCF10F, BP1E, BP1E-pSV2, BP1E-*neo* #145, BP1E-17*neo* D100 with their corresponding heated controls. Telomerase activity was absent only in BP1E-17*neo* D100 cells (reprinted with permission from: Yang, X., Huang, Y., Russo, I.H., Balsara, N.R., Barrett, C. and Russo, J. Functional roles of chromosomes 11 and 17 in the transformation of human breast epithelial cells in vitro. Int. J. Onc. 15:629–638, 1999)

reached a plateau by 172 h post-plating. Cell numbers remained unchanged up to 196 h, when the cell count was 50% that of the control cells (Fig. 8.15). BP1E-17*neo* D100 cells showed almost no growth at any of the time points tested and their total cell count at 196 h was approximately 10% of the control (Fig. 8.15). These results indicated that chromosome 11 partially inhibited the growth of the transformed cells, while chromosome 17 almost completely, suppressed the growth rate of the transformed cells.

Anchorage-independent growth in agar-methocel gel was reduced from 17% in control BP1E cells to 7% in the BP1E-11*neo* #145 cells, while BP1E-17*neo* D100 cells failed to form any colony (100% reduction), reflecting a more potent suppression of the BP1E cells by chromosome 17 than that by chromosome 11 (Fig. 8.16). These data indicated that the introduced chromosome 11 caused a partial growth inhibition, while chromosome 17 produced a nearly complete growth suppression of the BP1E cells [78]. Another phenotypic reversion induced by the chromosome transfer was the recovery of the ability of cells to form ductule-like structures in collagen gel, a property exhibited by BP1E-17*neo* D100 cells, similar to that of MCF-10F cells, while BP1E cells grew in loosely arranged clusters or as isolated cells. These observations confirmed the reversion of the trans-

formed phenotype by chromosome 17 transfer. The acquisition of mortality was also accompanied by inhibition of telomerase activity (Fig. 8.17).

Microsatellite analysis showed that the preexisting instability in the parental BP1E cells at loci D17S849 (17p13.3), TP53 (17p13.1), D17S786 (17p13.1), and D17S520 (17p12.0) was reverted in BP1E-17*neo* D100 cells, which acquired an allelic pattern similar to that of the mortal MCF-10 M cells (Figs. 8.18–8.21). In contrast, the instability of these markers was not restored in the BP1E-11*neo* #145 cells (Figs. 8.19, 8.22).

The acquisition of mortality, that was accompanied by inhibition of telomerase activity, the abrogation of the transformation phenotypes and the reversion of some of the MSI detected in chromosome 17 were associated with the insertion of two specific

Figure 8.18

A summary of microsatellite polymorphism[1] analysis of chromosome 17 in BP1E-17*neo* D100 cells. Marker, microsatellite markers along chromosome 17. [2]Retention, retention of donor copy in BP1E-17*neo* D100 cells from A9–17*neo* is indicated by a *solid circle* as positive, or by an *open circle* as negative. [3]Reversion, reversion of genomic instability

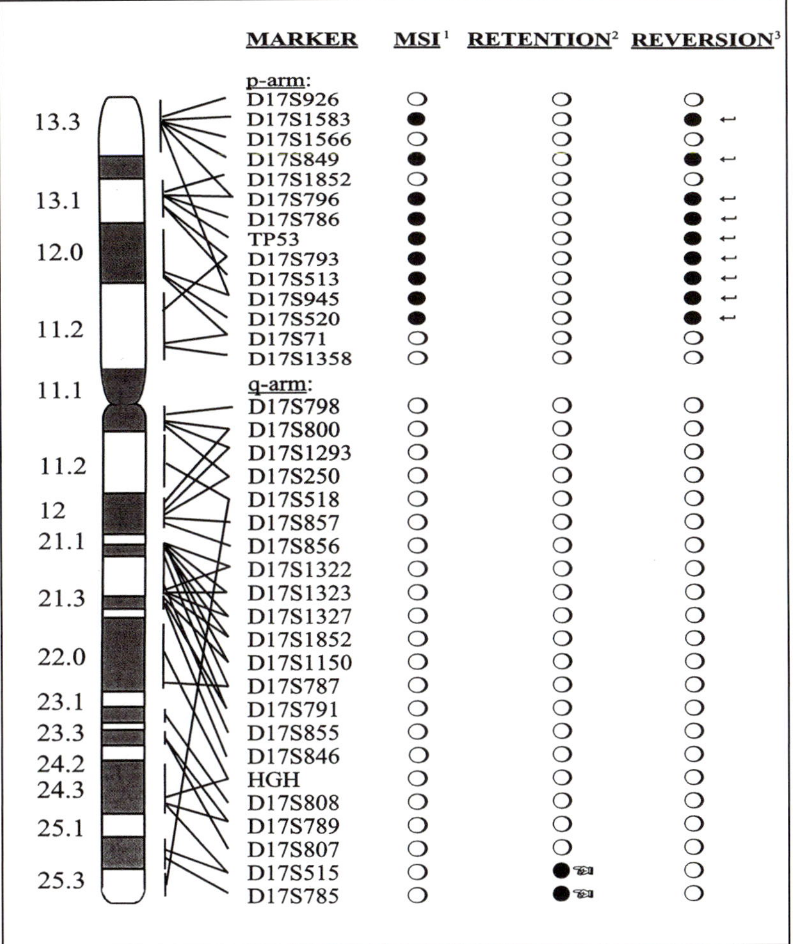

MARKER	MSI[1]	RETENTION[2]	REVERSION[3]
p-arm:			
D17S926	○	○	○
D17S1583	●	○	● ←
D17S1566	○	○	○
D17S849	●	○	● ←
D17S1852	○	○	○
D17S796	●	○	● ←
D17S786	●	○	● ←
TP53	●	○	● ←
D17S793	●	○	● ←
D17S513	●	○	● ←
D17S945	●	○	● ←
D17S520	●	○	● ←
D17S71	○	○	○
D17S1358	○	○	○
q-arm:			
D17S798	○	○	○
D17S800	○	○	○
D17S1293	○	○	○
D17S250	○	○	○
D17S518	○	○	○
D17S857	○	○	○
D17S856	○	○	○
D17S1322	○	○	○
D17S1323	○	○	○
D17S1327	○	○	○
D17S1852	○	○	○
D17S1150	○	○	○
D17S787	○	○	○
D17S791	○	○	○
D17S855	○	○	○
D17S846	○	○	○
HGH	○	○	○
D17S808	○	○	○
D17S789	○	○	○
D17S807	○	○	○
D17S515	○	● ☞	○
D17S785	○	● ☞	○

portions of chromosomes 17, 17q24.2–25.2 and 17q25.2 (markers D17S515 and D17S785 respectively) (Figs. 8.18–8.21). The transfer of chromosome 11, namely regions 11q13–23, 11q23.1 and 11q23.3 reduced the growth rate of BP1E cells and their colony formation in agar methocel. These data support the postulate that this chromosome hosts a putative tumor suppressor gene; in agreement with the reported reduction of tumorigenesis of MCF-7 breast cancer cells by 11q22-q23 transfer [79]. However, the transfer failed to revert the immortalized and transformation phenotypes, since the cells continued growing and telomerase activity was not affected in the transformed BP1E cells. Although a putative senescence gene has been mapped to chromosome 11p15, which caused in vitro growth arrest of rhabdomyosarcoma [80], and bladder carcinoma [81] cell lines, the donor chromosome 11 we transferred did not contain the 11p15 region, since it had a deletion of the majority of the p-arm and the distal q-arm.

The transfer of chromosome 17 suppressed the growth of BP1E cells by 90%, indicating that this chromosome hosts tumor suppressor gene(s), confirming studies in cancer cells reported by various authors [79, 82–89]. Significant senescence was observed in all BP1E-17*neo* clones obtained in this study, representing a novel finding, since senescence genes have not been reported in this chromosome.

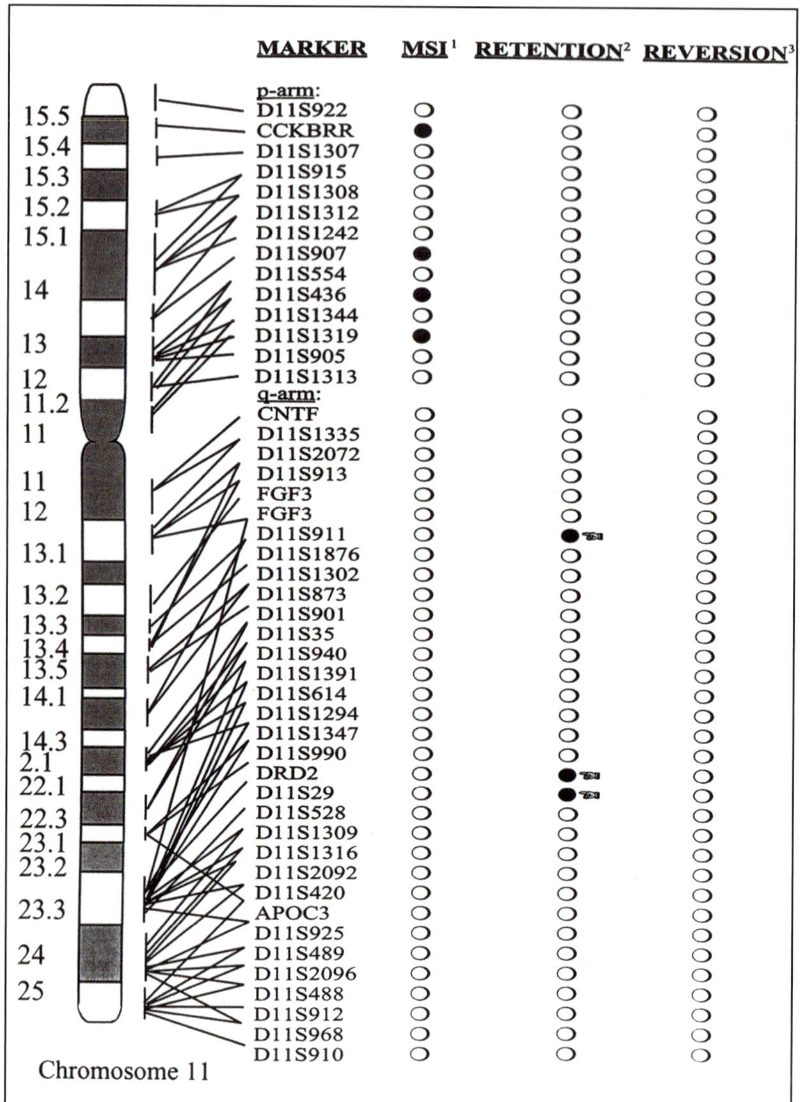

Figure 8.19

A summary of microsatellite polymorphism[1] analysis of chromosome 11 in BP1E-11*neo* #145 cells. Marker, microsatellite markers along chromosome 11. [2]Retention, retention of donor copy in BP1E-11*neo* #145 cells from A9-11*neo* is indicated by a *solid circle* as positive, or by an *open circle* as negative. [3]Reversion, reversion of genomic instability was not observed

Chromosome 17, in addition to *p53* and *BRCA1* genes that map to 17pl3.1 [84] and 17q21 [85], respectively, also hosts at least three more tumor suppressor genes, which have been located at 17pl3.3 [82, 86–89], central 17q, but distal to *BRCA1* [88, 89], and 17q24-q25 [83]. It is not clear whether the same tumor suppressor genes are involved in the suppression of growth of BP1E cells. In search for a mechanism of senescence in the hybrid cells, we measured telome-rase activity in various cells. It has been reported that repetitive TTAGGG sequences located at the telomeric ends of human chromosomes may act as a molecular mitotic clock [90]; each successive genome replication is accompanied by gradual 50–200 bp shortening due to incomplete replication of the 3' ends. Cellular senescence occurs when telomeres reach such a critically short length that the replication of the genome cannot be maintained [91]. The process of telo-

Figure 8.20

Drawing showing that the insertion of the chromosome 17q24.3–25.2 reverts the immortalization and transformation phenotypes

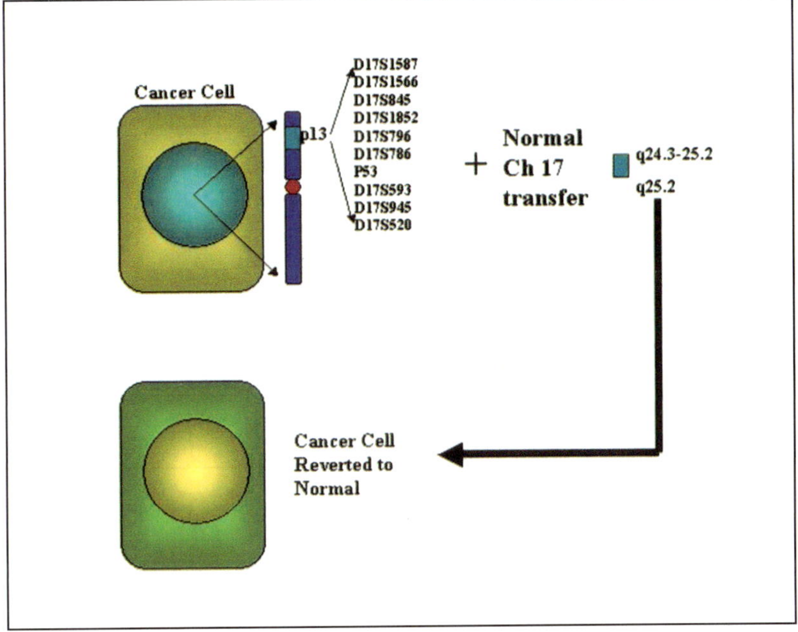

Figure 8.21

Drawing showing that the insertion of the chromosome 17q24.3–25.2 reverts the damaged area of chromosome 17p

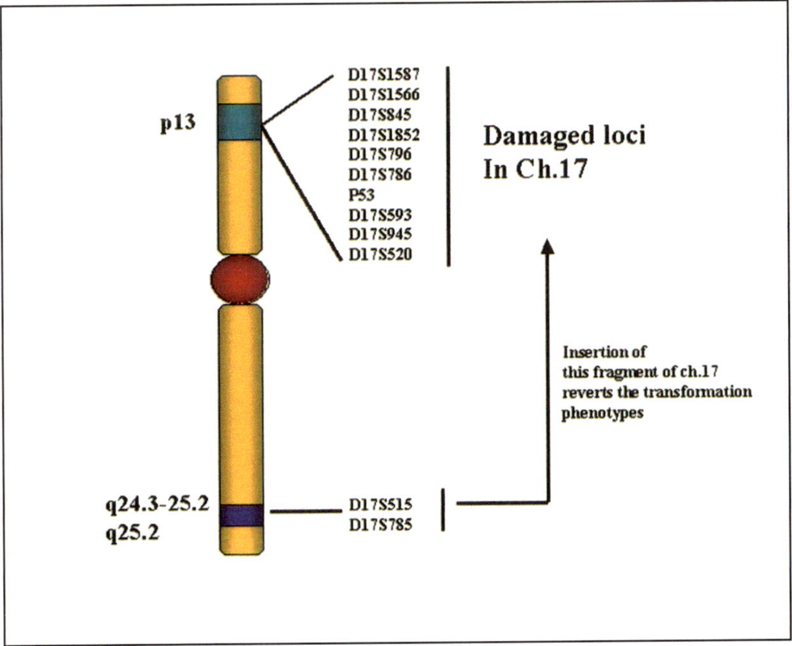

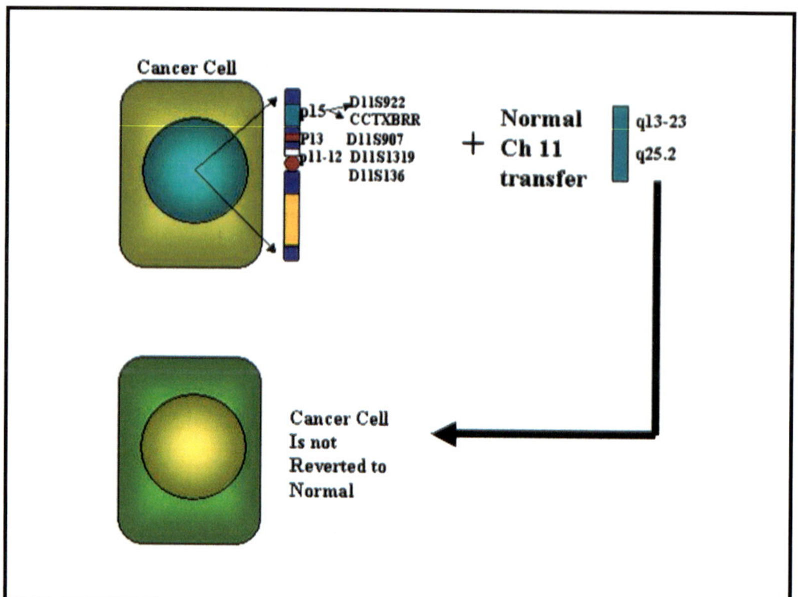

Figure 8.22

Drawing showing that the insertion of the chromosome 11 does not revert the immortalization and transformation phenotypes

meric stabilization involves the activation of telomerase, which adds TTAGGG repeats to the 3' ends of chromosomes [92, 93]. Thus, repression of telomerase is considered as a key element of cell immortalization [93], while elevated levels of telomerase activities is found in a number of immortal cell lines and human tumor tissues [94, 95–97]. The enzymatic activity was lost in BP1E-17*neo* D100 cells and it was not modified in BP1E11*neo* #145 cells. The data indicate that transfer of chromosome 17 abrogates the expression of immortalization and transformation phenotypes in BP1E cells. Although we have only detected retention of the regions 17q24.2–25.2 we cannot rule out the possibility that other regions of chromosomes 17 that have not been probed with the markers used might have played a role in the phenomena observed. The novelty of the observations lies in the fact that chromosome 17 hosts a gene or genes that controls the expression of immortalization phenotype in HBEC.

8.5.2 Reversion of the Transformation but Not Immortalization Phenotype

At difference of the region 17q24.3–25.2 [79] that is able to abrogate the immortalization phenotype and return all the characteristics of normal cells, the region 17p13.2 (D17S796) reverts the transformation phenotype as well as sensitivity to Fas mediated apoptosis but is unable to abrogate the immortalization phenotype. BP1E cells, derived from the immortalized MCF-10F cells transformed by the chemical carcinogen benzo(a)pyrene, express in vitro phenotypes indicative of neoplastic transformation such as resistance to Fas-mediated apoptosis, enhanced cell growth, anchorage independence, enhanced chemo invasiveness, and absence of ductulogenic capacity [30, 97, 98]. In the process of transformation, MCF10-F cells have lost genetic material from chromosome l7p13.2 encompassing the D17S796 locus (Fig. 8.23).

Chromosome transfer of 17q25.3 reverts the immortalization phenotype of BP1E cells [78] whereas in this experiment the transfer of 17p13.2 reverts the transformation phenotype. However, the immortalization phenotype persists based on our demonstration of telomerase analysis and the pattern of growth

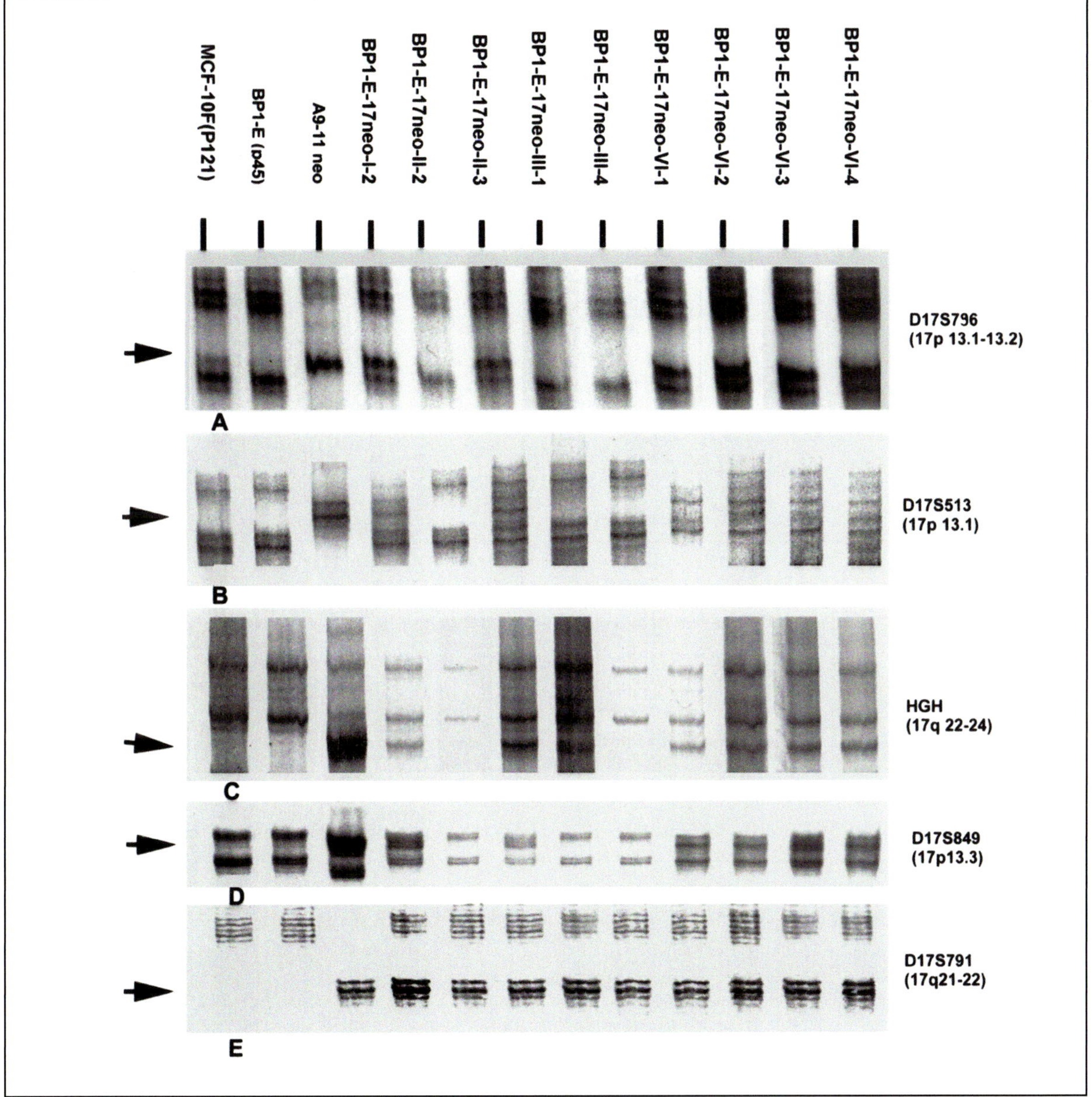

Figure 8.23 a–e

Representative gels showing retention of donor chromosome alleles in BP1E-17*neo* clones. **a** Retention of 17pl3.1–13.2 (Dl7S796). This panel also shows the loss of genetic material in the process of chemical transformation of MCF-10F cells; **b** 17p13.1 (D17S513); **c** 17q22–24 (HGH); **d** 17p13.3 (D17S849) and **e** 17q21–22 (D17S791). Data published in abstract form by: Lareef, M.H., Tahin, Q., Russo, I.H., Mor, G., Song, J., Mihaila, D., Slater, C.M., and Russo, J. Transfer of chromosome 17(p13.1) to chemically transformed human breast epithelial cells induces Fas-mediated apoptosis. Proc. Am. Assoc. Cancer Res. 42:1475a, 2001

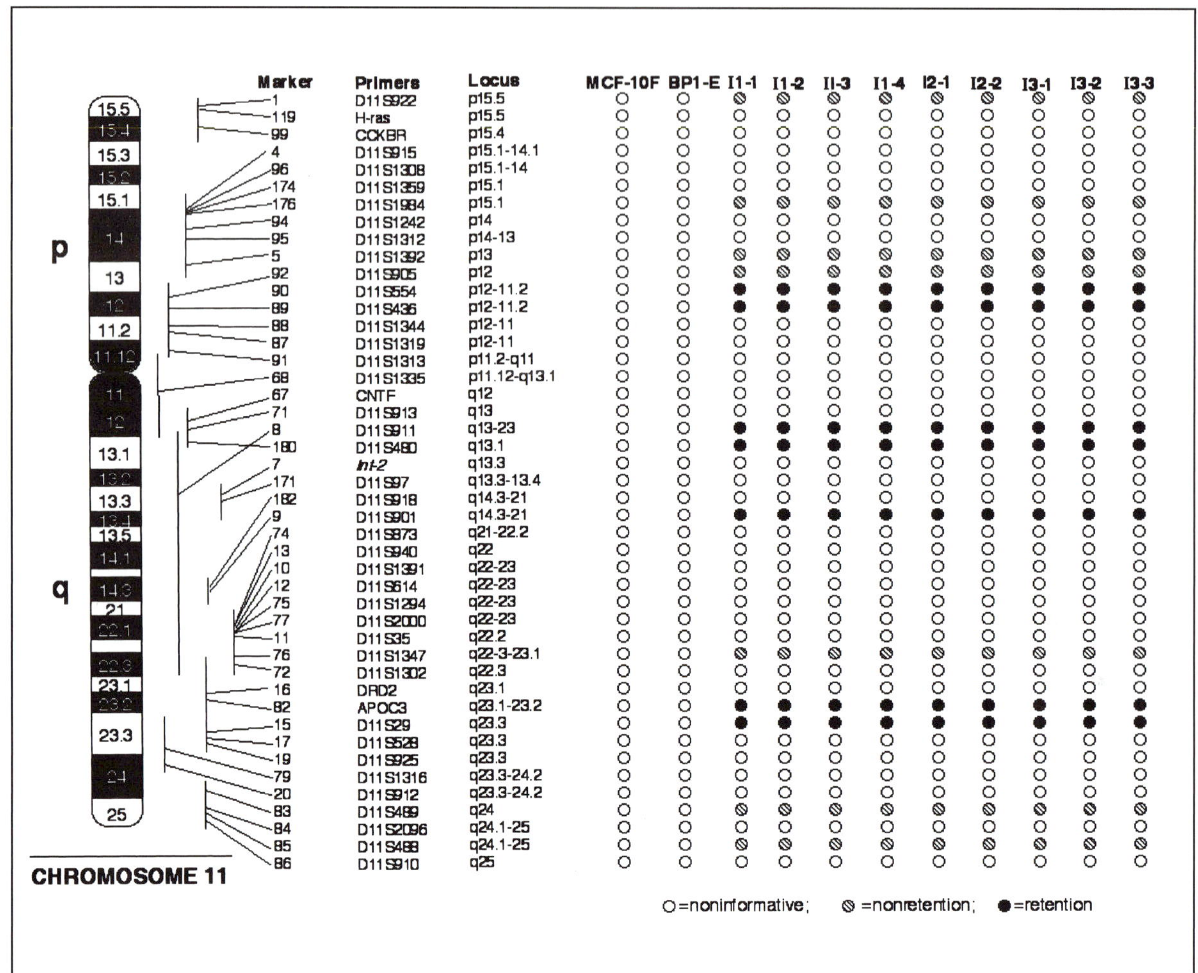

Figure 8.24

Ideogram of micro satellite polymorphism analysis of chromosome 11 transferred clones. Markers indicate micro satellite along chromosome 11. Retention of donor copy in BP1E-11*neo* clones from A9–11 *neo* indicated by a *solid circle* as positive, or by an *open circle* non informative. Data published in abstract form by: Lareef, M.H., Tahin, Q., Russo, I.H., Mor, G., Song, J., Mihaila, D., Slater, C.M., and Russo, J. Transfer of chromosome 17(p13.1) to chemically transformed human breast epithelial cells induces Fas-mediated apoptosis. Proc. Am. Assoc. Cancer Res. 42:1475a, 2001

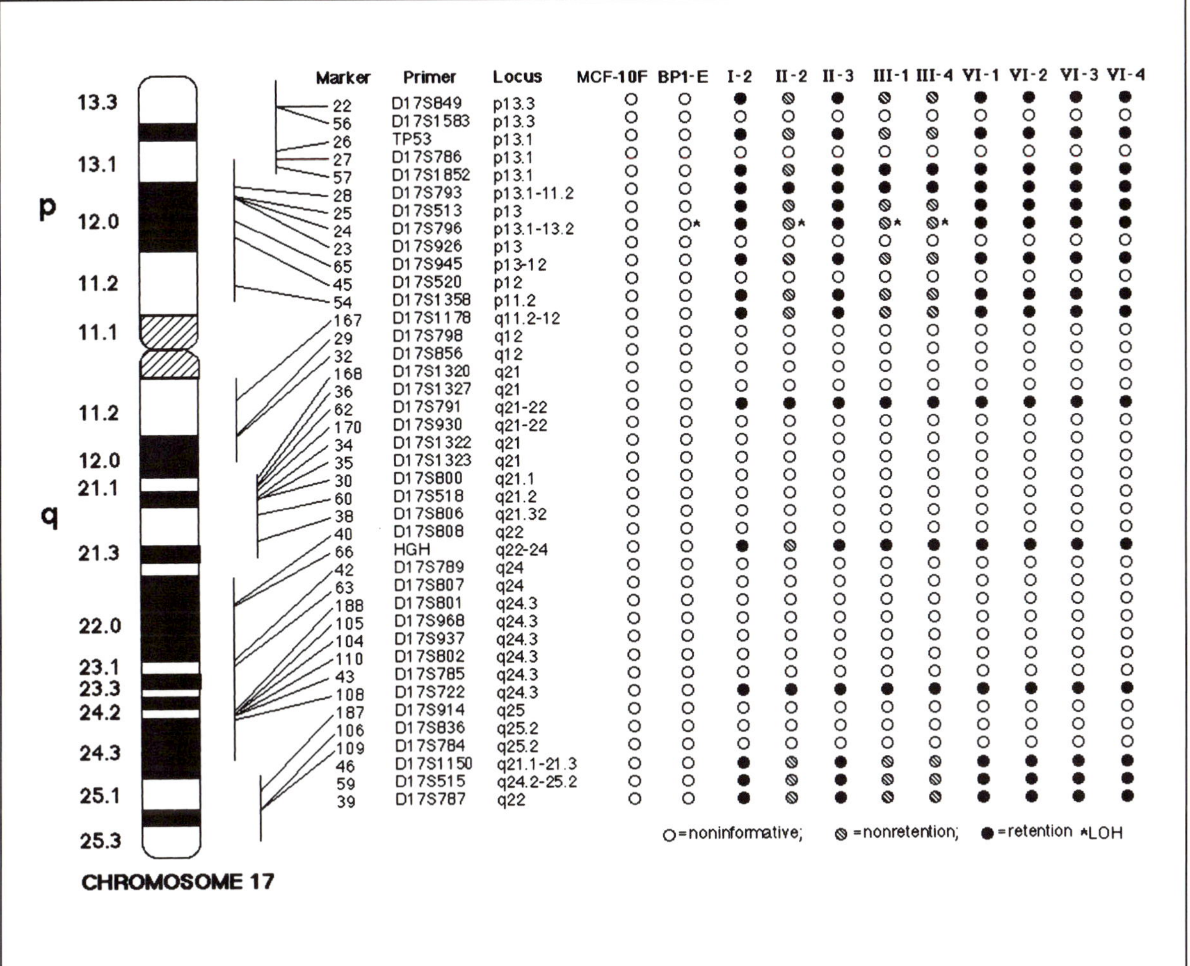

Figure 8.25

Ideogram of micro satellite polymorphism analysis of chromosome 17 transferred clones. Markers indicate the microsatellite along chromosome 17. Retention of donor copy in BP1E-17*neo* clones from A9–17*neo* indicated by a *solid circle* as positive, or by an *open circle* non informative. Data published in abstract form by: Lareef, M.H., Tahin, Q., Russo, I.H., Mor, G., Song, J., Mihaila, D., Slater, C.M., and Russo, J. Transfer of chromosome 17(p13.1) to chemically transformed human breast epithelial cells induces Fas-mediated apoptosis. Proc. Am. Assoc. Cancer Res. 42:1475a, 2001 in vitro. Colony formation in agar-methocel, a technique utilized as an in vitro assay for anchorage independent growth, a parameter indicative of neoplastic transformation [30, 78, 96–98], revealed that MCF-10F cells do not produce colonies whereas BP1E cells have a high CE. Importantly, this enhanced CE is abrogated after transfer of chromosome 17, but not with chromosome 11. All the clones of BP1E that did not retain the 17p13.2 maintain the same CE and growth rate than the transformed cells, even though they have retention of other fragments of chromosome 17 (Fig. 8.23). Assay of ductulogenic capacity in collagen matrix permits an assessment of the ability of cells to differentiate by providing evidence of whether transformed cells form tridimensional structures when grown in a collagen matrix [30, 98–100]. MCF-10F cells form ductules in collagen, whereas BP1E cells have lost their ductulogenic capacity. Out of 10 clones with chromosome 17 transfer 7 reverted ductulogenic capacity, producing duct like structures, forming ductules like MCF-10F immortal cells, wheras 3 clones produced spheroid structures similar to those seen in parental BP1E cells. All 10 clones in which chromosome 11 was transferred failed to produce ductules in collagen.

In order to further determine the specific region(s) of the donor chromosome retained in the microcell hybrids, 45 microsatellite markers for chromosome 11 (Fig. 8.24) and 41 markers for chromosome 17 (Fig. 8.25) were analyzed. The following chromosome 17 markers were retained: D17S849, TP53, D17S1852, D17S793, D17S513, D17S796, D17S945, D17S1358, D17S178, D17S791, HGH, D17S722, D17S1150, D17S515, and D17S787. Most of the other markers tested were non-informative (Figs. 8.23, 8.25). Among the 45 tested markers for chromosome 11, the following markers showed clear retention: D11S554, D11S436, D11S911, D11S480, D11S901, APOC3 and D11S29 (Fig. 8.24). Most of the other markers tested were non-informative.

Recent studies of the biochemical mechanisms evoked by conventional treatments for neoplastic diseases point to apoptosis as a key process for elimination of unwanted cells [101]. Impaired function of apoptosis-related genes is a crucial step in tumorigenesis [102–104]. Among the genes that control apoptosis is Fas (CD95/Apo-1) a cell membrane receptor that upon binding by its ligand (FasL) triggers a signal resulting in apoptotic cell death [103–105]. Fas is a cell-surface receptor that exists in two forms, transmembrane and soluble. The former induces apoptosis by ligation of FasL or agonistic anti-Fas antibody, whereas the latter inhibits Fas-mediated apoptosis by neutralizing its ligand [106, 107]. Harnessing the power of this complex molecule is expected to lead to the development of powerful chemotherapeutic advances. Our data establish a link between the Fas ligand-receptor complex in chemically transformed human breast epithelial cells and a gene/s located in chromosome 17p13.2.

Whereas gene transfer of Fas ligand (CD95L) using adenoviral vectors has been shown to generate apoptotic responses and potent inflammatory reactions that can be used to induce the regression of malignancies in vivo, there are significant unwanted reactions such as hepatotoxicity that may limit their clinical utility [107]. Several genes mapped in 17p13 locus are associated with cell death and apoptosis in different species, including those encoding cell death protein 4 (Ced4) [108], cell death protein 3 (Ced3) precursor [109], caspase 2 precursor, inhibitory of apoptosis protein (IAP) [110], caspase-4-precursor, caspase-13 precursor, caspase-5 precursor and caspase 11 precursor. Mutations in the gene encoding ced-4 block almost all programmed cell death that normally occurs during *C. elegans* development [111]. The fact that we have transferred the chromosome 17p13.2 region and regain Fas-mediated apoptosis suggests that in human breast cancer there may be a mutation in this gene that is rescued by chromosome 17 transfer. Abnormality of Ced-3 gene has been associated with cell death in nematodes in the effector mechanism of apoptotic cell death [109]. Viruses often express IAP which inhibits the host cell, thereby enhancing their infectivity [110]. This is supported by data indicating that breast cancer cells contain survivin, a cytoplasmic protein of the IAP family, whereas no expression of survivin was detected in adjacent normal breast tissue [112]. The fact that BP1E cells are resistant to apoptosis may indicate that in the process of transformation the human breast epithelial cells synthesize or acquired known or unknown protein of IAP as a property of cell transformation. The fact that MCF-10F is a spontaneously immortalized cell that is sensitive to apoptosis indicates that IAP is not involved in the immortalization process. This is confirmed by our studies of the telomerase activity and telomere length, which show that the chromosome17p13.2 region does not revert the immortalization phenotype. Immortalization is thought to be an essential event in the carcinogenic process [113]; immortalization involves abrogation of cellular programs for limiting the rate and the number of cell replications. This supports previous finding from our laboratory demonstrating that immortalization process in HBEC is associated with loss of 17q25.3 (D17S785) [78].

The phenotypic alterations indicative of neoplastic transformation induced by a chemical carcinogen in MCF-10F cells are not due to changes induced in the p53 gene [32, 114–115] as confirmed by microsatellite analysis of MCF-10F and BP1E cells with specific primers for p53, which revealed that neither LOH nor any other genetic alterations were observed in these two cell lines.

An important question that must be addressed is the relevance of these in vitro studies to the human situation. In hepatocellular carcinoma, LOH in 17p13, using the marker D17S796 has been found in 52.4 % of the cases studied [116]. LOH at this locus was associated significantly with a more aggressive tumorigenesis phenotype [116]. There is a significant amount of data pointing to LOH at17p13.2 in breast cancer [117, 118]. Few reports, however, have demonstrated LOH in 17p13.2 using the marker D17S796, although one report [119] has documented LOH at this locus in atypical ductal hyperplasia and in situ ductal carcinoma of the breast, suggesting this to be an early genomic change in the neoplastic process. Another report [120] indicated LOH and microsatellite instability involving D17S796 in benign proliferative diseases. Collectively, our data suggest that 17p13.2 may contain a gene(s) responsible for maintaining ductulogenic capacity in collagen, colony formation in agar-methocel, and most importantly controlling programmed cell death through the Fas/Fas L system. Therefore the identification of the critical 17p13.2 target gene(s) may provide insights into the regulation of the Fas/Fas L system [121–124] in human breast cancer.

8.6 The Role of Mismatch Repair in the Initial Event of Carcinogenesis

Although the cause of breast cancer remains largely unknown, and our understanding of the mechanisms responsible of cancer initiation and progression is limited, alterations in specific oncogenes [125], abnormalities in tumor suppressor genes [126], and microsatellite instability (MSI) [127–129] have been associated with the development of this disease. Alterations in the short interspersed tandem repeats, or MSI may be due to mispairing mediated by a slippage mechanism causing destabilization of DNA tracts during replication (genomic instability) [130, 131]. MSI, in turn, has been reported to be associated with alterations in known mismatch repair (MMR) genes [18, 132]. It was first observed in human colorectal carcinomas [133], and in aberrant colonic crypt foci [134]; more recently, MSI has been reported in breast lesions, such as ductal hyperplasia and carcinoma in situ [135, 136] as well as in advanced breast cancer [48, 137]. MMR genes in humans include the *Escherichia coli mutS* DNA homologues *hMSH2* (at *2p16*), *hMSH6* (G/T Binding Protein) (at *2p16*), and *hMSH3* (at *5q11-q12*), and the *MutL* homologues *hMLH1* (at *3p21*), *hPMS2* (at *7p22*), and *hPMS1* (at *2q 31–33*) [138]. Mutations in MMR genes have been detected in hereditary non-polyposis colorectal cancer (HNPCC) [139, 140], as well as in sporadic tumors, including those of stomach [141] and endometrium [142]. Mutations in these genes reflect certain tumor type specificities, as demonstrated by the high percentage of HNPCC cases exhibiting *hMLH1* and *hMSH2* mutations [138], whereas germline mutations in *hMSH6* lead to increased incidence of gynecological tumors in HNPCC families [143], and uterine carcinomas in homozygous *Msh6* mutant mice, although they also develop lymphomas and skin cancers [138]. Biochemical and genetic studies have revealed that heterodimers formed between hMSH2 and hMSH6 (MutSα) or hMSH2 and hMSH3 (MutSβ) are required for recognition of single bp mismatches, small insertion deletions, and single strand DNA loops, with some overlapping and some divergent specificities. The subsequent removal of these mismatched bases relies on a heterodimer formed by hMLH1 and hPMS2 [139, 144]. Although the current level of knowledge indicates that alterations in the MMR system could play a role in cancer causation, it remains to be clarified whether mutational mechanisms act either alone or in combination with other genes for causing cancer [145].

The experimental model developed in our laboratory revealed MSI at early stages of immortalization and transformation, whereas the expression of tumorigenesis is associated with allelic loss, or loss of heterozygosity (LOH) in different areas of the genome (Fig. 8.1). These data are supported by observations in other systems in which alterations in DNA replication or repair and in genomic stability have been reported to play a role in early stages of tumor growth and progression [129–131]. Of interest is the fact that genomic instability, which we [48] and other authors [135, 136] have reported in ductal carcinomas in situ, is manifested in chemically transformed cells before the tumorigenic phenotype is expressed, confirming the fact that loss of mismatch repair function can be a very early or initial event during the neoplastic transformation of mammalian cells [9, 146].

The mRNAs of the MMR genes *hMLH1*, *hMSH2*, *hPMS1*, *hPMS2*, and *hMSH6* are expressed in immortalized MCF-10F cells, in the transformed cells BP-1, in the tumorigenic cells BP-1Tras, and in all the tumor-derived cell lines. The levels of mRNA, as well as those of protein expression of hMSH2 and hMSH6 were significantly reduced in the tumoral cell lines. An association between downregulation of hMSH2 protein expression and cancer progression has been reported in invasive breast cancer [147]. In addition, hPMS2 protein expression was totally lost in BP-l-Tras and in all tumor cell lines derived from it. The reduction or loss of MMR protein expression has been also reported in prostate cancer [148], and in *Pms2*$^{-/-}$ mice [149]. We investigated if the variations observed in the transcriptional and translational levels of the MMR genes was a reflection of one or more mutations of the genes by DNA sequencing them using RT-PCR products. It was of interest to observe that

the *hPMS1* gene, that did not show mutations in any of the cells tested, did not exhibit significant changes in the levels of mRNA and protein expression at any of the various stages of cancer progression. These observations are in agreement with those of other authors that did not find mutations in the *hPMS1* gene to segregate in HNPCC and HNPCC-like families [150]. In *hMLH1* gene we found only silent mutations and no changes at protein expression levels with cancer progression. These observations contrast with the predominance of MLH1 and MSH2 genes mutations observed in HNPCC patients [151, 152]. In addition, *hMLH1* gene has been reported to be mutated and/or deleted in immortalized BPH-1 cells [153]. Although our observations suggest that mutations in the *hMLH1* gene might be specific for cell type, breast cancer has been reported to be to be present in 9 (1.66%) of *hMLH1* mutation-positive versus 2 (0.22%) *hMSH2* mutation-positive patients from 95 HNPCC families [154].

Our analysis of the *hMSH2* gene revealed that all the cell lines tested exhibited one polymorphism in codon 702 of exon 13. This mutation seems to be unique to our breast epithelial cell line system, since it differs from the *hMSH2* polymorphism reported in HNPCC (21%), and gastric cancer (23%) patients, as well as in 28% of normal individuals, which consists of a constitutional T to C transition in the intronic splice acceptor site at a position six base pairs upstream of the start of exon 13 [155, 156]. Our results demonstrated that the progressively increased malignancy of BP-transformed to tumorigenic cells was associated with an increased number of mutations in the *hMSH2* gene. It is possible to speculate that this increase is somewhat responsible/related to the decreased levels of mRNA and protein observed in the tumoral cell lines, as an expression of cancer progression [157].

The expression of mRNA transcripts and the MMR proteins for the *hPMS2* gene was detected only in the immortal MCF-10F and in BP-1 transformed cells. Although BP-1 cells exhibited a non-sense mutation in exon 10, no changes in protein expression were observed in relation to this mutation. Protein expression was lost in tumorigenic BP-1Tras and in tumor-derived cell lines, a phenomenon that was attributed to the presence of a non sense mutation in codon 470, exon 9 that resulted in a stop signal and premature truncation that was detected in all these cell lines. The confirmation of this truncation by Western blot analysis using antibodies specific for the hPMS2 amino terminal fragment revealed that the protein was also truncated in BP-1 cells. We further confirmed the hPMS2 protein truncation in 6 invasive ductal carcinomas. This is the first report of a truncated hPMS2 protein in human breast cells and in primary breast cancer. Our results are supported by the finding that 30% of hPMS2 cDNA products of Vaco481 colon cancer cell line demonstrate a G-T mutation at codon 279 within exon 8, which convert GGA (Gly) to a premature TGA stop codon [158]. In addition, the presence of a stop signal has been also reported in colorectal cancer and in HNPCC type 4 [159]. However, the G to A transition that has been reported in codon 20, which resulted in an arginine to glutamine change that codified the stop signal in 3 of 18 HNPCC patients has been interpreted to represent a polymorphism rather than a functional mutation [160].

In our results the *hMSH6*, *hMSH2* and *hPMS2* genes are mutated in transformed, tumorigenic and tumor-derived cell lines (Fig. 8.26). Heteroduplex analysis revealed that the efficiency of repair of G:A (TGA 89) and of T:G (GG88) mispairs was slightly reduced in BP-1 cell extracts in comparison with MCF-10F cells. In contrast, negligible or no repair occurred in the tumorigenic cells BP-1-Tras and in all the tumor derived cell lines due to the truncation of hPMS2 protein. We concluded that BP-induced transformation results in mutations in the MMR genes leading to impaired repair function, although enough functional activity is retained for repairing the mispairs G:A and T:G. Transfection of BP-1 cells with the mutated c-H-ras oncogene increased the number of MMR gene mutations resulting in a total loss of reparative activity. With the objective to demonstrate the hPMS2 role in the MMR activity during tumor progression, we incubated the DNA heteroduplex in vitro assay in the presence or absence of the hPMS2 wild type protein in complex with hMLH1 using the BP-1 Tras tumor cell line. We observed that the hPMS2-MLH1 normal complex repaired more than 52% of

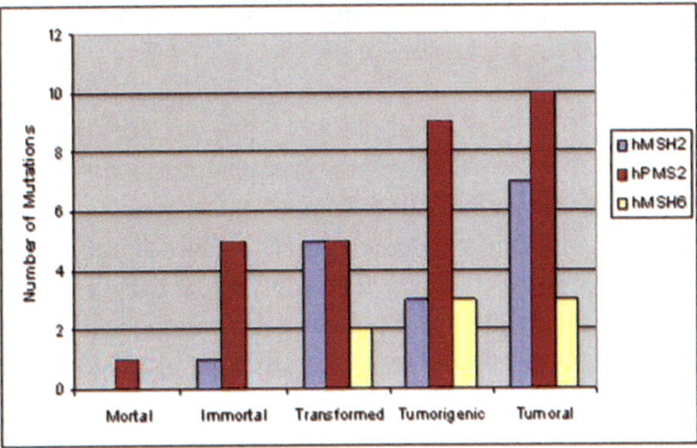

Figure 8.26

Total number of mutations in the MMR genes *hMSH2*, *hPMS2* and *hMSH6* in the mortal, immortal and the tumor cell lines. Data published in abstract form by: Balogh, G. A., Russo, IH, Clark, A., Kunkel, T. and Russo J. Role of truncation of the mismatch repair hPMS2 protein in the initiation and progression of breast cancer. Proc. Am. Assoc. Cancer Res. 43: 2002

the MMR deficiency in this tumor cell line. These data suggest that a major role in the impairment and loss of repair function could be attributed to the premature truncation of the hPMS2 protein, as supported by the findings that the somatic inactivation of hPMS2 protein can play a role in the development of the sporadic colon cancer, with expression of the full range of cancer phenotypes associated with inactivation of the MMR system [158].

Altogether our data clearly show that in this in vitro-in vivo system a chemical carcinogen like BP is able to induce mutations in MMR genes and that additional insult to the cells like the transfection with *cHa ras* results in a tumorigenic cell with further mutation and truncation of hMPS2 protein. These results acquired further relevance when the same level of truncation was detected in 2 out 6 invasive ductal carcinomas of the breast. This data strongly suggest that the MMR gene *hMPS2* is involved in human breast cancer.

8.7 Unifying Concepts

The model described above is a paradigm of the progressive nature of breast cancer. Although a step by step analogy with the pathogenesis of breast cancer, which is currently accepted starts as ductal hyperplasia, progressing to atypical ductal hyperplasia, intraductal carcinoma and invasive carcinoma, still needs to be done, there are several points in common with this in vitro model that deserve emphasis, namely:

1. The immortalization of MCF-10 M to MCF-10F cells may represent the stage of atypical ductal hyperplasia (ADH), since the cells composing these lesions are already clonal and with a higher proliferative activity
2. Alterations in several oncogenes have been detected in early carcinomas in situ, an indication that the phenomenon occurs early in the transformation process; in our in vitro model, we observed that amplification and overexpression of several oncogenes emerge as the result of clonal selection
3. The LOH observed in chromosomes 9, 11, 16 and 17 in tumorigenic cells is similar to what is observed in primary invasive breast cancer

The problem that clearly emerges is how to unify and make a rationale integration of this knowledge. For example p53 abnormalities have been shown by various measurements to be significantly associated with genetic instability. As a guardian of the genome, the p53 protein induces cell-cycle arrest at G_1 phase in response to DNA damage, thus allowing the cell to perform all necessary repairs. We previously found that a mutation in exon 7 of p53 gene is present in the immortalized and transformed HBECs. Interestingly, we showed here that the *TP53* locus was positive for MSI, as were other markers on chromosome 17p, indicating that these two alterations are associated, although it is not clear whether they occurred independently or one caused the other. Nevertheless, that mutation of TP53 occurred before several other genetic alterations in the oncogenes *cHa-ras*, *c-myc*, *erbB2*, *int-2*, and *mdm2* previously observed in these cells seems to suggest that the inactivation of *p53* at

least partially contributed to the genetic instability. This may be a characteristic of breast epithelial cells, as it has been reported that an inverse correlation exists between the replication error-prone phenotype and p53 mutation in colorectal cancer cell lines. In addition, it has been reported upregulation of human ferritin heavy chain mRNA in the immortalized MCF-10F cells and in the derived transformed BP1E cells, suggesting that an increased level of reactive iron in the cells may lead to an increase in oxygen free-radical generation, oxidative DNA damage, and mutation. This mechanism, together with mutation of *p53*, may contribute individually (or in concert with other changes) to genomic instability, as manifested by MSI in both the immortalized MCF-10F cells and the chemically transformed BP1, BP1E, D3, and D3-1 cells reported in this study. A manifestation of instability could well be the expression of MSI that has been associated with the initiation and progression of HBEC transformation in vitro. Specifically, chromosomes 11p and 17p were affected by MSI during the immortalization of MCF-10F cells. The accumulation of MSI in several other loci on chromosomes 11 and 13 was correlated with the progressive transformation induced by BP. The involvement of two loci on chromosomes 13 and 16 was implicated in the expression of the transformation phenotype induced by DMBA. Our observations of a correlation between MSI and HBEC immortalization and transformation indicate that defects in DNA replication and/or MMR are early factors contributing to the pathogenesis of immortalization and transformation of the human breast epithelium.

These findings support the notion that multiple genomic alterations are early events that initiate the multi stage process of breast carcinogenesis. However, it is not known whether any one of these changes is the driving force responsible for the ultimate expression of the transformed phenotype. The answer to this question can be sought by testing the functional role of specific genes on a chromosome. This phenomenon has been explored through the application of microcell-mediated chromosome transfer technique. This procedure has allowed us and other researchers to introduce specific genes into a target cell for testing putative tumor suppressor genes. For example, growth/tumor suppressor activities have been detected in chromosomes 1, 3, 5, 6, 7, 9, 11, 17 and X in various human tumor cell lines. Senescence genes have been found on chromosomes 1, 2, 3, 4, 6, 7, 10, 11, 18 and X. Putative tumor suppressor genes have been mapped to chromosomes 1q23-qter, 1, 3p, 6q21-q23 and/or 6q26-q27, 11, 17 and 17q. The technique of chromosome transfer provided an important tool to determine, if not the specific gene in a chromosome the area of the chromosome involving one or more known or unknown genes involved in the biologic process. The fact that in chromosome 17 transfer experiments we have identified areas in 17q that are able to abrogate both the transformation and immortalization phenotype of a transformed cells and that transfer of 17p abrogates only the transformation phenotypes related to the apoptotic function, but not the immortalization phenotype, clearly indicate that there is a hierarchy in which the genome control several process in the cell. This concept of genomic hierarchy, in which genes located in specific portion of a chromosome may have an organizing effect in the expression of other genes in another chromosomes needs further exploration.

References

1. Pillutla, R.C., Goldstein, N.I., Blume, A.J., Fisher, P.B. Target validation and drug discovery using genomic and protein-protein interaction technologies. Expert Opin. Ther. Targets 6(4): 517–531, 2002.
2. Voit, E.O. Metabolic modeling: a tool of drug discovery in the post- genomic era G. Discov. Today 7(11): 621–628, 2002.
3. Inoue, K., Lupski, J.R. Molecular mechanisms for genomic disorders. Annu. Rev. Genomics Hum. Genet. 3:199–203, 2002.
4. Bieche, I., Lidereau, R. Genetic alterations in breast cancer. Genes Chromosomes Cancer 14:227–251, 1995.
5. Coleman, W.B., Tsongalis, G.J. Multiple mechanisms account for genomic instability and molecular mutation in neoplastic transformation. Clin. Chem. 41:644–657, 1995.
6. Eshleman, J.R., Markowitz, S.D. Microsatellite instability in inherited and sporadic neoplasms. Current Opin. Oncol. 7:83–89, 1995.
7. Aldaz, C.M., Chen, T., Sahin, A., Cunningham, J., Bondy, M. Comparative allelotype of in situ and invasive human breast cancer: High frequency of microsatellite instability in lobular breast carcinomas. Cancer Res. 55:3976–3981, 1995.
8. Karnik, P., Plummer, S., Casey, G., et al. Microsatellite instability at a single locus (D11S988) on chromosome 11 pl5.5 as a late event in mammary tumorigenesis. Hum. Mol. Genet. 4:1889–1894, 1995.
9. Lakhani, S.R., Slack, D.N., Hamoudi, R.A., Collins, N., Stratton, M.R., Sloane, J.P. Detection of allelic imbalance indicates that a proportion of mammary hyperplasia of usual type are clonal, neoplastic proliferations. Lab. Invest. 74:129–135, 1996.
10. Shaw, J.A., Walsh, T., Chappell, S., Carey, N., Johnson, K., Walker, R.A. Microsatellite instability in early sporadic breast cancer. Br. J. Cancer 73:1393–1397, 1996.
11. Yang, X., Russo, I.H., Huang, Y., Russo, J. Microsatellite instability of D17S513 on chromosome 17 is associated with progression of breast cancer. Int. J. Oncol. 11:41–46, 1997.
12. Ionov, Y., Peinado, M.A, Malkhosyan, S., Shibata, D., Perucho, M. Ubiquitous somatic mutations in simple repeated sequences reveal a new mechanism for colonic carcinogenesis. Nature 363:558–561, 1993.
13. Boyer, J.C., Umar, A., Risinger, J., et al. Microsatellite instability, mismatch repair deficiency, and genetic defects in human cancer cell lines. Cancer Res. 55:6063–6070, 1995.
14. Boland, C.R. Roles of the DNA mismatch repair genes in colorectal tumorigenesis. Int. J. Cancer 69:47–49, 1996.
15. Eshleman, J.R., Markowitz, S.D. Mismatch repair defects in human carcinogenesis. Hum. Mol. Genet. 5:1489–1494, 1996.
16. Mellon, I, Rajpal, D.K., Koi, M., Boiand, C.R., Champe, G.N. Transcription-coupled repair deficiency and mutations in human mismatch repair genes. Science 272:557–560, 1996.
17. Sia, E.A., Links-Robertson, S., Petes, T.D. Genetic control of microsatellite stability. Mutat. Res. 383:61–70, 1997.
18. Loeb, L.A. Mutator phenotype may be required for multistage carcinogenesis. Cancer Res. 51:3075–3079, 1991.
19. Loeb, L.A. Many mutations in cancer. Cancer Surv. 28:329–342, 1996.
20. Loeb, L.A. Cancer cells exhibit a mutator phenotype. Adv. Cancer Res. 72:25–56, 1998.
21. Callahan, R., Cropp, C., Merlo, G.R., et al. Genetic and molecular heterogeneity of breast cancer cells. Clin. Chem. Acta 217:63–73, 1993.
22. Devilee, P., Cornelisse, C.J. Somatic genetic changes in human breast cancer. Biochem. Biophys. Acta 1198:113–130, 1994.
23. Tsuda, H., Hirohashi, S. Identification of multiple breast cancer of multicentric origin by histological observations and distribution of allele loss on chromosome 16q. Cancer Res. 55:3395–3398, 1995.
24. Radford DM, Fair KL, Phillips, N.J., et al. Allelotyping of ductal carcinoma in situ of the breast: Deletion of loci on 8p, 13q, 16p, 17p and 17q. Cancer Res. 55:3399–3405, 1995.
25. Devilee, P., Hermans, J., Eyfjord, J., et al. Loss of heterozygosity at 7q31 in breast cancer: Results from an international

collaborative study group. Genes Chromosomes Cancer 18:193–199, 1997.

26. Pandis, N., Bardi, G., Mitelman, F., Heim, S. Deletions of short arm of chromosome 3 in breast tumors. Genes Chromosomes Cancer 18:241–245, 1997.

27. Knudson, A.G., Jr. Genetics and etiology of human cancer. Adv. Hum. Genet. 8:1–66, 1977.

28. Soule, H.D., Maloney, T.M., Wolman, S.R., Peterson, W.D., Brenz, R., McGrath, C.M., Russo, J., Pauley, R.J., Jones, R.F. and Brooks, S.C.. Isolation and characterization of a spontaneously immortalized human breast epithelial cell line, MCF-10. Cancer Res. 50:607–086, 1990.

29. Calaf, G., Russo, J. Transformation of human breast epithelial cells by chemical carcinogens. Carcinogenesis 14:483–492, 1993.

30. Russo, J., Barnabas, N., Zhang, P.L., Adesina, K. Mini review: Molecular basis of breast cell transformation. Radiat. Oncol. Investig. 3:424–429. 1996.

31. Russo, J., Barnabas, N., Higgy, N., Salicioni, A.M., Wu, Y.L., Russo, I.H. Molecular basis of human breast epithelial cell transformation. In: Calvo, F., Crepin, M., Magdelenat, H., Editors. Breast cancer. Advances in biology and therapeutics, Paris, John Libbey Eurotext; 1996. pp. 33–43.

32. Barnabas, N., Moraes, R., Calaf, G., Estrada, S., Russo, J. Role of p53 in MCF-10F cell immortalization and chemically induced neoplastic transformation. Int. J. Oncol. 7:1289–1296, 1995.

33. Donehower, L.A. Effects of p53 mutation on tumor progression: Recent insights from mouse tumor models. Biochem. Biophys. Acta 1996;1242(3):171–176.

34. Zhang, P-L., Calaf, G., Russo, J. Allele loss and point mutation in codons 12 and 61 of the c-Ha-ras oncogene in carcinogen transformed human breast epithelial cells. Mol. Carcinog. 9:46–56, 1994.

35. Zhang, P.L., Chai, Y.L., Ho, T.H., Calaf, G., Russo, J. Activation of *c-myc*, *c-neu*, and *int-2* oncogenes in the transformation of HBEC MCFF treated with chemical carcinogens in vitro. Int. J. Oncol. 6:963–968, 1995.

36. Risinger, J.I., Umar, A., Boyer, J., et al. Microsatellite instability in gynecological sarcomas and in hMSH2 mutant uterine sarcoma cell lines defective in mismatch repair activity. Cancer Res. 55:5664–5669, 1995.

37. Murray, J.C., Buetow, K.H., Waber, J.L., et al. A comprehensive human linkage map with centimorgan density. Science 265:2049–2054, 1994.

38. Wu, Y.L., Barnabas, N., Russo, I.H., Yang, X., Russo, J. Microsatellite instability and loss of heterozygosity in chromosomes 9 and 16 in human breast epithelial cells transformed by chemical carcinogens. Carcinogenesis 18:1069–1074, 1997.

39. Habuchi, T., Ogawa, O., Kakehi, et al. Accumulated allelic losses in the development of invasive urothelial cancer. Int. J. Cancer 53:579–584, 1993.

40. Vertino, P.M., Spillare, E.A., Harris, C.C., Baylin, S.B. Altered chromosomal methylation patterns accompany oncogene-induced transformation of human bronchial epithelial cells. Cancer Res. 53:1684–1689, 1993.

41. Coles, C., Thompson, A.M., Elder, P.A., et al. Evidence implicating at least two genes on chromosomes 17p in breast carcinogenesis. Lancet 336:761–763, 1990.

42. Sato, T., Tanigami, A., Yamakawa, K., et al. Allelotype of breast cancer: Cumulative allele losses promote tumor progression in primary breast cancer. Cancer Res. 50:7184–7189, 1990.

43. Anderson, T.I., Gaustad, A., Ottestad, L., et al. Genetics alterations of the tumor suppressor gene regions 3p, 11 p, 13q, 17p, and 17q in human breast carcinomas. Genes Chromosomes Cancer 4:113–121, 1992.

44. Isomura, M., Tanigami, A., Saito, H., et al. Detailed analysis of loss of heterozygosity on chromosome band 17pl 3 in breast carcinoma on the basis of a high-resolution physical map with 29 markers. Genes Chromosomes Cancer 9:173–179, 1994.

45. Kirchweger, R., Zeillinger, R., Schneeberger, C., Speiser, P., Louason, G., Theillet, C. Patterns of allele losses suggest the existence of five distinct regions of LOH on chromosome 17 in breast cancer. Int. J. Cancer 56:193–199, 1994.

46. Theile, M., Hartmann, S., Scherthan, H., et al. Suppression of tumorigenicity of breast cancer cells by transfer of human chromosome 17 does not require transferred BRCA1 and p53 genes. Oncogene 10:439–447, 1995.

47. Gabra, H., Watson, J.E.V., Taylor, K.J., et al. Definition and refinement of region of loss of heterozygosity at 11q23.3-q24.3 in epithelial ovarian cancer associated with poor prognosis. Cancer Res. 56:950–954, 1996.

48. Tahin, Q., Russo, I.H., Russo, J. Genomic imbalance found in chromosome 11 of pre-invasive and invasive human breast cancer. Proceedings of the American Association for Cancer Research 39:341a, 1998.

49. Hamann, U., Herbold, C., Costa, S., et al. Allelic imbalance on chromosome 13q:Evidence for the involvement of BRCA2 and RB1 in sporadic breast cancer. Cancer Res. 56:1988–1990, 1996.

50. Bechmann, M.W., Picard, F., An, H.X., et al. Clinical impact of detection of loss of heterozygosity of BRCA1 and BRCA2 markers in sporadic breast cancer. Br. J. Cancer 73:1220–1226, 1996.

51. Gudmundsson, J., Johannesdottir, G., Bergthorsson, J.T., et al. Different tumor types from BRCA2 carriers show wild-type chromosome deletions on 13ql2-13. Cancer Res. 55:4830–4832, 1995.

52. Wooster, R., Bignel, G., Lancaster, J., et al. Identification of the breast cancer susceptibility gene BRCA2. Nature 378: 789–792, 1995.

53. Wooster, R., Cleton-Jansen, A.M., Collins, N., et al. Instability of short tandem repeats (microsatellites) in human cancers. Nat. Genet. 6:152–156, 1994.

54. Tavtigian, S.V., Simard, J., Rommens, J., et al. The complete BRCA2 gene and mutations in chromosome 13q-linked kindreds. Nat. Genet. 12:333–337, 1996.

55. Russo, I.H., Tahin, Q., Huang, Y. and Russo, J. Cellular and molecular changes induced by the chemical carcinogen benz (a) pyrene in human breast epithelial cells in association with smoking and breast cancer. J. of Women's Cancer 3:29–36, 2001.

56. Huang, Y., Bove, B., Wu, Y., Russo, I.H., Tahin, Q., Yang, X., Zekri, A., Russo, J. Microsatellite instability during the immortalization and transformation of human breast epithelial cells in vitro. Mol. Carcinog. 24:118–127, 1999.

57. Yee, C.J., Roodi, N., Verner, C.S., Parl, F.F. Microsatellite instability and loss of heterozygosity in breast cancer. Cancer Res. 54:1641–1644, 1994.

58. Toyama, T., Iwase, H., Iwata, H., et al. Microsatellite instability in in situ and invasive sporadic breast cancers of Japanese women. Cancer Lett. 108:205–209, 1996.

59. Toyama T, Iwase H, Yamashita H, et al. Microsatellite instability in sporadic human breast cancers. Int. J. Cancer 68: 447–451,1996.

60. Souvinos, G., Kiaris, H., Tsikkinis, A., Vassilaros, S., Spandidos, D.A. Microsatellite instability and loss of heterozygosity in primary breast tumours. Tumor Biol. 18:157–166, 1997.

61. Nelson, D.L., Warren, S.T. Trinucleotide repeat instability: When and where? Nat. Genet. 4:107–108, 1993.

62. Richards, R.I., Sutherland, G.R. Simple repeat DNA is not replicated simply. Nat. Genet. 6:114–116, 1994.

63. Ouyang, H., Shiwakum, H.O., Hagiwara, H., et al. The insulin-like growth factor II receptor gene is mutated in genetically unstable cancers of the endometrium, stomach and colorectum. Cancer Res. 57:1851–1854, 1997.

64. Thomas DC, Roberts JD, Kunkel TA. Measurement of hetero-duplex repair in human cell extracts. Methods 7:187–197, 1995.

65. Band, V., Dalal, S., Delmolino, L., Androphy, E. J. Enhanced degradation of p53 protein in HPV-6 and HPV-I-E6-immortalized human mammary epithelial cells. EMBO J. 12:1847–1852, 1993.

66. Shay, J. W., Tomlinson, G., Paityszek, M. A., Gollohoin, L. S. Spontaneous in vitro immortalization of breast epithelial cells from a patient with Li Fraumeni syndrome. Mol. Cell Biol. 15:425–432, 1995.

67. Chang, F., Syrjanen, S., Syrjanen, K. Implications of the p53 tumor-suppressor gene in clinical oncology. Clin. Oncol. 13:1009–22, 1995.

68. Barbacid, M. ras genes. Ann. Rev. Biochem. 56:779–827, 1987.

69. Rochlitz, C.F., Scott, G.K., Dodson, J.M., Liu, E., Dolibaum, C., Smith, H.S., Benz, C.C. Incidence of activating ras oncogene mutations associated with primary and metastatic human breast cancer. Cancer Res. 49:357–360, 1989.

70. Krontiris TG, DiMartino NA, Colb M, Parkinson DR. Unique allelic restriction fragments of the human Ha-ras locus in leukocyte and tumor- DNAs of cancer patients. Nature 313:369–74,1985.

71. Peters G, Brookers S, Smith R, Dickson C. Tumorigenesis by mouse mammary tumor virus: Evidence for common region for provirus integration in mammary tumors. Cell 33:369–77, 1983.

72. Guerin M, Barrois M, Terrier MJ: Overexpression of either c-myc or c-erbB-2 (neu) proto-oncogenes in human breast carcinomas: Correlation with poor prognosis. Oncogene Res 1988; 3:21–31.

73. Bartek, J., Iggo, R., Gannon, J., Lane, D.P. Genetic and immunochemical analysis of mutant p53 in human breast cancer cell lines. Oncogene 5:893–9,1990.

74. Callahan, R., and Campbell, A. Mutations in human breast cancer: an overview. J. Natl. Cancer Inst. 81:1780–1786,1989.

75. Devilee, P., Cornelisse, C.J. Genetics of human breast cancer. Cancer Survey 9:605–30,1990.

76. Kirchwerger, R., Zellinger, R., Schneeberger, C., Speiser, P., Lovason, G., Theillet, C. Patterns of allele losses suggest the existence of five distinct regions of LOH on chromosome 17 in breast cancer. Int. J. Cancer 6:193–199, 1994.

77. Barnabas, N., Bell, D., Calaf, G., Moraes, R.C.B., Testa, J., Russo, J. Loss of heterozygosity on chromosome 17p loci in transformed in vitro human breast epithelial cells treated with chemical carcinogens. Proc Am Assoc Cancer Res. 34:649a, 1993.

78. Yang, X., Huang, Y., Russo, I.H., Balsara, B.R., Barret, J.C., Russo, J. Functional roles of chromosomes 11 and 17 in the transformation of human breast epithelial cells in vitro. Int. J. Oncology 15:629–638, 1999.

79. Negrini, M., Sabbioni, S., Haldar, S., Possati, L., Castagnoli, A., Corallini, A., Barbanti-Brodano, G., and Croce, C.M. Tumor and growth suppression of breast cancer cells by chromosome 17associated functions. Cancer Res. 54:1818–1824, 1994.

80. Koi, M., Johnson, L.A., Kalikin, L.M., Little, P.F.R., Nakamura, Y., and Feinberg, A.P. Tumor cells growth arrest caused by subchromosomal transferable DNA fragments from chromosome 11. Science 260:361–364, 1993.

81. Oshimura, M., Shimizu, M. and Kugoh, H. Genetic regulation of telomerase in a multiple pathways model to cellular senescence. Hum, Cell 9:301–308, 1996.

82. Theile, M., Hartmann, S., Scherthan, H., Arnold, W., Deppert, W., Frege, R., Glaab, F., Hamsch, W., and Schemeck, S. Suppression of tumorigenicity of breast cancer cells by transfer of human chromosome 17 does not require transferred BRCA1 and p53 genes. Oncogene 10:439–447, 1995.

83. Plummer, S.J., Adams, L., Simmons, J.A., and Casey, G. Localization of a growth suppressor activity in MCF7 breast cancer cells to chromosome 17q24-q25. Oncogene 14:2339–2345, 1997.

84. Levine, A.J., Momand, J., and Finlay, C.A. The p53 tumor suppressor gene. Nature 351:453–456, 1991.

85. Albertsen, H., Plaetke, R., Ballard, L., Gufimoto, E., Connolly, J., Lawrence, E., Rodriguez, P., Robertson, M., Bradley, P., Miliner, B., Fuhrman, D., Marks, A., Sargent, R., Cartwright, P., Matsunami, N. and White, R. Genetic mapping of the BRCA1 region on chromosome 17q21. Am. J. Hum. Genet. 54:516–525, 1994.

86. Coles, C., Thompson, A.M., Elder, P.A., Cohen, B.B., Mackenzie, I.M., Granston, G., Ghetty, U., MacKay, J., MacDonald, M., Nakamura, Y., Hoyheim, B. and Steel, C.M. Evidence implicating at least two genes on chromosome 17p in breast carcinogenesis. Lancet 336:761–763, 1990.

87. Sato, T., Tanigami, A., Yamakawa, K., Akiyama, F., Kasumi, F., Sakamoto, G. and Kakamura, Y. Allelotype of breast cancer: cumulative allele losses promote tumor progression in primary breast cancer. Cancer Res. 50:7184–7189, 1990.

88. Andersenmm T,I, Gaustadm A, Ottestadm L, Farrants, G.W., Nesland, J.M., Tveit, K.M. and Borresen, A.L. Genetic alterations of the tumour suppressor gene regions 3p,11p, 13q, 17p and 17q in human breast carcinomas. Genes Chromosomes Cancer 4:113–121, 1992.

89. Isomura, M., Tanigami, A., Saito, H., Harada, Y., Katagiri, L., Ledbetter, D.H. and Nakamura, Y. Detailed analysis of loss of heterozygosity on chromosome band 17pq3 in breast carcinoma on the basis of a high-resolution physical map with 29 markers. Genes Chromosomes Cancer 9:173–179, 1994.

90. Harley, C.B. Telomere loss: mitotic clock or genetic time bomb? Mutat Res. 256:271–282, 1991.

91. Hopfer, U., Jacobberger, J.W., Gaenert, D.C., Eckert, R.L., Jat, R.S., Whitsett, J.A. Immortalization of epithelial cells. Am. J. Physiol. 270:CI-CII, 1996.

92. Blackburn, E. Telomerase. Annu. Rev. Biochem. 61:113–129, 1992.

93. Shay, J.W., Wright, W.E., Werbin, H. Toward a molecular understanding of human breast cancer: a hypothesis. Breast Cancer Res. Treat. 25:83–94, 1993.

94. Bacchetti, S., Counter, C.M. Telomeres and telomerase in human cancer. Int. J. Oncol. 7:423–432, 1995.

95. Avilion, A.A., Piatyszek, M.A., Gupta, J., Shay, J.W., Bacchetti, S., Greder, C.W. Human telomerase RNA and telomerase activity in immortal cells lines and tumor tissues. Cancer Res. 56:645–650, 1996.

96. Hu, Y-F, Russo, I.H., Slater, C.M., Russo, J. Down regulation of telomerase activity by extracellular calcium in normal human breast epithelial cells. Proc. Am. Assoc. Cancer Res. 40:1745a, 1999.

97. Russo, J., Calaf, G., Sohi N, Tahin, Q., Zhang, P.L., Alvarado, M.E., Estrada, S., Russo, I.H. Critical steps in breast carcinogenesis. The New York Academy of Sciences 698:1–20, 1993.

98. Russo, J., Reina, D., Frederick, J., Russo, I.H. Expression of phenotypical changes by human breast epithelial cells treated with carcinogens in vitro. Cancer Res. 48:2837–2857, 1988.

99. Russo, J., Russo, I.H. Role of differentiation on transformation on human breast epithelial cells. Medina, D., Kidwell, W., Heppner, G., Anderson, E. (eds.) Cellular, Molecular Biology of Mammary Cancer. New York: Plenum Publishing Co; pp 399–417, 1987.

100. Wu, Y., Barnabas, N., Russo, I.H., Xang, X., Russo, J. Microsatellite Instability, Loss of heterozygosity in chromosomes 9, 16 in human breast epithelial cells transformed by chemical carcinogens. Carcinogenesis 18:1069–1074, 1997.

101. Benjamin, C.W., Hiebsch, R.R., Jones, D.A. Caspase activation in MCF7 cells responding to etoposide treatment. Molecular Pharmacology. 53:446–450, 1998.

102. Mor, G., Kohen, F., Garcia-Velasco, J., Nilsen, J., Brown, W., Song, J., Naftolin, F. Regulation of fas ligand expression in breast cancer cells by estrogen: functional differences between estradiol, tamoxifen. J. Steroid Biochem. Molec. Biol. 73:185–194, 2000.

103. Mullauer, L., Mosberger, I., Grusch, M., Rudas, M., Chott, A. Fas ligand is expressed in normal breast epithelial cells, is frequently up-regulated in breast cancer. J. of Pathol. 190:20–30, 2000.

104. Shinoura, N., Muramatsu, Y., Yoshida, Y., Asai, A., Kirino, T., Hamada, H. Adenovirus-mediated transfer of caspase-3 with Fas ligand induces drastic apoptosis in U-373MG glioma cells. Experimental Cell Res. 256:423–433, 2000.

105. Buglioni, S., Bracalenti, C., Cardarelli, M.A., Ciabocco, L., Giannarelli, D., Botti, C., Natali, P.G., Concetti, A., Venanzi, F.M. Prognostic relevance of altered Fas (CD95)-system in human. Int. J. Cancer. 89:127–132, 2000.

106. Ueno, T., Toi, M., Tominaga, T. Circulating soluble Fas concentration in breast cancer patients. Clin. Cancer Res. 5:3529–3533, 1999.

107. Rubinchik, S., Ding, R., Qiu, A.J., Zhang, F., Dong, J. Adenoviral vector which delivers FasL-GFP fusion protein regulated by the tet-inducible expression system. Gene Therapy 7:875–885, 2000.

108. Chu, Z.L., Pio, F., Xie, Z., Welsh, K., Krajewska, M., Krajewski, S., Godzik, A., Reed, J.C. A novel enhancer of the Apaf1 apoptosome involved in cytochrome c-dependent caspase activation, apoptosis. J. Biol. Chem. 276:9239–9245, 2001.

109. Munday, N.A., Vaillancourt, J.P., Ali, A., Casano, F.J., Miler, D.K., Molineaux, S.M., Yamin, T.T., Yu, V.L., Nicholson, D.W. Molecular cloning, pro-apoptotic activity of ICEreIII, ICEreIIII, members of the ICE/CED-3 family of cysteine proteases. J. Biol. Chem. 270:15870–15876, 1995.

110. Digby, M.R., Kimpton, W.G., York, J.J., Connick, T.E., Lowenthal, J.W. ITA A vertebrate homologue of IAP that is in T lymphocytes. DNA Cell Biol. 15:981–988, 1996.

111. Yuan, J., Horvitz, H.R. The *Caenorhabditis elegans* cell death gene *ced-4* encodes a novel protein and is expressed during the period of extensive programmed cell death. Development 116:309–320, 1992.

112. Tanaka, K., Iwanto, S., Gon, G., Nohara, T., Iwamoto, M., Tanigawa, N. Expression of survivin, its relationship to loss of apoptosis in breast carcinomas. Clinical Can. Res. 6:127–134, 2000.

113. Bond, J.A., Willie, F.S., Wynford-Thomas, D. Escape from senescence in human diploid fibroblasts induced directly by mutant p53. Oncogene 7:1885–1888, 1994.

114. Soussi, T., Legros, Y., Lubin, R., Ory, K., Schlichtholz, B. Multifactorial analysis of p53 alterations in human cancer: a review. Int. J. Cancer 57:1–9, 1994.

115. Higgy, N.A., Salicioni, A.M., Russo, I.H., Zhang, P.L., and Russo, J. Differential expression of human ferritin H chain gene in immortal human breast epithelial MCF-10F cells. Molecular Carcinogenesis 20:332–339, 1997.

116. Suzuki, K., Hirooka, Y., Tsujitani, S., Yamane, Y., Ikeguechi, M., Kaibara, N. Relationship between loss of heterozygosity at microsatellite loci and computerized nuclear morphometry in hepatocellular carcinoma. Anti Cancer Res. 20:1257–1262, 2000.

117. Schultz, D.C., Vanderveer, L., Berman, D.B., Hamilton, T.C., Wong, A.J., Godwin, A.K. Identification of two candidate tumor suppressor genes on chromosome 17p13.3. Cancer Res. 56:1997–2002, 1996.

118. Cornelis, R.S., van Vliet, M., Vos, C.B.J., Cleto-Jansen, A.M., van der Vijver, M.J., Peterse, J.L., Khan, P.M., Borresen, A.L., Cornelisse, C.J., Devilee, P. Evidence for a gene on 17p13.3, distal to p53, as a target for allele loss in breast tumors without p53 mutations. Cancer Res. 54:4200–4206, 1994.

119. Lakhani, S.R., Collins, N., Stratton, M.R., Sloane, J.P. Atypical ductal hyperplasia of the breast: clonal proliferation with loss of heterozygosity on chromosomes 16q, 17p. J. Clin. Pathol. 48:611–615, 1995.

120. Kasami, M., Vnencak-Jones, C., Manning, S., Dupont, W., Page, D. Loss of heterozygosity and microsatellite instability in breast hyperplasia. No obligate correlation of these genetic alterations with subsequent malignancy. Am. J. Path. 150:1925–1932, 1997.

121. Owen-Schaub, L., Chan, H., Cusack, J.C., Roth, J., Hill, L.L. Fas, Fas ligand interactions in malignant disease. Intl. J. Oncol. 17:5–12, 2000.

122. Gutierrez, L., Eliza, M., Niven-Fairchild, T., Mor, G. Fas/Fas-Ligand system induced apoptosis in human breast carcinoma: A mechanism for immune evasion. Breast Cancer Research and Treatment 54:245–253, 1999.

123. Fan, L., Freeman, K.W., Khan, T., Pham, E., Spencer, D.M. Improved artificial death switches based on caspases, FADD. Human Gene Therapy 10:2273–2285, 1999.

124. Song, J., Sapi, E., Brown, WD., Nilsen, J., Naftolin, F., Mor, G. Mammary Gland Remodeling: Expression and Role of the Fas/Fas Ligand System during Pregnancy, Lactation and Involution. Journal of Clinical Investigation. 106:1209–1224, 2000.

125. Thomson, T.A. Her-2/neu in breast cancer, inter-observer variability performance of immunohistochemistry with 4 antibodies compared with fluorescent in situ hybridization. Mod. Pathol. 14:1079–1086, 2001.

126. Gudmundsdottir, K., Tryggvadottir, L. Eyfjord, J.E. GSTM1, GSTT1, GSTP1 Genotypes in Relation to Breast Cancer Risk Frequency of Mutations in the p53 Gene. Cancer Epidemiol Biomarkers Prev. 10:1169–1173, 2001.

127. Yee, C.J., Roodi, N., Verrier, C.S., Parl, F.F. Microsatellite instability loss of heterozygosity in breast cancer. Cancer. Res. 54:1641–1644, 1994.

128. Shaw, J.A., Walsh, T., Chappell, S.A., Carey, N., Johnson, K., Walker, R.A. Microsatellite instability in early sporadic breast cancer. Br. J. Cancer 73:1393–1397, 1996.

129. Loeb, L.A. Microsatellite instability, Marker of a mutator phenotype in cancer. Cancer Res. 54:5059–5063, 1994.

130. Strand, M., Prolla, TA., Liskay, R.M., Petes, T.D. Destabilization of tracts of simple repetitive DNA in yeast by mutation affecting DNA mismatch repair. Nature 365:274–276, 1993.

131. Liu, B., et al. Mismatch repair gene defects in sporadic colorectal cancers with microsatellite instability. Nature Gen. 9:48–55, 1995.

132. Glaab, W.E., Risinger, J.I., Umar, A., Kunkel, T.A., Barrett, J.C., Tindall, K.R. Characterization of distinct human endometrial carcinoma cell lines deficient in mismatch repair that originated from a single tumor. J. Biol. Chem. 273:26662–26669, 1998.

133. Peltomaki, P. Deficient DNA mismatch repair: a common etiologic factor for colon cancer. Hum. Mol. Genet. 10:735–740, 2001.

134. Augenlicht, L.H., Richards, C., Corner, G., Pretlow, T.P. Evidence for genomic instability in human colonic aberrant crypt foci. Oncogene 12:1767–1772, 1996.

135. Toyama, T et al. Microsatellite instability in sporadic human breast cancers. Int. J. Cancer 68:447–451, 1996.

136. Walker, R.A., Jones, J.L., Chappell, S., Walsh, T., Shaw, J.A. Molecular pathology of breast cancer and its application to clinical management. Cancer Metastasis Reviews 16:5–27, 1997.

137. Souvinos, G., Kiaris, H., Tsikkinis, A., Vassilaros, S., Spandidos, D.A. Microsatellite instability and loss of heterozygosity in primary breast tumors. Tumor Biol. 18:157–166, 1997.

138. Fishel, R. Signaling mismatch repair in cancer. Nature Medicine 5:1239–1241, 1999.

139. Nicholaides, NC et al. Mutations of two PMS homologues in hereditary non-polyposis colon cancer. Nature 371:75–80, 1994.

140. Papadopoulos, N., Lindblom, A. Molecular basis of HNPCC, Mutations MMR genes. Human Mutation 10:89–99, 1997.

141. Fleisher, A. S., et al. Hyper-methylation of the hMLH1 gene promoter in human gastric cancers with microsatellite instability. Cancer Res. 59:1090–1095, 1999.

142. Charames, G.S., Millar, A.L., Pal, T., Narod, S., Bapat, B. Do MSH6 mutations contribute to double primary cancers of the colo-rectum and endometrium? Hum. Genet. 107:623–629, 2000.

143. Kolodner, R.D. et al. Germ-line msh6 mutations in colorectal cancer families. Cancer Res. 59:5068–5074, 1999.

144. Xu, X.S., Narayanan, L., Dunklee, B., Liskay, R.M., Glazer. P.M. Hyper-mutability to ionizing radiation in mismatch repair-deficient, Pms2 knockout mice. Cancer Res. 61:3775–3780, 2001.

145. Ionov, Y., Peinado, M., Malkhosyan, S., Shibata, D. Perucho, M. Ubiquitous somatic mutations in simple repeated sequences reveal a new mechanism for colonic carcinogenesis. Nature 263:556–558, 1993.

146. Eshleman, J.R. Markowitz, S.D. Microsatellite instability in inherited and sporadic neoplasms. Current Opinion in Oncology 7:83–89, 1995.

147. Bock, N., Meden, H., Regenbrecht, M., Junemann, B., Wangerin, J. Marx, D. Expression of the mismatch repair protein hMSH2 in carcinoma in situ and invasive cancer of the breast. Anti Cancer Res. 20:119–124, 2000.

148. Yeh, C.C., Lee, C., Dahiya, R. DNA mismatch repair enzyme activity and gene expression in prostate cancer. Biochem. Biophys. Res. Commun. 285:409–413, 2001.

149. Winter, T. Altered spectra of hyper-mutation in antibodies from mice deficient for the DNA mismatch repair protein PMS2. Proc. Natl. Acad. Sci. USA. 95:69536–69538, 1998.

150. Liu, T. The Role of hPMS1 and hPMS2 in Predisposing to Colorectal Cancer. Cancer Res. 61:7798–7802, 2001.

151. Caluseriu, O. Four novel MSH2 and MLH1 frame-shift mutations and occurrence of a breast cancer phenocopy in hereditary nonpolyposis colorectal cancer. Hum. Mutat. 17:521, 2001.

152. Plaschke, J., Commer, T., Jacobi, C., Schackert, H.K., Chang-Claude, J. BRCA2 germline mutations among early onset breast cancer patients unselected for family history of the disease. J. Med. Genet. 37:E17, 2000.

153. Yeh, C.C., Lee, C., Huang, M.C., Dahiya, R. Loss of mismatch repair activity in simian virus 40 large T antigen-immortalized BPH-1 human prostatic epithelial cell line. Mol. Carcinog. 31:145–51, 2001.

154. Scott, et al. Hereditary nonpolyposis colorectal cancer in 95 families: differences and similarities between mutation-positive and mutation-negative kindreds. Am. J. Hum. Genet. 68:118–127, 2001.

155. Leach, F.S. et al. Mutations of a *muts* homolog in hereditary nonpolyposis colorectal cancer. Cell 75:1215–1225, 1993.

156. Sud, R., Wells, D., Talbot, I.C., Delhanty, J.D. Genetic alterations in gastric cancers from British patients. Cancer Genet. Cytogenet. 126:111–119, 2001.

157. Bock, N., Meden, H., Regenbrecht, M., Junemann, B., Wangerin, J., Marx, D. Expression of the mismatch repair protein hMSH2 in carcinoma in situ and invasive cancer of the breast. . Anti-Cancer Res. 20:119–124, 2000.

158. Ma, A.H. Somatic mutation of hPMS2 as a possible cause of sporadic human colon cancer with microsatellite instability. Oncogene 19:2249–2256, 2000.

159. Thomson, T.A. et al. Her-2/neu in breast cancer, inter-observer variability performance of immunohistochemistry with 4 antibodies compared with fluorescent in situ hybridization. Mod. Pathol. 14:1079–1086, 2001.

160. Nicholaides, N.C. Mutations of two PMS homologues in hereditary non-polyposis colon cancer. Nature 371:75–80, 1994.

Preventive Strategies in Breast Cancer

9.1 Introduction

Breast cancer is the most common neoplastic disease in women worldwide with an incidence of 750,000 new cases [1] and a mortality rate of 300,000 deaths annually [2]. In the United States, the incidence of breast cancer continues to rise and accounts for up to one third of all new cases of women's cancer [3]. In spite of advances in technologies for early detection and intervention of breast cancer, the mortality rate from this disease has remained almost unchanged in the past 5 decades, becoming second only to lung cancer as a cause of cancer deaths [4]. While success in the intervention of breast cancer largely depends on early detection by regular or even intensified mammography screening, prevention against the development of breast cancer, a national interest with a very high research priority, requires a better understanding of the specific agents or mechanisms that cause breast cancer.

Intensive epidemiological studies have identified a number of biological and social traits as risk factors associated with breast cancer, including evidence of *BRCA1* and *BRCA2* susceptibility genes, familiar history of cancer in the breast, ovary or endometrium, individual history of breast diseases, early onset of menstruation, nulliparity or delayed first childbirth, short duration of breast feeding, late menopause, advanced age, postmenopausal obesity, higher socio-economical status, tallness in adult life, consumption of alcohol, extended use of oral contraceptives, and prolonged estrogen replacement therapy (Table 9.1) [5]. However, these risk factors appear to account for only a third of all breast cancer cases [6, 7] with 5–10 % attributable to genetic predisposition. Other risk factors associated with the development of breast cancer include physical (e.g., excess ionizing radiation), chemical (e.g., carcinogens) and biological hazards (e.g., viral oncogenes) in the environment (Table 9.1). Even though chemical carcinogen is generally not considered as a significant risk factor influencing human breast cancer, a large number of environmental chemical carcinogens have been proven to be carcinogenic in in vitro cellular transformation and in vivo animal carcinogenesis models [8–12]. Environmental exposure to tobacco, whether in active smokers or in passive smokers, is clearly associated with an increased risk of breast cancer [13]. Given the large differences in the incidences of breast cancer between Western and Asian countries and changes in breast cancer incidence among migrant populations [14], diet has also been implicated as a factor influencing the risk of this disease [15]. Increased risk of breast cancer has been associated with an increase in fat intake [16], while a reduced risk of breast cancer has been related to increased consumption of vegetables and fruits [15, 17–23].

Disappointingly, the molecular mechanisms underlying each of these risk factors associated with development of breast cancer are not completely understood. Our current concepts of breast carcinogenesis are summarized schematically in Fig. 9.1. Initiation of breast carcinogenesis results from uncontrolled cellular proliferation and/or aberrant programmed cell death or apoptosis as a consequence of accumulative genetic damages that lead to activation of proto-oncogenes and inactivation of tumor suppressor genes. Genetic alterations can be either inherited as germline mutations or acquired as somatic mutations that occur as a result of exposure to environmental physical (e.g., excess ionizing radiation),

Table 9.1. Risk factors for human breast cancer

	Biomarkers	Odds ratio
Genetic	Evidence of susceptibility genes *BRCA1* or *BRCA2*	≥4.0
	Evidence of *p53* gene (in Li-Fraumeni syndrome)	≥4.0
	Evidence of *PTEN/MMAC1* (in Cowden syndrome)	≥4.0
	Heterozygosity for mutant alleles of *ATM* gene	≥4.0
	Premenopausal breast cancer in mother *and* sister	≥4.0
	Premenopausal breast cancer in mother *or* sister	2.0–4.0
	Postmenopausal breast cancer in first-degree relatives	≤2.0
	Individual history of cancer in one breast	2.0–4.0
	Individual history of ovarian or endometrial cancer	≤2.0
Clinical	Atypical hyperplasia in breast biopsy or aspirate	≥4.0
	Ductal or lobular carcinoma in situ	≥4.0
	Typical hyperplasia in breast biopsy or aspirate	2.0–4.0
	Predominantly nodular densities in mammogram	≤2.0
	Prolonged use of oral contraceptives in women under age 45	≤2.0
	Prolonged estrogen replacement therapy	≤2.0
Biological	Advanced age	2.0–4.0
	Early onset of menstruation (before age 12)	≤2.0
	Delayed first childbirth	≤2.0
	Nulliparity (in women under 40)	≤2.0
	Short duration of breast feeding	≤2.0
	Late onset of menopause (after age 49)	≤2.0
	Postmenopausal obesity	≤2.0
	Tallness in adult life	≤2.0
Social	Smoking	2.0–4.0
	Higher socio-economic status	≤2.0
	Low physical activity	≤2.0
Dietary	Higher alcohol consumption	≤2.0
	Higher fat/energy intake	≤2.0
	Xenobiotics	≤2.0
Environmental	Excess ionizing radiation to chest wall or breasts	≤2.0
	Exposure to chemical carcinogens	≤2.0
	Microbials or infectious agents	≤2.0

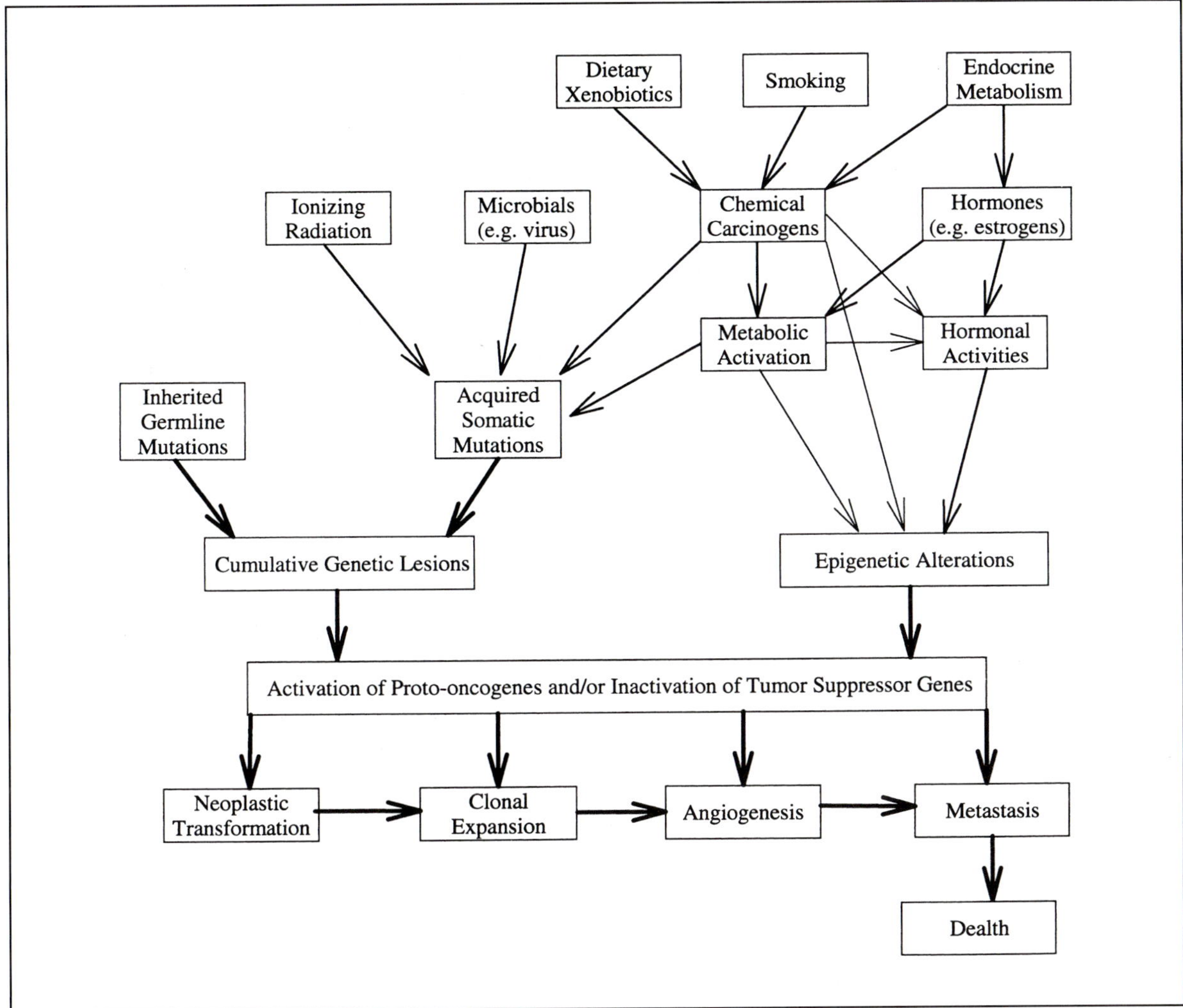

Figure 9.1

Schematic illustration of breast carcinogenesis

chemical (e.g., carcinogens) and biological carcinogens (e.g., virus). It is generally believed that the altered genotype of an initiated cell is irreversible, but the expression of transformed phenotypes requires further genetic or epigenetic changes. In the classical two-stage view of carcinogenesis that is primarily derived from animal models of chemical carcinogenesis, the second stage of tumorigenesis (i.e., promotion) involves epigenetic changes exclusively and is considered reversible [2]. Whether this is true in breast carcinogenesis remains to be determined, but it is safe to say that the model is oversimplified. Development of breast cancer entails multiple events [24–26]. The multistage nature of breast carcinogenesis presents a challenge for mechanistic studies of the disease, but it also provides ample opportunities for preventive intervention of the neoplastic process. Therefore, recent advances in our understanding of the genetic and molecular mechanisms of carcinogenesis have generated a tremendous amount of interest in the search for preventive measures and chemopreventive strategies that target on one or more of these risk factors to reverse, suppress, or prevent carcinogenesis before the development of invasive malignancy occurs.

There are many strategies that have been developed for the intervention of breast cancer. Removal of the whole target organ (i.e., breasts) constitutes a physical means of intervention that can be termed as physicoprevention. A large number of natural or synthetic compounds affecting various carcinogenic events have been exploited for use in the chemoprevention of breast cancer. Bioprevention of breast cancer employs active biomolecules (e.g., genes or gene products) or physiological processes (e.g., pregnancy) to reverse, suppress or prevent breast carcinogenesis, while socioprevention of breast cancer focuses on modulation of social behaviors to reduce the risk of developing breast cancer (e.g., exercise, cessation of smoking). Currently, most of the attention from the scientific and public communities has been paid to physicoprevention and chemoprevention of breast cancer. As a result, there is a very limited amount of information concerning the intervention of breast cancer by biological and social means. In this review, various preventive measures against the development of breast cancer will be discussed in the context of the multistage carcinogenic events.

9.2 Physicoprevention with Prophylactic Mastectomy

One of the most controversial procedures to prevent breast cancer in healthy women at a high risk of developing this disease is the surgical removal of bilateral noncancerous breast tissue, i.e., bilateral prophylactic mastectomy. Theoretically, removal of all the target tissues should provide maximum protection against the development of breast cancer and such a radical preventive measure can be described as physicoprevention of human breast cancer. Historically, bilateral prophylactic mastectomy has been recommended for women with severe cancerophobia and/or at a high risk of developing breast cancer, such as those with familial history of breast cancer, individual history of proliferative or deforming breast diseases and therapy-resistant gross cystic disease with intolerable pain [27, 28]. Currently, bilateral prophylactic mastectomy in combination with intensified breast cancer screening is offered as an option for those women with hereditary breast cancer [29]. However, psychological impact of the radical procedure presents a dilemma for a woman who is perceived as being at a higher risk [28]. Prophylactic mastectomy remains controversial considering the possible implications of genetic testing, attitudes and uptake of breast screening and accuracy of women's risk estimates [30]. In addition, the true preventive value of bilateral prophylactic mastectomy remains unsubstantiated. In fact, a survey of the results from animal and clinical studies led Stefanek [27] to urge prospective patient and physicians to consider the surgical option based on the fact that "prophylactic mastectomy, whether subcutaneous or total, may reduce, but likely not eliminate, the risk of breast cancer."

9.3 Bioprevention of Hereditary Breast Cancer

Hereditary breast cancer is characterized as relatively early onset of tumors, often in bilateral breasts or multiple primary sites of one breast, in multigenerational members of a family. Familial history of breast cancer confers an increased risk of developing this disease on all members of the family. Other tumors (e.g., ovarian and prostate cancers) often segregate within the same families. A major advance in the study of inherited forms of breast cancer occurred with the identification of two breast susceptibility genes, *BRCA1* and *BRCA2*, that may account for a majority of inherited forms (i.e., familial cluster with high penetrance) of breast cancer cases [31–35].

While an inherited risk of breast cancer has been associated with many other genes, such as *p53* gene in Li-Fraumeni syndrome, *PTEN/MMAC1* at 10q23 in Cowden syndrome and *ATM* gene at 11q22–23 in ataxia telangiectasia [36–38], there is little evidence that these or other dominant gene(s) are responsible for substantial numbers of breast cancer incidence. Therefore, genetic testing of mutations in *BRCA1* and *BRCA2* loci has allowed the identification of a cohort at a very high risk of developing breast cancer. Conceivably, introduction of these dominant breast cancer susceptibility genes or their gene products will offer the ultimate protection against the development of hereditary breast cancer in those individuals with the mutated genotypes. However, gene therapy is still in its embryonic stage and awaits further studies.

9.4 Chemoprevention Against Acquired Somatic Mutations

Somatic mutations occur frequently in individuals with intrinsic errors in DNA replication or deficiencies in mismatch repair machinery [39]. For instance, the risk of developing breast cancer increases fivefold in women who are apparently heterozygous for mutant alleles of the *ATM* gene that, in homozygous form, causes ataxia telangiectasia, a classic DNA repair disease [40, 41]. However, the vast majority of somatic mutations observed in sporadic breast cancer are likely to result from genetic damages caused by exposure to physical, chemical or microbial carcinogens. The influence of radiation, a physical carcinogen, on the development of breast cancer has been well documented from the Life Span Study (LSS) in the survivors of nuclear bombing in Japan [42]. Since adverse effects of external radiation are generally observed long after the initial exposure [43], young women should be advised to take precaution against excessive irradiation of their breasts.

Contribution of environmental microbial carcinogens to the breast cancer risk is not completely clear. It has been observed, though, that human breast carcinomas contain integrated viral DNA sequences [44, 45] homologous to mouse mammary tumor virus, a known inducer of mammary tumors in susceptible strains of mice [46, 47]. Based on the highly correlated geographical distributions of breast cancer and cytomegalovirus seropositivity, Richardson [48] has hypothesized that breast cancer results from late exposure to the common cytomegalovirus. In fact, interactions between viral carcinogen, genetics and hormonal factors carcinogen have been proposed to serve as key determinants of mammary carcinogenesis [49]. Nevertheless, the most well documented studies on acquired somatic mutations have been performed with chemical carcinogens. Therefore, chemoprevention against acquired somatic mutations has almost exclusively centered on the inhibition of chemical carcinogenesis.

Intensive studies have established that chemical carcinogens act through common mechanisms (Fig. 9.2). The ultimate carcinogenic forms of all the carcinogens are positively charged electrophiles or free radicals (e.g., O_2^-, OH) which interact directly with target DNA [39, 50, 51]. Some chemicals are positively charged electrophiles in nature, serving as direct acting carcinogens, while others require metabolic activation to assume their carcinogenic forms. For example, metabolic activation is essential for aromatic amines and amides to exert their chemical carcinogenic effects on humans and experimental animals [50, 51]. The reactive forms of carcinogens can be scavenged by physiological nucleophiles (e.g., reduced glutathione), and all the chemical carcinogens, regardless of their metabolic activation, can be detoxified by Phase II xenobiotics metabolizing enzyme systems consisting of NAD(P)H: quinone reductase, epoxide hydratase, glutathione-S-transferase and UDP-glucuronosyl transferase [52, 53].

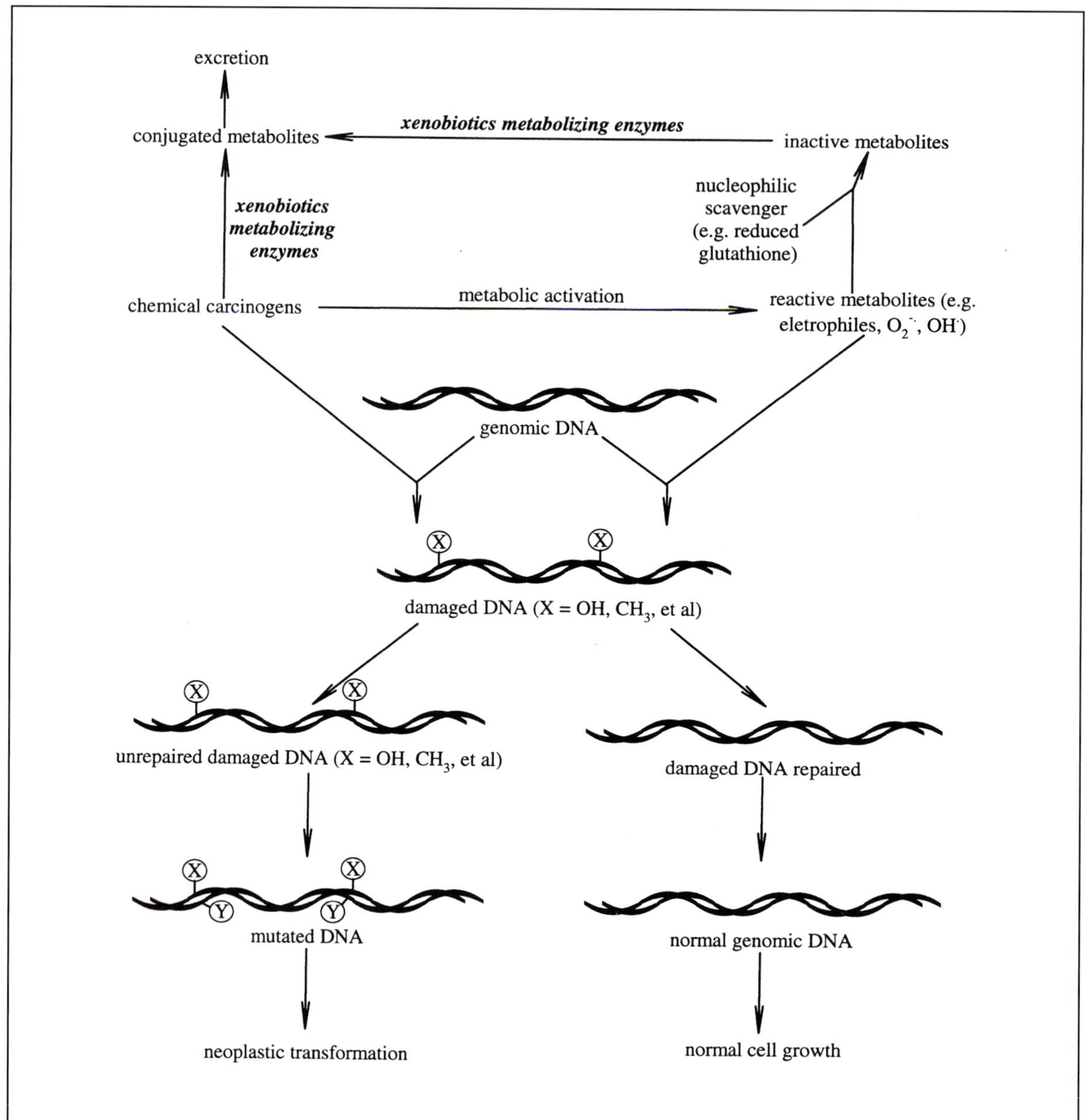

Figure 9.2

Common mechanisms of chemical carcinogenesis

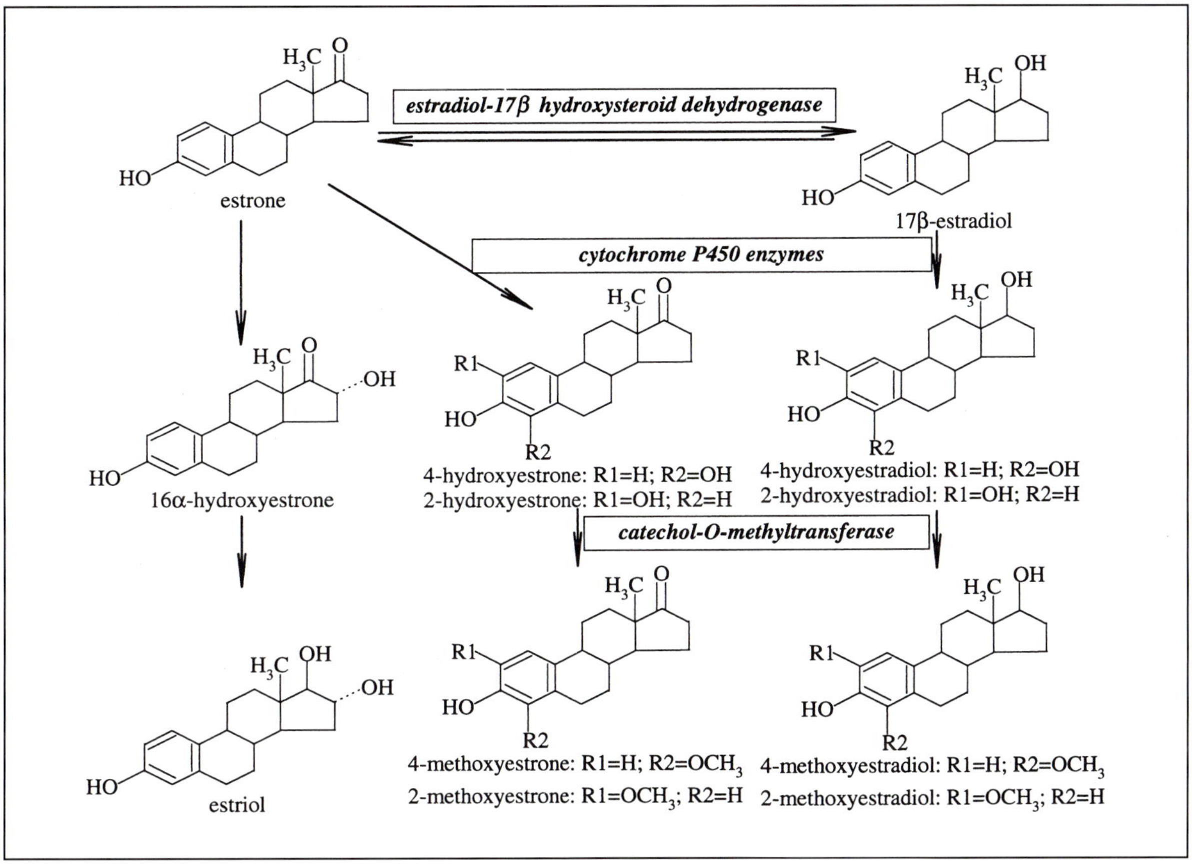

9.4.1 Limiting Accumulation of Chemical Carcinogens

Figure 9.3

Metabolic pathways leading to activation and inactivation of estrogens

Chemical carcinogens can be either produced endogenously or absorbed from an exogenous source. Most of the exogenous chemical carcinogens in the diet are converted to their carcinogenic forms by endogenous metabolisms. The major metabolic pathways that can produce endogenous chemical carcinogens are to some extent associated with catabolism of lipids (e.g., fat, arachidonic acids, steroids). Peroxidation of polyunsaturated membrane lipids and metabolism of arachidonic acid results in production of a direct-acting mutagen malondialdehyde [54–58]. Malondialdehyde is not only a product of normal metabolism, but is also present in a variety of fat-containing foodstuffs [59], which have been associated with forma-

tion of DNA adducts of malondialdehyde in human [60]. Clearly, a reduction in consumption of food containing procarcinogen or carcinogen will reduce the risk of breast cancer.

Essentially, all mutagenic events as a result of the oxidative catabolism of fatty acids and steroid estrogens occur via generation of reactive free radicals and intermediate metabolites that can cause oxidative stress and genomic damage directly. For instance, cytochrome P450-mediated hydroxylation of estrogens produces catechol estrogens that will easily be autooxidated to semiquinones and subsequently quinones, both of which are electrophiles capable of covalently binding to nucleophilic groups on DNA via a Michael addition and, thus, serve as the ultimate carcinogenic reactive intermediates in the peroxidatic activation of catechol estrogens [61]. In addition, a redox cycle consisting of the reversible formation of the semiquinones and quinones of catechol estrogens catalyzed by microsomal P450 and cytochrome P450-reductase can locally generate superoxide and hydroxyl radicals to produce additional DNA damage [62, 63]. Steady state concentrations of catechol estrogens are determined by the cytochrome P450-mediated hydroxylations of estrogens and monomethylation of catechols catalyzed by blood-borne catechol O-methyltransferase (Fig. 9.3) [64–67]. Increased formation of catechol estrogens as a result of elevated hydroxylations of estradiol-17β at C-4 [68] and C-16α [69–71] positions occurs in human breast cancer patients and in women at a higher risk of developing this disease (see Chapter 4). There is also evidence that lactoperoxidase, present in milk, saliva, tears and mammary glands, catalyzes the metabolism of estradiol-17β to its phenoxyl radical intermediates, with subsequent formation of superoxide and hydrogen peroxide that might be involved in estrogen-mediated oxidative stress [72]. A substantial increase in base lesions observed in the DNA of invasive ductal carcinoma of the breast [73, 74] has been postulated to result from the oxidative stress associated with metabolism of estradiol-17β [72]. Clearly, the ability of the mammary gland to metabolize estradiol-17β and/or to accumulate "genotoxic" metabolites could profoundly influence the neoplastic transformation of the epithelium [75]. Metabolic biotransformation of estradiol occurs in human mammary explant cultures [75, 76]. Treatment of normal mouse mammary epithelial cells with the mutagenic polycyclic hydrocarbon 7,12-dimethylbenz[α]anthracene (DMBA) results in production of 16α-hydroxy-estrone as the predominant metabolite of estrogens, which increases unscheduled DNA synthesis, cellular proliferation and anchorage-independent growth, indicative of preneoplastic transformation [77]. In experimental animals, catechols have been implicated as mediators of estrogen-induced carcinogenesis [78]. Elevated

metabolic conversion of estradiol-17β to catechol estrogens has been documented in a number of organs susceptible to estrogen-induced carcinogenesis, including hamster kidney [65, 79, 80], mouse uterus [81, 82] and rat pituitary [80, 83]. Modulation of catechol estrogen concentrations influences susceptibility to estrogen-inducible carcinogenesis. For instance, catecholamines, which are substrates and competitive inhibitors of the catechol O-methyltransferase, are present at much higher levels in the organs susceptible to estrogen-induced carcinogenesis [84]. Inhibition of the catechol O-methyltransferase-catalyzed O-methylation of 2- and 4-hydroxyl-estradiol-17β by quercetin, a flavonoid, increases accumulation of catechol estrogens [85] and augments the induction of estradiol-induced carcinogenesis [86].

However, intake and/or metabolism of dietary fat, estrogens and arachidonic acids have been frequently associated with alteration in hormonal profiles that induce epigenetic alterations [87, 88], chemoprevention targeting these metabolic pathways to maintain proper endocrine milieu will be discussed later. The following discussion will be focused on chemopreventive strategies that have been exploited to minimize chemical carcinogen-induced somatic mutations by enhancing its excretion and eliminating oxidative stress associated with metabolism of the xenobiotics.

9.4.2 Enhancing Excretion of Xenobiotics

9.4.2.1 Organosulfur Compounds

Organosulfur compounds, present in garlic and cruciferous vegetables (Brussels sprouts, cauliflower and cabbage), play an important role in the regulation of xenobiotics-metabolizing enzyme systems and, therefore, are the subject of extensive chemoprevention studies. There is epidemiological evidence that individuals on regular diet rich in garlic are at a lower risk of developing cancer [89, 90]. In laboratory animals, a variety of garlic sources have been shown to inhibit carcinogen-induced mammary carcinogenesis [91–93]. Garlic contains a complex mixture of water-soluble and lipid soluble organosulfur com-

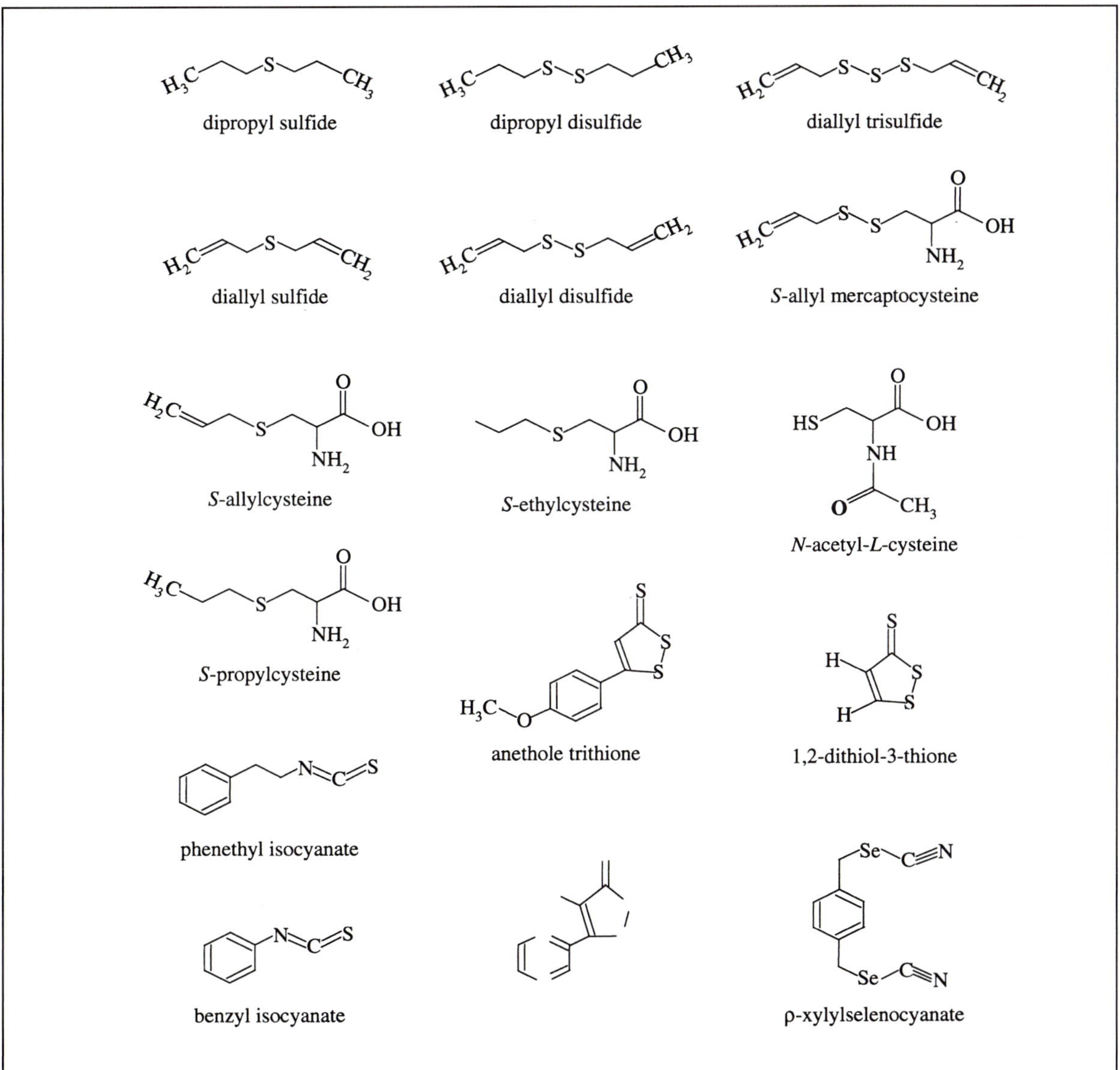

Figure 9.4

Chemical structures of organosulfur compounds

pounds. The water-soluble constituents consist of *S*-allylcysteine, *S*-ethylcysteine, *S*-propylcysteine and *S*-allylmercaptocysteine, while the lipid-soluble organosulfur compounds include diallyl sulfide, diallyl disulfide, diallyl trisulfide, dipropyl sulfide and dipropyl disulfide (Fig. 9.4) [94]. Experimental studies have shown that organosulfur constituents of garlic such as *S*-allylcysteine, *S*-allylmercaptocysteine and diallyl trisulfide are potent inhibitors of cell proliferation [95, 96]. Diallyl selenide, a volatile synthetic compound, and diallyl sulfide, a flavor component of garlic, show significant inhibitory effects on the development of DMBA-induced rat mammary tumor [97]. *S*-allylcysteine reduces the quantity of DMBA-induced DNA adducts in the mammary glands [98] and prevent chemically induced mammary carcinogenesis in experimental animals [91–93].

The organosulfur compound 1,2-dithiol-3-thione, present in cruciferous vegetables, and dithiolethione substitutes, such as anethole trithione and oltipraz [5-(2-pyrazinyl)-4-methyl-1,2-dithiole-3-thione] (Fig. 9.4), are potent activators of the carcinogen-detoxification enzymes glutathione S-transferase, NAD(P)H: quinone reductase, epoxide hydrolase and UDP-glucuronosyltransferase [99–101] and have shown chemopreventive activity against different classes of carcinogens targeting the small intestine, colon, urinary bladder, trachea, liver, mammary gland and skin [100, 102–104]. The 1,2-dithiole-3-thione can also increase the activity of DT-diaphorase, a Phase II detoxifying enzyme flavoprotein that catalyses two-electron reduction of quinones, quinone imines, and nitrogen oxides [105]. The chemopreventive activities of oltipraz can be accounted for, at least in part, by alteration of the metabolism and disposition of chemical carcinogens upon induction of several of these phase II enzymes, which is mediated through interaction with a 41-bp enhancer element common to the upstream regulatory regions of genes encoding these enzymes [106].

N-Acetyl-*L*-cysteine (Fig. 9.4) is one of the organosulfur compounds produced endogenously serving as precursor of the reduced glutathione [100] and has been shown to inhibit nitrosomethylurea (NMU)-induced mammary carcinogenesis [103, 107]. A number of mechanisms have been proposed to account for the chemopreventive action of *N*-acetyl-*L*-cysteine, including prevention of DNA adduct formation [108], suppression of oncogene expression [109], inhibition of malignant cell invasion and metastasis and other extracellular, cytoplasmic and nuclear effects [110].

Isothiocyanates occur naturally as glucosinolates (i.e., thioglycoside conjugates) in a variety of crucif-

erous vegetables such as watercress and broccoli [110]. Hydrolysis of glucosinates by myrosinase released from damaged vegetable cells results in production of bioactive isothiocyanates by a Lossen rearrangement [111]. Both naturally occurring and synthetic isothiocyanates can inhibit phase I and phase II carcinogen metabolism leading to increased carcinogen excretion or detoxification, and have been tested for their chemopreventive potentials against cancer of the mammary glands and other organs [111, 112]. Even though phenethyl isothiocyanate (Fig. 9.4), a naturally-occurring isothiocyanate, failed to affect mammary carcinogenesis induced by chemical carcinogens in one study [103], other studies have shown that phenethyl isothiocyanate prevents chemically-induced carcinogenesis of the mammary glands as well as lung, esophagus and forestomach [111, 113]. Benzyl isothiocyanate (Fig. 9.4) has also been reported to suppress chemically induced mammary carcinogenesis [114]. Sulforaphane, a naturally occurring aliphatic isothiocyanate is capable of mediating chemopreventive activity in animal models by modulation of drug-metabolizing enzymes [115].

9.4.2.2 Indole-3-Carbinol

Indole-3-carbinol (Fig. 9.5) is a derivative of indole glucosinate or glucobrassicin, a secondary plant metabolite rich in cruciferous vegetables [116]. Under normal physiological conditions, indole-3-carbinol, formed upon autolysis of glucobrassicins during maceration, rapidly dimerizes to form the biological-

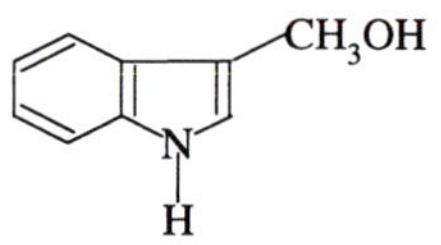

Figure 9.5

Chemical structure of indole-3-carbinol

ly active compound diindolylmethane [117, 118]. Administration of indole-3-carbinol in the diet has been associated with reduced incidence of spontaneous formation of estrogen-responsive mammary tumors in C3H/OuJ mice [119]. Indole-3-carbinol induces cytochrome P450 and glutathione-S-transferase activities, resulting in increased metabolism of chemical carcinogens and reduced mammary tumorigenic response to the carcinogens [103, 118, 120, 121]. Indole-3-carbinol in vitro prevents preneoplastic transformation of the mammary glands [122] and inhibits both the anchorage-dependent [123] and anchorage-independent growth of human breast cancer cells [118]. Indole-3-carbinol in vivo can prevent mammary carcinogenesis by direct and indirect acting carcinogens [121]. Administration of indole-3-carbinol at 400 mg/day for 3 months to human female volunteers alters estrogen metabolism in vivo, an indication of chemopreventive effects against human breast cancer, without producing any harmful side effects [118, 124]. Since all the dietary and biological responses associated with increased cancer risk decrease 2-hydroxylation and increase 16α-hydroxylation of estradiol along its metabolic pathways, the chemopreventive action of indole-3-carbinol is at least in part attributed to its induction of estradiol 2-hydroxylation, with a concomitant reduction in 16α-hydroxylation [118, 125]. Treatment of indole-3-carbinol also suppresses the perturbed molecular, endocrine and cellular biomarkers, such as persistent expression of oncogene specific mRNA transcripts, altered estradiol biotransformation and aberrant proliferation with concomitant induction of p53 dependent apoptosis [126, 127].

9.4.2.3 Phytoalexin

Brassinin [3-(S-methyldithiocarbamoyl)aminomethyl indole] (Fig. 9.6), a naturally occurring phytoalexin in cruciferous vegetables bearing both an indole nucleus and a dithiocarbamoyl-aminomethyl moiety structurally similar to indole-3-carbinol and benzyl isothiocyanate, induces a dose-dependent inhibition of DMBA-induced preneoplastic lesion formation of mouse mammary glands in organ culture [128]. Cyclobrassinin, a biologically derived product of the oxidative cyclization of brassinin, is as active as the parent compound in inhibiting the formation of preneoplastic mammary lesions in culture, suggesting oxidative cyclization may be an effective metabolic activation step [128]. Brassinin acts as an effective chemopreventive agent during both the initiation and promotion phases of carcinogenesis. A recently-synthesized novel cancer chemopreventive agent, (+/-)-4-methylsulfinyl-1-(S-methyldithiocarbamyl)-butane (trivial name, sulforamate), an aliphatic analogue of brassinin with structural similarities to sulforaphane (Fig. 9.6), has been shown to be a monofunctional inducer of NAD(P)H:quinone oxidoreductase [quinone reductase], a phase II enzyme and a potent inhibitor of preneoplastic lesion forma-

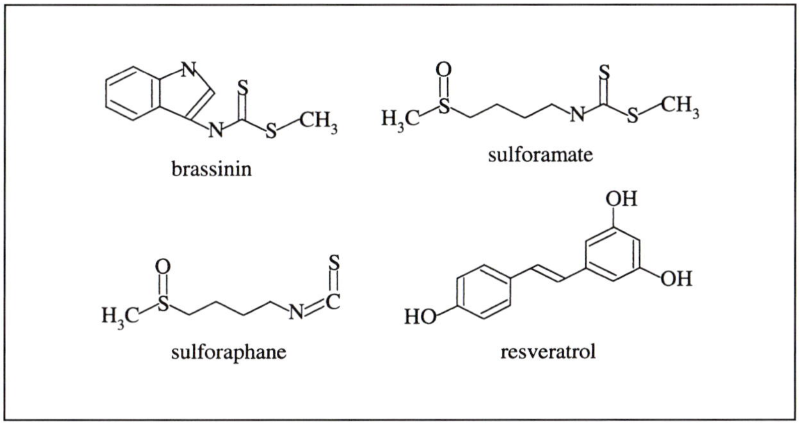

Figure 9.6

Chemical structures of phytoalexins

tion in carcinogen-treated mouse mammary glands in organ culture [115]. This analogue can be regarded as a readily available promising new cancer chemopreventive agent.

Resveratrol (3,5,4'-trihydroxy-trans-stilbene); (Fig. 9.6), a phytoalexin found in grapes and other food products, has shown potent anti-initiation, antipromotion and antiprogression activities [129, 130]. The anti-initiation activity is due to its antioxidant and antimutagen nature as well as induction of phase II drug-metabolizing enzymes [129]. The antipromotion activity results from its inhibition of cyclooxygenase and hydroperoxidase functions [129]. The antiprogression activity of resveratrol is mediated by mechanisms leading to cell differentiation [129]. In addition, it inhibits the development of preneoplastic lesions in carcinogen-treated mouse mammary glands in culture [129] and suppresses the growth of human breast epithelial cells independent of the estrogen receptor status [130]. These data suggest that resveratrol, a common constituent of the human diet, merits investigation as a potential cancer chemopreventive agent in humans.

9.4.2.4 Triterpenoids

Triterpenoids are widely distributed in nature and are the major components of some traditional medicinal herbs. Ursolic acid and oleanolic acid (Fig. 9.7) are pentacyclic triterpene acids that are potent enhancers of glutathione-S-transferase and quinone reductase activities [131], and inhibitors of neo-angiogenesis [132], indicative of chemopreventive potentials. In fact, rosemary and/or its constituents (e.g., carnosol, ursolic acid) (Fig. 9.7) have been shown to arrest human breast cancer cells at G1 [133], inhibit carcinogenesis in the skin [134], and to reduce DMBA-induced DNA adduct formation and tumorigenesis in the mammary glands [135].

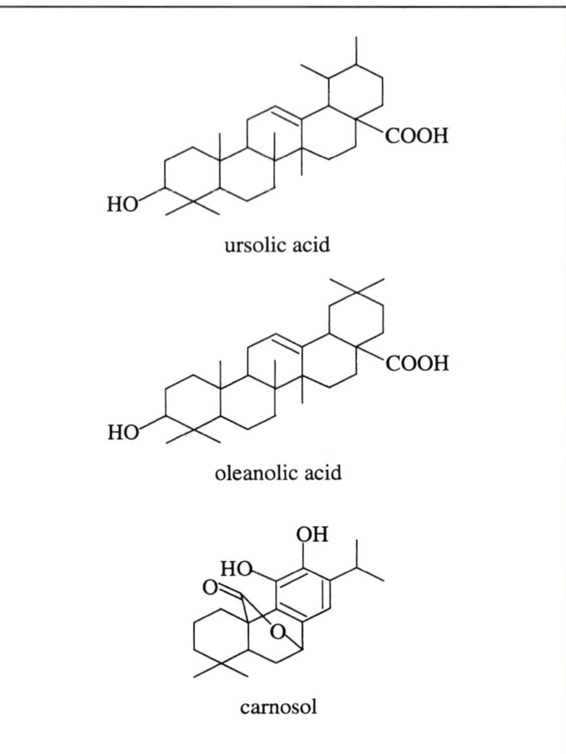

Figure 9.7

Chemical structures of triterpenoids

9.4.3 Eliminating Oxidative Stress

9.4.3.1 Carotenoids

Carotenoids (Fig. 9.8) constitute one of the most abundant groups of pigments present in the plant and animal kingdoms. There are more than seven hundred naturally-occurring carotenoids and up to 50 of the carotenoids from fruits and vegetables commonly consumed in the US can be absorbed and metabolized by humans [136, 137]. In plants, the conjugated polyene structure of carotenoids allows the molecule to absorb light, to quench and to inactivate singlet oxygen and free radicals in photosynthesis and photoprotection [138]. In human, there is epidemiological evidence that the intake of carotenoids

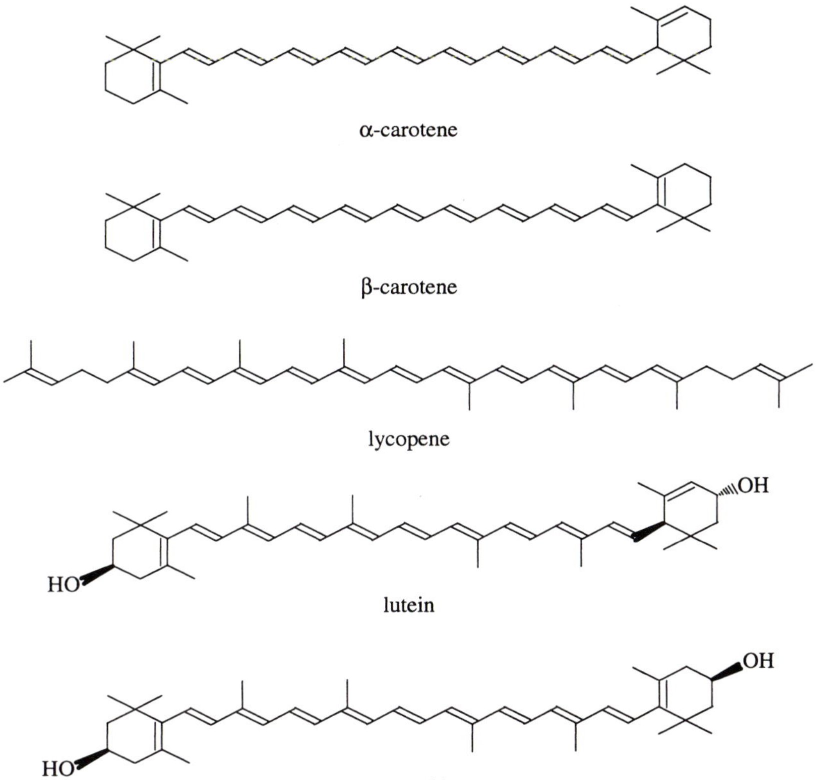

α-carotene

β-carotene

lycopene

lutein

zeaxanthin

Figure 9.8

Chemical structures of carotenoids

and other micronutrients is associated with protective effects of vegetable consumption for premenopausal and postmenopausal breast cancer [15, 19, 23, 139–144]. Results of a recent human intervention trial indicate that consumption of carotenoid-rich vegetables (e.g., tomatoes, carrots, spinach) reduces oxidative and other damage to genetic DNA in humans [145]. The potency of the protective effects varies with the type of products consumed probably depending on the respective type and levels of antioxidant ingredients [145].

β-Carotene (Fig. 9.8) is present in abundance in green and yellow vegetables (e.g., carrots, cantaloupes and broccoli) and has the highest provitamin A activity. Intake of β-carotene has been associated with a reduced risk of breast cancer [15, 140]. Accordingly, β-carotene has been proposed as the key cancer prevention agent, a notion that is supported by the experimental evidence that β-carotene inhibits chemically-induced carcinogenesis in salivary [146] and mammary [147–149] glands of experimental animals. However, the observation that dietary supplementation of β-carotene increases the incidence of lung cancer among heavy smokers [150] suggests that other natural carotenoids rather than β-carotene are responsible for the chemopreventive activities in green and yellow vegetables [151]. In a recent case-control study, Freudenheim et al. [15] have studied the risk of breast cancer in relation to intake of individual carotenoids and found that the protective effect of carotenoids against breast cancer is limited to α-carotene, β-carotene, and lutein + zeaxanthin. In contrast, Potischman et al. [140] have found no association of breast cancer risk with α-carotene or lycopene levels.

Lutein, a dihydroxycarotenoid, and lycopene, a hydrocarbon carotenoid, are two non-vitamin A active carotenoids abundant in most fruits and vegetables as well as in human serum [137]. Lycopene is the most abundant carotenoid found nearly exclusively in tomatoes and tomato-based food products [137]. It is an exceptionally active antioxidant, quenching singlet oxygen at a substantially higher capacity than β-carotene [152]. The biochemical properties of lycopene suggest that it possesses chemopreventive potential. In fact, lycopene has been shown to inhibit transformation of mammary organ cultures in vitro [149] and lycopene-enriched tomato oleoresin, but not β-carotene, inhibits DMBA-induced rat mammary carcinogenesis in a recent study [153]. Chronic ingestion of lycopene significantly suppresses the development of spontaneous mammary tumors in a high mammary tumor strain of SHN virgin mice

[154]. Chemopreventive effects against skin and lung carcinogenesis have been documented for α-carotene and lutein as well as β-carotene [137]. However, poor absorption and low levels of carotenoids that reach the target tissues complicate interpretation of data in rodent models of mammary carcinogenesis [155]. Very few animal studies are presently available in which purified carotenoids have been found effective against mammary carcinogenesis [155]. In human, no association has been observed between risk of breast cancer risk and intake of lycopene, vitamin C, α-tocopherol, folic acid and fiber [15]. Conceivably, further studies are warranted concerning the chemopreventive potential of α-carotene and lutein or other carotenoids that co-exist with β-carotene.

9.4.3.2 Vitamin E and Selenium

Vitamin E (Fig. 9.9), an essential nutrient for humans, is a lipophilic vitamin widely distributed in food (e. g., wheat germ, corn, sunflower seeds, rapeseeds, soybeans, alfalfa and lettuce) [149]. α-Tocopherol is a naturally-occurring product with vitamin E activity functioning as the major antioxidant present in all cell membranes [149]. Vitamin E induces differentia-

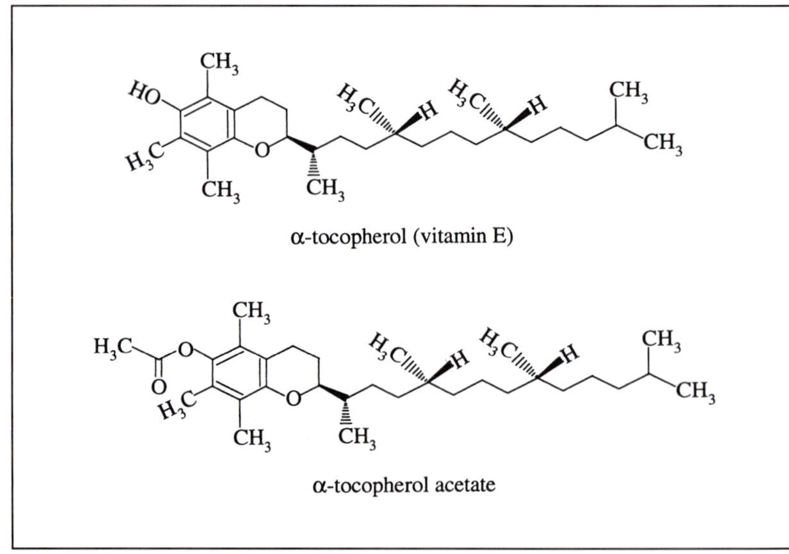

Figure 9.9

Chemical structures of compounds with vitamin E activity

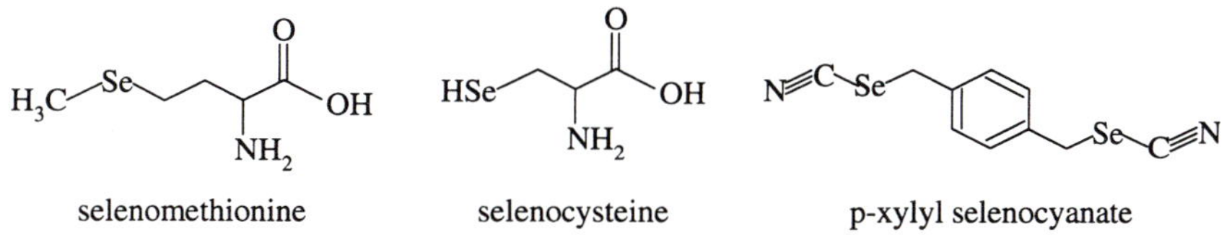

Figure 9.10

Chemical structures of organoseleniums

tion, inhibits proliferation, and blocks carcinogen adduct formation [146]. Supplementation of experimental animals with vitamin E inhibits DMBA-induced mammary carcinogenesis [156, 157]. The acetate derivative of vitamin E, such as α-tocopherol acetate, is also effective against chemically-induced mammary carcinogenesis [158–161]. In addition, vitamin E also potentiates the chemopreventive action of lower doses of other more toxic agents (e.g., selenium, fenretinide). In fact, there is epidemiological evidence that a higher risk for cancer development at several sites is correlated with a combination of low vitamin E and low selenium levels [162–164]. In experimental animals, a combination of α-tocopherol and selenium supplementation in the diet decreases the multiplicity and increases the latency of DMBA-induced mammary carcinogenesis [149, 165]. Considering the differences in the biologic mechanisms of breast carcinogenesis in women with or without a family history of breast cancer, alpha-tocopherol has been suggested as a potential chemopreventive agent for women with a family history of breast cancer particularly during the premenopausal period [166].

Selenium (Se) is an essential trace element, the deficiency of which is associated with an increased incidence of some human cancers [167]. Administration of selenium in its inorganic form (e.g., Na_2SeD_3) at levels above dietary requirement protects experimental animals from carcinogenesis in the mammary gland, liver, skin, colon, stomach, oral cavity, bladder and pancreas [103, 156, 157, 167–170]. Treatment of selenium is associated with a dose-dependent increase in cellular thioredoxin reductase activity, a newly discovered homodimeric selenocysteine-containing protein that catalyzes the NADPH-dependent reduction of the redox protein thioredoxin frequently overexpressed in human tumors [167]. To overcome the toxicity in animals fed with inorganic selenium at levels of greater than 5 ppm, a number of naturally occurring or synthetic novel selenium-containing organic compounds named as organoseleniums (Fig. 9.10) have been exploited as potential chemopreventive agents against human cancer [171]. Selenomethionine (Fig. 9.10) is one of the predominant organic forms of selenium in cereals, vegetables and grains [172] and can be as efficiently absorbed and utilized as inorganic selenium [173]. Studies in laboratory animals indicate that naturally-occurring organoseleniums such as selenomethionine and selenocysteine are often effective in chemoprevention of mammary carcinogenesis, even though in some cases they have a lower efficacy and higher toxicity than selenium [174, 175]. Supplementation of selenium-enriched garlic inhibits the post-initiation and early stages of mammary carcinogenesis [176]. A selenium-enriched garlic extract acts in part via the action of Se-methylselenocysteine to inhibit tumorigenesis by suppressing the proliferation and reducing the survival of the early transformed cells [177].

A number of novel organoseleniums that retain the chemopreventive activity of selenium but without its serious side-effects have been synthesized for use as chemopreventive agents against mammary carcinogenesis [171, 178–181]. Triphenylselenonium chloride, a novel synthetic organic selenium compound in which selenium is bonded to three unsubstituted benzene rings, possesses significant chemopreventive activity against chemically-induced mammary carcinogenesis without the toxic activities associated with selenite treatment [182]. Selenium homologs, such as aliphatic selenocyanates with increasing length of the alkyl side chain, effectively block DMBA-induced rat mammary carcinogenesis at the initiation phase [183]. The positively charged and amphiphilic triphenylselenonium has superior chemopreventive efficacy compared to the uncharged and lipophilic diphenylselenide [184]. One of the most effective synthetic organoseleniums, though, is xylyl selenocyanate or 1,4-phenylene-bis(methylene)selenocyanate, which inhibits human cytochrome P450-catalyzed oxidation of xenobiotics and procarcinogens [185], suppresses the formation of DMBA-DNA adduct in the mammary gland and reduces the multiplicity of mammary carcinomas [171, 179, 181]. The mechanisms of action of organoseleniums like xylyl selenocyanate include inhibition of thymidine kinase [186] and induction of apoptosis [181]. However, not all of these mechanisms are functional against each specific stage of mammary carcinogenesis. For instance, only chronic exposure to triphenylselenonium chloride can sustain its cancer inhibitory activity against the progression of *N*-methyl-*N*-nitrosourea (MNU)-induced premalignant to malignant mammary lesions in rats [187]. Further, triphenylselenonium can not induce regression of established mammary carcinomas or suppress the emergence of new tumors when it is given at the late stage of carcinogenesis [187]. These findings highlight the importance of understanding the range of activity of a given chemopreventive agent in order to maximize the probability of a successful outcome in the design of any future intervention trial.

9.4.3.3 Tea and Polyphenolic Antioxidants

Serving as a natural source of antioxidants, tea is one of the safest and most popular traditional beverages worldwide, second only to water [188]. There is epidemiological evidence that standardized mortality rates are low for all forms of cancer in the population of the Shizuoka area of Japan, where people drink large amounts of tea [189]. Although epidemiological studies found no associations between consumption of tea and risk of many cancers including breast cancer [190–192], polyphenolic components of tea have shown anticarcinogenic effects in the skin, lung, forestomach, esophagus, duodenum, colon, liver, pancreas and mammary glands [103, 193–195]. Tea is classified in two types, namely, green tea, which is made by steaming and drying fresh tea leaves, and black tea, which is produced by crushing the leaves to cause oxidative polymerization of the polyphenols in a polyphenol oxidase-dependent process known as "fermentation" [193]. Dried tea extract contains 25–40 % polyphenolic flavonols (catechins), of which the prevalent compound is epigallocatechingallate (EGCG) in green tea, and black tea polyphenols (BTP) thearubigens and theaflavins in black tea (Fig. 9.11), which are the oxidized products of catechins [193, 196]. Most experimental research has been conducted on the anticarcinogenic properties of green tea extracts and their major constituents because of the weaker anticarcinogenic activities of black tea extracts and their major constituents [193]. Among seven compounds isolated from the aqueous-alcoholic extract of green tea leaves, (+)-gallocatechin (GC), (-)-epicatechin (EC), (-)-epigallocatechin (EGC), (-)-epicatechingallate (ECG), (-)-epigallocatechin gallate (EGCG), caffeine and (+)-catechin, EGCG is the most potent green tea component against the growth of human breast cancer cells [197] and it prevents preneoplastic transformation of the mammary glands in vitro [122, 127]. Green tea catechins and other antioxidants such as 3-O-ethylascorbic acid, 3-O-dodecylcarbomethylascorbic acid, ellagic acid and, particularly 1-O-hexyl-2,3,5-trimethylhydroquinone, exert a potent chemopreventive action against 2-amino-1-methyl-6-phenylimidazo[4,5-b]pyridine-induced mammary carcinogenesis in rats [198]. Results from a recent study indicate that black tea, especially in combination with milk, decreases the incidence of chemical carcinogen-induced carcinogenesis in the rat mammary glands and colon [199]. Several mechanisms appear to be responsible for the antitumor properties of tea, including enhancement of antioxidant (glutathione peroxidase,

Figure 9.11

Chemical structures of tea polyphenols

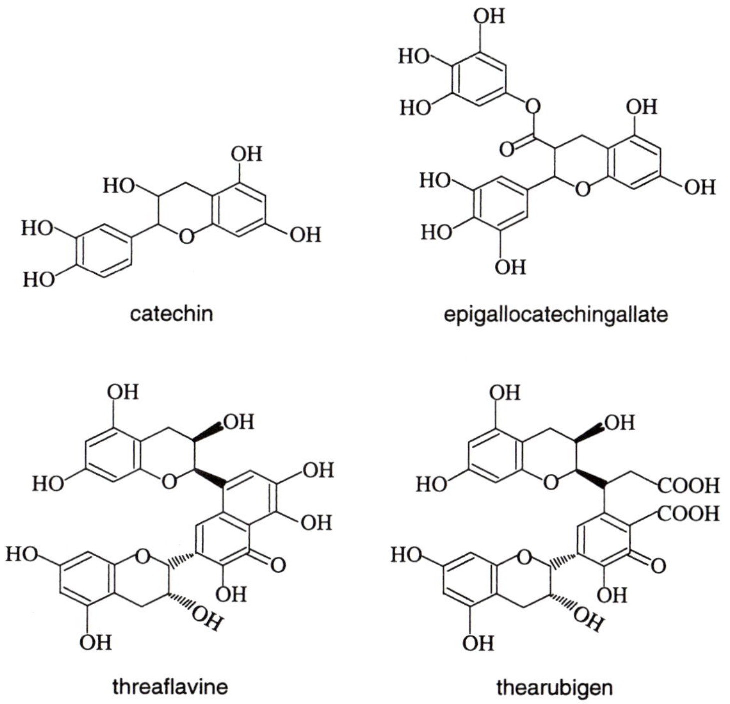

catalase and quinone reductase) and phase II (glutathione-*S*-transferase) enzyme activities, inhibition of chemically-induced lipid peroxidation, protein kinase C and cellular proliferation [195, 200].

9.4.3.4 Flavonoids

The flavonoids (e. g., quercetin, luteolin, genistein, kaempferol, myricetin, apigenin) comprise a large group of naturally-occurring low molecular weight substances that are rich in fruits, vegetables, leaves, flowers, seeds, nuts, stems, bark and roots of most plants, as well as tea, coffee and wine [201]. They are classified into several groups, such as flavones, isoflavones, flavanones, flavonols flavan-3-ol and coumarins, based on their chemical structures (Fig. 9.12, Table 9.2) [202]. Although flavonoids are generally not considered as nutritive agents, they have attracted

Table 9.2. Classification of flavonoids

Classes	Examples
Flavones	Apigenin, chrysin, luteolin
Isoflavone	Daidzein, genistein
Flavanones	Eriodictyol, hesperetin, naringenin
Flavonols	Baicalein, fisetin, galangin, myrisetin, quercetin
Flavan-3-ol	Catechin
Coumarin	Coumarin

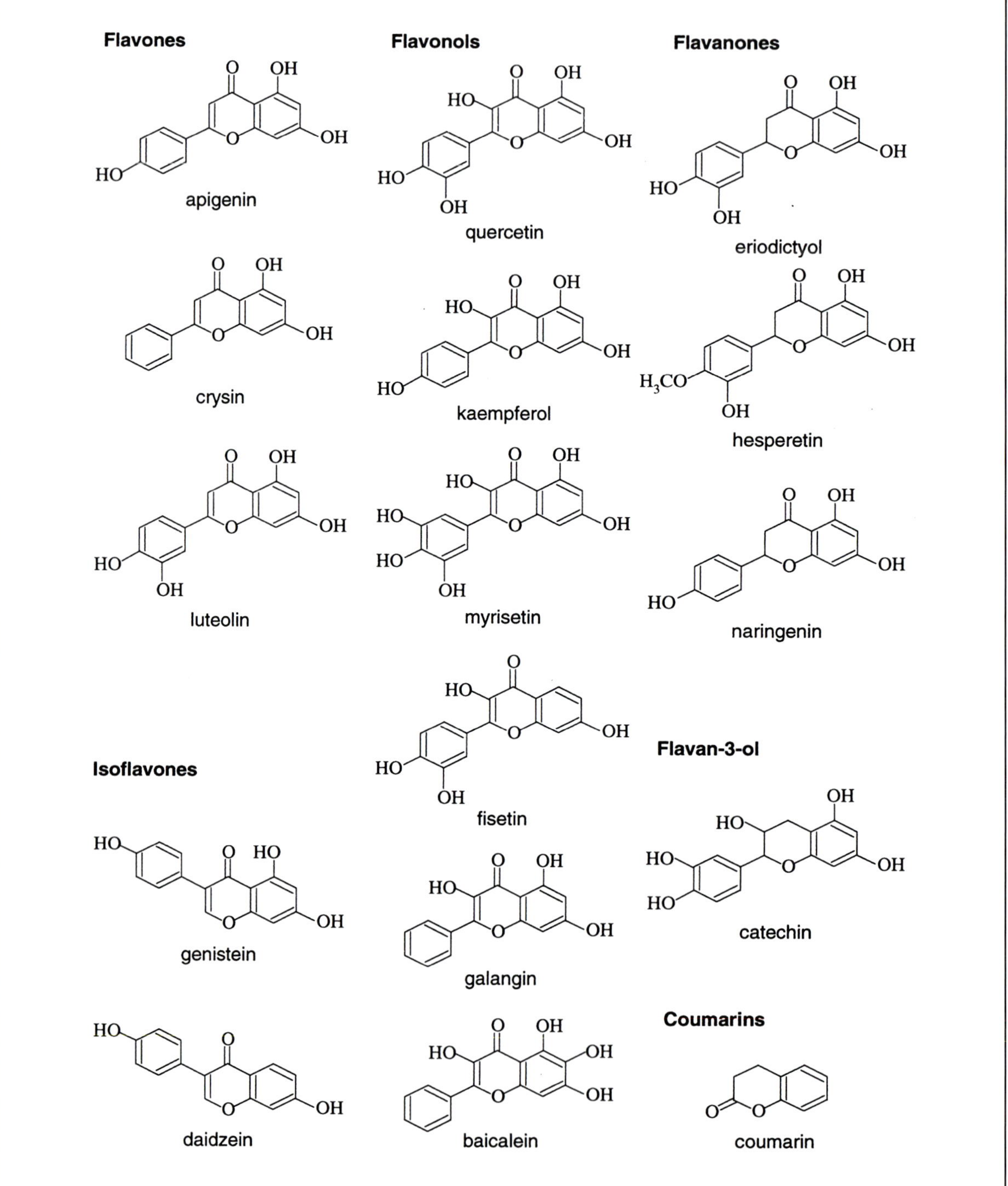

Figure 9.12

Classification and chemical structures of flavonoids

much of the attention due to their potential role in prevention of human cancer [203]. Dietary flavonoids have been shown to suppress lipid peroxidation, quench free radicals and reduce oxidative DNA damage in vitro [201, 202], and inhibit chemical carcinogen-induced carcinogenesis in vivo [204, 205]. Flavonoids also inhibit the growth of human breast cancer cells in vitro [206, 207]. The total content of all naturally-occurring flavonoids in a typical Western diet is estimated at 1 g/day [201], the dietary intake of flavonoids is presumably much higher in vegetarians than omnivores [208]. Therefore, the low incidence of cancer and mortality in vegetarians has been attributed to uptake of flavonoids in their diet [208].

9.5 Chemoprevention Against Epigenetic Alterations

9.5.1 Restricting Fat/Caloric Consumption

Epidemiological studies have documented the link between dietary intake of fatty acids and the risk of breast cancer, especially in the more industrialized Western world [209–211]. In experimental animals, a positive correlation between dietary intake of fatty acids and the incidence of chemical carcinogenesis or the rate of tumor growth has also been observed [212–216]. In fact, uptake of dietary fat even during the embryonic development stage affects the risk of developing mammary cancer later in life. For examples, the incidence of chemical carcinogen-induced mammary carcinomas is significantly higher in rats that have been exposed to isocaloric high dietary fat in utero via a maternal feed than in the low-fat group [217]. Chronic ingestion of an extract of coffee cherry, the residue left after removal of coffee beans, induced a marked suppression of spontaneous mammary tumor development in a high mammary tumor strain of SHN virgin mice mainly due to its inhibitory effects on the circulating level of free fatty acid [218].

However, mammary carcinogenesis is not influenced only by the total amount of fatty acids, but also by the types of fatty acids [87]. Various types of fatty acids exert different effects on mammary carcino-

genesis in experimental models of human breast cancer. For example, an elevated intake of linoleic acid stimulates the growth of human breast carcinoma cells in vitro [219], increases the incidence of chemical carcinogen-induced mammary carcinogenesis [220, 221] and enhances the growth of transplantable mammary tumors in experimental animals [222, 223]. In contrast, growth of mammary tumors can be inhibited in a dose-dependent manner by oleic acid [213–217, 219], decosahexaenoic acid [219] and arachidonic acid [224]. Results from a recent meta-analysis indicate that n-6 polyunsaturated fatty acids strongly promote the mammary carcinogenesis, saturated fatty acids slightly enhance the mammary tumorigenesis, while n-3 polyunsaturated fatty acids exhibit a small protective effects against the development of mammary cancer [87].

It should also be noted that caloric intake associated with the consumption of fat-containing food is known to increase mammary carcinogenesis independently [225]. In experimental animals, restricted caloric intake dramatically reduces the incidence of spontaneous, chemically- and viral-induced mammary tumorigenesis [225–232]. Even though increased physical activity (e.g., exercise) is generally observed to increase energy expenditure, reduce body weight gain and carcass fat [232, 233], excise has been reported to inhibit, stimulate or have no effects in animal models of breast cancer [234–239]. In human, both "overnutrition" and body mass have been associated with an increased risk of breast cancer [240, 241], and obesity appears related to a poor prognosis in cancer patients [242]. Physical activity during leisure time and at work has been associated with a reduced risk of breast cancer, especially in premenopausal women [243].

The mechanisms by which fatty acids or calorie influences mammary tumorigenesis remain to be established. Both fat intake and caloric restriction or exercise influence the endocrine milieu. In experimental animals, the influence of dietary fat on mammary carcinogenesis has been mainly attributed to their effects on the secretion of such hormones as prolactin and estrogen [244]. Caloric restriction per se is insufficient for protection against the development of mammary tumors [232]. Instead, modulation of the secretion of adrenal steroids by energy status is essential to the inhibitory effects of caloric restriction on mammary carcinogenesis [232]. In humans, reduction of fat content in a fiber-rich diet lowers the concentration of circulating estrogens in premenopausal and postmenopausal women [245–253]. Recent results from a randomized trial indicate that intervention with a low-fat, high-carbohydrate diet for two years reduces the area of mammographic density, a radiographic feature of the breast that is a risk factor for breast cancer [254]. Vigorous physical training [255–259] and even moderate exercise [260–262] can alter the endocrine milieu and interrupt the menstrual cycle. For instance, long-term physical activity at high or moderate levels can result in delayed menarche [258, 259], reduced steroidogenesis [251, 260, 263], shortened luteal phase [264, 265], anovulation [261, 263, 266] and secondary amenorrhea [256, 267]. A reduction in the cumulative exposure to cyclic steroids (e.g., estrogens and progesterone) has been proposed to account for the preventive effect of both leisure-time and work activity against the development of breast cancer [243].

Accordingly, women, especially those who are obese, should be advised to restrict their dietary intake of fat from dairy products, meats and partially hydrogenated oils, and replace sugar and highly refined carbohydrates in their diet with complex carbohydrates from fruits, vegetables, legumes and whole grains.

9.5.2 Maintaining Proper Endocrine Milieu

The risk of developing breast cancer can be profoundly influenced by an individual's history of reproductive functions such as menstruation, parity or childbirth, breast feeding and menopause. An increased risk has been associated with early onset of menstruation, nulliparity or delayed first childbirth, short duration of breast-feeding and late menopause [13, 268–270]. A principal culprit common for all these risk factors is the prolonged exposure to female sex hormones [271–273]. The hormonal influences have been mainly attributed to unopposed exposure to elevated levels of estrogens [274], as has been indi-

cated for a variety of female cancers, namely, vaginal, hepatic and cervical carcinomas [275–280]. In addition, both environmental and genetic factors are believed to exert their influence by a hormonal mechanism [281]. Therefore, a number of strategies have emerged to target on various aspects of hormonal actions.

9.5.2.1 Steroids

Although 67 % of breast cancers are manifested during the postmenopausal period, a vast majority, 95 %, are initially hormone-dependent, estrogens (Fig. 9.13) playing a crucial role in their development and evolution [274]. However, it is still unclear whether estrogens are carcinogenic to the human breast. Most of the current understanding of carcinogenicity of estrogens is based on studies in experimental animal systems and clinical observations of a greater risk of endometrial hyperplasia and neoplasia associated with estrogen supplementation or polycystic ovarian syndrome [278–280]. There are two mechanisms that have been considered to be responsible for the carcinogenicity of estrogens: a receptor-mediated hormonal activity, which has generally been related to stimulation of cellular proliferation, resulting in more opportunities for accumulation of genetic damages leading to carcinogenesis [282, 283], and cytochrome P450-mediated metabolic activation, which elicits direct genotoxic effects by increasing mutation rates [62, 63, 282]. There is also evidence that estrogen compromises the DNA repair system and allows accumulation of lesions in the genome essential to estrogen-induced tumorigenesis [284].

Estradiol-17β is biologically the most active estrogen in breast tissue. Circulating estrogens are mainly originated from ovarian steroidogenesis in premenopausal women and peripheral aromatization of ovarian and adrenal androgens in the postmenopausal women [270]. Early menopause prior to age 40, either occurring naturally or induced by bilateral ovariectomy, significantly reduces the risk of developing breast cancer [270, 285–287]. However, the uptake of estradiol-17β from the circulation does not appear to contribute significantly to the total content of estrogen in

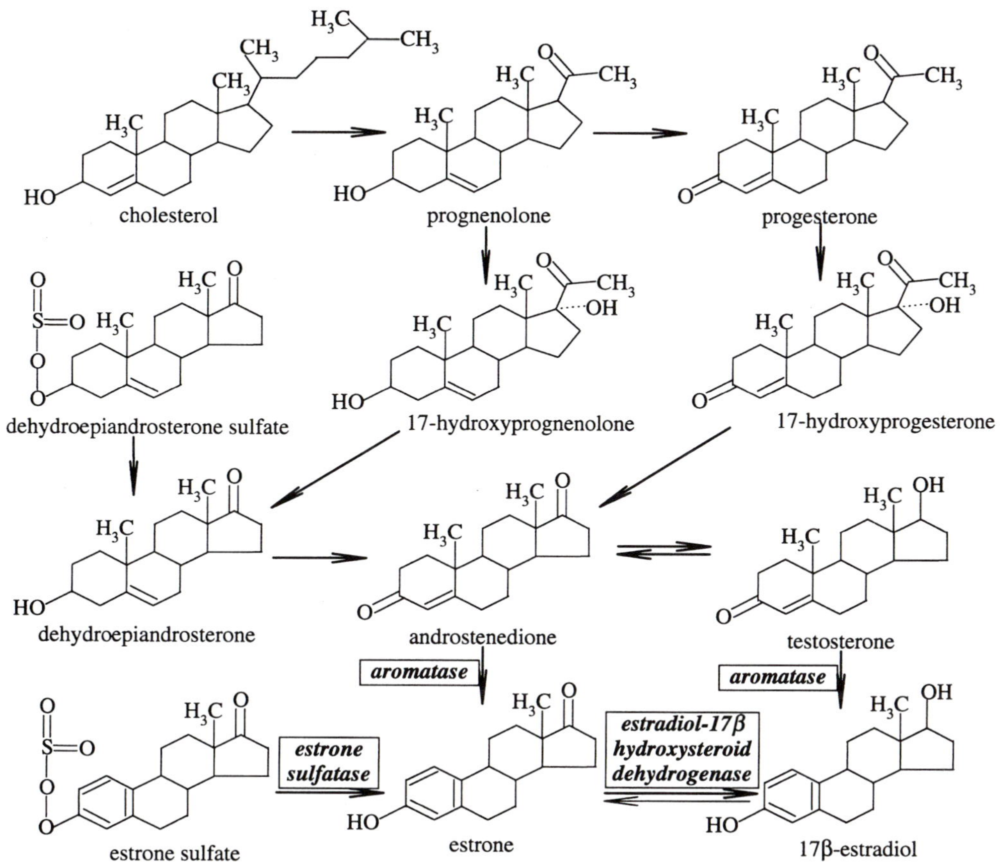

Figure 9.13

Metabolic pathways of estrogen production

breast tumors, the majority of estrogen present in the tumor tissues is derived from de novo biosynthesis [288–291]. In fact, there are no differences in the concentrations of estradiol-17β in breast cancer tissues between premenopausal and postmenopausal women, even though plasma levels of estradiol-17β decrease by 90% following menopause [292]. Three main enzyme complexes that are involved in the synthesis of biologically active estrogen (i.e., estradiol-17β) in the breast are:

1. The aromatase which converts androstenedione to estrone
2. Estradiol-17β hydroxysteroid dehydrogenase which preferentially reduces estrone to estradiol-17β in tumor tissues
3. Estrone sulfatase which hydrolyses the estrogen sulfate to estrone (Fig. 9.13) [293, 294]

Each of these pathways represents a potential target for chemoprevention of breast cancer. In addition, biosynthesis of estrogens can also be blocked by inhibiting the synthesis of androgens that serve as precursor for de novo steroidogenesis.

9.5.2.2 Aromatase Inhibitors

Aromatase (estrogen synthetase) is the enzyme complex responsible for the final step in estrogen synthesis – the conversion of androstenedione and testosterone to estrone and estradiol, respectively (Fig. 9.13). Inhibitors of this enzyme have been shown to be clinically effective in the treatment of advanced breast cancer in postmenopausal women, in whom the major source of estrogen production derives from aromatization of adrenal androgens in peripheral tissues, such as muscle, liver, and fat [295, 296]. A number of steroidal (e.g., 4-hydroxyandrostendione) and non-steroidal (e.g., fadrozole, liarozole, vorozole) aromatase inhibitors (Fig. 9.14) have been synthesized and subjected to clinical and pharmacological studies. Most of the synthetic inhibitors of aromatase have been extensively evaluated for their efficacy of obliterating the peripheral aromatase activity to justify their use as potential optimal post-tamoxifen, second-line agents for the treatment of advanced breast cancer [296]. Since increased breast cancer susceptibility has been associated with aberrant aromatase activities [297, 298] and a genetic polymorphism in the aromatase gene [296], inhibition of aromatase activity has emerged as a valid strategy in the prevention of breast cancer. Indeed, inhibitors of aromatase have shown promising potential in various experimental models. For instance, fadrozole can almost completely prevent spontaneous mammary tumorigenesis in a highly susceptible strain of rats at a dosage below that required to exert a maximal antiproliferative effect on established tumors [299]. Similarly, vorozole, a triazole derivative with potent and highly specific inhibitory activity against aromatase, effectively blocks the development of chemical carcinogen-induced mammary carcinogenesis in the rats [300]. However, total suppression of aromatase may have adverse effects including increased osteoporosis, cardiovascular disease, and urogenital atrophy, as is evident in postmenopausal women [301]. One possibility is to obtain chemopreventive effects without total suppression of aromatase and circulating estrogen levels. Another alternative is to suppress local estrogen production by drugs targeting on the unique transcriptional promoter of aromatase gene expression, I.4, in breast adipose tissue [301].

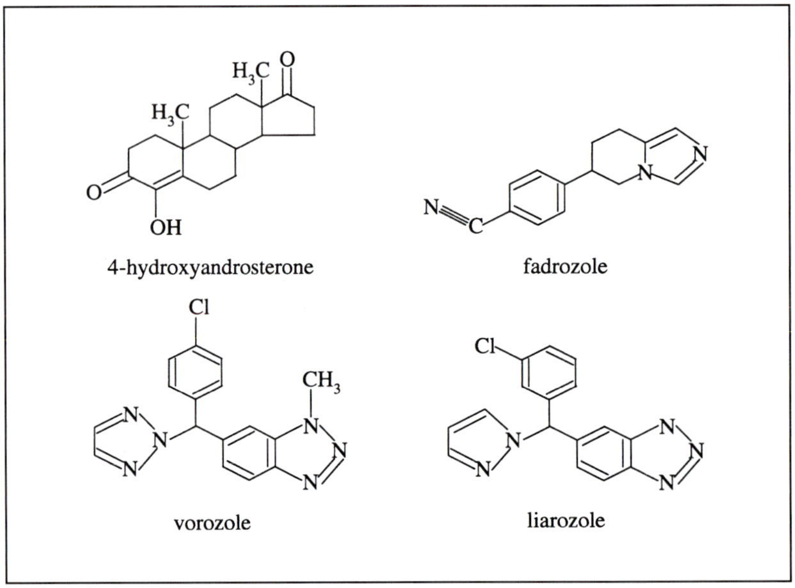

Figure 9.14

Chemical structures of aromatase inhibitors

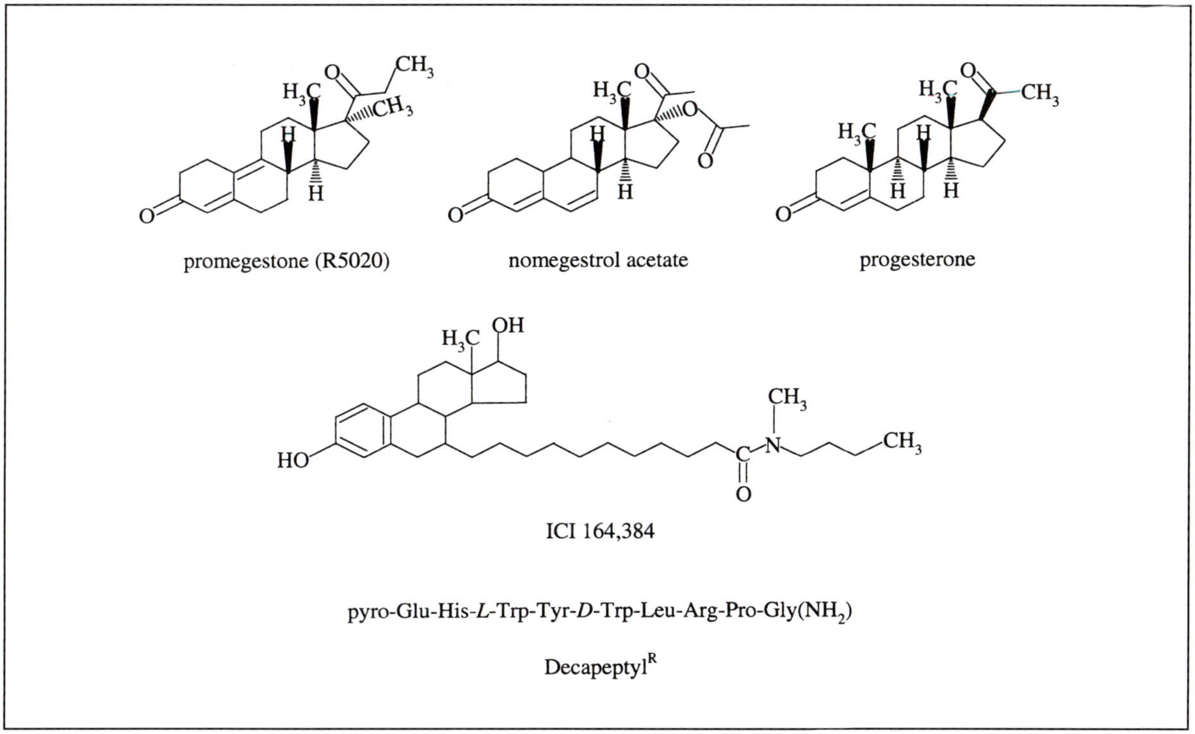

Figure 9.15

Chemical structures of estrone sulfatase inhibitors

9.5.2.3 Estrone Sulfatase Inhibitors

Even though the major pathway of estrone synthesis is via aromatization of the precursor androgens in the ovary or peripheral tissue, much of the estrone synthesized is converted to estrone sulfate, which can be converted back to estrone by estrone sulfatase-mediated hydrolysis [302]. Sulfation is an important process in the metabolism and inactivation of steroids, including estrogens, because the addition of the charged sulfonate group prevents the binding of the steroid to its receptor [303]. It has been postulated that the main pathway for the formation of estrone is through the hydrolysis of estrone sulfate in breast cancer tissues, which contain 10–100 times higher sulfatase activity than the aromatase activity [293]. Thus, estrone sulfate is quantitatively the most important circulating estrogen in women and acts as a large reservoir for the formation of estrone [304, 305]. A large amount of estrone sulfate and estrone sulfatase activity have been observed in breast tumor tissues, especially in those from postmenopausal women [293]. Substances that have been explored as anti-sulfatase agents include natural progesterone and synthetic analogs (e.g., Nomegestrol acetate, Promegestone or R-5020), the GnRH agonist Decapeptyl and the pure antiestrogen ICI 164,384 (Fig. 9.15) [293]. TAP-144-SR biodegradable microcapsules of copoly (DL-lactic/glycolic acid) copolymer containing a potent LHRH agonist, TAP-144 (D-Leu6-(des-Gly10-NH2)-LHRH ethylamide, leuprolide acetate) reduce tumor incidence and multiplicity of DMBA-induced rat mammary carcinogenesis [306]. While daidzein does not affect sterol sulfatase, its sulfoconjugates are potent inhibitors of this enzyme [307], providing a biochemical basis for the putative chemopreventive role of dietary isoflavones against breast cancer.

9.5.2.4 Dehydroepiandrosterone

Circulating free and conjugated dehydroepiandrosterone (DHEA) (Fig. 9.16) are the major steroid precursors for estrogen synthesis in the peripheral tissue, especially in postmenopausal women. The plasma concentration of DHEA sulfate is highest in the second decade of life and declines markedly during adulthood [308]. Concentrations of circulating DHEA are inversely correlated with the risk of breast cancer [309–311], an epidemiological observation that has generated a great deal of interest in studies of DHEA as a chemopreventive agent against breast cancer. DHEA inhibits DNA synthesis [312, 313] and spontaneous [314] or chemically-induced [103, 315–318] carcinogenesis in mammary tissue. Dietary DHEA at a dose as low as 5 ppm is effective, decreasing tumor multiplicity and increasing tumor latency in a dose-dependent manner [318]. Even limited exposure to DHEA for a period of 7 weeks profoundly decreases final tumor incidence and multiplicity [318]. But use of the chemopreventive DHEA at pharmacological doses is limited due to its potent androgenic activity and liver toxicity [319]. To eliminate these side effects, Schwartz et al. [319, 320] have designed several DHEA analogues, one of which is DHEA analog 8354 (fluasterone) that produces reduced side effects without compromising the chemopreventive potential against MNU-induced mammary carcinogenesis [103, 315–317, 319]. Recently, an exceptional chemopreventive activity against chemically-induced mammary carcinogenesis in the rat has been achieved by low-dose DHEA which also induces massive lobular-alveolar proliferation and mammary gland differentiation [321].

9.5.2.5 Genistein

There is increasing evidence that differences in the diet may account for the wide variations in breast cancer incidence between American and Southeast Asia populations (e.g., China, Indonesia, Japan, Korea, Singapore). A remarkable difference in the diet is the consumption of soy foods. A review of epidemiological data has revealed an association between soy intake and reduction in cancer risk in nearly two-thirds of the studies reported [322]. This epidemiological observation is supported by experimental evidence that dietary supplementation of whole soybeans reduces the incidence of mammary tumors induced by x-ray irradiation [323] and chemical carcinogens [324, 325]. Soya products have also been found to have antitumoral effects in many other organs of experimental animals [326]. Consumption of soya diets for one month by premenopausal women reduces circulating levels of adrenal androgens and ovarian steroids implicated in the etiology of breast cancer [327]. Many compounds of diverse structure present in soybeans exhibit pleiotropic biological effects that have implications in the chemoprevention of cancer. Biochanin A, an isoflavone derivative, inhibits the development of MNU-induced rat mammary carcinogenesis [325]. Protease inhibitors of soybean origin have been shown to suppress mammary carcinogenesis induced by chemical carcinogen, radiation and mouse mammary tumor virus in experimental ani-

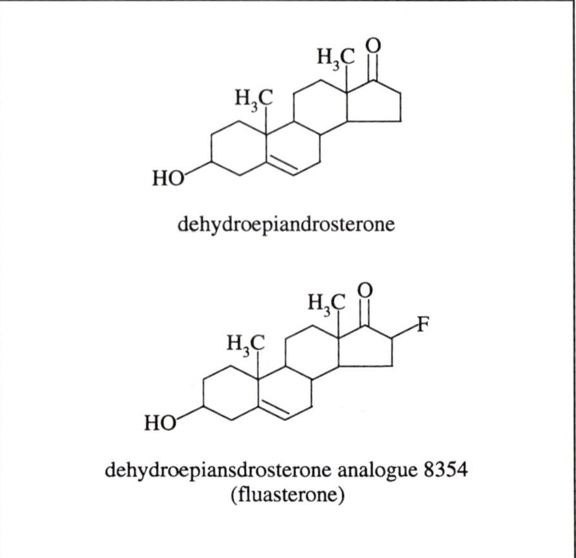

Figure 9.16

Chemical structures of dehydroepiandrosterone and fluasterone mals [328]. Of all soya-derived chemopreventive compounds, only the phytoestrogens daidzein and genistein (Fig. 9.12), which combine to represent over 90% of the soybean isoflavone content [329], have been detected in human urine and blood [330–332]. The isoflavone genistein was discovered in 1987 as a naturally occurring tyrosine kinase inhibitor in soy [333]. The concentration of genistein in most soy food materials ranges from 1–2 mg/g. Oriental populations, who have low rates of breast and prostate cancer, consume 20–80 mg of genistein/day, almost entirely derived from soy, whereas the dietary intake of genistein in the US is only 1–3 mg/day [333]. Genistein strongly inhibits the growth of human breast cancer cells in vitro [334, 335], blocks DMBA-induced genetic damage in vivo [336] and protects animals from experimentally-induced mammary carcinogenesis [329, 337]. The mechanism of genistein's preventive action is in part dependent on its estrogenic activity, which causes a more rapid differentiation of terminal ductal structures, alters the endocrine system to reduce cell proliferation in the mammary gland as occurs during early pregnancy [338, 339]. In fact, administration of genistein to laboratory animals during the neonatal or prepubertal period induces precocious maturation of undifferentiated terminal end buds to more differentiated lobules and reduces the incidence and multiplicity of chemically-induced mammary cancer [338, 340]. At physiological concentrations, genistein exerts its effect by modulating estrogenic pathways, as a result of either direct competition with estrogen by binding to its receptor, or down regulating estrogen receptor expression [341]. Genistein and coumestrol are able to reduce the conversion of [³H]estrone to [³H] estradiol-17β catalyzed by estrogen-specific 17β-hydroxysteroid oxidoreductase Type 1 in vitro [342]. Inhibition of 17β-hydroxysteroid oxidoreductase Type 1 enzyme could lead to a decrease in the availability of the highly active endogenous estrogen estradiol-17β. At pharmacological doses, genistein is an inhibitor of tyrosine kinase activity essential to the signal transduction mediated by receptors for both growth factors (e.g., epidermal growth factor (EGF), platelet-derived growth factor (PDGF), insulin, IGF) and oncogene products (e.g., pp60v-src, pp110gag-fes) [333,

343]. Genistein inhibits cell proliferation similarly in estrogen receptor (ER)-positive and ER-negative human breast carcinoma cell lines in vitro [344]. Its chemopreventive action involves blockage of critical checkpoints of cell cycle control (e.g., specific G2/M arrest) and induction of apoptosis [127; 335, 344].

9.6 Melatonin

Melatonin (Fig. 9.17), the hormone produced and secreted by the pineal gland during the night in virtually all mammalian species including men, has been implicated in such human reproductive processes as puberty and menstrual cycle [345, 346]. It inhibits the secretion of GnRH in the hypothalamus and the responsiveness to GnRH in the pituitary, leading to "hypothalamic gonadectomy" [347, 348]. In experimental animals, administration of melatonin results in reduction of ovarian weight, blockade of ovulation and estrous cycle [349, 350]. Melatonin exerts oncostatic effects on breast cancer and a variety of other neoplasms [351, 352]. The chemopreventive potential of melatonin against breast cancer is suggested by experimental studies showing that melatonin significantly suppresses the incidences and the growth of chemical carcinogen-induced rat mammary tumors [351, 353]. A combination of melatonin and tamoxifen has been considered as "the most likely candidate in achieving the ultimate goal of total suppression of mammary carcinogenesis" [353].

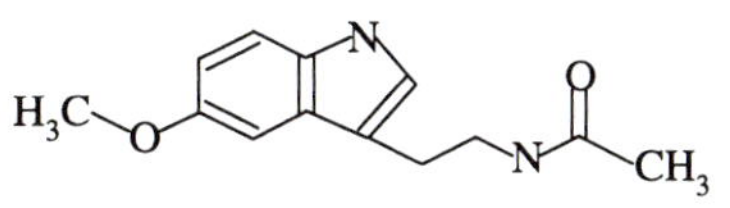

Figure 9.17

Chemical structure of melatonin

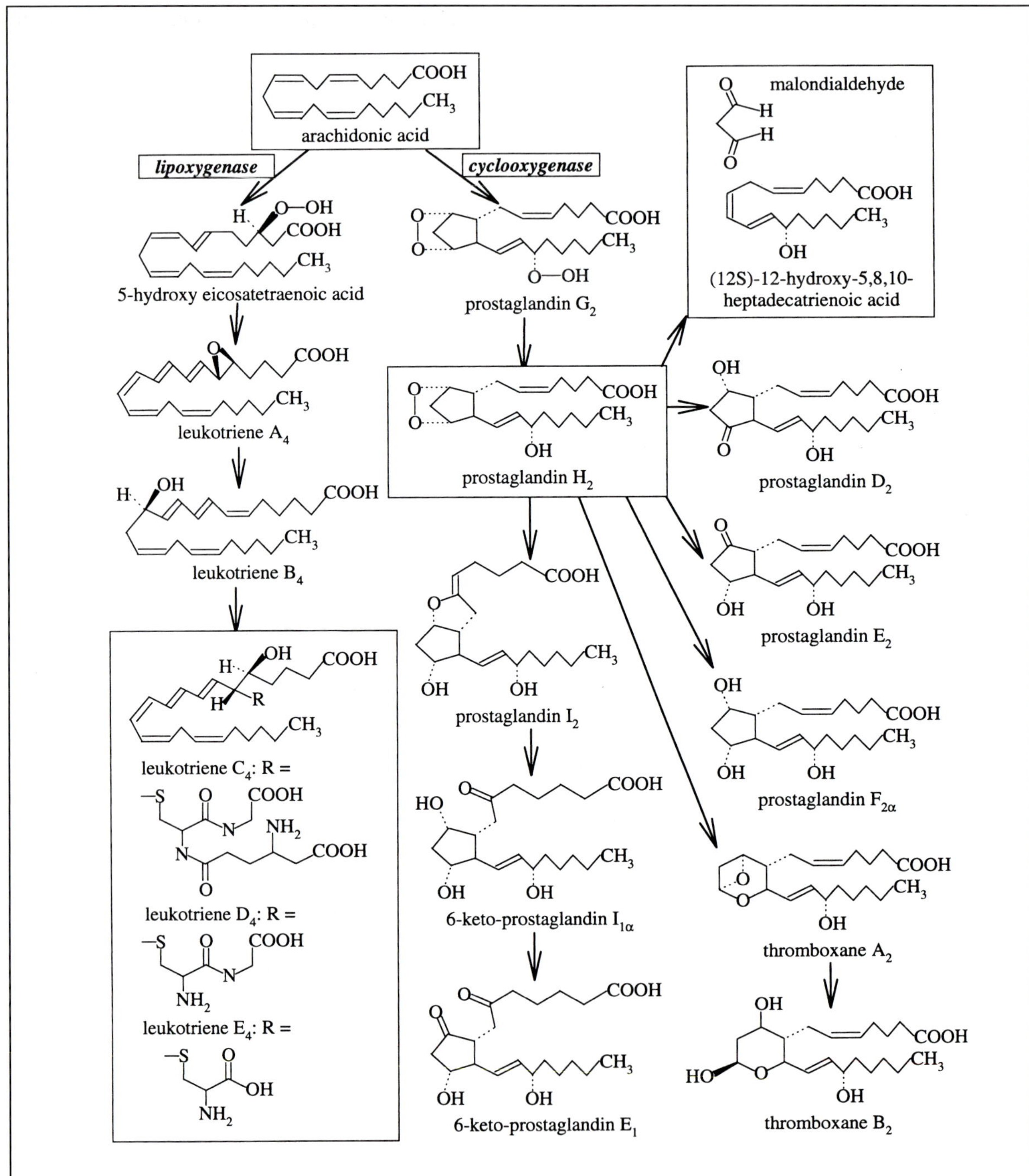

Figure 9.18

Metabolic pathways of eicosanoids

9.7 Eicosanoids

Eicosanoids, such as prostaglandins, leukotrienes and thromboxanes (Fig. 9.18), are known to promote neoplastic growth, suppress immune surveillance and facilitate tumor cell invasion and metastasis [55–58, 354]. The carcinogenic effects of eicosanoids are attributed to the production of free radicals and of a direct-acting mutagen malondialdehyde from the metabolism of arachidonic acid [55–58]. In addition, eicosanoids are believed to play a role in mammary carcinogenesis as influenced by dietary fat [355–357]. It has been demonstrated that breast cancers contain higher levels of several eicosanoids, namely prostaglandins and thromboxane B2, than benign breast tumors or normal mammary tissue [358, 359]. Eicosanoids levels are also elevated in chemically-induced mammary tumors [360, 361].

Eicosanoids result from the metabolism of arachidonic acid by one of two pathways, the cyclooxygenase or the lipoxygenase pathways [354]. Clearly, the inhibition or modification of these pathways constitutes a promissory strategy for intervention in mammary cancer control.

Eicosapentaenoic acid (EPA) and docosahexaenoic acid (DHA) (Fig. 9.19), which are n-3 polyunsaturated fatty acids rich in fish oil, function as competitive inhibitors of cyclooxygenase-mediated prostaglandin synthesis [362]. There is also an inverse relationship between the incidence of breast cancer and the level of fish consumption [363]. In particular, the incidences of breast cancer are considerably lower in rural Japanese [364] and Greenland Eskimos [365] who consume a larger amount of dietary n-3 polyunsaturated fatty acids, as compared to the high-risk Americans [365, 366]. EPA inhibits neoplastic transformation of mammary explant culture in response to chemical carcinogens or virus [122, 367]. Dietary supplementation of fish oil [368], EPA or DHA [369] inhibits chemical carcinogen-induced mammary carcinogenesis in vivo.

The inhibition of cyclooxygenase activity by non-steroidal anti-inflammatory drugs (NSAIDs) (Fig. 9.20) may have a role in the chemoprevention of breast cancer. Indomethacin [355–357], flurbiprofen [370], ibuprofen [103, 371], piroxicam [372, 373], sulindac [374] and the antioxidant phytochemical curcumin [103, 375, 376] are NSAIDs that have been shown to suppress mammary carcinogenesis and/or breast cancer growth in experimental model systems. Aspirin, another NSAID that is capable of inhibiting prostaglandin synthetase activity, has been associated with reduced incidence of breast cancer in some epidemiological studies [377, 378]. However, aspirin and piroxicam did not show significant effects on certain epidemiological studies [379], or in chemically induced mammary carcinogenesis [103], respectively. It should also be noted that not all of the inhibitory effects of NSAIDs on mammary cancer could be accounted for by their actions on arachidonic acid metabolism. Sulindac sulfoxide, a commonly prescribed anti-inflammatory drug, has cancer chemopreventive activity [374]. During its metabolism, the inactive prodrug sulindac sulfoxide undergoes either reduction to the active anti-inflammatory metabolite sulindac sulfide or irreversible oxidation to sulindac sulfone, which lacks prostaglandin synthetase inhibitory activity [374]. Interestingly, sulindac sulfone has been reported to have chemopreventive activity by induction of apoptosis against mammary carcinogenesis, especially against carcinogenesis involving alterations in the Ha-ras-associated signal transduction cascade [374]. Clearly, more studies are needed for clarifying the chemopreventive potential of NSAIDs against human breast cancer.

Nordihydroguaiaretic acid (Fig. 9.21) is a major component of "chaparral tea" prepared from the desert shrub *Larrea divaricata* [380]. Nordihydroguaiaretic acid, a polyhydroxyphenolic antioxidant, was once used at 100–200 ppm to prevent oxidation of unsaturated fats in fat-containing products to preserve their flavor and nutrients [381]. The anticarcinogenic potential of nordihydroguaiaretic acid is suggested by its effects against oxidation leading to formation of mutagenic free radicals [381]. However, there is much stronger evidence for its use in chemoprevention. Nordihydroguaiaretic acid is a potent inhibitor of the lipoxygenase pathway of arachidonic acid metabolism [355, 382]. It also suppresses induction of ornithine decarboxylase activity by prolactin in the mammary glands [383]. Administration of

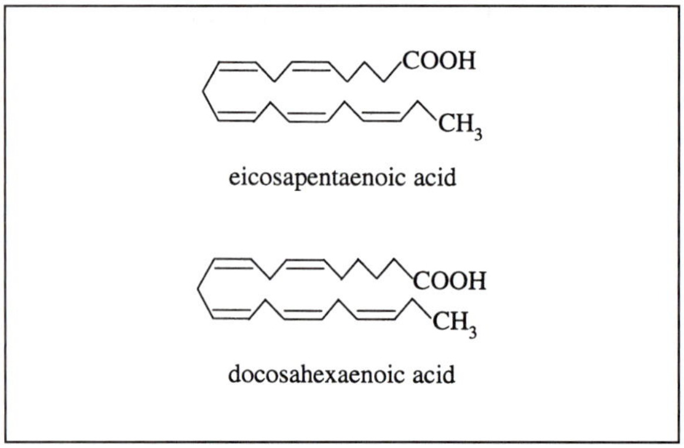

Figure 9.19

Chemical structures of eicosapentaenoic acid and docosahexaenoic acid

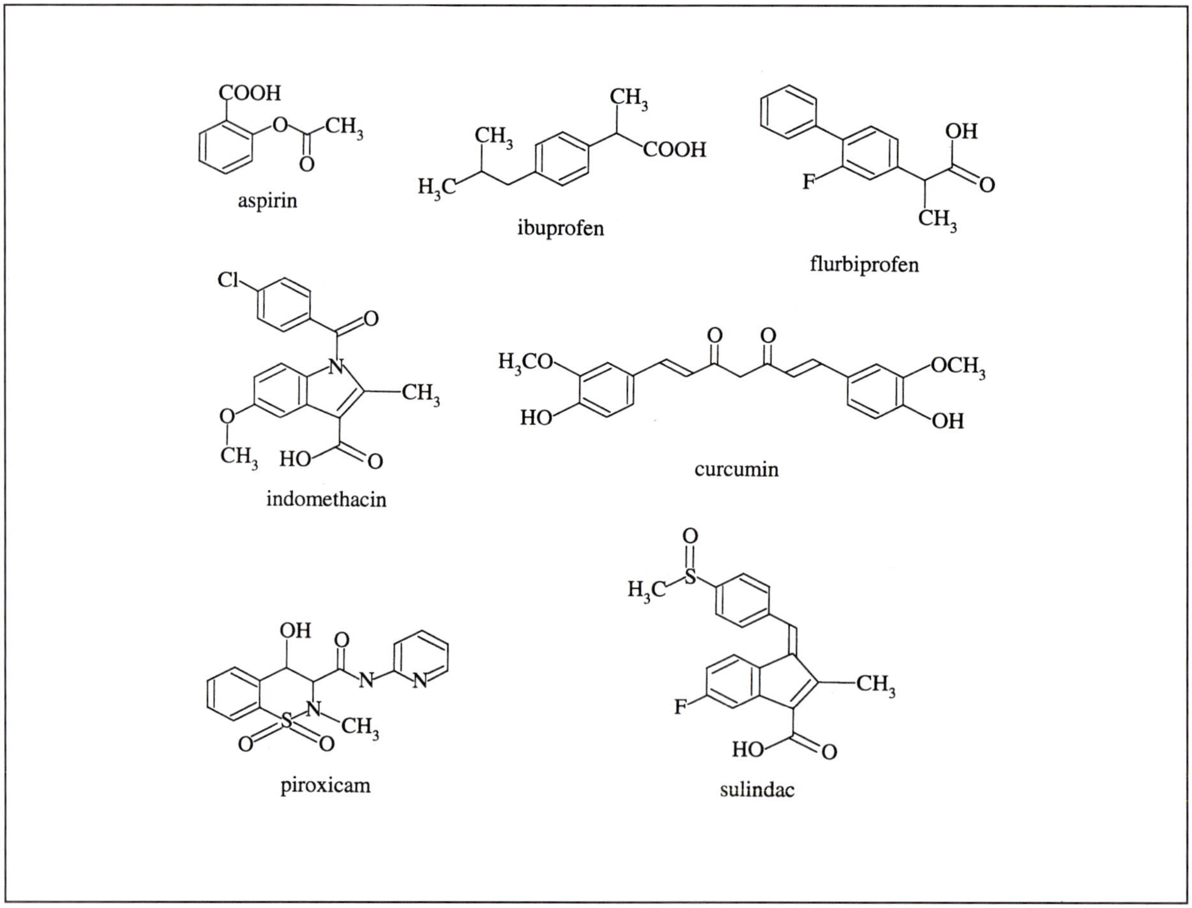

Figure 9.20

Chemical structures of non-steroidal anti-inflammatory drugs

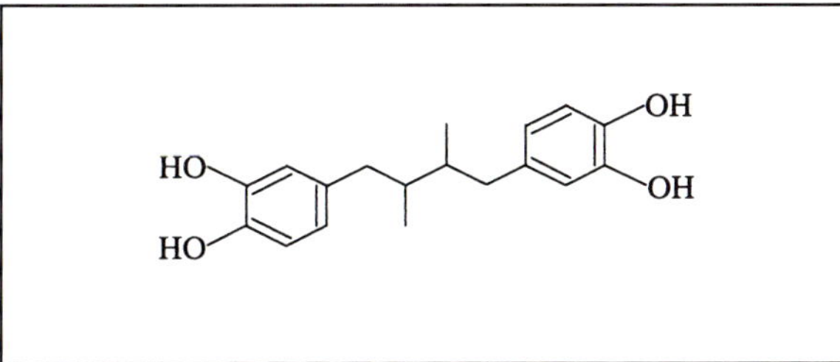

Figure 9.21

Chemical structure of nordihydroguaiaretic acid

nordihydroguaiaretic acid to experimental animals can prevent MNU-induced mammary carcinogenesis on one study [382], but not in another [103].

9.8 Estrogen Antagonists

Estrogen acts on its cognate nuclear receptors to elicit biological responses that are mediated, at least in part, by the production of autocrine and paracrine growth factors from the epithelium and the stroma in the breast [384, 385]. The action of estrogens can be blocked by antiestrogens that bind to the estrogen receptor but elicit minimal or no estrogenic responses.

9.8.1 Antiestrogens

Tamoxifen (Fig. 9.22), a prototype triphenylethylene antiestrogen in the breast [386], has been used for the treatment of advanced breast cancer in the United States since 1978 [387]. Thanks to its remarkable efficacy against breast cancer mortality [388, 389], it is currently the most prescribed medicine for breast cancer patients, becoming the endocrine treatment of choice for all stages of breast cancer as described by the World Health Organization [387]. The prevention of breast cancer with tamoxifen was first documented more than twenty years ago in an experimental animal model of chemical carcinogen-induced mammary carcinogenesis [390, 391]. Tamoxifen showed a strong, long-lasting chemopreventive effect on mammary benign tumors and cancers as well as other tumors such as pituitary adenomas, adrenal pheochromocytomas, islet cell pancreatic tumors, Leydig cell testicular tumors, and polyps of the uterus [392]. Subsequently, it has been observed that adjuvant use of tamoxifen in women with cancer in one breast reduces the incidence of tumors in the contralateral breast [281, 388]. Tamoxifen reduces the risk of developing breast cancer [393] and reduces mammographic density [394]. Three clinical trials – one in the United States and Canada, one in Italy and an international trial coordinated in the United Kingdom – are currently ongoing to study tamoxifen as a preventive agent against the development of breast cancer in healthy women [395, 396]. In addition, tamoxifen has been shown to confer protection against myocardial infarction [397–400] and osteoporosis [401–403]. However, tamoxifen treatment is associated with a significant loss of bone mineral density in premenopausal women, whereas it prevents bone loss in postmenopausal women [404]. More importantly, breast and uterus respond differently to the mitogenic stimuli of steroid hormones [405], use of tamoxifen as a breast preventive agent is facing strong challenges due to its various side-effects, most notably, an increased endometrial cancer risk [406–409]. Whether tamoxifen serves as an antagonist or an agonist of the estrogen receptor depends upon the estrogen receptor complex present in a particular cell or tissue [410]. If a cell type requires activating factors 1 and 2 of the estrogen receptor to be functioning concurrently, tamoxifen is antagonistic. However, if a cell or tissue requires only activating factor 1 to interact with transcription factors at the promoter, tamoxifen is agonistic [410]. Even though long-term dosing of tamoxifen leads to DNA damage detectable by ^{32}P-postlabeling and the development of hepatocellular tumors in rats, no evidence has been observed for tamoxifen-induced DNA damage in the livers of seven women taking this drug therapeutically [411]. Nevertheless, tamoxifen has been recently classified as a carcinogen by the International Agency for Research on Cancer [387]. Therefore, the search for new drugs with no serious side-effects is already in progress. A number of tamoxifen analogues have been synthesized and evaluated, but they

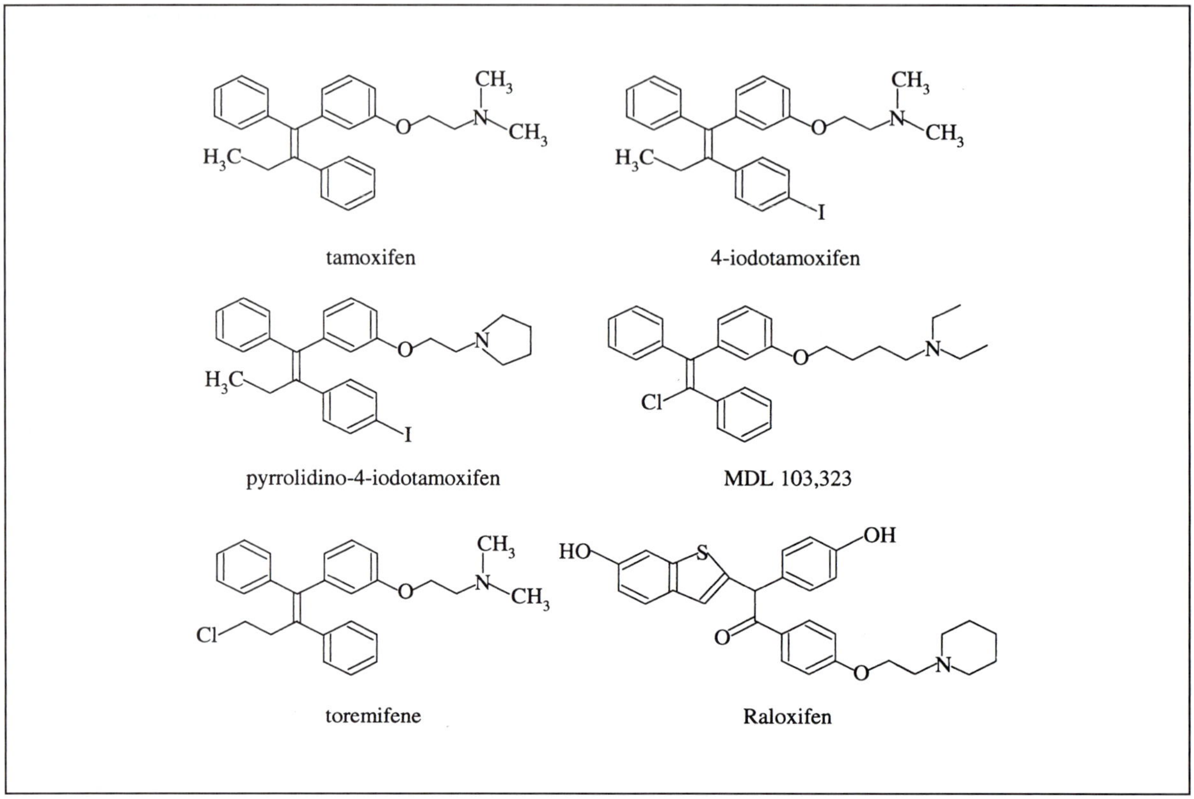

Figure 9.22

Chemical structures of antiestrogens

share the same agonistic properties with tamoxifen in the endometrium, which would prevent their broad application in the prevention of human breast cancer [396]. Idoxifene is a more potent antiestrogen than tamoxifen and is as effective against mammary carcinogenesis as tamoxifen in the rat while causing only very low levels of DNA adducts in liver tissue [412]. MDL 103,323, an enclomiphene analog with an affinity for the human estrogen receptor that is 5–6 fold greater than either tamoxifen or enclomiphene, inhibits the growth of breast cancer cells in vitro and tumor xenografts in vivo and prevents n-ethylnitrosourea-induced rat mammary carcinogenesis [413]. One of the more promising candidates is raloxifene, a

drug used in worldwide trials for the prevention of osteoporosis [414]. Raloxifene (Fig. 9.22) is known to possess little or no estrogenic activity [415, 416], yet it prevents chemical carcinogen-induced mammary carcinogenesis in experimental animals [417].

9.8.2 Aryl Hydrocarbon Receptor Agonists

Estrogen receptor-mediated response can also be influenced by agonists for aryl hydrocarbon receptor (AhR) via interactions between the AhR- and ER-mediated response pathways [418]. Natural AhR agonists, such as indole-3-carbinol and related compounds in cruciferous vegetables, inhibit the estrogenic response in various experimental models [419–421]. Environmental pollutant, 2,3,7,8-tetrachlorodibeno-ρ-dioxin (TCDD) (Fig. 9.23), activates AhR and elicits inhibitory actions on a broad spec-

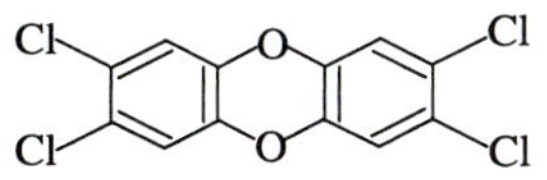

2,3,7,8-tetrachlorodibenzo-p-dioxin

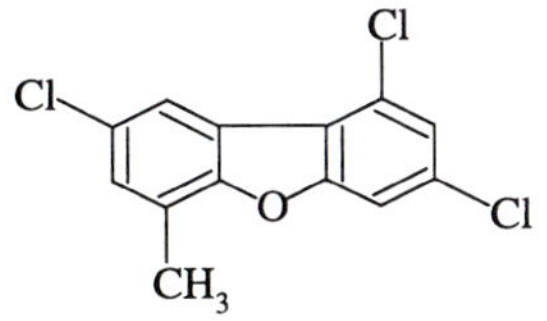

6-methyl-1,3,8-trichlorodibenzofuran

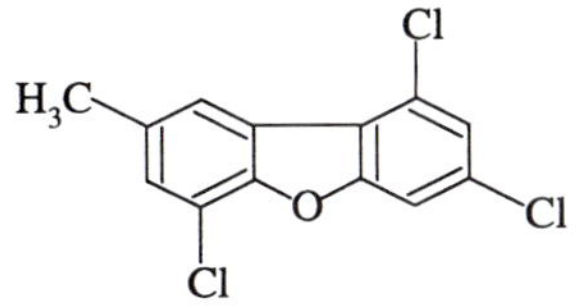

8-methyl-1,3,6-trichlorodibenzofuran

Figure 9.23

Chemical structures of aryl hydrocarbon receptor inhibitors

trum of estrogenic responses in human breast cancer cells [422]. To avoid the toxic side-effects of TCDD, Safe et al. [423–426] have developed a series of relatively non-toxic AhR agonists as potential chemotherapeutic agents for the clinical treatment of human breast cancer. Two alkyl substituted chlorinated dibenzofurans, 6-methyl-1,3,8-trichlorodibenzofuran and 8-methyl-1,3,6-trichlorodibenzofuran (Fig. 9.23), exhibit dose-dependent inhibition of DMBA-induced rat mammary tumor growth [418]. The chemopreventive potential of this new class of indirect-acting antiestrogens is not clear and warrants further studies.

9.9 Interrupting Carcinogenic Signal Transduction

9.9.1 Inhibitors of Receptor Tyrosine Kinases

Biological responses to extracellular or intracellular stimuli involve changes in transcriptional activation mediated through a complicated network of signal transduction pathways (Fig. 9.24) [427]. Key components of these pathways are protein tyrosine kinases that catalyze the phosphorylation of tyrosine residues on a variety of proteins [428]. In general, protein tyrosine kinases are classified as either receptor tyrosine kinases, which receive signals directly through their extracellular structural domain, or cellular tyrosine kinases, which are involved in the intracellular signal transduction [429]. Neoplastic cells differ significantly from their normal counterparts in that they display various alterations in the signal transduction pathways [430]. In fact, many of the oncogenes encode for protein tyrosine kinases [431]. For example, the products of the c-erbB-1 proto-oncogene are EGF receptor tyrosine kinases [432]. One of the alterations frequently observed in breast cancer cells is the loss of regulatory mechanisms involving EGF receptor tyrosine kinases [433]. Accordingly, this deregulated signaling pathway has been targeted as a potential site for chemoprevention of human cancer. A number of chemopreventive agents have been shown to interfere with the EGF receptor tyrosine kinase pathway, including flavonoids quercetin and genistein, other naturally occurring products (e.g., erbstatin, herbimycin A, lavendustin A, (++)-areaplysinin-1) and numerous synthetic tyrosine phosphorylation inhibitors collectively known as tyrphyostins (e.g., benzylidene malonitrile RG-14620, dianilinophthalimides DAPH1 and DAPH2, quinazolins PD 153035 and AG 1478, [(alkylamino)methyl]acrylophenone EGFR inhibitor 18, endollactone BE-23372 M, dihydroxybenylaminosalicylates, 2-thioindole PD 146568, aminoflavone 6-hydroxy-3',5,7-triaminoflavone, tyrosine analogue-containing peptides) (Fig. 9.25) [135, 433, 434]. Unfortunately, many of these tyrosine kinase inhibitors are not specific for the catalytic domain of EGF receptor tyrosine kinase,

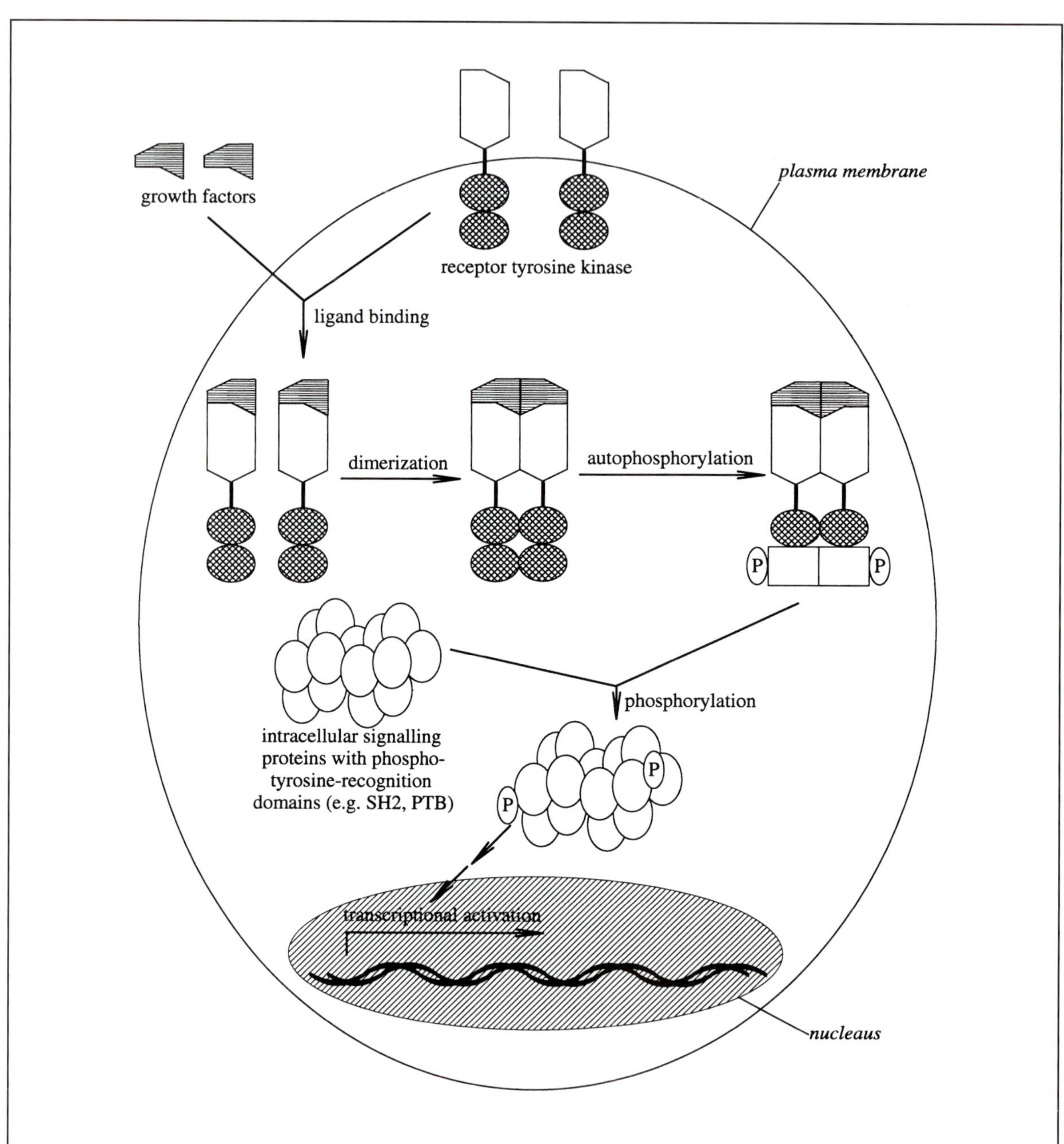

Figure 9.24

Pathways of tyrosine kinases-mediated signal transduction

Figure 9.25 ▶

Chemical structures of receptor tyrosine kinase inhibitors

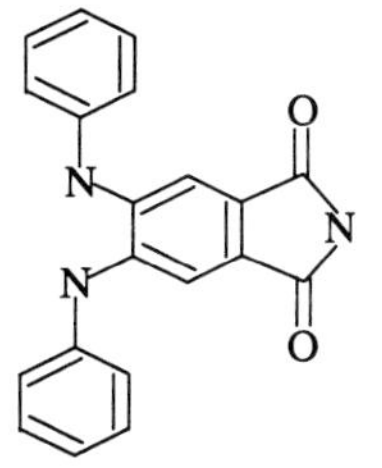

DAPH1

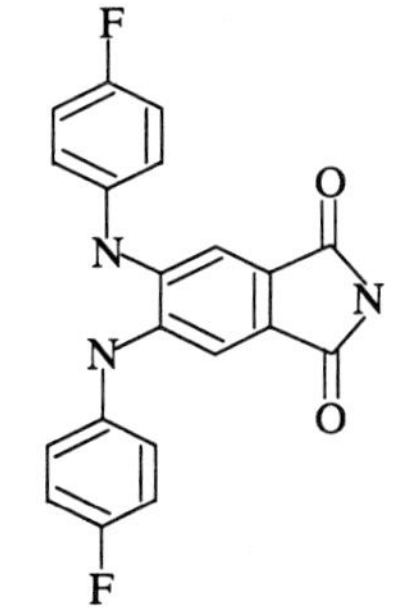

DAPH1

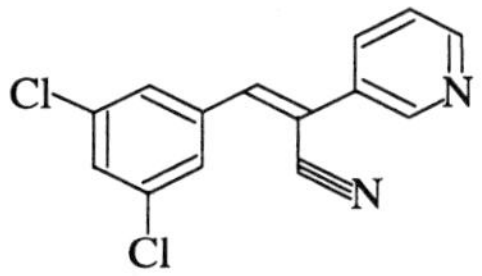

RG 14620

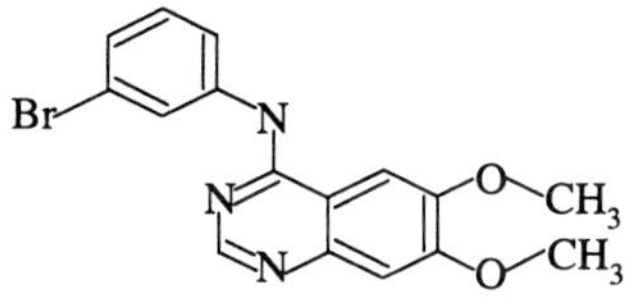

PD 153035

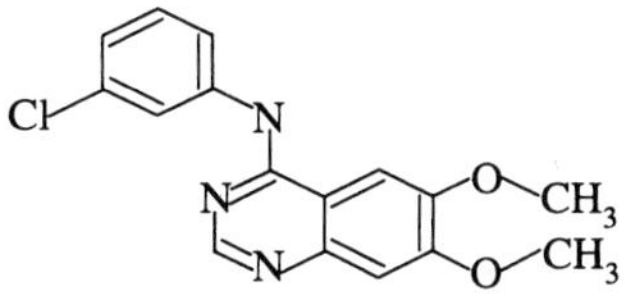

AG 1478

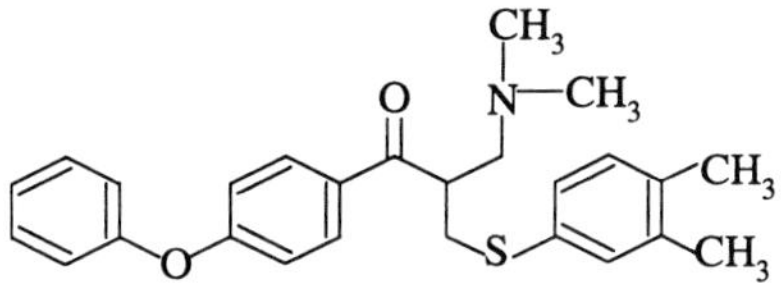

EGFR inhibitor 18

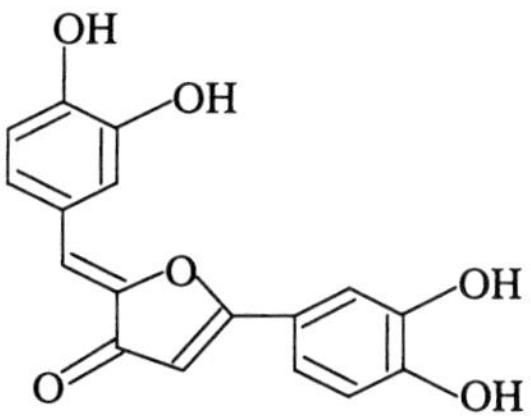

BE-23372M

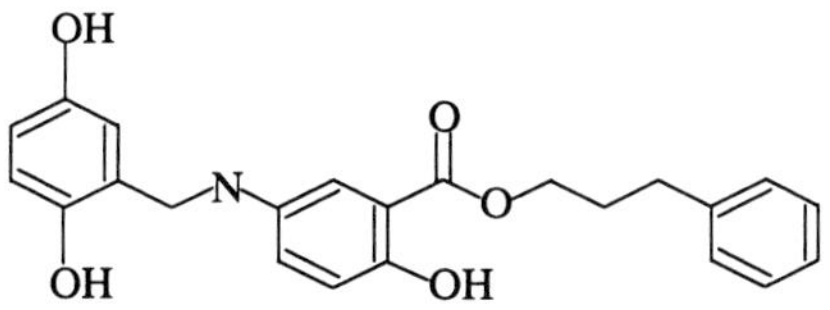

2-hydroxy-5-{N-[2,5-dihydroxyphenyl)methyl]
amino}benzoic acid 3- phenylpropyl ester

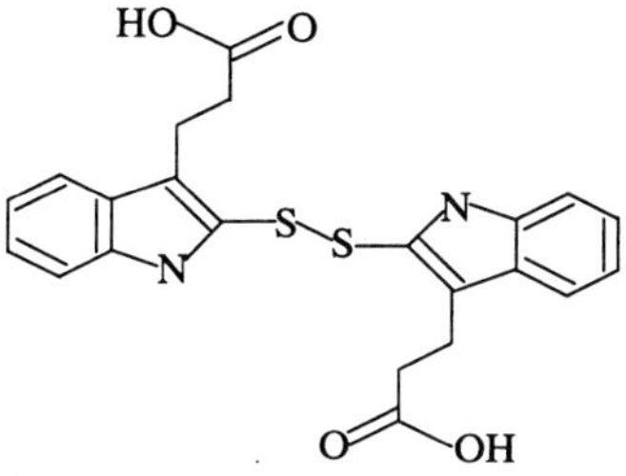

PD 146568

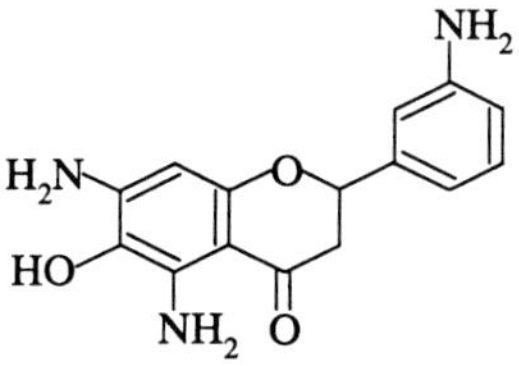

6-hydroxy-3',5,7-triaminoflavone

more understanding of the three-dimensional structure of the tyrosine kinases is clearly required before specific inhibition of a signal pathway is available for use in the prevention of human breast cancer.

9.9.2 Inhibitors of p21^{ras} Farnesylation

Mutational or transcriptional activation of *ras* oncogene has been documented in mammary tumors of rats [435], mice [436) and human [437]. Transfer of a farnesyl group from farnesyl pyrophosphate to p21^{ras} proteins, the *ras* gene product (Fig. 9.26), is a universal posttranslational modification necessary for the cellular p21^{ras} proteins to be localized to the cytoplasmic membrane to exert their growth-promoting and transforming activities [438–440]. There are at least two major strategies that have been developed to block p21^{ras} farnesylation, one employing depletion of the substrate for p21^{ras} farnesylation by inhibiting the 3-hydroxy-3-methylglutaryl coenzyme A (HMG-CoA) reductase that catalyzes the conversion of HMG-CoA to mevalonate, the precursor of isoprenoid formation, and the other targeting inhibition of the enzyme farnesyl protein transferase that catalyzes the p21^{ras} farnesylation reaction [441]. The first strategy has been accomplished by lovastatin and its synthetic derivatives [442, 443], while the second strategy has been successful with a number of novel RAS and farnesyl pyrophosphate analogs such as benzodiazepine peptidomimetics [444–446] and monoterpenes [447].

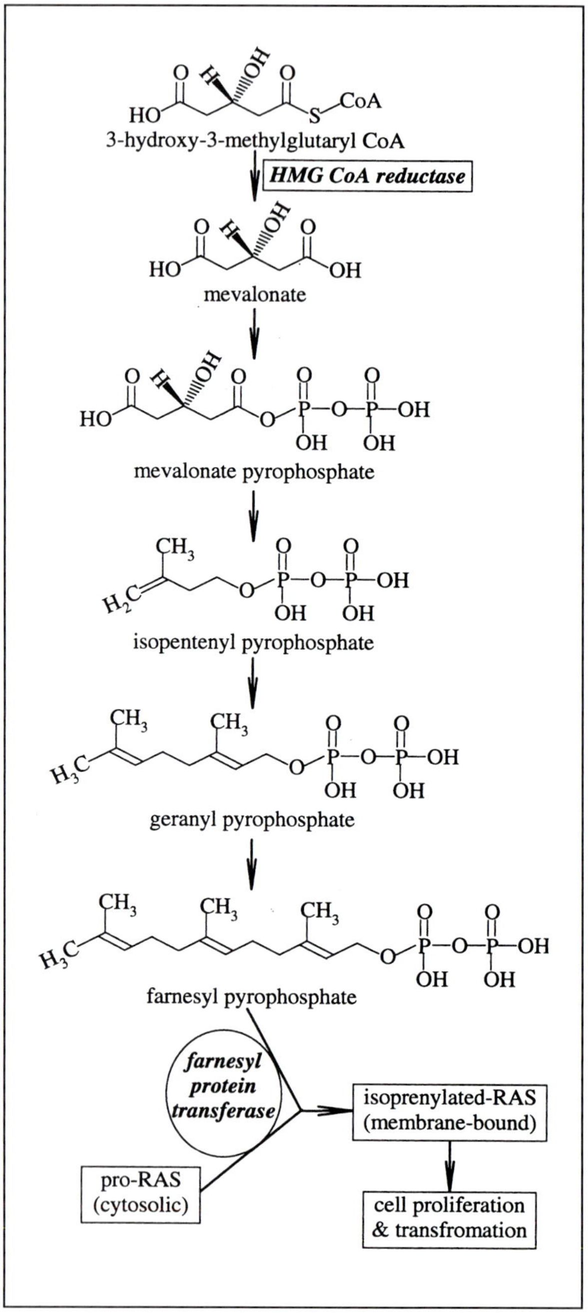

Figure 9.26

Pathways of *ras* farnesylation

Figure 9.27

Chemical structures of HMG-CoA reductase inhibitors

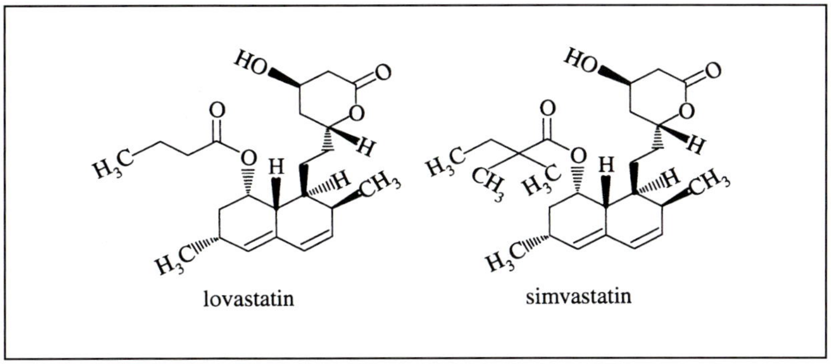

lovastatin   simvastatin

9.9.3 Inhibitors of HMG-CoA Reductase

HMG-CoA reductase is the rate-limiting enzyme of cholesterol biosynthesis [448]. Mevalonate, the product of HMG-CoA reductase [448], is then converted sequentially to geranyl pyrophosphate and farnesyl pyrophosphate, the substrate for farnesyl protein transferase (Fig. 9.26) [441]. Naturally occurring lovastatin (Fig. 9.27) isolated from the culture filtrate of *Aspergillus terreus* [442, 449], its synthetic derivative simvastatin (Fig. 9.27) [443] are potent inhibitors of HMG-CoA reductase. Simvastatin induces G1 arrests and growth inhibition in human breast cancer cells in vitro [450, 451] and exhibits anticarcinogenic activity during the promotion phase of radiation-induced mammary tumorigenesis in rats [452].

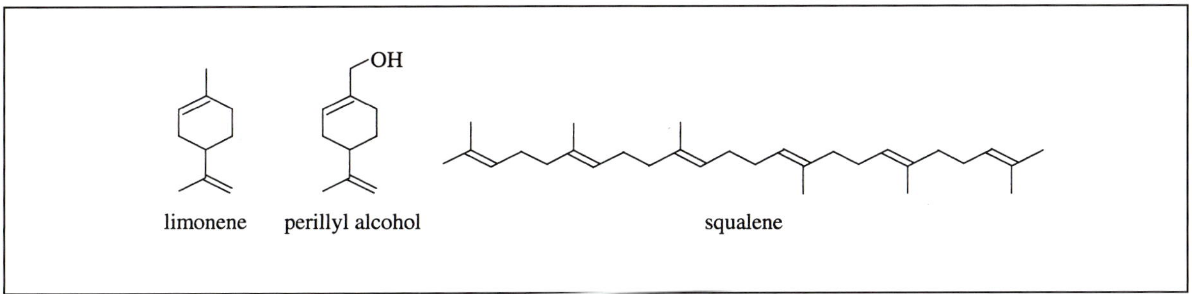

9.9.4 Monoterpenes

Monoterpenes in monocyclic, bicyclic and acyclic forms (Fig. 9.28) are naturally occurring products contained in human food such as fruits (e.g., citrus fruits), vegetables and food flavoring such as mint [453]. Administration of monoterpenes (e.g., limonene) to laboratory animals results in a reduction of chemically-induced mammary tumors [454, 455]. It also prevents induction of mammary carcinogenesis by direct in situ transfer of *v-Ha-ras* into rat mammary epithelial cells [456]. Limonene inhibits the isoprenylation of small G-proteins at 21 to 26 kDa, including p21[ras], essential to signal transduction and carcinogenesis [457]. In search of natural and synthetic analogs of limonene for use as chemopreventive agents, Crowell et al. [447] have found perillyl alcohol, a hydroxylated analog of limonene, which is more than five times more effective at inhibiting the isoprenylation of small G-proteins and cell proliferation than limonene. Perillyl alcohol has been shown

Figure 9.28

Chemical structures of monoterpenes

limonene   perillyl alcohol   squalene

to prevent preneoplastic transformation of the mammary glands in vitro [122] and induce regression of mammary carcinomas in vivo [458]. Squalene, a potent inhibitor of p21^{ras} farnesylation abundant in shark liver oil and olive oil, has been to prevent preneoplastic transformation of the mammary glands in vitro [122]. However, there is also evidence that the chemopreventive activity of (+)-limonene (d-limonene) and related monoterpenes against mammary is independent of inhibition of p21^{ras} function [459]. Monoterpenes prevent tumorigenesis at both initiation and promotion/progression stages and are also potential therapeutic agents for human breast cancer [453].

9.9.5 Eicosapentaenoic Acid

Eicosapentaenoic acid (EPA) (Fig. 9.19) is a potent inhibitor of p21^{ras}-GTPase as well as a competitive inhibitor of cyclooxygenase-mediated prostaglandin synthesis [362]. EPA or EPA-rich fish oil prevents chemical carcinogen-induced mammary carcinogenesis in vitro [122, 367] and in vivo [368].

9.10 Inducing Breast Cell Differentiation

9.10.1 Retinoids

Retinoids are a large family of compounds including the natural and synthetic vitamin A (Fig. 9.29) [460]. Retinoids are potent modulators of development, differentiation, morphogenesis, growth, metabolism and homeostasis [461]. Their action is mediated by nuclear receptors, retinoic acid (RA) receptors (RAR alpha, RAR beta, RAR gamma) and retinoid X receptors (RXR alpha, RXR beta, RXR gamma) and modulated by cellular retinol binding proteins [462]. All-trans-RA and 9-cis-RA are equipotent activators of RAR, but 9-cis-RA is expected to activate RXR at physiological concentrations of retinoids [463]. N-(4-Hydroxyphenyl)retinamide (4-HPR or fenretinide), a synthetic retinoid, is a highly selective activator of RAR [464], while another synthetic retinoid, LGD1069 (or Targretin), is a selective RXR ligand that

is devoid of significant RAR binding and transactivation of RAR-responsive genes [465].

Both malignant and benign breast tissues may be targets for retinoids, justifying the use of natural and synthetic vitamin A derivatives in the chemoprevention of breast disease [462]. In animals, various retinoids have shown significant chemopreventive activity against carcinogenesis in mammary glands, bladder, head and neck, lung, cervix, skin and prostate [466, 467]. Several retinoids have shown promise as chemopreventive agents against chemically induced mammary carcinogenesis in mice and especially in rats [155]. For instance, both DMBA and NMU-induced mammary tumors can be inhibited by fenretinide, whereas NMU-induced mammary carcinogenesis can be prevented by other retinoids such as Ro 16–9100, Ro 19–296, BASF-47851, 9-cis RA and LGD1069 or Targretin [113, 465, 466, 468]. Recently, it has been shown that inhibition of cell growth by retinoic acid occurs only in cells that are able to metabolize retinoic acid to unidentified polar and very polar products [469]. The non-polar metabolites of RA include 13-cis-RA, 9-cis-RA, 4-OH-RA and 4-oxo-RA, not all of which are able to mediate RA function [470, 471].

The anti-proliferative effects of RAs are mediated by various mechanisms including induction of apoptosis in some cells and induction of differentiation without apoptosis in others [472, 473]. Unlike natural RAs, the synthetic fenretinide is a potent inducer of programmed cell death or apoptosis and does not induce cell differentiation [464]. In addition, even though fenretinide is a highly selective activator of retinoid receptors [464], the chemopreventive actions of fenretinide involve retinoid receptor-independent pathways in human breast carcinoma [474]. Similarly, two C-linked analogs, retinamidobenzyl glucuronide and retinamidobenzyl glucose, despite poor binding to the nuclear RAR, are more potent than the parent fenretinide and its less stable natural O-glucuronide analog in inhibiting tumor incidence and multiplicity of DMBA-induced rat mammary tumor [475]. In contrast, chemoprevention of chemically-induced mammary carcinoma by LGD1069 or Targretin has been attributed to its selective activation of the RXR pathway [465]. LGD1069 treatment

Figure 9.29

Chemical structures of retinoids

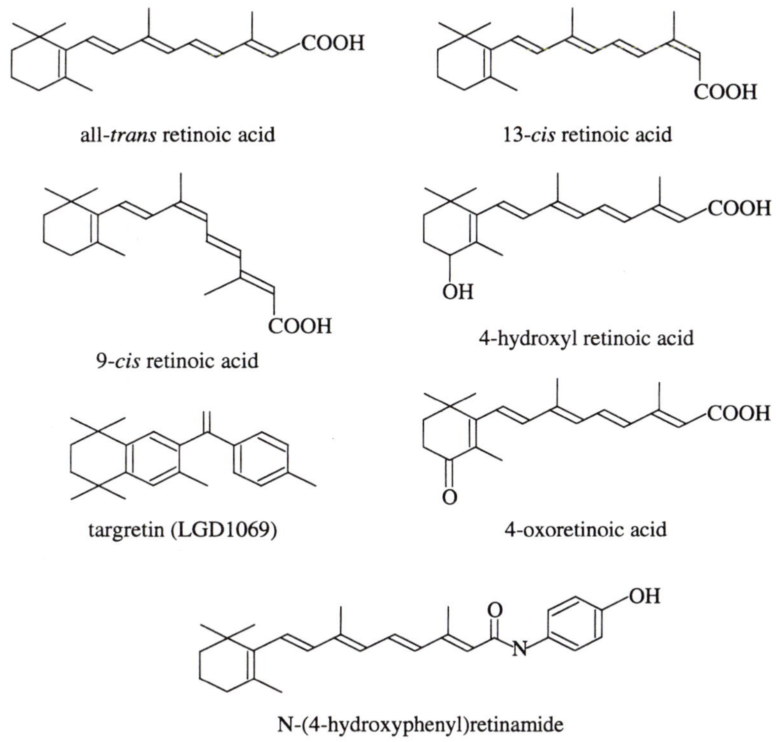

results in a reduction in tumor malignancy, an increase in differentiation, and a sharp decrease in cellular proliferation without classic signs of "retinoid-associated" toxicities during 13 weeks of chronic therapy [476]. It also enhances the activity of tamoxifen as an efficacious therapeutic agent for mammary carcinoma [476]. Ironically, RXR overexpression is associated with an increased risk for the development of invasive breast cancer in human breast lesions [477]. Clearly, further studies are warranted to determine the role of each receptor pathway in the control of cell proliferation, differentiation and apoptosis. Nevertheless, the combination of fenretinide with tamoxifen not only is more effective in suppressing breast cancer than either agent alone, but also inhibits the appearance of subsequent cancers following the surgical removal of the first tumor [155]. These studies suggest that retinoids, like tamoxifen,

may be applicable to the prevention of contralateral breast cancer in women who underwent breast cancer surgery. Currently, a randomized multicenter clinical trial is in progress to evaluate the effectiveness of the synthetic retinoid fenretinide, at a dose of 200 mg per os every day for 5 years, in reducing the incidence of contralateral breast cancer in a population of patients previously operated on for breast cancer [478, 479].

Some of the other chemopreventive agents modulate the effects of retinoic acid. For instance, liarozole, an imidazole-derived high-affinity inhibitor of mammalian cytochrome P450-dependent enzymes [480], inhibits mammalian androgen biosynthesis and reduces the growth of androgen-dependent transplantable R3327-G prostatic carcinoma in the rat to the same extent as castration [481]. Encouraging results have been obtained in treatment of advanced prostatic cancer with liarozole [482]. However, inhibition of androgen does not appear to be responsible for liarozole action because the inhibition of prostate cancer growth by liarozole can not be reversed with testosterone supplementation and liarozole also inhibits the growth of androgen-independent R3327-Dunning prostatic adenocarcinomas [483]. Liarozole inhibits the activity of cytochrome P450-dependent 4-hydroxylase, the enzyme involved in metabolism of retinoic acid [480, 484]. Oral administration of liarozole results in an increase in the plasma levels of retinoic acid in experimental animals [484] and human prostate cancer patients [482]. The potential chemopreventive effect of liarozole against breast cancer is suggested by the evidence that liarozole augments the antiproliferative action of retinoic acid in MCF-7 human breast cancer cells [485].

9.10.2 Pregnancy and Human Chorionic Gonadotropin

This topic is discussed at length in Chapter 10. Briefly, there is epidemiological and clinical evidence that full-term pregnancy offers protection against the development of human breast cancer [272, 486–488]. There is also experimental evidence that parity is an important modulator of the susceptibility of human breast epithelial cells to chemical carcinogen-induced neoplastic transformation [489]. In experimental animals, full-term pregnancy protects the mammary glands from subsequent chemical carcinogen-induced tumor development [490–493]. For instance, the polycyclic hydrocarbon DMBA induces maximal mammary tumor incidence in young virgin rats [490, 494, 495], but its effect is significantly reduced or almost completely abolished in parous rats between 3 and 9 weeks post-delivery with or without lactation [492, 493, 496, 497–517]. However, this protection is minimized or nullified if pregnancy is interrupted [492, 493].

9.11 N-Chemoprevention Against Growth of Neoplasms: Suppressing the Growth of Neoplastic Cells

9.11.1 Vitamin D and Calcium

Vitamin D is a secosteroid of a steroid hormone family and contains a series of compounds (e.g., D_2, D_3, D_4, D_5, D_6) with very similar chemical structures (Fig. 9.30) [518]. It binds to specific nuclear vitamin D receptors and activates the expression of genes that contain vitamin D-response elements [519]. The vitamin D-responsive genes include the p21[waf 1] and p27[kip 1] cyclin-dependent kinase inhibitors and bax, which are essential to vitamin D-induced cell cycle arrest in G_1 and apoptosis, respectively [519, 520]. In normal and malignant breast tissues, vitamin D elicits diverse biological responses, such as inhibition of cell proliferation and induction of differentiation [519, 521–523]. The biologically active form 1α,25-dihydroxy vitamin D_3 [1α,25(OH)$_2$D$_3$] of the vitamin D_3 series has attracted almost all the attention because it serves as a key regulator of serum calcium [518, 519]. Not surprisingly, calcium becomes the focal point in some of the studies on vitamin D as a chemopreventive agent. An inverse relationship has been observed between the consumption of calcium and colon cancer risk, leading to extensive studies of calcium in relation to colon cancer prevention [103, 524]. The effects of calcium on colon epithelial cells include decreased cell proliferation, enhanced cell differentiation, and reduced incidence of carcinogen-induced colon tumor in experimental animals [524, 525]. An inverse association between dietary calcium intake and breast cancer risk has been demonstrated in one study [526], but not in others [527]. Nevertheless, decreased intake of calcium and vitamin D in a nutritional stress diet, which contains four components of a Western-style diet, has been shown to expand the size of proliferative compartment, increase the number of proliferating epithelial cells and stimulate growth or hyperplasia in the mammary glands [528]. Most of these changes occur in the terminal end buds [528], the site of origin of chemically-induced mammary carcinomas [490–493]. Decreased

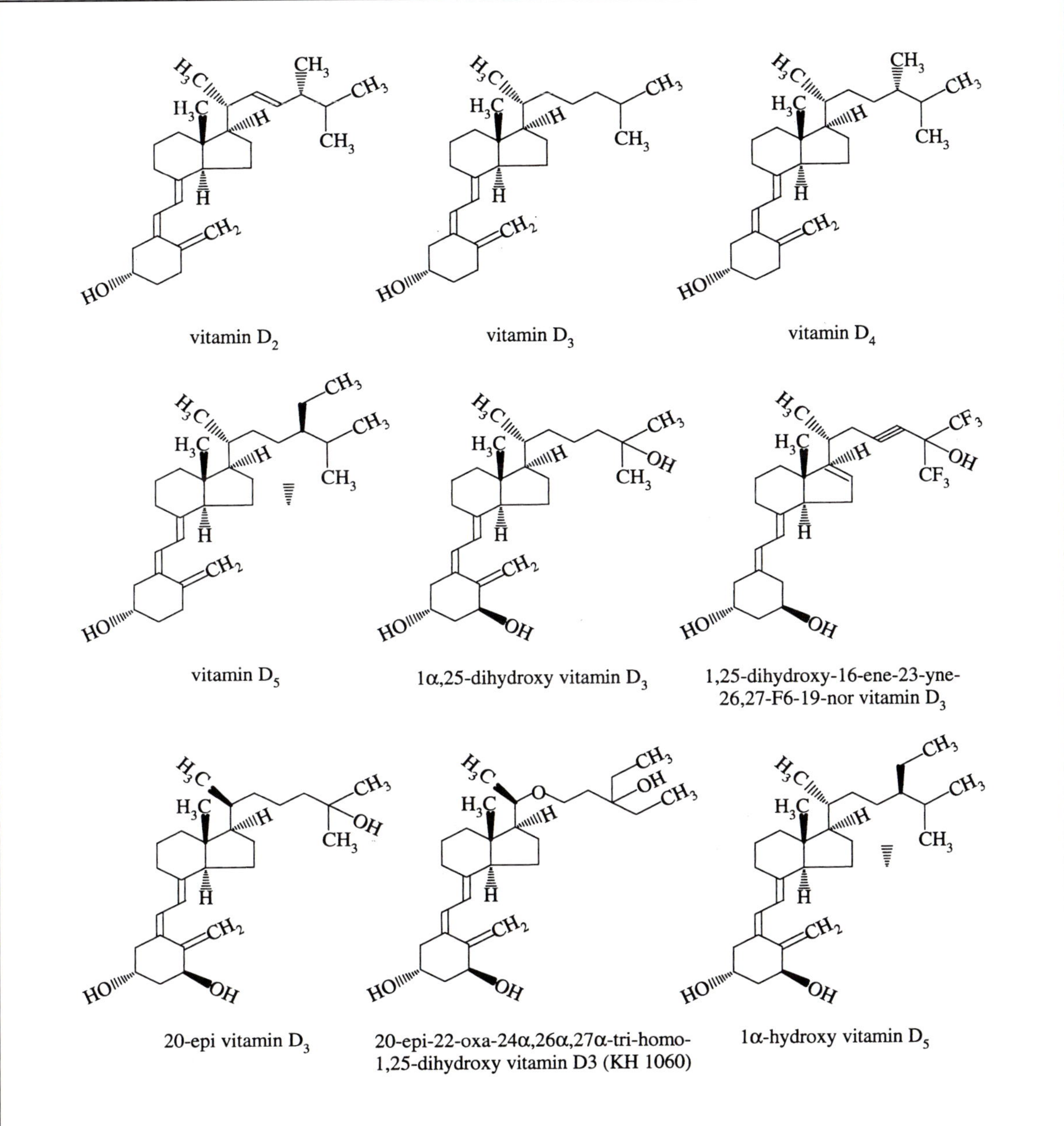

Figure 9.30

Chemical structures of vitamin D and its analogues

intake of calcium and vitamin D also increases the ability of a high fat diet to promote mammary growth and DMBA-induced mammary tumorigenesis in female Sprague-Dawley rats [529]. In contrast, dietary supplement of calcium has been reported to attenuate the growth-promoting effects of a high-fat diet in the mammary glands of young mice [530]. Calcium glucarate, which may both change the internal hormonal milieu and also directly detoxify any environmental agents responsible for breast cancer, has been suggested as an agent in the chemoprevention of breast cancer [531].

It should be noted, however, that vitamin D is assumed to function solely on calcium homeostasis in these experimental studies involving depletion of vitamin D. Ironically, one of the limiting factors in the successful use of vitamin D_3 in cancer prevention is its calcemic activity because growth of neoplastic cells in vivo can only be suppressed by supplementation of vitamin D_3 at concentrations that cause hypercalcemia and death [518]. A major focus of current research on vitamin D as a chemopreventive agent is the search for synthetic analogues of 1α-25(OH)$_2$D$_3$ that lack hypercalcemic properties, but retain prominent antiproliferative and differentiating effects against cancer cells [519]. A new class of synthetic vitamin D analogues (see Fig. 9.32) has emerged as deltanoids due to their lack of the classical actions of enhancing intestinal absorption or immobilizing calcium in bone matrix [522]. Deltanoids can inhibit human breast cancer cell growth in vitro and suppress chemically-induced mammary carcinogenesis in experimental animals [522]. While one deltanoid is a novel vitamin D_5 analogue 1α-hydroxyvitamin D_5 [518], almost all of the other deltanoids synthesized are specific vitamin D_3 analogues, including many hexafluoro derivatives [520, 522], 20-epi-vitamin D_3 analogues [523] and the 22-oxa-calcitriol [532]. Initial clinical trials of breast cancer prevention are under way for some of these deltanoids [519]. Undoubtedly, more deltanoids of various vitamin D series (e. g., D_2, D_3, D_4, D_5, D_6) will be synthesized for further studies of chemoprevention against breast cancer.

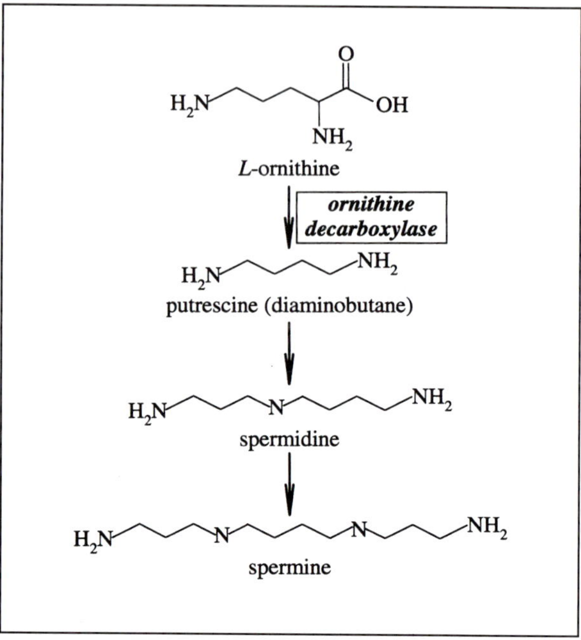

Figure 9.31

Pathways of polyamine biosynthesis

9.11.2 Ornithine Decarboxylase Inhibitors

Cancer cells of nearly all types are characterized by having elevated levels of ornithine decarboxylase (ODC) [533–535]. This rate-limiting enzyme decarboxylates the amino acid ornithine, leading to the synthesis of putrescine, spermidine and spermine (Fig. 9.31), polyamine cations ubiquitously distributed throughout prokaryotic and eukaryotic organisms [533]. Polyamines play such a key role in the S-phase of the cell cycle and in a number of other biochemical processes that their depletion inhibits cell growth and suppresses carcinogenesis in essentially all the experimental models studied [534, 535]. Difluoromethylornithine (DFMO) (Fig. 9.32), first synthesized in the mid-1970s, is an irreversible suicide substrate inhibitor of ODC that has been shown to inhibit the growth of normal and neoplastic cells [536]. DFMO inhibits mammary epithelial cell proliferation [535], suppresses chemically-induced mammary carcino-

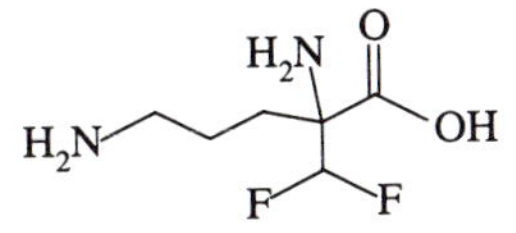

Figure 9.32

Chemical structure of ornithine decarboxylase inhibitor difluoromethylorthinine

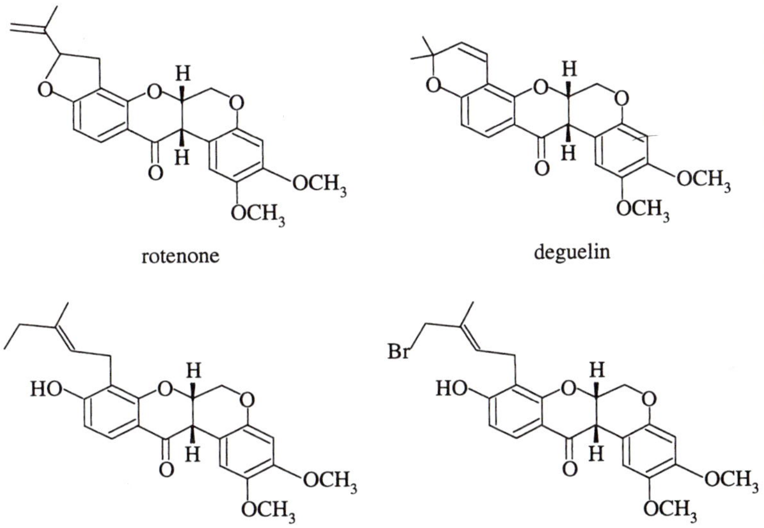

Figure 9.33

Chemical structures of rotenoids

genesis [103, 537, 538], and when combined with retinyl acetate, results in enhanced chemopreventive efficacy [538]. Alterations in epithelial cell-extracellular matrix interactions have been postulated to account in part for the chemopreventive effects of DFMO plus RA [538]. Other agents that have shown to inhibit ODC activity include rotenoids (e.g., rotenone, deguelin) present in plant extracts of *Derris, Lonchocarpus* or *Tephrosia* species that has long been used as insecticides and fish poisons in South America and East Africa [539, 540] (Fig. 9.33). Four active rotenoids, obtained from the African plant *Mundulea sericea* (*Leguminosae*), are highly potent in inhibiting chemically induced preneoplastic lesions in mamma-

ry organ culture [541]. The toxic action of rotenone is attributed to inhibition of NADH:ubiquinone oxidoreductase activity and the purported cancer chemopreventive effect of deguelin analogs has been associated with inhibition of phorbol ester-induced ODC activity [542]. Rotenoids, flavonoids, stilbenoids, genistein and resveratrol all contained molecular features of essential to inhibit NADH:ubiquinone oxidoreductase activity and ODC induction, indicating that inhibition of NADH:ubiquinone oxidoreductase activity lowers the level of induced ODC activity leading to the antiproliferative effect and anticancer action [542]. However, their chemopreventive potential against breast cancer awaits to be determined.

9.12 O-Inhibiting Neovascularization or Angiogenesis

Neovascularization or angiogenesis, the process of generating new capillaries from preexisting vessels, occurs naturally only in a very limited number of physiological processes such as wound healing, luteal formation and embryonic development. It occurs frequently in pathological conditions, most notably, during the development of solid malignant tumors [543]. Use of inhibitors of angiogenesis represents one of the most efficient strategies for prevention of breast cancer. Many of the compounds that possess potent antiproliferative activities against the development of breast cancer, as described in the previous sections, have also been shown to be anti-angiogenic. A diverse group of anti-angiogenic compounds identified so far include naturally-occurring flavonoids (e.g., quercetin, kaempferol, myricetin, apigenin, luteolin) (Fig. 9.12) or isoflavonoids (e.g., genistein) (Fig. 9.16) [208, 544], synthetic vitamin D_3 analogues (Fig. 9.30) [532], ursodeoxycholic acid and its derivatives (Fig. 9.7) [545]. Linomide, a low molecular weight, water-soluble agent with excellent p.o. absorption and bioavailability, has antiangiogenic abilities against a series of rat and human prostatic cancer xenografts growing in vivo and inhibit by both MNU- and DMBA-induced mammary carcinogenesis in female rats [546]. In addition, linomide blocks vascular endothelial growth factor (VEGF)-dependent angiogenesis in vivo in the absence of a growing tumor mass and its antiangiogenic effect is both angiosuppressive and angiostatic, creating a persistently unfavorable conditions for capillary progression [547].

9.13 Socioprevention of Breast Cancer

As a endocrine related process, development of breast cancer is profoundly influenced by the degree of lobular differentiation and hormonal exposure of the breast epithelium, which are, in turn, influenced by the occurrence of a full-term pregnancy and a spectrum of lifestyle factors, respectively [272, 486–488, 548]. Manipulation of these processes by technologically simple and practical means is a major goal of research. Modulation of preneoplastic growth of breast epithelial cells by chemopreventive agents remains challenging due to the absence of target-organ specificity and frequent toxicity. With the emergence of well-supported breast carcinogenesis models, behavioral and social strategies are likely to be key to achieving the ultimate goal of preventing the development of breast cancer [548]. Many laboratory studies and human epidemiological data suggest that mortality from most cancer including breast cancer is attributable to lifestyle, including nutritional factors and tobacco and alcohol consumption [5, 9, 13, 549]. Correction of the high-risk habits and exercise of healthy options will certainly constitute an effective measure that can be classified as socioprevention of breast cancer. Conceivably, the risk of developing breast cancer can be reduced by cessation of smoking, consumption of low-fat, high-fiber healthy food, reduction of alcohol consumption, exercise and weight control. Plan on early childbearing might also be an option, but full-term pregnancy does not necessarily confer protection against the development of breast cancer in women with a family history of the disease [550]. Further understanding lifestyle factors that may be involved in the etiology of breast cancer and are amenable to preventive intervention thus remains a top priority, with diet and physical activity of greatest interest [551]. More physical activity during leisure time and at work has been associated with lower risk of developing breast cancer, especially in premenopausal women [243]. With respect to early detection, regular mammography screening for women aged 50 years and older is clearly associated with a significant reduction in breast cancer mortality, but mammography among women aged 40 to 49 remains controversial [552]. The "earliest" detection of a lump by palpation or imaging frequently fails to recognize the precancerous state of the mammary tissue as a whole in cancer cases, where a gross excess of focal hyperplasia is associated with a six-fold increase in the risk of further primary carcinogenesis [553].

Table 9.3. A summary of strategies for prevention of human breast cancer. *NSAIDS* non-steroidal anti-inflammatory drugs, *hCG* human chorionic gonadotropin

Strategies	Mechanisms	Examples
Physicoprevention	Removal of target organ	Prophylactic mastectomy
Bioprevention	Supply of defected genes/products	*BRCA1* gene therapy
Chemoprevention	Limiting accumulation of carcinogens	Low fat/calorie diet
	Enhancing excretion of xenobiotics	Garlic, cruciferous vegetables
	Eliminating oxidative DNA damage	Carotenoids, vitamin E, tea
	Maintaining proper endocrine	Soya, genistein, NSAIDS
	Antiestrogen	Tamoxifen, raloxifen
	Interrupting signal transduction	Citrus fruits, vegetables
	Inducing breast differentiation	Retinoids, pregnancy, hCG
	Suppressing neoplastic growth	Vitamin D, rotenone
	Inhibiting angiogenesis	Flavonoids, linomide
Socioprevention	Promoting low-risk lifestyle	No smoking, diet, exercise

9.14 Summary and Future Perspectives

Continued advances in our understanding of the temporal sequencing of relevant exposures promises to shed light on the design of numerous physical, chemical and sociological strategies for prevention of human breast cancer (Table 9.3). Even though the risks associated with *BRCA1* and *BRCA2* mutations may be less than previously estimated [551], the biological and molecular mechanisms of breast carcinogenesis are very likely to be different in women with or without a family history of this disease [166]. In a population perceived as being at a higher risk, prophylactic mastectomy remains controversial considering the possible implications of genetic testing, attitudes and uptake of breast screening and accuracy of women's risk estimates [30]. Chemoprevention of malignancies is still in the early stages of development. Many different classes of agents have been exploited as chemopreventives, including antimutagens (*N*-acetylcysteine, oltipraz), antiproliferatives (DFMO, DHEA, selenomethionine), antioxidants (vitamin E, curcumin), anti-inflammatories (aspirin, piroxicam, ibuprofen, sulindac, sulfone) and hormonally active agents (tamoxifen, finasteride), among others [554]. Even though there are over 500 compounds that have been proven to be chemopreventive in animals, there are around 20 chemopreventive trials in progress in the United States. Evaluation of the results of large randomized trials for some of these substances such as β-carotene and tamoxifen [555] indicate that further studies are warranted and that new agents with different mechanisms of action need to be tested for the prevention of breast cancer. Most of the interventives have been discovered by epidemiological studies and their mechanisms of action largely remain to be determined. The mechanism-based design of preventive agents has shown promising results. Ultimate prevention of breast cancer depends upon further understanding of the etiology of breast cancer at the cellular, molecular and physico-chemical levels.

References

1. Parkin, D.M., Psiani, P. and Ferlay, J. Estimates of the world-wide incidence of eighteen major cancers in 1985. Int. J. Cancer 54: 594–606, 1993.
2. Pisani, P., Parkin, D.M. and Ferlay, J. Estimates of the world-wide mortality of eighteen major cancers in 1985. Implication for prevention and projections of future burden. Int. J. Cancer 54: 891–903, 1993.
3. American Cancer Society. Cancer Facts and Figures. American Cancer Society, Atlanta. 1993.
4. Harris, J.R., Lippman, M.E., Veronesi, U. and Willet, W. Breast cancer. N. Engl. J. Med. 327: 319–328, 1992.
5. Stoll, Reducing Breast Cancer Risk in Women. Kluwer Academic Publishers, 1995. pp 3–9.
6. Henderson, B.E., Ross, R.G. and Pike, M.C. Hormonal prevention of cancer in women. Science 259: 633–638, 1993.
7. Marshall, E. Search for a killer: Focus shifts from fat to hormones. Science 259:618–621, 1993.
8. Commoner B., Vithayathil, A.J., Delora, P., Sabhadra, N., Madyastha, P., and Cuca, G.C. Formation of mutagens in beef and beef extract during cooking. Science (Washington, DC) 201: 913–916, 1978.
9. Surgeon General's Report. Smoking and Health, USPHS Publication No. 79–50066. Government Printing Office, Washington, DC, 1979.
10. Stampfer, M.R. and J.C. Bartley: Induction of Transformation and Continuous Cell Lines from Normal Human Mammary Epithelial Cells After Exposure to Benzo[a]pyrene. Proc. Natl. Acad. Sci. USA, 82: 2394–2398, 1984.
11. Russo, J., Reina, D., Frederick, J. and Russo, I.H. Expression of phenotypical changes by human breast epithelial cells treated with carcinogens in vitro. Cancer Res. 48:2837–2857, 1988.
12. Russo, J., Gusterson, B.A., Rogers, A.E., Russo, I.H., Wellings, S.R. and Van Zwieten, M.J. Comparative study of human and rat mammary tumorigenesis. Lab. Invest. 62: 1–32, 1990.
13. Morabia, A., Bernstein, M., Ruiz, J., Heritier, S. et al. Relation of smoking to breast cancer by estrogen status. Int. J. Cancer. 75: 339–342, 1998.
14. Kelsey, J.L. and Horn-Ross, P.L. Breast cancer: magnitude of the problem and descriptive epidemiology. Epidemiol. Rev. 15: 7–16, 1993.
15. Freudenheim, J.L., Marshall, J.R., Vena, J.E., Laughlin, R., et al. Premenopausal breast cancer risk and intake of vegetables, fruits, and related nutrients. J. Natl. Cancer Inst. 88: 340–348, 1996.
16. Hunter, D.J. and Willet, W.C. Diet, body size and breast cancer. Epidemiol. Rev. 15: 110–132, 1993.
17. Katsouyanni, K., Trichopoulous, D., Boyle, P., Xirouchaki, E., Trichoopoulou, A., Lisseos, B., et al. Diet and breast cancer, a case-control study in Greece. Int. J. Cancer 38: 815–20, 1986.
18. La Vecchia, C., Decarli, A., Franceschi, S., Gentile, A., Negri, E. and Parazzini, F. Dietary factors and the risk of breast cancer. Nutr. Cancer 10: 205–214, 1987.
19. Iscovich, J.M., Iiscovich, R.B., Howe, G., Shiboski, S. and Kaldor, J.M. A case-control study of diet and breast cancer in Argentina. Int. J. Cancer 44: 770–776, 1989.
20. Ingram, D.M., Nottage, E., Roberts, T. The role of diet in the development of breast cancer: a case-control study of patients with breast cancer, benign epithelial hyperplasia and fibrocystic disease of the breast. Br. J. Cancer 64: 187–191, 1991.
21. Pawlega, J. Breast cancer and smoking, vodka drinking and dietary habits, A case-control study. Acta Oncol. 31: 387–92, 1992.
22. Rohan, T.E., Howe, G.R., Friedenreich, C.M., Jain, M. and Miller, A.B. Dietary fiber, vitamins A, C, and E and risk of breast cancer: a cohort study. Cancer Causes Control 4: 29–37, 1993.
23. Levi, F., La Vecchia, C., Gulie, C. and Negri, E. Dietary factors and breast cancer risk in Vaud, Switzerland. Nutr. Cancer 19: 327–335, 1993.
24. Murray, A.W., Edwards, E.M. and Hii, C.S.T. Tumor Promotion: Biology and Molecular Mechanisms. In: Chemical Carcinogenesis and Mutagenesis II (Cooper, C.S. and Grover, P.L. eds), Springer Verlag, Berlin. 1990. pp 135–149.
25. Russo, J., Calaf, G., and Russo, I.H. A critical approach to the malignant transformation of human breast epithelial cells. CRC Crit. Rev. Oncogenesis. 4: 403–417, 1993.
26. Russo, J., Barnabas, N., Zhang, P.L. and Adesina, K. Molecular Basis of breast cell transformation. Radiat. Oncol. Invest. 3: 424–429, 1996.
27. Stefanek, M.E. Bilateral prophylactic mastectomy: Issues and concerns. J. Natl Cancer Inst. Monogr. 17: 37–42, 1995.
28. Simmons, R.M. and Osborne, M.P. Prophylactic mastectomy. Breast J. 3: 372–379, 1997
29. Weber, B.L., Giusti, R.M. and Liu, E.T. Developing strategies for intervention and prevention in hereditary breast cancer. Monogr. Natl Cancer Inst 17: 99–102, 1995.
30. Hopwood, P. Psychological issues in cancer genetics: current research and future priorities. Patient Edu. Counsel. 32: 19–31, 1997.
31. Hall, J.M., Lee, M.K., Newman, B. et al., Linkage of early-onset familial breast cancer to chromosome 17q21. Science 250: 1684–1689, 1990.
32. Miki, Y., Swensen, J., Shattuck-Eidens, D. et al. A strong candidate for the breast and breast-ovarian cancer susceptibility gene *BRCA1*. Science 266: 66–71, 1994.
33. Futreal, P.A., Liu, Q., Shattuck-Eidens, D., et al. BRCA1 mutations in primary breast and ovarian carcinomas. Science 266: 120–122, 1994.
34. Wooster, R., Bignell, G., Lancaster, J., et al. Identification of the breast cancer susceptibility gene *BRCA2*. Nature (London) 378: 789–792, 1995.
35. Marcus, J.N., Watson, P., Page, D.L. Hereditary breast cancer: Pathobiology, prognosis and *BRCA1* and *BRCA2* gene linkage. Cancer 77: 697–709, 1996.

36. Jones, K.A., Brown, M.A. and Solomon, E. Molecular genetics of sporadic and familial breast cancer. Cancer Survey 25: 315–334, 1995.

37. Rhei, E., Kang, L., Bogomolniy, F., Federici, M.G. et al. Mutation analysis of the putative tumor suppressor gene PTEN/MMAC1 in primary breast carcinomas. Cancer Res. 57: 3657–3659, 1997.

38. Wolman, S.R., Heppner, G.H. and Wolman, E. New directions in breast cancer research. FASEB J. 11: 535–543, 1997.

39. Loeb, L.A. Many mutations in cancers. Cancer Survey 28: 329–342, 1996.

40. Swift, M., Morrell, D., Massey, R.B. and Chase, C.L. Incidence of cancer in 161 families affected by ataxia-telangiectasia. N. Engl. J. Med. 325: 1831–1836, 1991.

41. Weinberg, P.A. Prospects for cancer genetics. Cancer Survey 25: 3–12, 1995.

42. Land, C.E. Studies of cancer and radiation dose among atomic bomb survivors. The example of breast cancer. J.A.M.A. 274: 402–407, 1995.

43. Miller, R.W. Delayed effects of external radiation exposure: a brief history. Radiation Res. 144: 160–169, 1995.

44. Wang, Y., Holland, J.F., Bleiweiss, I.J., Melana, S. et al. Detection of mammary tumor virus env gene-like sequences in human breast cancer. Cancer Res., 55: 5173–5179, 1995.

45. Pogo, B.G. and Holland, J.F. Possibility of a viral etiology of human breast cancer, A review. Biol. Trace Element Res. 56: 131–142, 1997.

46. Bittner, J.J. Some possible effects of nursing on the mammary gland tumor incidence in mice. Science 84: 162–164, 1936.

47. Callahan, R. MMTV-induced mutations in mouse mammary tumors: their potential relevance to human breast cancer. Breast Cancer Res. Treat. 39: 33–44, 1996.

48. Richardson, A. Is breast cancer caused by late exposure of a common virus? Med. Hypothesis 48: 491–497, 1997.

49. Bradlow, H.L., Hershcopf, R., Martucci, C.P. and Fishman, J. Estradiol 16α-hydroxylation in the mouse correlates with mammary tumor incidence and presence of murine mammary tumor virus: A possible model for the hormonal etiology of breast cancer in humans. Proc. Natl. Acad. Sci. U.S.A. 82: 6295–6299, 1985.

50. Miller, J.A. and Miller, E.C. The metabolic activation of carcinogenic aromatic amines and amides. Prog. Exp. Tumor Res. 11: 273–301, 1969.

51. Miller, E.C. Some current perspectives on chemical carcinogenesis in human and experimental animals. Cancer Res. 38: 1479–1496, 1978.

52. Wattenberg, L.W. Chemoprevention of cancer. Cancer Res. 45: 1–8, 1985.

53. Kensler, T.W., Helzlsouer, K.J. Oltipraz: clinical opportunities for cancer prevention. J. Cell. Biochem. Suppl. 22: 101–107, 1995.

54. Vaca, C.E., Wihelm, J. and Harms-Ringdahl, M. Interaction of lipid peroxidation products with DNA, A review. Mutat. Res. 195: 137–149, 1988.

55. Eling, T.E., Thompson, D.C., Foureman, G.L., Curtis, J.F. and Hughes, M.F. Prostaglandin H synthetase and xenobiotic oxidation. Ann. Rev. Pharmacol. Toxicol. 30: 1–45, 1990.

56. Chen, Y.Q., Liu, B., Tang, D.G. and Honn, K.V. Fatty acid modulation of tumor cell-platelet-vessel wall interaction. Cancer Metastasis Rev. 11: 389–409, 1992.

57. Marnett, H.J. Aspirin and the potential role of prostaglandins in colon cancer. Cancer Res. 52: 5575–5589, 1992.

58. Liu, X.H., Connolly, J.M. and Rose, D.P. Eicosanoids as mediators of linoleic acid-stimulated invasion and type IV collagenase production by a metastatic human breast cancer cell line. Clin. Exp. Metastasis 14: 145–152, 1996.

59. IARC. IARC Monographs on the Evaluation of the Carcinogenic Risk of Chemicals to Humans: Alkyl Compounds, Aldehydes, Epoxides and Peroxides. IARC, Lyon, France, vol 36, pp163–177, 1988.

60. Fang, J.-L., Vaca, C.E., Valsta, L.M. and Mutanen, M. Determination of DNA adducts of malonaldehyde in humans: effects of dietary fatty acid composition. Carcinogenesis 17: 1035–1040, 1996.

61. Dwivedy, I., Devanesan, P., Cremonesi, P., Rogan, E. and Cavalieri, E. Synthesis and characterization of estrogen 2,3- and 3,4-quinones. Comparison of DNA adducts formed by the quinones versus horseradish peroxidase-activated catechol estrogens. Chem. Res. Toxicol. 5: 828–833, 1992.

62. Liehr, J.G., Ulubelen, A.A. and Strobel, H.W. Cytochrome P-450-mediated redox cycling of estrogens. J. Biol. Chem. 261: 16865–16870, 1986.

63. Roy, D. and Liehr, J.G. Temporary decrease in renal quinone and reductase activity induced by chronic administration of estradiol to male Syrian hamsters: increased superoxide formation by redox cycling of estrogen. J. Biol. Chem. 263: 3646–3651, 1988.

64. Ball, P. and Knuppen, R. Catecholestrogens (2- and 4-hydroxy-oestrogens). Chemistry, biosynthesis, metabolism, occurrence and physiological significance. Acta Endocr. (Copenh.) 232(suppl.): 1–127, 1980.

65. Ashburn, S.P., Han, X. and Liehr, J.G. Microsomal hydroxylation of 2- and 4-fluoroestradiol to catechol metabolites and their conversion to methyl ethers: Catechol estrogens as possible mediators of hormonal carcinogenesis. Mol. Pharmacol. 43: 534–541, 1993.

66. Knuppen, R., Ball, P. and Emons, G. Importance of A-ring substitution of estrogens for the physiology and pharmacology of reproduction. J. Steroid Biochem. 24: 193–198, 1986.

67. Creveling, C.R. and Inoue, K. Catechol-O-methyltransferase: Factors relating to the carcinogenic potential of catecholestrogens. Polycyclic Aromat. Compd. 6: 253–259, 1994.

68. Liehr, J.G. and Ricci, M.J. 4-Hydroxylation of estrogens as a marker of human mammary tumors. Proc. Natl. Acad. Sci. USA 93: 3294–3296, 1996.

69. Schneider, J., Kinne, D., Fracchia, A., Pierce, V., Anderson, K.E., Bradlow, H.L. and Fishman, J. Abnormal oxidative metabolism of estradiol in women with breast cancer. Proc. Natl. Acad. Sci. USA. 79: 3047–3051, 1982.

70. Bradlow, H.L., Hershcopf, J., Martucci, C. and Fishman, J. 16α-Hydroxylation of estradiol: a possible risk marker for breast cancer. Ann. N.Y. Acad. Sci. 464: 138–151, 1986.

71. Osborne, M.P., Bradlow, H.L., Wong, G.Y.C. and Telang, N.T. Upregulation of estradiol 16α-hydroxylation in human breast tissue: a potential biomarker of human breast cancer risk. J. Natl. Cancer Inst. 85: 1917–1920, 1993.

72. Sipe, H.J. Jr., Jordan, S.J., Hanna, P.M. and Mason, R.P. The metabolism of 17β-estradiol by lactoperoxidase: a possible source of oxidative stress in breast cancer. Carcinogenesis 15: 2637–2643, 1994.

73. Malins, D.C. and Haimanot, R. Major alterations in the nucleotide structure of DNA in cancer of the female breast. Cancer Res. 51: 5430–5432, 1990.

74. Malins, D.C., Holmes, E.H., Polissar, N.L. and Gunselman, S.J. The etiology of breast cancer: characteristic alterations in hydroxyl radical-induced DNA base lesions during Oncogenesis with potential for evaluating incidence risk. Cancer 71: 3036–3043, 1993.

75. Telang, N.T., Axelrod, D.M., Bradlow, H.L. and Osborne, M.P. Metabolic biotransformation of estradiol in human mammary explant cultures. Ann. N.Y. Acad. Sci. 586: 70–78, 1990.

76. Fishman, J., Osborne, M.P. and Telang, N.T. The role of estrogen in mammary carcinogenesis. Ann. N.Y. Acad. Sci. 768: 91–100, 1995.

77. Telang, N.T., Suto, A., Wong, G.Y., Osborne, M.P. and Bradlow, H.L. Induction by estrogen metabolite 16α-hydroxyestrone of genotoxic damage and aberrant proliferation in mouse mammary epithelial cells. J. Natl. Cancer Inst. 84: 634–638, 1992.

78. Stalford, A.C., Maggs, J.L., Gilchrist, T.L. and Park, B.K. Catecholestrogens as mediators of carcinogenesis: correlation of aromatic hydroxylation of estradiol and its fluorinated analogs with tumor induction in Syrian hamsters. Mol. Pharmacol. 45: 1259–1267, 1994.

79. Zhu, B.T., Bui, Q.D., Weisz, J. and Liehr, J.G. Conversion of estrone to 2- and 4-hydroxyestrone by hamster kidney and liver microsomes: Implications for the mechanism of estrogen-induced carcinogenesis. Endocrinology 135: 1772–1779, 1994.

80. Weisz, J., Bui, Q.D., Roy, D. and Liehr, J.G. Elevated 4-hydroxylation of estradiol by hamster kidney microsomes: a potential pathway of metabolic activation of estrogens. Endocrinology 131: 655–661, 1992.

81. Bunyagidj, C. and McLachlan, J.A. Catechol estrogen formation in mouse uterus. J. Steroid Biochem. 31: 795–801, 1988.

82. Paria, B.C., Chakraborty, C. and Dey, S.K. Catechol estrogen formation in the mouse uterus and its role in implantation. Mol. Cell. Endocrinol. 69: 25–32, 1990.

83. Bui, Q.D. and Weisz, J. Identification of microsomal, organic hydroperoxide-dependent catechol estrogen formation: Comparison with NADPH dependent mechanisms. Pharmacology 36: 356–364, 1988.

84. Zhu, B.T. and Liehr, J.G. Inhibition of the catechol-*O*-methyltransferase catalyzed *O*-methylation of 2- and 4-hydroxyestradiol by catecholamines: Implications for the mechanism of estrogen-induced carcinogenesis. Arch. Biochem. Biophys. 304: 248–256, 1993.

85. Zhu, B.T. and Liehr, J.G. Inhibition of the catechol-*O*-methyltransferase-catalyzed *O*-methylation of 2- and 4-hydroxyestradiol by quercetin: Possible role in estradiol-induced carcinogenesis. J. Biol. Chem. 271: 1357–1363, 1996.

86. Zhu, B.T. and Liehr, J.G. Quercetin increases the severity of estradiol-induced tumorigenesis in hamster kidney. Toxicol. Appl. Pharmacol. 125: 149–158, 1994.

87. Fay, M.P., Freedman, L.S., Clifford, C.K. and Midthune, D.N. Effect of different types and amounts of fat on the development of mammary tumors in rodents: a review. Cancer Res. 57: 3979–3988, 1997.

88. El-Sohemy, A. and Archer, M.C. Regulation of mevalonate synthesis in rat mammary glands by dietary n-3 and n-6 polyunsaturated fatty acids. Cancer Res. 57: 3685–3687, 1997.

89. Buiatti, E., Palli, D., Decarli, A., Amadori, D., Avellini, C., Bianchi, S., Biserni, R., Cipriani, F., Cocco, P., Giacosa, A., et al. A case-control study of gastric cancer and diet in Italy. Int. J. Cancer 44: 611–616, 1989.

90. You, W.C., Blot, W.J., Chang, Y.S., Ershow, A., et al. Allium vegetables and reduced risk of stomach cancer. J. Natl. Cancer Inst. 81: 162–164, 1989.

91. Ip, C., Lisk, D.J. and Stoewsand, G.S. Mammary cancer prevention by regular and selenium-riched garlic. Nutr. Cancer 17:279–286, 1992.

92. Liu, J.Z., Lin, R.I. and Milner, J.A. Inhibition of 7,12-dimethylbenz(α)anthracene-induced mammary tumors and DNA adducts by garlic powder. Carcinogenesis 13: 1847–1851, 1992.

93. Schaffer, E.M., Liu, J.Z., Green, J., Dangler, C.A. and Milner, J.A. Garlic and associated allyl sulfur compounds inhibits N-methyl-N-nitrosourea induced rat mammary carcinogenesis. Cancer Lett. 102: 199–204, 1996.

94. Weinberg, D.S., Manier, M.L., Richardson, M.D. and Haibach, F.G. Identification and quantification of organosulfur compliance markers in a garlic extract. J. Agric. Food Chem. 41: 37–41, 1993.

95. Sundaram, S.G. and Milner, J.A. Impact of organosulfur compounds in garlic on canine mammary tumor cells in culture. Cancer Lett. 74: 85–90, 1993.

96. Lee, E.S., Steiner, M. and Lin, R. Thioally compounds: potent inhibitors of cell proliferation. Biochim Biophys. Acta 1221: 73–77, 1994.

97. El-Bayoumy, K., Chae, Y.H., Upadhyaya, P. and Ip, C. Chemoprevention of mammary cancer by diallyl selenide, a novel organoselenium compound. Anticancer Res. 16: 2911–2915, 1996.

98. Amagase, H. and Milner, J.A. Impact of various sources of garlic and their constituents on 7,12-dimethylbenz(α)anthracene binding to mammary cell DNA. Carcinogenesis 14: 1627–1631, 1993.

99. Ansher, S.S., Dolan, P. and Bueding, E. Biochemical effects of dithiothiones. Food Chem. Toxicol. 24: 405–415, 1986.

100. Reddy, B.S., Rao, C.V., Riverson, A. and Kelloff, G. Chemoprevention of colon carcinogenesis by organosulfur compounds. Cancer Res. 53: 3493–3498, 1993.

101. Egner, P.A., Kensler, T.W., Prestera, T., Talalay, P., et al. Regulation of phase 2 enzyme induction by oltipraz and other dithiolethiones. Carcinogenesis 15: 177–181, 1994.

102. Kensler, T.W. and Helzlsouer, K.J. Oltipraz: clinical opportunities for cancer prevention. J. Cell. Biochem. Suppl. 22: 101–107, 1995.

103. Steele, V.E., Moon, R.C., Lubet, R.A., Grubbs, C.J., et al. Preclinical efficacy evaluation of potential chemopreventive agents in animal carcinogenesis models: methods and results from the NCI Chemoprevention Drug Development Program. J. Cell. Biochem. Suppl. 20: 32–54, 1994.

104. Lubet, R.A., Steele, V.E., Eto, I., Juliana, M.M., Kelloff, G.J. and Grubbs, C.J. Chemopreventive efficacy of anethole trithione, N-acetyl-L-cysteine, meconazole and phenethylisothiocyanate in the DMBA-induced rat mammary cancer model. Int. J. Cancer 72: 95–101, 1997.

105. Begleiter, A., Leith, M.K., Curphey, T.J. and Doherty, G.P. Induction of DT-diaphorase in cancer chemoprevention and chemotherapy. Oncol. Res. 9: 371–382, 1997.

106. Egner, P.A., Kensler, T.W., Prestera, T., Talalay, P., et al. Regulation of phase 2 enzyme induction by oltipraz and other dithiolethiones. Carcinogenesis 15: 177–181, 1994.

107. De Flora, S., Cesarone, C.F., Balansky, R.M., Albini, A., et al. Chemopreventive properties and mechanism of N-acetylcysteine. The experimental background. J. Cell. Biochem. Suppl. 22: 33–41, 1995.

108. Balansky, R., Izzotti, A., Scatolini, L., D'Agostini, F. and De Flora, S. Induction by carcinogens and chemoprevention by N-acetylcysteine of adducts to mitochondrial DNA in rat organs. Cancer Res. 56: 1642–1647, 1996.

109. Janssen, Y.M., Heintz, N.H. and Mossman, B.T. Induction of c-fos and c-jun proto-oncogene expression by asbestos is ameliorated by N-acetyl-L-cysteine in mesothelial cells. Cancer Res. 55: 2085–2089, 1995.

110. Sones, K., Heaney, R.K. and Fenwick, G.R. An estimate of the mean daily intake of glucosinates from cruciferous vegetables in the U.K. J. Sci. Food. Agri. 35: 712–720, 1984.

111. Hecht, S.S. Chemoprevention by isothiocyanates. J. Cell. Biochem. Suppl. 22: 195–209, 1995.

112. Zhang, Y., Kensler, T.W., Cho, C.D., Posner, G.H. and Talalay, P. Anticarcinogenic activities of sulforaphane and structurally related synthetic norbonyl isothiocyanates. Proc. Natl Acad. Sci. USA 91: 3145–3150, 1994.

113. Wattenberg, L.W. Inhibition of carcinogenic effects of polycyclic hydrocarbons by benzyl isothiocyanate and related compounds. J. Natl Cancer Inst. 58: 395–398, 1977.

114. Wattenberg, L.W. Inhibition of carcinogen-induced neoplasia by sodium cyanate, tert-butyl isocyanate, and benzyl isothiocyanate administered subsequent to carcinogen exposure. Cancer Res., 41: 2991–2994, 1981.

115. Gerhauser, C., You, M., Liu, J., Moriarty, R.M., Hawthorne, M., Mehta, R.G., Moon, R.C. and Pezzuto, J.M. Cancer chemopreventive potential of sulforamate, a novel analogue of sulforaphane that induces phase 2 drug-metabolizing enzymes. Cancer Res. 57: 272–278, 1997.

116. McDanell, R., McLean, A.E.M., Hanley, A.B., Heaney, R.K. and Fenwick, G.R. Chemical and biological properties of indole glucosinate (glucobrassicins): a review. Food Chem. Toxicol. 26: 59–70, 1986.

117. Niwa, T., Swaneck, G. and Bradlow, H.L. Alterations in estradiol metabolism in MCF-7 cells induced by treatment with indole-3-carbinol and related compounds. Steroids. 59: 523–527, 1994.

118. Bradlow, H.E., Sepkovic, D.W., Telang, N.T. and Osborne, M.P. Indole-3-carbinol. A novel approach to breast cancer prevention. Ann. N.Y. Acad. Sci. 768: 180–200, 1995.

119. Bradlow, H.L., Michnovicz, J.J., Telang, N.T. and Osborne, M.P. Effects of dietary indole-3-carbinol on estradiol metabolism and spontaneous mammary tumors in mice. Carcinogenesis 12: 1571–1574, 1991.

120. Wattenberg, L.W. and Loub, W.D. Inhibition of polycyclic hydrocarbon-induced neoplasia by naturally occurring indoles. Cancer Res. 38: 1410–1413, 1978.

121. Grubbs, C., Steele, V.E., Casebolt, T., Juliana, M.M., et al. Chemoprevention of chemically-induced mammary carcinogenesis by indole-3-carbinol. Anticancer Res. 15: 709–716, 1995.

122. Katdare, M., Singhal, H., Newmark, H., Osborne, M.P. and Telang, N.T. Prevention of mammary preneoplastic transformation by naturally-occurring tumor inhibitors. Cancer Lett. 111: 141–147, 1997.

123. Tiwari, R.K., Guo, L., Bradlow, H.L., Teleng, N.T. and Osborne, M.P. Selective responsiveness of human breast cancer cells to indole-3-carbinol, a chemopreventive agent. J. Natl. Cancer Inst. 86: 126–131, 1994.

124. Bradlow, H.L., Michnovicz, J.J., Halper, M., Miller, D.G., Wong, G.Y.C. and Osborne, M.P. Long-term responses of women to indole-3-carbinol or a high fiber diet. Cancer Epidemiol. Biomarkers Prev. 3: 591–595, 1994.

125. Michnoviz, J.J., Adlercreutz, H. and Bradlow, H.L. Changes in levels of urinary estrogen metabolites after oral indole-3-carbinol treatment in humans. J. Natl. Cancer Inst. 89: 718–723, 1997.

126. Telang, N.T., Inoue, S., Bradlow, H.L. and Osborne, M.P. Negative growth regulation of oncogene-transformed mammary epithelial cells by tumor inhibitors. Adv. Exp. Med. Biol. 400A: 409–18, 1997.

127. Katdare, M., Osborne, M.P. and Telang, N.T. Inhibition of aberrant proliferation and induction of apoptosis in preneoplastic human mammary epithelial cells by natural phytochemicals. Oncol. Report 5: 311–315, 1998.

128. Mehta, R.G., Liu, J., Constantinou, A., Thomas, C.F., Hawthorne, M., You, M., Gerhuser, C., Pezzuto, J.M., Moon, R.C. and Moriarty, R.M. Cancer chemopreventive activity of brassinin, a phytoalexin from cabbage. Carcinogenesis 16: 399–404, 1995.

129. Jang, M., Cai, L., Udeani, G.O., Slowing, K.V., Thomas, C.F., Beecher, C.W., Fong, H.H., Farnsworth, N.R., Kinghorn, A.D., Mehta, R.G., Moon, R.C. and Pezzuto, J.M. Cancer che-

mopreventive activity of resveratrol, a natural product derived from grapes. Science 275: 218–220, 1997.

130. Mgbonyebi, O.P., Russo, J. and Russo, I.H. Antiproliferative effect of synthetic resveratrol on human breast epithelial cells. Int. J. Oncol. 12: 865–869, 1998.

131. Singletary, K.W. Rosemary extract and carnosol stimulate liver glutathione-S-transferase and quinone reductase activities. Cancer Lett. 100: 139–144, 1996.

132. Sohn, K.H.S., Lee, H.Y., Chung, H.Y., Young, H.S., Yi, S.Y. and Kim, K.W. Anti-angiogenic activity of triterpene acids. Cancer Lett. 94: 213–218, 1995.

133. Es-Saddy, D., Simon, A., Jayat-Vignoles, C., Chulia, A.J. and Delage, C. MCF-7 cell cycle arrested at G1 through ursolic acid, and increased reduction of tetraazolium salts. Anticancer Res. 16: 481–486, 1996.

134. Huang, M.T., Ho, C.H., Wang, Z.Y., Ferraro, T., et al. Inhibition of skin tumorigenesis by rosemary and its constituents carnosol and ursolic acid. Cancer Res. 54: 701–708, 1994.

135. Singletary, K. and Nelshoppen, J. Inhibition of 7,12-dimethylbenz(α)anthracene (DMBA)-induced mammary tumorigenesis and of in vivo formation of mammary DMBA-DNA adducts by rosemary extract. Cancer Lett. 60: 169–175, 1991.

136. Khachik, F., Beecher, G.R., Goli, M.B. and Lusby, W.R. Separation, identification and quantification of carotenoids in fruits, vegetables and human plasma by high performance liquid chromatography. Pure Appl. Chem. 63: 71–80, 1991.

137. Khachik, F., Beecher, G.R. and Smith, J.C. Lutein, lycopene, and their oxidative metabolites in chemoprevention of cancer. J. Cell. Biochem. Suppl. 22: 236–246, 1995.

138. Krinsky, N.I. Actions of carotenoids in biological systems. Ann. Rev. Nutr. 13: 561–587, 1993.

139. Rohan, T.E., McMichael, A.J. and Baghurst, P.A. A population-based case-control study of the diet and breast cancer in Austria. Am. J. Epidemiol. 128: 478–489, 1988.

140. Potischman, N., McCulloch, C.E., Byers, T., Nemoto, T., et al. Breast cancer and dietary and plasma concentrations of carotenoids and vitamin A. Am. J. Clin. Nutr. 52: 909–915, 1990.

141. Graham, S., Hellann, R., Marshall, J., Freudenheim, J., et al. Nutritional epidemiology of postmenopausal breast cancer in Western New York. Am. J. Epidemiol. 134: 552–566, 1991.

142. Lee, H.P., Courley, L., Duffy, S.W., Esteve, J., Lee, J. and Day, N.E. Dietary effects on breast cancer risk in Singapore. Lancet 337: 1197–1200, 1991.

143. Hunter, D.L., Manson, J.E., Colditz, G.A., Stampfer, M.J., et al. A prospective study of the intake of vitamins C, E, and A and the risk of breast cancer. N. Engl. J. Med. 329: 234–240, 1993.

144. Holmberg, L., Ohlander, E.M., Byers, T., Zack, M., et al. Diet and breast cancer risk. Results from a population-based, case-control study in Sweden. Arch. Intern. Med. 154: 1805–1811, 1994.

145. Pool-Zobel, B.L., Bub, A., Muller, H., Wollowski, I. and Rechkemmer, G. Consumption of vegetables reduces genetic damage in humans: first results of a human intervention trial with carotenoid-rich foods. Carcinogenesis 18: 1847–1850, 1997.

146. Alam, B.S. and Alam, S.Q. The effect of different levels of dietary β-carotene on DMBA-induced salivary gland tumors. Nutr. Cancer 9: 93–101, 1987.

147. Rettura, G., Duttagupta, C., Listowski, P., Levenson, S.M. and Seifter, E. Dimethylbenz(α)-anthracene (DMBA)-induced tumors: prevention by supplemental β-carotene (BC). Fed. Proc. 42: 786 (abstr. No. 2891), 1983.

148. Rettura, G., Levenson, S.M. and Seifter, E. 7,12-Dimethylbenz(α)-anthracene carcinogenicity: Moderation by supplemental beta-carotene (B-Car) and vitamin A (Vit A). Fed. Proc., 41:67 (abstr. No. 11), 1982.

149. Kelloff, G.J., Crowell, J.A., Boone, C.W., Steele, V.E., et al. Strategy and planning for chemopreventive drug development: clinical development plan. J. Cell. Biochem. Suppl. 20: 55–299, 1994.

150. The α-Tocopherol, β-Carotene Cancer Prevention Study Group. The effect of vitamin E and β-carotene on the incidence of lung cancer and other cancers in male smokers. N. Engl. J. Med. 330: 1029–1035, 1994.

151. Nishino, H. Cancer chemoprevention by natural carotenoids and their related compounds. J. Cell. Biochem. Suppl. 22: 231–235, 1995.

152. Di Mascio, P., Murphy, M.E. and Sies, H. Antioxidant defense systems: the role of carotenoids, tocopherols and thiols. Am. J. Clin. Nutr. 53: 194S-200S, 1991.

153. Sharoni, Y., Giron, E., Rise, M. and Levy, J. Effects of lycopene-enriched tomato oleoresin on 7,12-dimethyl-bnz[a] anthracene-induced rat mammary tumors. Cancer Detect. Prev. 21: 118–123, 1997.

154. Nagasawa, H., Mitamura, T., Sakamoto, S. and Yamamoto, K. Effects of lycopene on spontaneous mammary tumour development in SHN virgin mice. Anticancer Res. 15: 1173–1178, 1995.

155. Moon, R.C. and Constantinou, A.I. Dietary retinoids and carotenoids in rodent models of mammary tumorigenesis. Breast Cancer Res. Treat. 46: 181–189, 1997.

156. Ip, C. The chemopreventive role of selenium in carcinogenesis. Adv. Exp. Med. Biol. 206: 431–447, 1986.

157. Ip, C. Selenium and experimental cancer. Ann. Clin. Res. 18: 22–29, 1986.

158. Wang, Y.M., Howell, S.K., Tsai, C.C. and van Eyss, J. Daunorubicin-induced mammary tumors in female Sprague-Dawley rats and the role of α-tocopherol as a modifier to the carcinogenesis. Proc. Am. Assoc. Cancer Res. 22: 190 (abstr. no. 352), 1983.

159. King, M.M. and McCoy, P.B. Modulation of tumor incidence and possible mechanisms of inhibition of mammary carcinogenesis by dietary antioxidants. Cancer Res. 43(suppl.): 2485–2490, 1983.

160. Grubbs, C.J., Eto, I., Juliana, M.M. and Witaker, L.M. Effect of canthaxanthin on chemically induced mammary carcinogenesis. Oncology 48: 239–245, 1991.

161. Thompson, H.J. Effects of combined deficiencies of felenium (Se) and vitamin E (Vit E) on the initiation and promotion phases of 7,12-dimethylbenz(a)anthracene (DMBA)-induced mammary tumorigenesis. Proc. Am. Assoc. Cancer Res. 32: 146 (abstr. no. 877), 1993.

162. Willett, W.C., Polk, B.F., Underwood, B.A., Stampfer, M.J., et al. Relation of serum vitamins A and E and carotenoids to the risk of cancer. N. Engl. J. Med. 310: 430–434, 1983.

163. Willett, W.C., Morris, J.S., Pressel, S., Taylor, J.O., et al. Prediagnostic serum selenium and the risk of cancer. Lancet 2: 130–134, 1983.

164. Salonen, J.T., Salonen, R., Lappetetainen, R., Maenpaa, PH., Alfthan, G. and Puska, P. Risk of cancer in relation to serum concentrations of selenium and vitamins A and E: matched case-control analysis of prospective data. Br. Med. J. 290: 417–420, 1985.

165. Takada, H., Hirooka, T., Hatano, T., Hamada, Y. and Yamamoto, M. Inhibition of 7,12-dimethyl-benz(a)anthracene-induced lipid peroxidation and mammary tumor development in rats by vitamin E in conjunction with selenium. Nutr. Cancer 17: 115–122, 1992.

166. Ambrosone, C.B., Marshall, J.R., Vena, J.E., Laughlin, R., Graham, S., Nemoto, T. and Freudenheim, J.L. Interaction of family history of breast cancer and dietary antioxidants with breast cancer risk. Cancer Cause Control 6: 407–415, 1995.

167. Gallegos, A., Berggren, M., Gasdaska, J.R. and Powis. G. Mechanisms of the regulation of thioredoxin reductase activity in cancer cells by the chemopreventive agent selenium. Cancer Res. 57: 4965–4970, 1997.

168. Medina, D., Lane, H.W. and Tracey, C.M. Selenium and mouse mammary tumorigenesis, an investigation of possible mechanisms. Cancer Res. 43: 2460s-22464 s, 1983.

169. Ip, C. and Medina, D. Current concepts of selenium and mammary tumorigenesis. In: Cellular and Molecular Biology of Mammary Cancer (Medina, C., Kidwell, W., Heppner, G.H. and Anderson, E. eds), Plenum Press, New York. 1987. pp 479–494.

170. El-Bayoumy, K. The role of selenium in cancer prevention. In: Cancer Principles and Practice of Oncology (De Vita, V., Hellman, S. and Rosenberg, S.A. eds) (4th ed), J.B. Lippinncott., Philadelphia. 1991. pp 1–15.

171. El-Bayoumy, K., Upadhyaya, P., Chae, Y.H., Sohn, O.S., et al. Chemoprevention of cancer by organoselenium compounds. J. Cell. Biochem. Suppl. 22: 92–100, 1995.

172. Young, V.R., Nahapetian, A. and Janghorbami, M. Selenium bioavailability with reference to human nutrition. Am. J. Clin. Nutr. 35: 1076–1088, 1982.

173. Thomson, C.D., Stewart, R.D.H. and Robinson, M.J. Metabolic studies in rats of [75Se]selenomethionine and of 75Se incorporated in vivo into rabbit kidney. Br. J. Nutr. 33: 45–54, 1975.

174. Thompson, H.J., Meeker, L.D. and Kokoska, E. Effect of an inorganic and organic form of dietary selenium on the promotional stage of mammary carcinogenesis in the rat. Cancer Res. 44: 2803–2806, 1984.

175. Ip, C. and Hayes, C. Tissue selenium levels in selenium-supplemented rats and their relevance in mammary cancer protection. Carcinogenesis 10: 921–925, 1989.

176. Ip, C., Lisk, D.J. and Thompson, H.J. Selenium-enriched garlic inhibits the early stage but not the late stage of mammary carcinogenesis. Carcinogenesis 17: 1979–1982, 1996.

177. Lu, J., Pei, H., Ip, C., Lisk, D.J., Ganther, H. and Thompson, H.J. Effect on an aqueous extract of selenium-enriched garlic on in vitro markers and in vivo efficacy in cancer prevention. Carcinogenesis 17: 1903–1907, 1996.

178. Nayini, J., El-Bayoumy, K., Sugie, S., Cohen, L.A. and Reddy, B.S. Chemoprevention of experimental mammary carcinogenesis by the synthetic organoselenium compound, benzylselenocyanate, in rats. Carcinogenesis 10: 509–512, 1989.

179. El-Bayoumy, K., Chae, Y.H., Upadhyaya, P., Meschter, C., Cohen, L.A. and Reddy, B.S. Inhibition of 7,12-dimethylbenz(a)anthracene-induced tumors and DNA adduct formation in the mammary glands of female Sprague-Dawley rats by the synthetic organoselenium compound, 1,4-phenylenebis(methylene)-selenocyanate. Cancer Res. 52: 2402–2407, 1992.

180. Ip, C., El-Bayoumy, K., Upadhyaya, Ganther, H., Vadhanavikit, S. and Thompson, H. Comparative effect of inorganic and organic selenocyanate derivatives in mammary cancer chemo-prevention. Carcinogenesis 15: 191–196, 1994.

181. Thompson, H.J., Wilson, A., Lu, J., Singh, M., Jiang, C., Upadhyaya, P., El-Bayoumy, K. and Ip, C. Comparison of the effects of an organic and an inorganic form of selenium on a mammary carcinoma cell line. Carcinogenesis 15: 183–186, 1994.

182. Lu, J., Jiang, C., Kaeck, M., Ganther, H., Ip, C. and Thompson, H. Cellular and metabolic effects of triphenylselenonium chloride in a mammary cell culture model. Carcinogenesis 16: 513–517, 1995,

183. Ip, C., Vadhanavikit, S. and Ganther, H. Cancer chemoprevention by aliphatic selenocyanates: effect of chain length on inhibition of mammary tumors and DMBA adducts. Carcinogenesis 16: 35–38, 1995.

184. Ip, C., Lisk, D.J., Ganther, H. and Thompson, H.J. Triphenylselenonium and diphenylselenide in cancer chemoprevention: comparative studies of anticarcinogenic efficacy, tissue selenium levels and excretion profile. Anticancer Res. 17: 3195–3199, 1997.

185. Shimada, T., El-Bayoumy, K., Upadhyaya, P., Sutter, T.R., Guengerich, F.P. and Yamazaki, H. Inhibition of human cytochrome P450-catalyzed oxidations of xenobiotics and procarcinogens by synthetic organoselenium compounds. Cancer Res. 57: 4757–4764, 1997.

186. Tillotson, J.K., Upadhyaya, P. and Ronai, Z. Inhibition of thymidine kinase in cultured mammary tumor cells by the chemopreventive organoselenium compound, 1,4-phenylenebis(methylene)-selenocyanate. Carcinogenesis 15: 607–610, 1994.

187. Ip, C., Thompson, H.J. and Ganther, H.E. Cytostasis and cancer chemoprevention: investigating the action of tri-

phenylselenonium chloride in in vivo models of mammary carcinogenesis. Anticancer Res., 18(1A): 9–12, (1998).

188. Weisburger, J.H. Tea and health: a historical perspective. Cancer Lett. 114: 315–317, 1997.

189. Oguni, I., Nasu, K., Kanaya, S., Ota, Y., Yamamoto, S. and Nomura, T. Epidemiological and experimental studies on the antitumor activity of green tea extracts. Jpn. J. Nutr. 47: 93–102, 1989.

190. Yang, C.S. and Wang, Z.Y. Tea and Cancer. J. Natl. Cancer Inst. 85: 1038–1049, 1993.

191. Ewertz, M. Breast cancer in Denmark. incidence, risk factors and characteristics of survival. Acta Oncol. 32:595–615, 1993.

192. Goldbohm, R.A., Hertog, M.G., Brants, H.A.M., van Proppel, G. and van den Brandt, P.A. Consumption of black tea and cancer risk: a prospective cohort study. J. Natl. Cancer Inst. 88: 93–100, 1996.

193. Wang, Z.Y., Hong, J.Y., Huang, M.T., Reuhl, K.R., Conney, A.H. and Yang, C.S. Inhibition of N-nitrosodiethylamine- and 4-(methylnitrosamino)-11-(3-pyridyl)-1-butanone-induced tumorigenesis in A/J mice by green tea and black tea. Cancer Res. 52: 1943–1947, 1992.

194. Hirose, M. Hoshiya, T., Akagi, K., Futakuchi, M. and Ito, N.Inhibition of mammary gland carcinogenesis by green tea catechins and other naturally occurring antioxidants in female Sprague-Dawley rats pretreated with 7,12-dimethylbenz(a)anthracene. Cancer Lett. 83: 149–156, 1994.

195. Stoner, G.D. and Mukhtar, H. Polyphenols as cancer chemopreventive agents. J. Cell. Biochem. Suppl. 22: 169–180, 1995.

196. Balentin, D.A. Manufacturing and chemistry of tea. In: Phenolic compounds in food and their effects on health. I. Analysis, occurrence and chemistry (Ho, C.T., Lee, C.Y. and Huang, M.T. eds). American Chemical Society, Washington DC. 1992. pp 102–117.

197. Valcic, S., Timmermann, B.N., Alberts, D.S., Wachter, G.A., Krutzsch, M., Wymer, J. and Guillen, J.M. Inhibitory effect of six green tea catechins and caffeine on the growth of four selected human tumor cell lines. Anti-Cancer Drugs 7: 461–468, 1996.

198. Hirose, M., Akagi, K., Hasegawa, R., Yaono, M., Satoh, T., Hara, Y., Wakabayashi, K. and Ito, N. Chemoprevention of 2-amino-1-methyl-6-phenylimidazo[4,5-b]-pyridine (PhIP)-induced mammary gland carcinogenesis by antioxidants in F344 female rats. Carcinogenesis 16: 217–221, 1995.

199. Weisburger, J.H., Rivenson, A., Carr, K. and Aliaga, C. Tea, or tea and milk, inhibit mammary gland and colon carcinogenesis. Cancer Lett. 114: 323–327, 1997.

200. Yu, R., Jiao, J.-J., Duh, J.-L., Gudehithlu, K., Tan, T.-H. and Kong, A.-N.T. Activation of mitogen-activated protein kinases by green tea polyphenols: potential signaling pathways in the regulation of antioxidant-responsive element-mediated phase II enzyme gene expression. Carcinogenesis 18: 451–456, 1997.

201. Cai, Q., Rahn, R.O. and Zhang, R. Dietary flavonoids, quercetin, luteolin and genistein, reduce oxidative DNA damage and lipid peroxidation and quench free radicals. Cancer Lett. 119: 99–107, 1997.

202. Mora, A., Paya, M., Rois, J.L. and Alcaraz, M.J. Structure-activity relationships of polymethoxyflavones and other flavonoids as inhibitors of non-enzymatic lipid peroxidation. Biochem. Pharmacol. 40: 793–797, 1990.

203. Hertog, M.G.L, Hollman, P.C.H., Katan, M.B. and Kromhout, D. Intake of potentially anticarcinogenic flavonoids and their determinants in adults in the Netherlands. Nutr. Cancer 20: 21–29, 1993.

204. Elangovan, V., Sekar, N. and Govindasamy, S. Chemopreventive potential of dietary bioflavonoids against 20-methylcholanthrene-induced tumorigenesis. Cancer Lett. 87: 107–113, 1994.

205. Das, A., Wang, J.H. and Lien, E.L. Carcinogenicity, mutagenicity and cancer preventing activities of flavonoids: a structure-system-activity relationship (SSAR) analysis. In: Progress in Drug Research (Jucker E. ed), Birkhaeuser Verlag., Basel. 1995. pp 133–166.

206. Scambia, G., Ranelletti, F.O., Benedetti, P., Piantelli, M., et al. Quercetin inhibits the growth of a multidrug-resistant estrogen-receptor-negative MCF-7 human breast cancer cell line expressing type II estrogen-binding sites. Cancer Chemother. Pharmacol. 28: 255–258, 1991.

207. Albert, Y., Herenyiova, M. and Weber, G. Quercetin: synergistic action with carboxyamidotriazole in human breast carcinoma cells. Life Sci. 57: 1285–1292, 1995.

208. Fotsis, T., Pepper, M.S., Aktas, E., Breit, S., et al. Flavoids, dietary-derived inhibitors of cell proliferation and in vitro angiogenesis. Cancer Res. 57: 2916–2921, 1997.

209. Boyd, N.F., Martin, L.J., Noffel, M., Lockwood, G.A., et al. A meta-analysis of studies of dietary fat and breast cancer risk. Br. J. Cancer 68: 627–636, 1993.

210. Gaard, M., Tretli, S. and Loken, E.B. Dietary fat and the risk of breast cancer: A prospective study of 25892 Norwegian women. Int. J. Cancer 63: 13–17, 1995.

211. Yuan, J.M., Wang, Q.S., Ross, R.K., Henderson, B.E. and Yu, M.C. Diet and breast cancer in Shanghai and Tianjin, China. Br. J. Cancer 71: 1353–1358, 1995.

212. Sylvester, P.W., Russel, M., Ip, M.M. and Ip, C. Comparative effects of different animal and vegetable fats fed before and during carcinogen administration on mammary tumorigenesis, sexual maturation and endocrine function in rats. Cancer Res. 46: 757–762, 1986.

213. Cohen, L.A., Thompson, D.O., Maeura, Y., Choi, K., Blank, M.E. and Rose, D.P. Dietary fat and mammary cancer. I. Promoting effects of different dietary fats on N-nitrosomethylurea-induced mammary tumorigenesis. J. Natl. Cancer Inst. 77: 33–42, 1986.

214. Freedman, L.S., Clifford, C. and Messina, M. Analysis of dietary fat, calories, body weight, and the development of mammary tumors in rats and mice: a review. Cancer Res. 50: 5710–5719, 1990.

215. Welsch, C.W. Relationship between dietary fat and experimental mammary tumorigenesis: A review and critique. Cancer Res. 52: 2040s-2048 s, 1992.

216. Lu, J., Jiang, C., Fontains, S. and Thompson, H.J. Ras may mediate mammary promotion by high fat. Nutr. Cancer 23: 283–290, 1995.

217. Hilakivi-Clarke, L., Cho, E., Raygada, M., Onojafe, I., et al. Early life affects the risk of developing breast cancer. Ann. N.Y. Acad. Sci. 768: 327–330, 1995.

218. Nagasawa, H., Yasuda, M., Sakamoto, S. and Inatomi, H. Protection by coffee cherry against spontaneous mammary tumour development in mice. Anticancer Res. 15: 141–146, 1995.

219. Rose, D.P. and Connolly, J.M. Effects of fatty acids and inhibitors of eicosanoid synthesis on the growth of a human breast cancer cell line in culture. Cancer Res. 50: 7139–7144, 1990.

220. Ip, C., Carter, C.A. and Ip, M.M. Requirement of essential fatty acid for mammary tumorigenesis in the rat. Cancer Res. 45: 1997–2001,1985.

221. Fischer, S.M., Leyton, J., Lee, M.L., Locniskar, M. et al. Differential effects of dietary linoleic acid on mouse skin-tumor promotion and mammary carcinogenesis. Cancer Res. 52: 2049s-2054 s, 1992.

222. Hillyard, L.A. and Abraham, S. Effect of dietary polysaturated fatty acids on growth of mammary adenocarcinomas in mice and rats. Cancer Res. 39: 4430–4437, 1979.

223. Abraham, S. and Hillyard, L.A. Effect of dietary 18-carbon fatty acids on growth of transplantable mammary adenocarcinomas in mice. J. Natl Cancer Inst. 71: 601–605, 1983.

224. Rao, G.A. and Abraham, S. Reduced growth rate of transplantable mammary adenocarcinoma in C3H mice fed eicosa-5,8,11,14-tetraynoic acid. J. Natl. Cancer Inst. 58: 445–447, 1983.

225. Kritchevsky, D., Weber, M.M. and Klurfeld, D.M. Dietary fat versus caloric content in initiation and promotion of 7,12-dimethylbenz[α]anthracene-induced mammary tumorigenesis in rats. Cancer Res. 44: 3174–3177, 1984.

226. Sylvester, P.W., Aylsworth, C.F., van Vugt, D.A. and Meites, J. Influence of underfeeding during the critical period or after on carcinogen-induced mammary tumors in rats. Cancer Res. 42: 4943–4947, 1982.

227. Klurfeld, D.M., Weber, M.M. and Kritchevsky, D. Inhibition of chemically induced mammary and colon tumor promotion by caloric restriction in rats fed increased dietary fat. Cancer Res. 47: 2759–2761, 1987.

228. Ip, C. Quantitative assessment of fat and calories as risk factors in mammary carcinogenesis in an experimental model. Prog. Clin. Biol. Res. 346: 107–117, 1990.

229. Kritchevsky, D. Caloric restriction and experimental carcinogenesis. Adv. Exp. Med. Biol. 322: 134–141, 1992.

230. Welsch, C.W. Dietary fat, calories and mammary gland tumorigenesis. Adv. Exp. Med. Biol. 322: 203–222, 1992.

231. Zhu, Z., Haegele, A.D. and Thompson, H.J. Effect of caloric restriction on pre-malignant and malignant stages of mammary carcinogenesis. Carcinogenesis 18: 1007–1012, 1997.

232. Gillette, C.A., Zhu, Z., Westerlind, K.C., Melby, C.L., Wolfe, P. and Thompson, H.J. Energy availability and mammary carcinogenesis: effects of calorie restriction and exercise. Carcinogenesis 18: 1183–1188, 1997.

233. Pitts, G.C. Body composition in the rat: interactions of exercise, age, sex, and diet. Am. J. Physiol. 246: R495-R501, 1984.

234. Thompson, H.J., Ronan, A.M., Ritacco, K.A., Tagliaferro, A.R. and Meeker, L.D. Effect of exercise on the induction of mammary carcinogenesis. Cancer Res. 48: 2720–2723, 1988.

235. Thompson, H.J., Ronan, A.M., Ritacco, K.A. and Tagliaferro, A.R. Effect of type and amount of fat on the enhancement of rat mammary tumorigenesis by exercise. Cancer Res. 49: 1904–1908, 1989.

236. Shephard, R.J. Physical activity and cancer. Int. J. Sports. Med. 11: 413–420, 1990.

237. Cohen, L.A. Physical activity and cancer. Cancer Prev. June: 1–10, 1991.

238. Thompson, H.J., Westerlind, K.C., Snedden, J., Briggs, S. and Singh, M. Inhibition of mammary carcinogenesis by treadmill exercise. J. Natl. Cancer Inst. 87: 453–455, 1995.

239. Thompson, H.J., Westerlind, K.C., Snedden, J., Briggs, S. and Singh, M. Exercise intensity dependent inhibition of 1-methyl-1-nitrourea induced mammary carcinogenesis in female F-344 rats. Carcinogenesis 16: 1783–1786, 1995.

240. De Waard, F. Breast cancer incidence and nutritional status with particular reference to body weight and height. Cancer Res. 35: 3351–3356, 1975.

241. Wynder, E.L. Nutrition and Cancer. Fed. Proc. 35: 1309–1315, 1976.

242. Tartter, P.I., Papatestas, A.E., Ioannovich, J., Mulvihill, M.N., Lesnick, G. and Aufses, A.H. Jr. Cholesterol and obesity as prognostic factors in breast cancer. Cancer 47: 2222–2227, 1981.

243. Thune, I., Brenn, T., Lund, E. and Gaard, M. Physical activity and the risk of breast cancer. N. Engl. J. Med. 336: 1269–1275, 1997.

244. Inano, H., Suzuki, K. and Wakabayashi, K. Chemoprevention of radiation-induced mammary tumors in rats by benafibrate administered together with diethylstilbestrol as a promoter. Carcinogenesis 17: 2641–2646, 1996.

245. Goldin, R.B., Adlercreutz, H., Gorbach, S.L., Warram, H., et al. Estrogen excretion patterns and plasma levels in vegetarian and omnivorous women. N. Engl. J. Med. 307: 1542–1547, 1982.

246. Ingram, D.M., Bennet, F.C., Willcox, D. and de Klerk, N. Effect of low-fat diet on female sex hormone levels. J. Natl. Cancer Inst. 79: 1225–1229, 1987.

247. Longcope, C., Gorbach, S.L., Goldin, B.R., Woods, M.N., et al. The effect of a low fat diet on estrogen metabolism. J. Clin. Endocrinol. Metab. 64: 1246–1250, 1987.

248. Rose, D.P., Boyar, A.P., Cohen, C. and Strong, L.E. Effect of a low-fat diet on hormone levels in women with cystic

breast disease. I. Serum steroids and gonadotropins. J. Natl. Cancer Inst. 78: 623–626, 1987.

249. Woods, M.N., Gorbach, S.L., Longcope, C., Goldin, B.R., et al. Low-fat, high-fiber diet and estrone sulfate in premenopausal women. Am. J. Clin. Nutr. 49: 1179–1183, 1989.

250. Prentice, R., Thompson, D., Clifford, C., Gorbach, S., et al. Dietary fat reduction and plasma estradiol concentration in healthy postmenopausal women. The Women's Health Trial Study Group. J. Natl. Cancer Inst. 82: 129–134, 1990.

251. Rose, D.P., Goldman, M., Connolly, J.M. and Strong, L.E. High-fiber diet reduces serum estrogen concentrations in premenopausal women. Am. J. Clin. Nutr. 54: 520–525, 1991.

252. Schaefer, E.J., Lamon-Fava, S., Spiegelman, D., Dwyer, J.T., et al. Changes in plasma lipoprotein concentrations and composition in response to a low-fat, high-fiber diet are associated with changes in serum estrogen concentrations in premenopausal women. Metabolism 44: 749–756, 1995.

253. Goldin, B.R., Woods, M.N., Spiegelman, D.L., Longcope, C., et al. The effect of dietary fat and fiber on serum estrogen concentrations in premenopausal women under controlled dietary conditions. Cancer 74: 1125–1131, 1994.

254. Boyd, N.F., Greenberg, C., Lockwood, G., Little, L., et al. Effects of two years of a low-fat, high-carbohydrate diet on radiologic features of the breast: results from a randomized trial. J. Natl. Cancer Inst. 89: 488–496, 1997.

255. Warren, M.P. The effects of exercise on pubertal progression and reproductive function in girls. J. Clin. Endocrinol. Metab. 51: 1150–1157, 1980.

256. Frisch, R.E., Gotz-Welbergen, A.V., McArthus, J.W. et al. Delayed menarche and amenorrhea of college athletes in relation to age at onset of training. J.A.M.A., 246: 1559–1563, 1981.

257. Bullen, B.A., Skrinar, G.S., Beitins, I.Z., von Mering, G., Turnbull, B.A. and McArthur, J.W. Induction of menstrual disorders by strenuous exercise in untrained women. N. Engl. J. Med. 312: 1349–1353, 1985.

258. Moisan, J., Meyer, F. and Gingras, S. Leisure physical activity and age at menarche. Med. Sci. Sports. Exerc. 23: 1170–1175, 1991.

259. Merzenich, H., Boeing, H. and Wahrendorf, J. Dietary fat and sports activity as determinants for age at menarche. Am. J. Epidemiol. 138: 217–224, 1993.

260. Ellison, P.T. and Lager, C. Moderate recreational running is associated with lowered salivary progesterone profiles in women. Am J. Obstet. Gynecol. 154: 1000–1003, 1986.

261. Bernstein, L., Ross, R.K., Lobo, R.A., Hanisch, R., Krailo, M.D. and Henderson, B.E. The effects of moderate physical activity on menstrual cycle patterns in adolescence: implications for breast cancer prevention. Br. J. Cancer 55: 681–685, 1987.

262. Harlow, S.D. and Matanoski, G.M. The association between weight, physical activity, and stress and variation in the length of the menstrual cycle. Am. J. Epidemiol. 133: 38–49, 1991.

263. Broocks, A., Pirke, K.M., Schweiger, U. et al. Cyclic ovarian function in recreational athletes. J. Appl. Physiol. 68: 2083–2086, 1990.

264. Loucks, A.B., Mortola, J.F., Girton, L. and Yen, S.S.C. Alterations in the hypothalamic-pituitary-ovarian and the hypothalamic-pituitary-adrenal axes in athletic women. J. Clin. Endocrinol. Metab., 68: 402–411, 1989.

265. Beitins, I.Z., McArthur, J.W., Turnbull, B.A., Skrinar, G.S. and Bullen, B.A. Exercise induces two types of human luteal dysfunction: confirmation by urinary free progesterone. J. Clin. Endocrinol. Metab. 72: 1350–1358, 1991.

266. Russell, J.B., Mitchell, D., Musey, P.I. and Collins, D.C. The relationship of exercise to anovulatory cycles in female athletes: hormonal and physical characteristics. Obstet. Gynecol. 63: 452–456, 1982

267. Henderson, B.E., Ross, R.K., Judd, H.L., Krailo, M.D. and Pike, M.C. Do regular ovulatory cycles increase breast cancer risk? Cancer 56: 1206–1208, 1985.

268. Pike, M.C., Spicer, D.V., Dahmoush, L. and Press, M.F. Estrogens, progesterone, normal breast cell proliferation and breast cancer risk. Epidemiol. Rev. 15: 17–35, 1993.

269. Kelsey, J.L., Gammon, M.D. and John, E.M. Reproductive factors and breast cancer. Epidemiol. Rev. 15: 36–47, 1993.

270. Bernstein, L. and Ross, R.K. Endogenous hormones and breast cancer risk. Epidemiol. Rev. 15: 48–65, 1993.

271. Henderson, B.E., Ross, R.K., Pike, M.C. and Casagrande, J.T. Endogenous hormones as a major factor in human cancer. Cancer Res. 42: 3232–3239, 1982.

272. Henderson, B.E., Ross, R.K. and Pike, M.C. Hormonal chemoprevention of cancer in women. Science 259: 633–638, 1993.

273. Spencer-Feigelson, H., Ross, R.K., Yu, M.C., Coetzee, G.A., Reichardt, J.K.V. and Henderson, B.E. Genetic susceptibility to cancer from exogenous and endogenous exposures. J. Cell. Biochem. 25S: 15–22, 1996.

274. Henderson, B.E., Ross, R. and Bernstein, L. Estrogens as a cause of human cancer: the Richard and Hinda Rosenthal Foundation Award Lecture. Cancer Res. 48: 246–253, 1988.

275. Greenwald, P., Barolom, J.J. and Nasca, P.C. Vaginal cancer after maternal treatment with synthetic estrogens. N. Engl. J. Med. 285: 390–392, 1971.

276. Nissen, E.D. and Kent, D.R. Liver tumours and oral contraceptives. Obst. Gynecol. 46: 460–467, 1975.

277. Herbst, A.L. Clear cell adenocarcinoma and current status of DES-exposed females. Cancer 48: 484–488, 1981.

278. Shaw, R.W. Adverse long term effects of oral contraceptives– a review. Br. J. Obst. Gynecol. 94: 724–730, 1987.

279. Chivers, C. Mant, D. and Pike, M.C. Cervical adenocarcinoma and oral contraceptives. Br. Med. J. 295: 1446–1447, 1987.

280. Beral, V., Hannaford, P. and Kay, C. Oral contraceptive use and malignancies of the genital tract. Lancet ii: 1331–1334, 1988.

281. Cuzick, J. and Baum, M. Tamoxifen and contralateral breast cancer. Lancet 2: 28, 1985.

282. Adlercreutz, H., Gorbach, S.L., Goldin, B.R., Woods, M.N. and Hamalainen, E. RE: Estrogen metabolism and excretion in Oriental and Caucasian women– Response. J. Natl. Cancer Inst. 86: 1644–1645, 1994.

283. Nandi, S., Guzman, R.C. and Yang, J. Hormones and mammary carcinogenesis in mice, rats and humans: A unifying hypothesis. Proc. Natl. Acad. Sci. USA 92: 3650–3657, 1995.

284. Yan, Z-J. and Roy, D. Mutations in DNA polymerase β mRNA of stilbene estrogen-induced kidney tumors in Syrian hamster. Biochem. Mol. Biol. Int. 37: 175–183, 1995.

285. Feinleib, M. Breast cancer and artificial menopause: A cohort study. J. Natl. Cancer Inst. 41: 315–329, 1968.

286. Trichopouloos, D., MacMahon, B. and Cole, P. Menopause and breast cancer risk. J. Natl. Cancer Inst. 48: 605–613, 1972.

287. Nissen-Meyer, R. Primary breast cancer: the effect of ovarian irradiation. Ann. Oncol. 2: 343–346, 1991.

288. McNeill, J.M., Reed, M.J., Beranek, P.A., Bonney, R.C., et al. Comparison of the in vivo uptake and metabolism of 3H-oestrone and 3H-oestradiol by normal breast and breast tumor tissue in postmenopausal women. Int. J. Cancer 38: 193–196, 1986.

289. Reed, M.J., Owen, A.M., Lai, L.C., Coldham, N.G., et al. In situ oestrone synthesis in normal breast and breast tumour tissues: effect of treatment with 4-hydroxyanndrostenedione. Int. J. Cancer 44: 233–237, 1989.

290. Blankenstein, M.A., Maitimu-Smeele, I., Donker, G.H., Daroszewski, J. et al. On the significance of in situ production of oestrogens in human breast cancer tissue. J. Steroid Biochem Mol. Biol. 41: 891–896, 1992.

291. Duncan, L.J. and Reed, M.J. The role and proposed mechanism by which oestradiol 17β-hydroxysteroid dehydrogenase regulates breast tumour oestrogen concentrations. J. Steroid Biochem Mol. Biol. 55: 565–572, 1995.

292. van Landeghem, AA.J., Poortman, J., Nabuurs, M. and Thijssen, J.H.H. Endogenous concentration and subcellular distribution of estrogens in normal and malignant human breast tissue. Cancer Res. 45: 2900–2906, 1985.

293. Pasqualini, J.R., Chetrite, G., Nguyen, B.L., Maloche, C. et al. Estrone sulfate-sulfatase and 17β-hydroxysteroid dehydrogenase activities: a hypothesis for their role in the evolution of human breast cancer from hormone-dependence to hormone-independence. J. Steroi Biochem. Mol. Biol. 53: 407–412, 1995.

294. Reed, M.J., Purohit, A., Duncan, L.J., Singh, A. et al. The role of cytokines and sulfatase inhibitors in regulating oestrogen synthesis in breast tumours. J. Steroid Biochem Mol. Biol. 53: 413–420, 1995.

295. Goss, P.E. and Tye, L.M. Anastrozole: a new selective non-steroidal aromatase inhibitor. Oncology 11: 1697–1703; discussion 1707–1708, 1997.

296. Dowsett, M. Future use of aromatase inhibitors in breast cancer. J. Steroid Biochem Mol. Biol. 61: 261–266, 1997.

297. Miller, W.R. and O'Neill, J. The importance of local synthesis of oestrogen with the breast. Steroids 50: 537–548, 1987.

298. Bulun, S.E., Price, T.M. and Aitken, J. A link between breast cancer and local oestrogen synthesis suggested by quantification of breast tissue aromatase cytochrome P450 transcripts using polymerase chain reaction. J. Clin. Endocr. Metab. 77: 1622–1628, 1993.

299. Gunson, D.E., Steele, R.E. and Chau, R.Y., Prevention of spontaneous tumours in female rats by fadrozole hydrochloride, an aromatase inhibitor. Br. J. Cancer 72: 72–75, 1995.

300. Grubbs, C.J., Decoster, R., Bowden, C.R., Steele, V.E. et al. Vorozole, an aromatase inhibitor, as a chemopreventive agent in methylnitrosourea (MNU)-induced mammary cancer model. Proc Am. Assoc. Cancer Res. 37: 274, 1996.

301. Kelloff, G.J., Lubet, R.A., Lieberman, R., Eisenhauer, K., Steele, V.E., Crowell, J.A., Hawk, E.T., Boone, C.W. and Sigman, C.C. Aromatase inhibitors as potential cancer chemopreventives. Cancer Epidemiol. Biomarker Prevent. 7: 65–78, 1998.

302. Reed, M.J. and Purohit, A. Sulfatase inhibitors: the rationale for the development of a new endocrine therapy. Rev. Endocrine-Related Cancer 45: 51–62, 1993.

303. Falany, J.L. and Falany, C.N. Expression of cytosolic sulfotransferases in normal mammary epithelial cells and breast cancer cell lines. Cancer Res. 56: 1551–1555, 1996.

304. Loriaux, D.L., Ruder, H.J. and Lipsett, M.B. The measurement of estrone sulfate in plasma. Steroids 18: 463–472, 1971.

305. Roberts, K.D., Rochefort, J.G., Bleau, G. and Chapdelaine, A. Plasma estrone sulfate levels in postmenopausal women. Steroids 35: 179–187, 1980.

306. Inada, K., Tominaga, T., Toi, M., Yamamoto, Y., Abe, M., Yamashita, J. and Ogawa, M. Protective effect of leuprolide acetate on 7,12-dimethylbenz(a)anthracene (DMBA)-induced mammary carcinogenesis in rats. Eur. J. Surg. Oncol. 22: 583-587, 1996.

307. Wong, C.K. and Keung, W.M. Daidzein sulfoconjugates are potent inhibitors of sterol sulfatase (EC 3.1.6.2). Biochem. Biophys. Res. Commun. 233: 579–583, 1997.

308. Orentreich, N., Brind, J.L. and Rizer, R.L. Age changes and sex differences in serum dehydroepiandrosterone sulfate concentrations throughout adulthood. J. Clin. Endocrinol. Metab. 59: 551–555, 1984.

309. Gordon, C.B., Shantz, L.M. and Talalay, P. Modulation of growth, differentiation and carcinogenesis by dehydroepiandrosterone. Adv. Enzyme Regul. 26: 355–382, 1987.

310. Gordon, G.B., Bush, T.L., Helzlsouer, K.J., Miller, S.R. and Constock, G.W. Relationship of serum levels of dehydroepiandrosterone and dehydroepiandrosterone sulfate to the risk of developing postmenopausal breast cancer. Cancer Res. 50: 3859–3862, 1990.

311. Secreto, G., Toniolo, P., Berrino, F., Recchione, C., et al. Serum and urinary androgens and risk of breast cancer in postmenopausal women. Cancer Res. 51: 2572–2576, 1991.

312. Pashko, L.L., Schwartz, A.G., Abou-Gharbia, M. and Swern, D. Inhibition of DNA synthesis in mouse epidermis and

breast epithelium by dehydroepiandrosterone and related steroids. Carcinogenesis 2: 717–721, 1981.

313. Boccuzzi, G., Brignardello, E., DiMonoco, M., Forte, C., Leonardi, L. and Pizzini, A. Influence of dehydroepiandrosterone and 5-en-androstene-3β, 17β-diol on the growth of MCF-7 human breast cancer cells induced by 17β-estradiol. Anticancer Res. 12: 799–804, 1992b.

314. Schwartz, A.G. Inhibition of spontaneous breast cancer formation in C3H-A^{vy}/a mice by long-term treatment with dehydroepiandrosterone. Cancer Res. 39: 1129–1132, 1979.

315. Ratko, T.A., Mehta, R.G., Detrisac, C.J., Kelloff, G.J. and Moon, R.C. Inhibition of rat mammary gland chemical carcinogenesis by dietary dehydroepiandrosterone or a fluorinated analogue of dehydroepiandrosterone. Cancer Res. 51: 481–486, 1991.

316. Boccuzzi, G., Aragno, M., Brignardello, E., Tamagno, E., et al. Opposite effects of dehydroepiandrosterone on the growth of 7,12-dimethyl-benz(a)anthracene-induced rat mammary carcinomas. Anticancer Res. 12: 1479–1484, 1992a.

317. Li, S., Yan, X., Belanger, A. and Labrie, F. Prevention by dehydroepiandrosterone of the development of mammary carcinoma induced by 7,12-dimethylbenz(a)anthracene (DMBA) in the rat. Breast Cancer Res. Treat. 29: 203–217, 1993.

318. Lubet, R.A., Gordon, G.B., Prough, R.A., Lei, X.D., You, M., Wang, Y., Grubbs, C.J., Steele, V.E., Kelloff, G.J., Thomas, C.F. and Moon, R.D. Modulation of methylnitrosourea-induced breast cancer in Sprague Dawley rats by dehydroepiandrosterone: dose-dependent inhibition, effects of limited exposure, effects on peroxisomal enzymes, and lack of effects on levels of Ha-Ras mutations. Cancer Res. 58: 921–926, 1998.

319. Schwartz, A.G., Lewbart, M.L. and Pashko, L.L. Novel dehydroepiandrosterone analogues with enhanced biological activity and reduced side effects in mice and rats. Cancer Res. 48: 4817–4822, 1988.

320. Schwartz, A.G. and Pashko, L.L. Cancer prevention with dehydroepiandrosterone and non-androgenic structural analogs. J. Cell. Biochem. Suppl. 22: 210–217, 1995.

321. McCormick, D.L., Rao, K.V.N., Johnson, W.D., Bowman-Gram, T.A., et al. Exceptional chemopreventive activity of low-dose dehydroepiandrosterone in the rat mammary gland. Cancer Res. 56: 1724–1726, 1996.

322. Messina, M., Persky, V., Setchell, K.D.R. and Barnes, S. Soy intake and cancer risk: a review of in vitro and in vivo data. Nutr. Cancer 21: 113–131, 1994.

323. Troll, W., Wiesner, R., Shellabarger, C.J., Holtzman, S. and Stone, J.P. Soybean diet lowers breast cancer incidence in irradiated rats. Carcinogenesis 1: 469–472, 1980.

324. Barnes, S., Grubbs, C., Setchell, K.D.R. and Carlson, J. Soybeans inhibits mammary tumors in models of breast cancer. In: Mutagens and Carcinogens in the Diet (Pariza, M. ed). Wiley-Liss, New York. 1990. pp 239–253.

325. Gotoh, T., Yamada, K., Yin, H., Ito, A., Kataoka, T. and Dohi, K. Chemoprevention of N-nitroso-N-methylurea-induced rat mammary carcinogenesis by soy foods or biochanin A. Jpn J. Cancer Res. 89: 137–142, 1998.

326. Messina, M. and Barnes, S. The role of soy products in reducing risk of cancer. J. Natl. Cancer Inst. 83: 541–546, 1991.

327. Lu, L.J.W., Anderson, K.E., Grady, J.J. and Nagamani, M. Effects of soya consumption for one month on steroid hormones in premenopausal women: Implication for breast cancer risk reduction. Cancer Epidemiol. Biomarkers Prevent. 5: 63–70, 1996.

328. Fernandes, A.O. and Banerji, A.P. Long-term feeding of field bean protein containing protease inhibitors suppresses virus-induced mammary tumors in mice. Cancer Lett. 116: 1–7, 1997.

329. Constantinou, A., Mehta, R.G. and Vaughan, A. Inhibition of N-methyl-N-nitrosourea-induced mammary tumors in rats by the soybean isoflavones. Anticancer Res. 16: 3293–3298, 1996.

330. Adlercreutz, H. Quantitative determination of lignans and isoflavonoids in plasma of omnivorous and vegetarian women by isotope dilution gas chromatography-mass spectrometry. Scand. J. Clin. Lab. Invest. 53(suppl. 215): 5–18, 1993.

331. Adlercreutz, H., Fotsis, T., Bannwart, C., Wahala, K., Brunow, G. and Hase, T. Isotope dilution gas chromatographic-mass spectrometric method for the determination of lignans and isoflavonoids in human urine, including identification of genistein. Clin. Chim. Acta 199: 263–278, 1991.

332. Lu, L.J.W., Hokanson, J.A., Anderson, K.E., Marchall, M.V., et al. Urinary excretion of isflavones in healthy subjects after soymilk consumption. Proc. Am. Assoc. Cancer Res. 34: 556, 1993.

333. Barnes, S., Peterson, T.G. and Coward, L. Rationale for the use of genistein-containing soy matrices in chemoprevention trials for breast and prostate cancer. J. Cell. Biochem. – Supplement 22: 181–187, 1995.

334. Peterson, G. and Barnes, S. Genistein inhibits the growth of human breast cancer cells: independence from estrogen receptors and the multi-drug resistance gene. Biochem. Biophys. Res. Commun. 179: 661–667, 1991.

335. Pagliacci, M.C., Smacchia, M., Migliorati, G., Grignani, F., Riccardi, C. and Nicoletti, I. Growth-inhibitory effects of the natural phytoestrogen genistein in MCF-7 human breast cancer cells. Eur. J. Cancer 30A: 1675–1682, 1994.

336. Giri, A.K. and Lu, L.J.W. Genetic damage and the inhibition of 7,12-dimethylbenz[a]anthacene-induced genetic damage by the phytoestrogens, genistein and daidzein, in female ICR mice. Cancer Lett. 95: 125–133, 1995.

337. Fotsis, T., Pepper, M., Aldercreutz, H., Fleischmann, G., et al. Genistein, a dietary-derived inhibitor of in vitro angiogenesis. Proc. Natl. Acad. Sci. USA 90: 2690–2694, 1993.

338. Lamartiniere, C.A., Moore, J., Brown, N.M., Thompson, R., Hardin, M.J. and Barnes, S. Genistein suppresses mammary cancer in rats. Carcinogenesis 16: 2833–2840, 1995.

339. Barnes, S. The chemopreventive properties of soy isoflavonoids in animal models of breast cancer. Breast Cancer Res. Treat. 46: 169–179, 1997.

340. Lamartiniere, C.A., Moore, J., Holland, M. and Barnes, S. Neonatal genistein chemoprevents mammary cancer. Proc. Soc. Exp. Biol. Med. 208: 120–123, 1995.

341. Wang, T.T.Y., Sathyamoorthy, N. and Phang, J.M. Molecular effects of genistein on estrogen receptor mediated pathways. Carcinogenesis 17: 271–275, 1996.

342. Makela, S., Poutanen, M., Lehtimaki, J., Kostian, M.L., Santti, R. and Vihko, R. Estrogen-specific 17 beta-hydroxysteroid oxidoreductase type 1 (E.C. 1.1.1.62) as a possible target for the action of phytoestrogens. Proc. Soc. Exp. Biol. Med. 208: 51–59, 1995.

343. Akiyama, T., Ishida, J., Nakagawa, S., Ogawara, H., et al. Genistein, a specific inhibitor of tyrosine-specific protein kinases. J. Biol. Chem. 262: 5592–5595, 1987.

344. Shao, Z.M., Alpaugh, M.L., Fontana, J.A. and Barsky, S.H. Genistein inhibits proliferation similarly in estrogen receptor-positive and negative human breast carcinoma cell lines characterized by P21WAF1/CIP1 induction, G2/M arrest, and apoptosis. J. Cell. Biochem. 69: 44–54, 1998.

345. Waldhuser, F., Weissenbacher, G., Zeitlhuber, U., Waldhuser, M. and Wurtman, R.J. Fall in nocturnal serum melatonin levels during prepuberty and pubescence. Lancet 1: 362–365, 1984.

346. Hariharasubramanian, N., Nair, N.P.V. and Piplil, C. Circadian rhythm of plasma melatonin and cortisol during the menstrual cycle. In: The Pineal Gland: Endocrine Aspects (Bown, G.M. and Wainwright, S.D. eds), Pergamon Press, Toronto. 1984. Vol. 1, pp. 131–135.

347. Martin, J.E. and Sattler, C. Selectivity of melatonin pituitary inhibition for luteinizing hormone-releasing hormone. Neuroendocrinology 34: 112–116, 1982.

348. Walker, R.F., McCamant, S. and Timiras, P.S. Melatonin and the influence of the pineal gland on the timing of the LH surge in rats. Neuroendocrinology 35: 37–42, 1982.

349. Wurtman, R.J., Axelrod, J. and Chu, E.W. Melatonin, a pineal substance: effect on the rat ovary. Science 141: 277–278, 1963.

350. Ying, S.Y. and Greep, Y.O. Inhibition of ovulation by melatonin in the cyclic rat. Endocrinology 93: 333–335, 1973.

351. Blask, D. Melatonin in oncology. In: Melatonin Biosynthesis, Physiological Effects and Clinical Applications (Yu, H.S. and Reiter, R.J. eds). CRC Press, Boca Raton, FL. 1993. pp 447–475.

352. Blask, D.E., Wilson, S.T., Zalatan, F. Physiological melatonin inhibition of human breast cancer cell growth in vitro: evidence for a glutathione-mediated pathway. Cancer Res. 57: 1909–1914, 1997.

353. Kothari, A., Borges, A., Ingle, A. and Kothari, L. Combination of melatonin and tamoxifen as a chemoprophylaxis against N-nitroso-N-methylurea-induced rat mammary tumors. Cancer Lett. 111: 59–66, 1997.

354. Higgs, G.A. and Vane, J.R. Inhibition of cyclooxygenase and lipoxygenase. Br. Med. Bull. 39: 265–270, 1983.

355. Carter, C.A., Milholland, R.J., Shea, W. and Ip, M.M. Effect of the prostaglandin synthase inhibitor indomethacin on 7,12-dimethylbenz(a)anthracene-induced mammary tumorigenesis in rats fed different levels of fat. Cancer Res. 43: 3559–3562, 1983.

356. Fulton, A.M. In vivo effects of indomethacin on the growth of murine mammary tumors. Cancer Res. 44: 2416–2420, 1984.

357. McCormick, D.L., Madigan, M.J. and Moon, R.C. Modulation of rat mammary carcinogenesis by indomethacin. Cancer Res. 45: 1803–1808, 1985.

358. Karmali, R.A., Welt, S., Thaler, H.T. and Lefevre, F. Prostaglandins in breast cancer: Relationship to disease stage and hormone status. Br. J. Cancer 48: 689–696, 1983.

359. Watson, J. and Chuah, S.Y. Prostaglandins, steroids and human breast cancer. Eur. J. Cancer Clin. Oncol. 21: 1051–1055, 1985.

360. Karmali, R.A., Thaler, H.T. and Cohen, L.A. Prostaglandin concentrations and prostaglandin synthase activity in N-nitrosamethylurea-induced rat mammary carcinoma. Eur. J. Cancer Clin. Oncol. 19: 817–823, 1983.

361. Tan, W.C., Privett, O.S. and Goldyne, M.E. Studies of prostaglandins in rat mammary tumors induced by 7,12-dimethylbenz(a)anthracene. Cancer Res. 34: 3229–3231, 1974.

362. Karmali, R.A. Eicosanoids in neoplasia. Prev, Med. 16: 483–502, 1987.

363. Kaizer, F., Boyd, N.F., Kriukow, V. and Trichler, D. Fish consumption and breast cancer risk: an ecological study. Nutr. Cancer 12: 61–68, 1989.

364. Iso, H., Sato, S., Folsom, A.R., Shimamoto, T., et al. Serum fatty acids and fish intake in rural Japanese, urban Japanese, Japanese American and Caucasian American men. Int. J Epidemiol. 18: 374–381, 1989.

365. Sinclair, H.M. The relative importance of essential fatty acids of the linoleic and linolenic families: studies with an Eskimo diet. Prog. Lipid Res. 20: 897–899, 1981.

366. Cohen, L.A., Chen-Backlund, J.Y., Sepkovic, D.W. and Sugie, S. Effect of varying proportions of dietary menhaden and corn oil on experimental rat mammary tumor proliferation. Lipids 28: 449–456, 1993.

367. Telang, N.T., Bradlow, H.L. and Osborne, M.P. Molecular and endocrine biomarkers in non-involved breast: relevance to cancer chemoprevention. J. Cell. Biochem. 16G: 161–169, 1992.

368. Gabor, H. and Abraham. Effect of dietary menhaden oil on tumor cell loss and accumulation of the mass of a transplantable mammary adenocarcinoma in BALB/c mice. J. Natl. Cancer Inst. 76: 1223–1229, 1986.

369. Noguchi, M., Minami, M., Yagasaki, T., Kinoshita, K., et al. Chemoprevention of DMBA-induced mammary carcinogenesis in rats by low-dose EPA and DHA. Br. J. Cancer 75: 348–353, 1997.

370. McCormick, D.L. and Moon, R.C. Inhibition of mammary carcinogenesis by flurbiprofen, an non-steroidal antiinflammatory agent. Br. J. Cancer 48: 859–861, 1983.

371. Lee, P.P. and Ip. M.M. Regulation of proliferation of rat mammary tumor cells by inhibitors of cyclooxygenase and

lipoxygenase. Prostaglandins Leukot Essent Fatty Acids 45: 21–31, 1992.

372. Kitagawa, H. and Noguchi, M. Comparative effects of piroxicam and escueletin on incidence, proliferation and cell kinetics of mammary carcinomas induced by 7,12-dimethylben(a)anthracene in rats on high and low fat diets. Oncology 51: 401-410, 1994.

373. Earashi, M., Noguchi, M. and Tanaka, M. In vitro effects of eicosanoid synthesis inhibitors in the presence of linoleic acid on MDA-MB-231 human breast cancer cells. Breast Cancer Res. Treat. 37: 29–37, 1996.

374. Thompson, H.J., Briggs, S., Paranka, N.S., Piazza, G.A., Brendel, K., Gross, P.H., et al., Inhibition of mammary carcinogenesis in rats by sulfone metabolites of sulindac. J. Natl Cancer Inst. 87: 1259–1260, 1995.

375. Pereira, M.A., Grubbs, C.J., Barnes, L.H., Li, H., Olson, G.R., Eto, I., Juliana, M., Whitaker, L.M., Kelloff, G.J., Steele, V.E. and Lubet, R.A. Effects of the phytochemicals, curcumin and quercetin, upon azoxymethane-induced colon cancer and 7,12-dimethylbenz(a)anthracene-induced mammary cancer in rats. Carcinogenesis 17: 1305–1311, 1996.

376. Deshpande, S.S., Ingle, A.D. and Maru, G.B. Chemopreventive efficacy of curcumin-free aqueous turmeric extract in 7,12-dimethylbenz[a]anthracene-induced rat mammary tumorigenesis. Cancer Lett. 123: 35–40, 1998.

377. Harris, R.E., Nambodiri, K.K., Stellman, S.D. and Wynder, E.L. Breast cancer and NSAID use: heterogeneity of effect in a case-control study. Prev. Med. 24: 119–120, 1995.

378. Harris, R.E., Nambodiri, K.K. and Farrar, W.B. Non-steroidal anti-inflammatory drugs and breast cancer. Epidemiology 7: 203–205, 1996.

379. Egan, K.M., Stampfer, M.J., Giovannucci, E., Rosner, B.A. and Colditz, G.A. Prospective study of regular aspirin use and the risk of breast cancer. J. Natl Cancer Inst. 88: 988–993, 1996.

380. Sathyamoorthy, N., Wang, T.Y. and Phang, J.M. Stimulation of pS2 expression by diet-derived compounds. Cancer Res. 54: 957–961, 1994.

381. Johnson, F.C. A critical review of the safety of phenolic antioxidants in food. CRC Crit. Rev. Food Technol. 2: 267–304, 1971.

382. McCormick, D.L. and Spicer, A.M. Nordihydroguaiaretic acid suppression of rat mammary carcinogenesis induced by N-methyl-N-nitrosourea. Cancer Lett. 37: 139–146, 1987.

383. Rillema, J.A. Effects of NDGA, a lipoxygenase inhibitor, on prolactin actions in mouse mammary gland explants. Prostaglandins, Leukotriene Med. 16: 89–94. 1984.

384. Dickson, R.B., Johnson, M.D., Bano, M., Shi, E., et al. Growth factors in breast cancer: mitogenesis to transformation. J. Steroid Biochem. Mol. Biol. 43: 69–78, 1992.

385. Rosen, J.M., Humphreys, R., Krnacik, S., Juo, P. et al. The regulation of mammary gland development by hormones, growth factors, and oncogenes. Prog. Clin. Biol. Res. 387: 95–111, 1994.

386. Furr, B. and Jordan, C. The pharmacology and clinical uses of tamoxifen. Pharmac. Ther. 25: 127–205, 1984.

387. Jordan, V.C. Tamoxifen: the herald of a new era of preventive therapeutics. J. Natl. Cancer Inst. 89: 747–749, 1997.

388. Early Breast Cancer Trialists' Group. Systemic treatment of early breast cancer by hormonal, cytotoxic, or immune therapy. 133 randomised trials involving 31,000 recurrences and 24,000 deaths among 75,000 women. Lancet 339: 1–15, 1992.

389. Swedish Breast Cancer Cooperative Group. Randomized trial of two versus five years of adjuvant tamoxifen for postmenopausal early stage breast cancer. J. Natl. Cancer Inst. 88: 1543–1549, 1996.

390. Jordan, V.C. Antitumor activity of the antiestrogen ICI 46,474 (tamoxifen) in the dimethylbenzanthracene (DMBA)-induced rat mammary carcinoma model. J. Steroid Biochem. 5: 354, 1974.

391. Jordan, V.C. Effect of tamoxifen (ICI 46,474) on the initiation and growth of DMBA-induced rat mammary carcinoma. Eur. J. Cancer 12: 419–424, 1976.

392. Maltoni, C., Minardi, F., Pinto, C., Belpoggi, F. and Bua, L. Results of three life-span experimental carcinogenicity and anticarcinogenicity studies on tamoxifen in rats. Ann. N.Y. Acad. Sci. 837: 469–512, 1997.

393. Cook, L.S., Weiss, N.S., Schwartz, S.M., White, E., et al. Population-based study of tamoxifen therapy and subsequent ovarian, endometrial and breast cancers. J. Natl. Cancer Inst. 87: 1359–1364, 1995.

394. Ursin, G., Pike, M.C., Spicer, D.V., Porrath, S.A. et al. Can mammographic densities predict effects of tamoxifen on the breast [letter]. J. Natl. Cancer Inst. 88: 128–129, 1996..

395. Jordan, V.C. (ed) Tamoxifen: a guide for clinicians and patients. PRR Inc., Huntington, NY. 1996.

396. Cuzick, J. Chemoprevention of breast cancer with tamoxifen. IARC Scientif. Pub. 136: 95–109, 1996.

397. McDonald, C.C. and Stewart, H.J., The Scottish Breast Cancer Committee. Fetal Myocardial infarction in the Scottish tamoxifen trial. B. M. J. 303: 435–437, 1991.

398. Rutqvist, L.E., Mattson, A. and The Stockholm Breast Cancer Study Group. Cardiac and thromboembolic morbidity among postmenopausal women with early-stage breast cancer in a randomized trial of adjuvant tamoxifen. J. Natl. Cancer Inst. 85: 1398–1406, 1993.

399. McDonald, C.C., Alexander, F.E., Whyte, B.W., Forrest, A. P. and Stewart, H.J. Cardiac and vascular morbidity in women receiving with adjuvant tamoxifen for breast cancer in a randomized trial. B.M.J. 311: 977–980, 1995.

400. Costantino, J.P., Kuller, L.H., Ives, D.G., Fisher, B. and Diagnam, J. Coronary heart disease mortality and adjuvant tamoxifen therapy. J. Natl. Cancer Inst. 89: 776–782, 1997.

401. Turken, S., Siris, E., Seldin, d., Flaster, E., Hyman, G. and Lindsay, R. Effects of tamoxifen on spinal bone density in women with breast cancer. J. Natl. Cancer Inst. 81: 1086–1088, 1989.

402. Love, R.R., Mazess, R.B., Barden, H.S., Epstein, S., et al. Effects of tamoxifen on bone mineral density in postmenopausal women with breast cancer. New Engl. J. Med. 326: 852–856, 1992.

403. Chang, J., Powles, T.J., Ashley, S.E., Gregory, R.K., et al. The Effects of tamoxifen and hormone replacement therapy on serum cholesterol, bone mineral density and coagulation factors in healthy postmenopausal women participating in a randomized controlled tamoxifen prevention study. Am. Oncol. 7: 671–675, 1996.

404. Powles, T.J., Hickish, T., Kanis, J.A., Tidy, A. and Ashley, S. Effect of tamoxifen on bone mineral density measured by dual-energy x-ray absorptiometry in healthy premenopausal and postmenopausal women. J. Clin. Oncol. 14: 78–84, 1996.

405. Anderson, T.J. Normal breast: myths, realities, and prospects. Modern Pathol. 11: 115–119, 1998.

406. Fornander, T., Rutqvist, L.E., Wilking, N., Carlstrom, K. and Schoultz, B. Oestrogenic effects of adjuvant tamoxifen in postmenopausal breast cancer. Enr. J. Cancer 29A: 497–500, 1993.

407. Van Leevwen, F.E., Benraadt, J., Coebergh, J.W.W., et al. Risk of endometrial cancer after tamoxifen treatment of breast cancer. Lancet 343: 448–452, 1994.

408. Magriples, U., Naftolin, F., Schwartz, P.E., Carcangiu, M.L., et al. High-grade endometrial carcinoma in tamoxifen-treated breast cancer patients. J. Clin. Oncol. 11: 485–490, 1993.

409. Assikis, V.J., Neven, P., Jordan, V.C. and Vergote, I. A realistic clinical perspective of tamoxifen and endometrial carcinogenesis. Eur. J. Cancer 32A: 1464–1476, 1996.

410. Gallo, M.A. and Kaufman, D. Antagonistic and agonistic effects of tamoxifen: significance in human cancer. Sem. Oncol. 24(Suppl 1): S1–71–S1–80, 1997.

411. Smith, L.L. and White, I.N. Chemoprevention of breast cancer by tamoxifen: risks and opportunities. Toxicol. Lett. 82–83: 181–186, 1995.

412. Pace, P., Jarman, M., Phillips, D., Hewer, A., Bliss, J. and Coombes, R.C. Idoxifene is equipotent to tamoxifen in inhibiting mammary carcinogenesis but forms lower levels of hepatic DNA adducts. Br. J. Cancer 76: 700–704, 1997.

413. Bitonti, A.J., Baumann, R.J., Bush, T.L., Cashman, E.A., Wright, C.L. and Prakash, N.J. Antitumor and chemopreventive effects of a clomiphene analog, MDL 103,323, in mammary carcinoma. Anticancer Res. 16: 2553–2557, 1996.

414. Draper, M.W., Flowers, D.E., Huster, W.J., Neild, J.A., et al. A controlled trial of raloxifene (LY139481) HCl: impact on bone turnover and serum lipid profile in healthy postmenopausal women. J. Bone. Miner. Res. 11: 835–842, 1996.

415. Black, L.J., Jones, C.D. and Falcones, J.F. Antagonism of estrogen action with a new benothiophene derived antiestrogen. Life Sci. 32: 1031–1036, 1983.

416. Black, L.J., Sato, M., Rowley, E.R., Magee, D.E., et al. Raloxifene (LY139481 HCl) prevents bone loss and reduces serum cholesterol without causing uterine hypertrophy in ovariectomized rats. J. Clin. Invet. 93: 63–69, 1994.

417. Gottardis, M.M. and Jordan, V.C. Antitumor actions of keoxifene and tamoxifen in the N-nitrosomethylurea-induced rat mammary carcinoma model. Cancer Res. 47: 4020–4024, 1987.

418. McDougal, A., Wilson, C. and Safe, S. Inhibition of 7,12-dimethylbenz[a]anthracene-induced rat mammary tumor growth by aryl hydrocarbon receptor agonists. Cancer Lett. 120: 53–63, 1997

419. Liu, H., Wormke, M., Safe, S. and Bjeldanes, L.F. Indolo[3,2-b]carbazole, a dietary factor which exhibits both antoestrogenic and estrogenic activity. J. Natl. Cancer Inst 86: 1758–1765, 1994.

420. Tiwari, R.K., Guo, L., Bradlow, H.L., Telang, N.T., and Osborne, M.P. Selective responsiveness of breast cancer cells to indole-3-carbinol, a chemopreventive agent. J. Natl. Cancer Inst. 86: 126–131, 1994.

421. Grubbs, C.J., Steele, V.E., Casebolt, T., Juliana, M.M. et al. Chemoprevention of chemically-induced mammary carcinogenesis by indole-3-carbinol. Anticancer Res. 15: 709–716, 1995.

422. Safe, S. Modulation of gene expression and endocrine response pathways by 2,3,7,8-tetrachlorodibenzo-r-dioxin and related compounds. Pharmacol. Ther. 67: 247–281, 1995.

423. Astroff, B. and Safe, S. Comparative antiestrogenic activities of 2,3,7,8-tetrachlorodibenzo-r-dioxin and 6-methyl-1,3,8-trichlorodibenzofuran in the female rat. Toxicol. Appl. Pharmacol. 95: 435–443, 1988.

424. Astroff, B. and Safe, S. 6-Alkyl-1,3,8-trichlorodibenzofuran as antiestrogens in female Sprague-Dawley rats. Toxicology 69: 187–197, 1991.

425. Zaccharewski, T., Harris, M., Biegel, L., Morrison, V., Merchant, M. and Safe, S. 6-Methyl-1,3,8-trichlorodibenzofuran (MCDF) as an antiestrogen in human and rodent cancer cell lines: evidence for the role of Ah receptors. Toxicol. Appl. Pharmacol. 113: 311–318, 1992.

426. Dickerson, R., Howie-Keller, L. and Safe, S. Alkyl polychlorated dibenzofurans and related compounds as antiestrogens in the female rat uterus: structure-activity studies. Toxicol. Appl. Pharmacol. 135: 287–298, 1995.

427. Hill, C.S. and Treisman, R. Transcriptional regulation by extracellular signals: mechanisms and specificity. Cell 80: 199–211, 1995.

428. Karin, M. and Hunter, T. Transcriptional control by protein phosphorylation: signal transmission from the cell surface to nucleus. Curr. Biol. 5: 747–757, 1995.

429. Levitzki, A. and Gazit, A. Tyrosine kinase inhibition: an approach to drug development. Science 267: 1782–1788, 1995.

430. Cooper, G.M. Oncogenes and growth factors. In: Oncogenes. Jones and Barlett Publishers, Boston. 1990. pp 163–173.

431. Powis, G. Signaling pathways as targets for anticancer drug development. Pharmacol. Ther. 62: 57–95, 1994..

432. Kumar, V., Bustin, S.A. and McKay, I.A. Transforming growth factor α. Cell Biol. Int. 19: 373–388, 1995.

433. Kelloff, G.J., Fay, J.R., Steele, V.E., Lubert, R.A., et al. Epidermal growth factor tyrosine kinase inhibitors as potential cancer chemopreventives. Cancer Epidemiol Biomarker Prev. 5: 657–666, 1996.

434. Levitzki, A. Tyrphostins: tyrosine kinase blockers as novel antiproliferative agents and dissectors of signal transduction. FASEB J., 6: 3275–3282, 1992.

435. Zarbl, H., Sukumar, S., Arthur, A.V., Martin-Zanca, D. and Barbacid, M. Direct mutagenesis of Ha-ras-1 oncogenes in N-nitroso-N-methylurea during initiation of mammary carcinogenesis in rats. Nature (Lond.) 315: 382–385, 1985.

436. Dandekar, S., Sukumar, S., Zarbl, H., Young, L.J.T. and Cardiff, R.D. Specific activation of the cellular Harvey-ras oncogene in dimethylbenzanthracene-induced mouse mammary tumours. Mol. Cell. Biol. 6: 4104–4108, 1986.

437. Ohuchi, N., Thor, A., Page, D.L., Hand, P.H., Halter, S.A. and Schlom, J. Expression of the 21,000 molecular weight ras protein in a spectrum of benign and malignant human mammary tissues. Cancer Res. 46: 2511–2519, 1986.

438. Schafer, W.R., Kim, R., Sterne, R., Thorner, J., Kim, S.H. and Rine, J. Genetic and pharmacological suppression of oncogenic mutations in ras genes of yeast and humans. Science 245: 379–385, 1989.

439. Hancock, J.F., Magee, A.I., Childs, J.E. and Marshall, C.J. All ras proteins are polyisoprenylated and only some are palitoylated. Cell 57: 1167–1177, 1989.

440. Jackson, J.H., Cochrane, C.G., Bourne, J.R., Solski, P.A., Buss, J.E. and Der, C.J. Farnesol modification of Kirsten-ras exon 4B protein is essential for transformation. Proc. Natl. Acid. Sci. U.S.A. 87: 3042–3046, 1990.

441. Hohl, R.J. and Lewis, K. Differential effects of monoterpenes and lovastatin on RAS processing. J. Biol. Chem. 270: 17508–17512, 1995.

442. Sinensky, M., Beck, L.A., Leonard, S. and Evans, R. Differential inhibitory effects of lovastatin on protein isoprenylation and sterol synthesis. J. Biol. Chem. 265: 19937–19941, 1990.

443. Puppo, M.D., Rauli, S. and Kienle, M.D. Inhibition of cholesterol synthesis and hepatic 3-hyoy-3-mehtylglutaryl-CoA reductase in rats by simvastatin and pravastatin. Lipids 30: 1057–1061, 1995.

444. James, G.L., Goldstein, J.L., Brown, M.S., Rawson, T.E., et al. Benzodiazepine peptidomimetics: potent inhibitors of Ras farnesylation in animal cells. Science 260: 1937–1942, 1993.

445. Garcia, A.M., Rowell, C., Ackermann, K., Kowalczyk, J.J. and Lewis, M.D. Peptidomimetic inhibitors of Ras farnesylation and function in whole cells. J. Biol. Chem. 268: 18415–18418, 1993.

446. Gibbs, J.B., Pompliano, D.L., Mosser, S.D., Rands, E. et al. Selective inhibition of farnesyl transferase blocks ras processing in vivo. J. Biol. Chem. 268: 7617–7620, 1993.

447. Crowell, P.L., Ren, Z., Lin, S., Vedejs, E. and Gould, M.N. Structure-activity relationships among novel monoterpene inhibitors of small G protein isoprenylation and cell proliferation. Biochem. Pharmacol. 47: 1405–1415, 1994.

448. Goldstein, J.L. and Brown, M.S. Regulation of the mavalonate pathway. Nature (Lond.) 343: 425–430, 1990.

449. Alberts, A.W., Chen, J., Kuron, G., Hunt, V., et al. Mevinolin, a highly potent competitive inhibitor of hydroxymethyl-glutaryl-coenzyme A reductase and a cholesterol-lowering agent. Proc. Natl. Acad. Sci. U.S.A. 77: 3975–3961, 1980.

450. Addeo, R., Altuci, L., Battista, T., Bonapace, I.M., et al. Stimulation of human breast cancer MCF-7 cells with oestrogen prevents cell cycle arrest by HMG-CoA reductase inhibitors. Biochem. Biophys. Res. Commun. 220: 864–870, 1996.

451. Bonapace, I.M., Addeo, R., Altuci, L., Ciatiello, L., et al. 17β-Estradiol overcomes a G1 block induced by HMG-CoA reductase inhibitors and fosters cell cycle progression without inducing ERK-1 and –2 MAP kinases activation. Oncogene 12: 753–776, 1996.

452. Inano, H., Suzuki, K., Onoda, M. and Wakebayashi, K. Anticarcinogenic activity of simvastatin during the promotion phase of radiation-induced mammary tumorigenesis of rats. Carcinogenesis 18: 1723–1727, 1997.

453. Gould, M.N. Prevention and therapy of mammary cancer by monoterpenes. J. Cell. Biochem. Suppl. 22: 139–144, 1995.

454. Wattenberg, L.W. Inhibition of neoplasia by minor dietary constituents. Cancer Res. 43: 2448–2453, 1983.

455. Elgbede, J.A., Elson, C.E., Qureshi, A., Tanner, M.A. and Gould, M.N. Inhibition of DMBA-induced mammary cancer by the momoterpene d-limonene. 1984.

456. Gould, M.N., Moore, C.J., Zhang, R., Wang, B., Kennan, W.S. and Haad, J.D. Limonene chemoprevention of mammary carcinoma induction following direct in situ transfer of v-Ha-ras into rat mammary epithelial cells using replication-defective retroviral vectors. Cancer Res. 54: 3540–3543, 1994.

457. Crowell, P.L., Chang, R.R., Ren, Z., Elson, C.E. and Gould, M.N. Selective inhibition of isoprenylation of 21026 kda proteins by the anticarcinogen d-limonene and its metabolites. J. Biol. Chem. 266: 17679–17685, 1991.

458. Haag, J.D. and Gould, M.N. Mammary carcinoma regression induced by perillyl alcohol, a hydroxylated analog of limonene. Cancer Chemother. Pharmacol. 34: 477–483, 1994.

459. Karlson, J., Borg-Karlson, A.K., Unelius, R., Shoshan, M.C., Wilking, N., Ringborg, U. and Linder, S. Inhibition of tumor cell growth by monoterpenes in vitro: evidence of a Ras-independent mechanism of action. Anti-Cancer Drugs 7: 422–429, 1996.

460. Smith, M.A., Parkinson, D.R., Cheson, B.D. and Friedman, M.A. Retinoids in cancer therapy. J. Clin. Oncol. 10:839–864, 1992.

461. Sporn, M.B., Roberts, A.B. and Goodman, O.S. The Retinoids: Biology, Chemistry and Medicine (2nd ed), Raven Press, Ltd. New York, 1994

462. Pasquali, D., Bellastella, A., Valente, A., Botti, G., Capasso, I., del Vecchio, S., Salvatore, M., Colantuoni, V. and Sinisi, A.A. Retinoic acid receptors alpha, beta and gamma, and

cellular retinol binding protein-I expression in breast fibrocystic disease and cancer. Eur. J. Endocrinol. 137: 410–4, 1997.

463. Heyman, R.A., Mangelsdorf, D.J., Dyck, J.A., Stein, R.B., Evans, R.M. and Thaller, C. 9-cis-Retinoic acid is a high affinity ligand for the retinoic X receptor. Cell 68: 397–406, 1992.

464. Fanjul, A.N., Delia, D., Pierotti, M.A., Rideout, D., Qiu, J. and Pfahl, M. 4-Hydroxyphenyl retinamide is a highly selective activator of retinoid receptors. J. Biol. Chem. 271: 22441–22446, 1996.

465. Gottardis, M.M., Bischoff, E.D., Shirley, M.A., Wagoner, M.A., Lamph, W.W. and Heyman, R.A. Chemoprevention of mammary carcinoma by LGD1069 (Targretin): an RXR-selective ligand. Cancer Res. 56: 5566–5570, 1996.

466. Anzano, M.A., Byers, S.W., Smith, J.M., Peer, C.W., Mullen, L.T., Brown, C.C., et al. Prevention of breast cancer in the rat with 9-cis-retioid acid as a single agent or in combination with tamoxifen. Cancer Res. 54: 4614–4617, 1994.

467. Lippman, S.M., Heyman, R.A., Kurie, J.M., Benner, S.E., Hong, W.K. Retinoids and chemoprevention: Clinical and basic studies. J. Cell. Biochem. Suppl. 22: 1–10, 1995.

468. Anzano, M.A., Peer, C.W., Smith, J.M., Mullen, L.T., et al. Chemoprevention of mammary carcinogenesis in the rat: Combined use of Raloxifene and 9-cis-retioid acid. J. Natl. Cancer Inst. 88: 123–125, 1996.

469. Takatsuka, J., Takahashi, N. and De Luca, L.M. Retinoic acid metabolism and inhibition of cell proliferation: an unexpected liaison. Cancer Res. 56: 675–678, 1996.

470. Frolik, C.A., Roberts, T.E., Tavela, P.P., Newton, D. and Sporn, M.B. Isolation and identification of 4-hydroxy- and 4-oxoretinoic acid: in vitro metabolites of all-trans– retinoic acid in hamster trachea and liver. Biochemistry 18: 2092–2097, 1979.

471. Leo, M.A., Iida, S. and Lieber, C.S. Retinoid metabolism by a system reconstituted with cytochrome P-450. Arch. Biochem. Biophys. 234: 305–312, 1984.

472. Lee, P.P., Lee, M.T., Darcy, K.M., Shudo, K. and Ip, M.M. Modulation of normal mammary epithelial cell proliferation, morphogenesis, and functional differentiation by retinoids: a comparison of the retinobenzoic acid derivative RE80 with retinoic acid. Endocrinology 136: 1707–1717, 1995.

473. Toma, S., Isnardi, L., Raffo, P., Dastoli, G., De Francisci, E., Riccardi, L., Palumbo, R. and Bollag, W. Effects of all-trans-retinoic acid and 13-cis-retinoic acid on breast-cancer cell lines: growth inhibition and apoptosis induction. Int. J. Cancer 70: 619–627, 1997.

474. Sheikh, M.S., Shao, Z.M., Li, X.S., Ordonez, J.V., et al. N-(4-hydroxyphenyl)retinamide (4-HPR)-mediated biological actions involve retinoid receptor-independent pathways in human breast carcinoma. Carcinogenesis 16: 2477–2486, 1995.

475. Curley, R.W. Jr., Abou-Issa, H., Panigot, M.J., Repa, J.J., Clagett-Dame, M. and Alshafie, G. Chemopreventive activities of C-glucuronide/glycoside analogs of retinoid-O-glucuronides against breast cancer development and growth. Anticancer Res. 16: 757–763, 1996.

476. Bischoff, E.D., Gottardis, M.M., Moon, T.E., Heyman, R.A. and Lamph, W.W. Beyond tamoxifen: the retinoid X receptor-selective ligand LGD1069 (TARGRETIN) causes complete regression of mammary carcinoma. Cancer Res. 58: 479–484, 1998.

477. Lawrence, J.A., Merino M.J., Simpson, J.F., Manrow, R.E., Page, D.L. and Steeg, P.S. A high-risk lesion for invasive breast cancer, ductal carcinoma in situ, exhibits frequent overexpression of retinoid X receptor. Cancer Epidemiol. Biomarker Prevent. 7: 29–35, 1998.

478. Veronesi, U., De Palo, G., Coasta, a., Formelli, F. and Decensi, A. Chemoprevention of breast cancer with fenretinide. IARC Scientific. Pub. 136: 87–94, 1996.

479. De Palo, G., Camerini, T., Marubini, E., Costa, A., Formelli, F., Del Vecchio, M., Mariani, L., Miceli, R., Mascotti, G., Magni, A., Campa, T., Di Mauro, M.G., Attili, A., Maltoni, C., Del Turco, M.R., Decensi, A., D'Aiuto, G. and Veronesi, U. Chemoprevention trial of contralateral breast cancer with fenretinide. Rationale, design, methodology, organization, data management, statistics and accrual. Tumori 83: 884–894, 1997.

480. Bruynseels, J., De Coster, R., van Rooy, P., Wouters, W., et al. R75251, a new inhibitor of steroid biosynthesis. Prostate 16: 345–359, 1990.

481. van Ginckel, R., De Coster, R., Wouters, W., Vanherck, W., et al. Antitumoral effects of R 85251 on the growth of transplantable R3327 prostatic adenocarcinoma in rats. Prostate 16: 313–323, 1990.

482. Mahler, c., Verhelst, J. and Denis, L. Ketoconazole and liarozole in the treatment of advanced prostatic cancer. Cancer 71: 1068–1073, 1992.

483. Dijkman, G.A., van Moorselaar, R.J.A., van Ginckel, R., van Stratum, P., et al. Antitumoral effects of liarozole in androgen-dependent and independent R3327-Dunning prostate adenocarcinomas. J. Urol. 151: 217–222, 1994.

484. Van Wauwe, J.P., Coene, M.C., Goossens, J., Cools, W. and Monbaliu, J. Effects of cytochrome P-450 inhibitors on the metabolism of all-trans-retinoic acid in rats. J. Pharmacol. Exp. Ther. 252: 365–369, 1990.

485. Wouters, W., van Dun, J., Dillen, A., Coene, M.C., Cools, W. and De Coster, R. Effects of liarozole, a new antitumoral compound, on retinoic acid-induced inhibition of cell growth and on retinoic acid metabolism in MCF-7 human breast cancer cells. Cancer Res. 52: 2841–2846, 1992.

486. De Waard, F. and Trichopoulos, D. A unifying concept of the aetiology of breast cancer. Int. J. Cancer 41: 666–669, 1988.

487. Trichopoulos, D., Li, F.P. and Hunter, D.J. What causes cancer? Scientific American 275: 80–87, 1996.

488. MacMahon, B., Cole, P., Liu, M., Lowe, C.R., et al. Age at first birth and breast cancer risk. Bull. World Health Organ. 34: 209–221, 1970.

489. Russo, J. and Russo, I.H. Role of differentiation on transformation of human epithelial cells. In: Cellular and Molecular Biology of Mammary Cancer. (D. Medina et al., Eds.) Plenum Press, New York, 1987. pp. 399–417.

490. Russo, J. and Russo, I.H. Biological and Molecular Bases of Mammary Carcinogenesis. Lab. Invest 57: 112–137, 1987.

491. Russo, J., Saby, J., Isenberg, W. and Russo, I.H. Pathogenesis of mammary carcinomas induced in rats by 7,12-dimethylbenz(a)anthracene. J. Natl. Cancer Inst. 59:435–445, 1977.

492. Russo, J. and Russo, I.H. Susceptibility of the mammary gland to carcinogenesis. II. Pregnancy interruption as a risk factor in tumor incidence. Am. J. Pathol. 100: 497–512, 1980.

493. Russo, J. and Russo, I.H. Influence of differentiation and cell kinetics on the susceptibility of the mammary gland to carcinogenesis. Cancer Res. 40: 2677–2687, 1980.

494. Russo, I.H. and Russo, J. Developmental stage of the rat mammary gland as determinant of its susceptibility to 7,12-dimethylbenz(a)anthracene. J. Natl. Cancer Inst. 61: 1439–1449, 1978.

495. Russo, J., Wilgus, G. and Russo, I.H. Susceptibility of the mammary gland to carcinogenesis. I. Differentiation of the mammary gland as determinant of tumor incidence and type of lesion. Am. J. Pathol. 96: 721–734, 1979.

496. Russo, J. and Russo, I.H. Is Differentiation the Answer in Breast Cancer Prevention? Internat Res Com (IRCS) 10: 935–945, 1982.

497. Russo, J. and Russo, I.H. Physiological basis of breast cancer prevention. European J. Cancer Prev. 2: 101–111, 993.

498. Russo, I.H. and Russo, J. Hormone prevention of mammary carcinogenesis: a new approach in anticancer research. Anticancer Res. 8: 1247–1264, 1988.

499. Russo, I.H. and Russo, J. Hormone prevention of mammary carcinogenesis by norethynodrel-mestranol. Breast Cancer Res. Treat. 14: 43–56, 1989.

500. Alvarado, M.V., Russo, J. and Russo, I.H. Immunolocalization of inhibin in the mammary gland of rats treated with hCG. J. Histochem. Cytochem. 41: 29–34, 1992.

501. Matzuk, M.M., Finegold, M.J., Su, S.G.J., Husueh, A.J.W. and Bradley, A. Inhibin is tumour-suppressor gene with gonadal specificity in mice. Nature 360: 313–319, 1992.

502. Alvarado, M.V., Alvarado, N.E., Russo, J. and Russo, I.H. Human chorionic gonadotropin inhibits proliferation and induces expression of inhibins in human breast epithelial cells in vitro. In Vitro Cell Rev. Biol. 30A: 4–8, 1994.

503. Russo, J., Tay, L.K. and Russo, I.H. Differentiation of the mammary gland and susceptibility to carcinogenesis: a review. Breast Cancer Res. Treat. 2:5–73, 1982.

504. Berenblum, I. A speculative review: the probable nature of promoting action, its significance in the understanding of the mechanism of carcinogenesis. Cancer Res. 14: 471–476, 1976.

505. Frei, J.V. and Harsano, T. Increased susceptibility to low doses of carcinogen of epidermal cells in stimulated DNA synthesis. Cancer Res. 27: 1482–1491, 1967.

506. Marquardt, H., Baker, S., Tierney, B., Grover, P.L. and Sims, P. Comparison of mutagenesis and malignant transformation by dihydrodiols of 7,12-dimethylbenz(a)anthracene. Br. J. Cancer 9: 540–547, 1979.

507. Ciocca, D.R., Parente, A. and Russo, J. Endocrinological milieu and susceptibility of the rat mammary gland to carcinogenesis. Am. J. Pathol. 109: 47–56, 1982.

508. Tay, L.K. and Russo, J. 7,12-Dimethylbenz(a)anthracene (DMBA)-induced DNA binding and repair synthesis in susceptible and non-susceptible mammary epithelial cells in culture. J Natl Cancer Inst . 67: 155–161, 1981.

509. Tay, L.K. and Russo, J. Formation and removal of 7,12- dimethylbenz(a)anthracene nucleic acid adducts in rat mammary epithelial cells with different susceptibility to carcinogenesis. Carcinogenesis 2: 1327–1333, 1981.

510. Tay, L.K. and Russo, J. Effect of human chorionic gonadotropin on 7, 12-dimethylbenz (a)anthracene-induced DNA binding and repair synthesis by rat mammary epithelial cells. Chem.-Biol. Interact. 55: 13–21, 1985.

511. Russo, I.H., Koszalka, M.S. and Russo, J. Protective effect of chorionic gonadotropin on DMBA-induced mammary carcinogenesis. British Journal of Cancer 62: 243–247, 1990.

512. Chan, P.C. and Dao T.L. Effects of dietary fat on age-dependent sensitivity to mammary carcinogenesis. Cancer Lett. 18: 245–253, 1983.

513. Welsch, C.W. Host factors affecting the growth of carcinogen-induced rat mammary carcinomas; a review and tribute to Charles Brenton Huggins. Cancer Res. 45: 3415–3443, 1985.

514. Thompson, H.J. and Ronan, A. Effect of L-a-difluoromethylornithine and endocrine manipulation on the induction of mammary carcinogenesis by 1-methyl-1- nitrosourea. Carcinogenesis 57: 2003–2009, 1987.

515. Russo, I.H., Koszalka, M. and Russo, J. Comparative study of the influence of pregnancy and hormonal treatment on mammary carcinogenesis. Brit. J. Cancer 64: 481–484, 1991.

516. Russo, J. and Russo, I.H. Hormonally-induced differentiation; A novel approach to breast cancer prevention. J. Cell Biochem. 22: 58–64, 1995.

517. Srivastava, P., Russo, J. and Russo, I.H. Chorionic gonadotropin inhibits rat mammary carcinogenesis through activation of programmed cell death. Carcinogenesis 18: 1799–1808. 1997.

518. Mehta, R.G., Moriarty, R.M., Metha, R.A., Penmasta, R., et al. Prevention of preneoplastic lesion development by a novel vitamin D analogue, 1α-hydroxyvitamin D_5. J. Natl. Cancer Inst. 89: 212–218, 1997.

519. Campbell, M.J. and Koeffler, H.P. Toward therapeutic intervention of cancer by vitamin D compounds. J. Natl. Cancer Inst. 89: 182–185, 1997.

520. Koike, M., Elstner, E., Campbell, M.J., Asou, H., et al. 19-nor-Hexafluoride analogue of vitamin D_3: a novel class of potent inhibitors of proliferation of human breast cell lines. Cancer Res. 57: 4545–4550, 1997.

521. James, S.Y., Mackay, A.G., Binderup, L. and Colstton, K.W.

Effects of a new synthetic vitamin D analogue, EB1089, on the oestrogen-responsive growth of human breast cancer cells. J Endocrinol. 141: 555–563, 1994.

522. Anzano, M.A., Smith, J.M., Uskokovic, M.R., Peer, C.W., et al. 1α,25-dihydroxy-16-ene-23-yne-26,27-hexafluorocholecalciferol (Ro24-5531), a new deltanoid (vitamin D analogue) for prevention of breast cancer in rat. Cancer Res. 54: 1653–1656, 1994.

523. Elstner, E., Linker-Israel, M., Said, J., Umeil, T., et al. 20-epi-Vitamin D_3 analogues: a novel class of potent inhibitors of proliferation and inducers of differentiation of human breast cancer cell lines. Cancer Res. 55: 2822–2830, 1995.

524. Lipkin, M. and Newmark, H. Calcium and the prevention of colon cancer. J. Cell. Biochem Suppl. 22: 65–73, 1995.

525. Whitfield, J.F., Bird, R.P., Chakravarthy, B.R., Iaacs, R.J. and Morley, P. Calcium– Cell cycle regulator, differentiator, killer, chemopreventor, and maybe, tumor promotor. J. Cell. Biochem. Suppl. 22: 74–91, 1995.

526. Knekt, P., Jarninen, R., Seppanen, R., Pukkala, E. and Aromaa, A. Intake of dairy products and the risk of breast cancer. Br. J. Cancer 73: 687–691, 1996.

527. Katsouyanni, K., Trichopoulos, D., Boyle, P., Xirouchaki, E., et al. Diet and breast cancer: a case-control study in Greece. Int. J. Cancer 38: 815–820, 1986.

528. Khan, N., Yang, K., Newmark, H., Wong, G., Telang, N., Rivlin, R. and Lipkin, M. Mammary ductal epithelial cell hyperproliferation and hyperplasia induced by a nutritional stress diet containing four components of a Western-style diet. Carcinogenesis 15: 2645–2648, 1994.

529. Jacobson, E.A., James, K.A., Newmark, H.L. and Carroll, K.K. Effects of dietary calcium and Vitamin D on growth and mammary tumorigenesis induced by 7,12-dimethylbenz(a)anthracene in female Sprague-Dawley rats. Cancer Res. 49: 6300–6303, 1989.

530. Zhang, L., Bird, R.P. and Bruce, W.R. Proliferative activity of murine mammary epithelium as affected by dietary fat and calcium. Cancer. Res. 47: 4905–4908, 1987.

531. Heerdt, A.S., Young, C.W. and Borgen, P.I. Calcium glucarate as a chemopreventive agent in breast cancer. Israel J. Med. Sci. 31:101–105, 1995.

532. Oikawa, T., Yoshida, Y., Shimamura, A., Ashino-Fuse, H., et al. Antitumor effect of 22-oxa-1α,25dihydroxyvitamin D_3, a potent angiogenesis inhibitor, on rat mammary tumors induced by 7,12-dimethylbenz[α]anthracene. Anticancer Res. 2: 475–80, 1991.

533. Tabor, C.W. and Tabor, H. Polyamines. Ann. Rev. Biochem. 53: 749–790, 1984.

534. Scalbrino, G. and Ferioli, M.E. Polyamines in mammalian tumors: part II. Adv. Cancer Res. 36: 1–102, 1982.

535. Pegg, A.E. Polyamine metabolism and its importance in neoplastic growth and a target for chemotherapy. Cancer Res. 48: 759–774, 1988.

536. Sjoerdsma, A. and Schechter, J. Chemotherapeutic implications of polyamine biosynthesis inhibition. Clin. Pharmacol. Ther. 35: 287–300, 1984.

537. Ratko, T.A., Detrisac, C.J., Rao, C.V., Thomas, C.F., Kelloff, G.J. and Moon, R.C. Interspecies analysis of the chemopreventive efficacy of dietary α-difluoromethylornithine. Anticancer Res. 10: 67–72, 1990.

538. Schedin, P., Strange, R., Singh, M., Kaeck, M.R., Fontaine, S.C. and Thompson, H.J. Treatment with chemopreventive agents, difluoromethylornithine and retinyl acetate, results in altered mammary extracellular matrix. Carcinogenesis 16: 1787–1794, 1995.

539. Udeani, G.O., Gerhauser, C., Thomas, C.F., Moon, R.C., et al. Cancer chemopreventive activity mediated by deguelin, a naturally occurring rotenoid. Cancer Res. 57: 3424–3428, 1997.

540. Gerhauser, C., Lee, S.K., Kosmeder, J.W., Moriarty, R. M., et al. Regulation of ornithine decarboxylase induction by deguelin, a natural product cancer chemopreventive agent. Cancer Res. 57: 3429–3435, 1997.

541. Gerhauser, C., Mar, W., Lee, S.K., Suh, N., Luo, Y., Kosmeder, J., Luyengi, L., Fong, H.H., Kinghorn, A.D., Moriarty, R.M. et al., Rotenoids mediate potent cancer chemopreventive activity through transcriptional regulation of ornithine decarboxylase [published erratum appears in Nat Med 6:598, 1995]. Nature Med. 1: 260–266, 1995.

542. Fang, N. and Casida, J.E. Anticancer action of cube insecticide: correlation for rotenoid constituents between inhibition of NADH:ubiquinone oxidoreductase and induced ornithine decarboxylase activities. Proc. Natl Acad. Sci. USA, 95: 3380–3384, 1998.

543. Folkman, J. Tumor angiogenesis. Adv. Cancer Res. 43: 175–203, 1985.

544. Fotsis, T., Pepper, M., Adlercreutz, H., Fleischmann, G., et al. Genistein, a dietary-derived inhibitor of in vitro angiogenesis. Proc. Natl. Acad. Sci. USA 90: 2690–2694, 1993.

545. Suh, H., Jung, E.J., Kim, T.H., Lee, H.Y., et al. Anti-angiogenic activity of ursodeoxycholic acid and its derivatives. Cancer Lett. 113: 117–122, 1997.

546. Joseph, I.B., Vukanovic, J. and Isaacs, J.T. Antiangiogenic treatment with linomide as chemoprevention for prostate, seminal vesicle, and breast carcinogenesis in rodents. Cancer Res. 56: 3404–3408, 1996.

547. Ziche, M., Donnini, S., Morbidelli, L., Parenti, A., Gasparini, G. and Ledda, F. Linomide blocks angiogenesis by breast carcinoma vascular endothelial growth factor transfectants. Br. J. Cancer 77: 1123–1129, 1998.

548. Love, R.R. and Vogel, V.G. Breast cancer prevention strategies. Oncology 11: 161–173, 1997.

549. El-Bayoumy, K., Chung, F.L., Richie, J. Jr., Reddy, B.S., Cohen, L., Weisburger, J. and Wynder, E.L. Dietary control of cancer. Proc. Soc. Exp. Biol. Med. 216: 211–223, 1997.

550. Colditz, G.A., Rosner, B.A. and Speizer, F.E., Risk factors for breast cancer according to family history of breast cancer. J. Natl. Cancer Inst. 88: 365–371, 1996.

551. Alberg, A.J. and Helzlsouer, K.J. Epidemiology, prevention, and early detection of breast cancer. Curr. Opinion Oncol. 9: 505–511, 1997.

552. Daudt, A., Alberg, A.J. and Helzlsouer, K.J. Epidemiology, prevention, and early detection of breast cancer. Curr. Opinion Oncol. 8: 455–461, 1996.

553. Simpson, H.W. Sir James Young Simpson Memorial Lecture 1995. Breast cancer prevention: a pathologist's approach. J. Royal College Surg. Edinburgh 41: 359–70, 1996.

554. Boone, C.W. and Kelloff, G.J. Biomarker end-points in cancer chemoprevention trials. IARC Sci. Pub. 142: 273–280, 1997.

555. Russo, J. and Russo, I.H. Toward a physiological approach to breast cancer prevention. Cancer Epidemiol. Biomarkers Prev. 3: 353–364, 1994.

The New Paradigm in Breast Cancer Prevention

10.1 Rationale for a New Paradigm

Sporadic breast cancer is the fatal disease most frequently diagnosed in American women from all ethnic groups [1, 2]. It has been increasing at a rate of approximately 6% per year [1, 2]. Similar trends are observed worldwide, even in countries characterized by their low breast cancer incidence [3, 4]. Although lower in frequency, genetic cancer represents a definitive threat to women carrying germline mutations in the BRCA1 and BRCA2 genes, who are at an 85% lifetime risk of developing breast cancer, with a significantly earlier age of onset of the disease [5]. Improved detection methods and diagnosis at an early stage have resulted in a decline in breast cancer mortality in the United States [1–3]. Nearly one third of lymph node negative and more than one half of lymph node positive women that will eventually develop metastatic disease, as well as all women with metastatic disease from the time of diagnosis will die of breast cancer [6]. The incurability of the disease, in association with the worldwide increase in incidence indicates that primary prevention is the ultimate goal for breast cancer control [6–9].

The possibility of developing strategies for preventing the initiation of cancer are hindered by the multistep nature of the process, and the facts that only inheritance of cancer-predisposing genes [6, 10–17], and radiation exposure at a young age [18–22] have been identified as a mechanism or causal agent associated with cancer initiation. Current strategies to prevent breast cancer focused on dietary changes advocate trials with reduced fat intake designed to mimic the diets of countries with low breast cancer incidence. Opponents of this approach argue that only a lifetime dietary change can decrease the risk of breast cancer, and therefore major dietary changes undertaken now may not alter breast cancer incidence for another generation [23]. Another strategy capitalizes in a unique feature of breast cancer, its endocrine, namely estrogen, dependence, which can be manipulated to control growth or prevent tumor development utilizing either selective estrogen receptor modulators (SERMs), such as tamoxifen (see Chapter 9) [10, 12, 24–26], or aromatase inhibitors (AIs), such as Arimidex, Letrozole and Exemestane [22, 23]. The inability to predict precisely who will develop breast cancer has required the implementation of broad, population-based strategies utilizing preventative measures that have significant side effects and require a protracted treatment. These drawbacks have made these strategies not widely acceptable to a majority of treated women who would not have develop breast cancer even if untreated [27]. Therefore what is needed is to precisely identify that woman that should take a preventive agent, sparing the other 7 that will not develop the disease during their lifetime. It is in this stage of knowledge that we have developed a new paradigm for breast cancer prevention.

10.2 The New Paradigm

Our paradigm has emerged from epidemiological observations of a direct association of breast cancer risk with nulliparity and of protection conferred by an early first full-term pregnancy [28–34]. *Why have we chosen this specific angle and no other?* Because it is a window of opportunity that nature offers us for learning how a physiological event produces in a significant percentage of women (25%) a complete protection against cancer. We are cognizant that this physiological event does not explain all the questions about this complex disease but it provides a blueprint for a new paradigm in breast cancer prevention. *The novelty of this paradigm does not arise from the knowledge that an early first full-term pregnancy protects the breast against neoplastic transformation, but from our studies [35–46]. We have been the first ones to unravel the biological principle underlying the protection conferred by an early first full-term pregnancy and by demonstrating experimentally that it induces in the breast the expression of a specific signature that results from the completion of a cycle of this organ's differentiation driven by the reproductive process.* This signature, in turn, is a biomarker associated with lifetime decreased breast cancer risk. More importantly, *we have harnessed this biological principle* by demonstrating in an experimental model that a short treatment with human chorionic gonadotropin (hCG), a placental hormone secreted during pregnancy, induces the same genomic signature than pregnancy, inhibiting not only the initiation but also the progression of mammary carcinomas, stopping the development of early lesions, such as intraductal proliferations, and carcinomas in situ (CIS). These observations indicate that hCG administered for a very short period of time has significant potential as a chemopreventive agent, protecting the normal cell from becoming malignant [35–46]. *This new biological concept also implies that when the genomic signature of protection or refractoriness to carcinogenesis is acquired, the hormonal treatment with hCG is no longer required.* This is a novel concept that contraposes the current knowledge that a chemopreventive agent needs to be given for a long period to suppress a metabolic pathway or abrogate the function of an organ [10, 12].

10.3 Epidemiological and Clinical Basis for the New Paradigm

Epidemiological and clinical evidences indicate that endocrinological and reproductive influences play major roles in breast cancer. It has long been known that the incidence of breast cancer is greater in nulliparous than in parous women [33, 34, 47]. Changes in lifestyle, that in turn influence the endocrinology of women, have been observed during the last decades in American women, namely a progressive decrease in the age of menarche [33] and a progressive increase in the age at which a woman bears her first child [34]. The significance of these changes is highlighted by the reduction in breast cancer risk associated with late menarche and the completion of a full term pregnancy before age 24, with further reduction in the lifetime breast cancer risk as the number of pregnancies increases [33, 34, 47]. Women who undergo their first full term pregnancy after age 30, on the other hand, appear to be at higher risk of breast cancer development than nulliparous women, suggesting that parity-induced protection against breast cancer is related to the *timing* of a first full-term pregnancy. Although pregnancy appears to have a dual effect on breast cancer risk, a transient increase (relative to nulliparous women) lasting 10–15 years, followed thereafter by a decreased risk, the protection conferred lasts a lifetime [34]. Of interest is the fact that women from different countries and ethnic groups exhibit a similar degree of parity-induced protection from breast cancer, regardless of the endogenous incidence of this malignancy [48, 49]. This observation suggests that the reduction in breast cancer risk associated with early first full-term pregnancy does not result from factors specific to a particular environmental, genetic, or socioeconomic setting, but rather from an intrinsic effect of parity on the biology of the breast (which nevertheless may be modified by environmental, genetic, or other factors) [33, 34, 47–52]. These observations indicate that an early first full-term pregnancy modifies, through mechanisms still poorly understood, specific biological characteristics of the breast that result in a lifetime decreased risk of cancer development. This protection, nevertheless, is being attributed in great part to the induction of terminal differentiation of the mammary gland, a mechanisms that has been found to reduce the susceptibility of the mammary epithelium to carcinogenesis [47, 48, 53–59]. These observations indicate that the terminally differentiated state of lactation should be reached for attaining protection, although other mechanisms have been proposed for the protective effect of early first full-term pregnancy, including the occurrence of sustained changes in the level or regulation of hormones that affect the breast [60, 61]. Regardless the intervening mechanism, the end result of the first pregnancy is a dramatic modification of the architecture of the breast [57, 58]. The direct association of breast cancer risk with nulliparity, as well as the protection afforded by early first full term pregnancy have been in great part explained by experimental studies [47, 53, 56, 59–62].

10.4 Data from Experimental Animal Studies

10.4.1 Pregnancy

Pregnancy alone or followed by lactation, induces in the mammary gland a permanent protective effect from chemically induced carcinogenesis, since administration of a carcinogen to parous rats when the glands have regressed to a resting stage either fails to induce carcinomas or considerably lowers their incidence [63, 64]; in addition, mammary glands showing gestational or lactational hyperplasia are moderately refractory to DMBA induced carcinogenesis [65, 66]. This indicates that it is not the transient hormonal status occurring during pregnancy and lactation that protects the mammary gland, but the permanent changes induced in the gland structure and in the biological properties of the glandular epithelium by the reproductive phenomenon [67].

These changes consist of complete differentiation of all terminal end buds (TEBs) to lobules, which show active secretary activity during lactation [68]. Those glands that have regressed to a pregestational condition, such as occurs after several weeks of weaning, do not appear extremely different in morpholo-

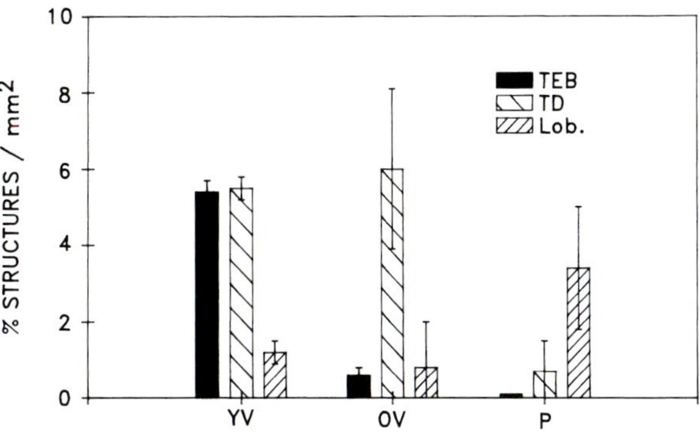

Figure 10.1

Number of structures/mm² (ordinate) in young virgin (*YV*; 55 days of age), old virgin (*OV*; 180 days of age) and parous (*P*; 180 days of age) (reprinted with permission from: Russo J., and Russo, I.H. Cancer Epidemiology, Biomarker and Prevention, 3:353–364, 1994). *TEB* terminal end buds, *TD* terminal duct, *Lob.* lobule

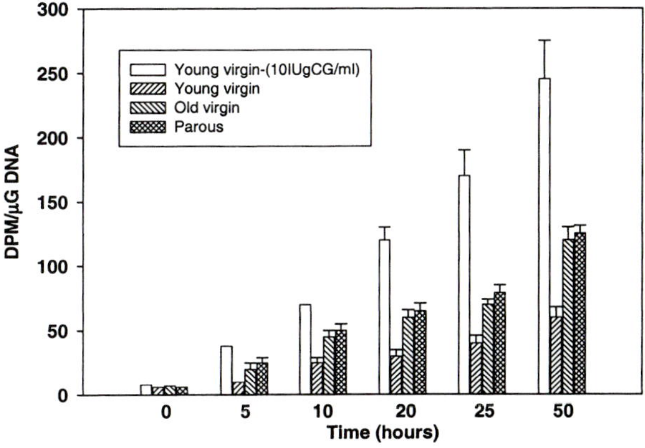

Figure 10.2

DNA excision repair in rat mammary epithelial cells treated with 0.1 μg of DMBA/ml of medium, expressed as disintegrations per minute per μg DNA (ordinate)

gy from the glands of virgin animals except for the absence of TEBs, fewer terminal ducts (TDs), and more alveolar buds (ABs) and lobules (Fig. 10.1) [54, 64]. These structures, however, show a marked diminution of growth fraction (GF) and a lengthening of

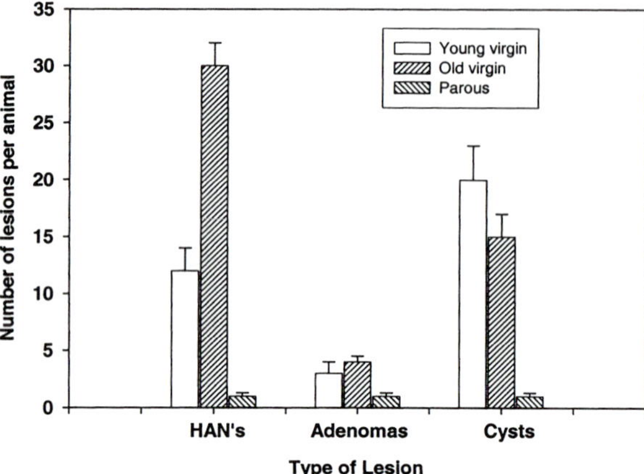

Figure 10.3

Histogram depicting the type of lesions identified in the mammary glands of virgin and parous rats. *HANs* hyperplastic alveolar nodules

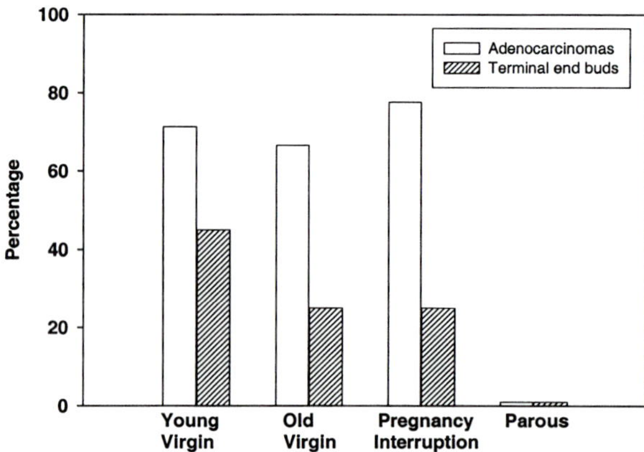

Figure 10.4

Effect of pregnancy and pregnancy interruption in tumor incidence

Tc at the expense of the GI phase of the cell cycle [54]. Very few TDs show active DNA synthesis, having only occasional cells labeled with [^{3}H] thymidine. The DNA-LI of ABs, that is 7.9% and 10.9% in young (55-day-old) and old (180-day-old) virgin rats, respectively, diminishes to 0.3% in parous rats (see Figs. 6.9, 6.19, and 6.20 in Chapter 6). Parous rat mammary epithelial cells also have a lower binding of DMBA to DNA and a more efficient DNA repair (Fig. 10.2) [68–71].

In addition to tumor incidence, tumor type correlates with the degree of differentiation of the mammary gland at the time of exposure to the carcinogen. All of the tumors developed by young virgin rats are carcinomas of ductal origin (see Chapter 6). Both young and old virgin rats present a higher incidence of hyperplastic alveolar nodules, adenomas, and cysts than multiparous rats [72]. Fibroadenomas on the other hand are twice as frequent in multiparous rats as in age matched old virgin rats (Fig. 10.3) [64, 69, 72]. Importantly, in order for pregnancy to be protective if must be complete, because pregnancy interruption in this animals is not associated with protection and the animals developed the same number of tumors and malignant lesions that those virgin controls (Fig. 10.4) [73].

10.4.2 Placental Hormones

The observation that pregnancy before carcinogen administration seems to be the only truly protective factor in chemically induced mammary gland carcinogenesis, suggests that placental hormones play an important role in mammary growth and development during pregnancy [61, 67–70, 74, 75]. The main placental hormone, human chorionic gonadotropin (hCG) has a stimulatory effect on the mammary gland when administered exogenously, producing either a gestational or a lactational type of mammary development that considerably reduces the incidence of tumors, [61, 66]. The fact that the hormonal changes of pregnancy accelerate DMBA-induced mammary tumor growth when mating occurs after carcinogen administration [65–77] indicates that *the most important event in determining the role that this*

Table 10.1. Incidence of DMBA-induced adenocarcinomas in rats pretreated with human chorionic gonadotropin (*hCG*) and human placental lactogen (*hPL*)

Group	Treatment[a]	Dose	Animals/ animals with tumors[d]		Tumor/ animal	Animals with adeno- carcinomas		Adeno- carcinomas per animal
			n	%		n	%	
I	Control		19/9	47.0	2.33	8	42.0	2.25
II	hCG	1 IU	14/3	21.4	0.85	2	14.0	0.14
III	hCG[b]	5 IU	8/1	12.5	0.12	1	12.5	0.12
IV	hCG[b]	10 IU	8/1	12.5	0.12	1	12.5	0.12
V	hCG[c]	10 IU	18/3	17.0	2.00	2	11.0	1.50
VI	hCG[c]	100 IU	20/6	30.0	1.16	0	0.0	0.00
VII	hCG+hPL	1 IU+0.5 mg	5/3	60.0	1.20	3	60.0	1.00
VIII	hPL	0.5 mg	7/4	57.1	1.42	4	57.5	1.14

[a] Chorionic gonadotropin was administered daily for 21 days, starting when the animals were 50 days old. All animals received 10 mg of DMBA/100 g body weight at 21 days after the last injection. Tumorigenesis was evaluated after 22 weeks
[b] National Institutes of Health, Bethesda, Maryland
[c] Sigma Chemical Company, St. Louis, Missouri
[d] Tumor incidence represented the addition of benign (adenomas, fibroadenomas) plus adenocarcinomas

nother placentol hormones plays in either preventing initiation or in promoting tumor growth is the sequence in which it they reach the mammary gland.

DMBA administration at 21 days after the termination of hCG inoculation in doses of 1, 5, 10, or 100 IU/day for 21 days, starting when the rats are 50 days old, markedly reduces the incidence of tumors from 42.0% in control to 14.0%, 12.5%, 12.5% and 0% respectively in animals treated with the above listed doses (Table 10.1). Furthermore, the number of carcinomas per animal diminishes from 3 in the control to 0 in the experimental group treated with 100 IU, and the number of benign lesions reduces from 8.7 in controls to 2.6 per gland in animals thus treated [74].

Treatment of 50-day-old rats with 0.5 mg/day of placental lactogen alone or in combination with 1 IU of hCG for 21 days before DMBA administration significantly increases the incidence of carcinomas with regards to control animals (Table 10.1). The effect of these hormones on tumor incidence is explained by their influence on mammary gland development. hCG induces a greater differentiation of the gland, resulting in a greater number of ABs and lobules, and with a consequently decreased number of TEBs and TDs. These changes are accompanied by a decreased DNA-LI [74]. Placental lactogen administration, either alone or in combination with hCG fails to stimulate gland differentiation and glands from animals thus treated have more TEBs and TDs and fewer ABs and lobules than do glands of control animals. The DNA-LI in all of these terminal structures is similar or slightly higher than that of control animals [74].

Altogether these studies have revealed that the susceptibility of the mammary gland to be transformed by a chemical carcinogen is modulated by specific biological conditions of the host and of the target organ [63, 74, 76]. Tumor incidence and number of tumors per animal, which are the biological endpoints when evaluating tumorigenic response, are maximal when the carcinogen is administered to young but cycling virgin rats. Cancer incidence is di-

Table 10.2. Effect of hCG on DMBA-induced mammary carcinogenesis. *AdCa* adenocarcinoma

Group	Treatment	Tumors					Adenocarcinoma				
		Total number of animals	Number of animals with tumor	%	Total number of tumors	Number of tumors/ animal	Number of animals with AdCa	%	Total number AdCa	Number of AdCa/ animal[a]	Latency period (days)
Protocol 1											
I	–/DMBA[b]	80	49	61.3*	101	1.26	35	48.30**	73	0.91	55–191
II	Pregnancy/DMBA	18	1	5.6*	1	0.06	1	5.6**	1	0.06	91
III	hCG(100 IU)/DMBA	65	19	29.2*	27	0.41	4	6.15**	4	0.06	90–195
Protocol 2											
IV	–/DMBA	27	12	44.4*	18	0.67	5	18.52**	5	0.18	52–153
V	Pregnancy/DMBA	21	3	14.2S*	4	0.19	2	9.52**	2	0.09	52–210
VI	hCG(100 IU)/DMBA	27	7	25.92*	7	0.25	2	7.40**	2	0.07	52–210

a Number of adenocarcinomas per animal per total number of animals at risk
b DMBA – 7,12-dimethylbenz(a)anthracene, 8 mg/100 g body weight
* Tumor incidence Chi-square with df = 3, value 22.4118 and sample size 254, probability is $p = 5.35 \times 10^{-5}$
** Carcinoma incidence Chi-square with df = 3, value 31.6775 and sample size 254 probability is $p = 6.12 \times 10^{-7}$

Figure 10.5

Experimental protocol to study the effect of human chorionic gonadotropin (hCG) and pregnancy in DMBA induced mammary carcinogenesis

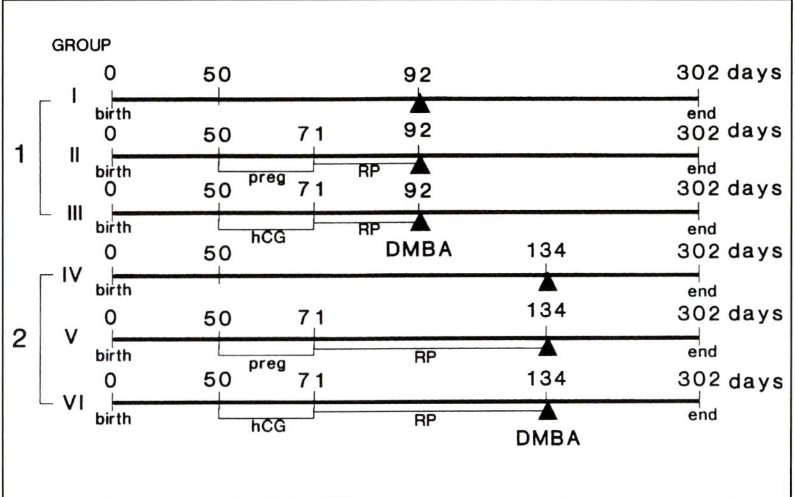

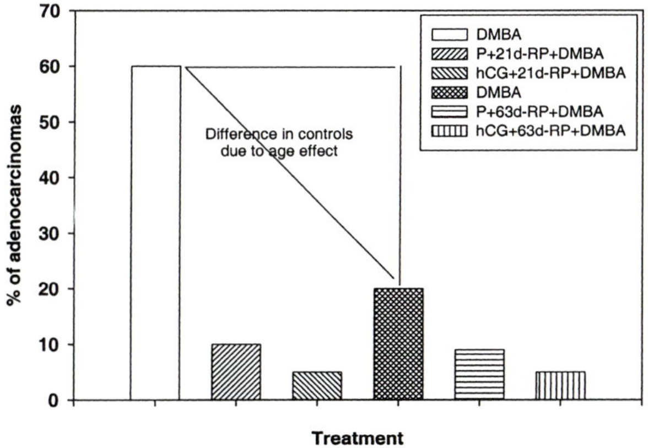

Figure 10.6

Adenocarcinoma incidence (ordinate): percentage of animals developing mammary adenocarcinomas. *DMBA* 7,12 dimethylbenz(a)anthracene. *P* pregnancy, *RP* resting period post pregnancy or hCG; *hCG* human chorionic gonadotropin

such as it occurs during pregnancy, or after completion of a 21-day treatment of virgin rats with hCG, reduce the susceptibility of the mammary epithelium to be transformed by the carcinogen (Table 10.2). The reduction in cancer incidence is permanent, as demonstrated by the similar degree of reduction when DMBA is administered after a delay of 21, 42, or 63 days after termination of hCG treatment (Figs. 10.5, 10.6).

10.4.3 Estrogenic and Progestagenic Agents

The observation that estrogenic and progestagenic agents used with the purpose of contraception modify the mammary gland structure, thus modulating its susceptibility to carcinogenesis [76, 78, 79], and the fact that most studies report that their use does not result in increased breast cancer risk [80], led us to test the use of contraceptives in breast cancer prevention, which implies that the hormones have to be administered to nulliparous females of young age in order to drive mammary gland development enough to be protective, without altering the basic physiology of the gland, its potential to respond with lactation to a full-term pregnancy late in life, and without altering the endocrinologic profile and physiology of the host.

rectly proportional to the number of terminal end buds (TEBs) that are at their peak of cell proliferation [63, 74, 76, 77]. Stimulation of the development and differentiation of the gland, resulting in profuse lobular development and depression of DNA synthesis,

The administration of the hormone combination norethynodrel-mestranol, and of the progestagenic agent medroxyprogesterone acetate (MPA), to virgin rats led to several important discoveries. These two agents differ in their mechanism of action; norethynodrel has a weak progestagenic activity and is considered to be atypical since it induces perinuclear vacuolization of endometrial epithelium, an effect similar to that of estrone [81], and in addition it is administered in conjunction with the estrogenic compound mestranol. MPA is an acetoxyprogesterone derivative more potent than progesterone [81] that significantly reduces estradiol receptor levels in human endometrium [82] and cervical epithelium [83]; however, when both agents are administered at the same dose used for contraception, they induce a degree of mammary gland development which suffices to reduce cancer incidence by more than 85% (Fig. 10.7). However, maximal protection is achieved only when the hormones are administered to young but sexually mature animals ranging in age from 55 to 65 days old (Fig. 10.7) [84, 85].

We call this period the "protection window" which overlaps with the "risk window" since the same age range represents the peak of susceptibility to neoplastic transformation [56, 69]. Treatment at a younger age, but after puberty and after 65 days of age, either diminishes the protective effect of the combination contraceptive or increases the risk of breast cancer development when the progestagenic contraceptive is used (Fig. 10.8) [84, 85]. The selective susceptibility of the mammary gland's TEBs to respond with either differentiation under hormonal stimuli, or transformation under a carcinogenic stimulus, at that specific age indicates that both systems act on the same target and probably utilize the same receptors. Of greater concern is the effect of MPA, which when administered to postpubertal females or to old virgin females stimulates the TEBs of the young animals or reactivates the quiescent TDs of old animals, thus expanding the "risk window' for carcinogenesis. These observations are confirmed by data demonstrating that prolonged treatment with progestogens results in development of mammary nodules [86, 87] and malignant neoplasms in the bitch [86–89]. Epidemiological observations concur with these findings, as a

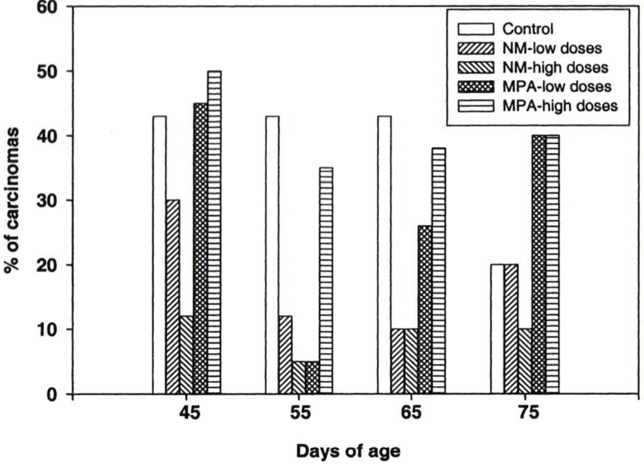

Figure 10.7

Histogram showing the effect of norethynodrel-mestranol (*NM*) and medroxyprogesterone (*MPA*) in DMBA induced mammary carcinogenesis in relation to age

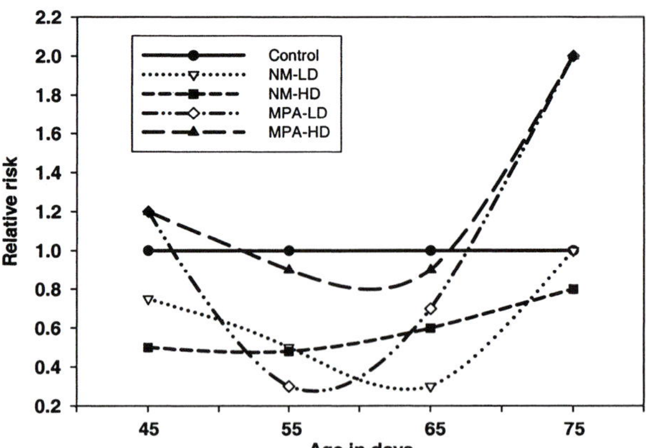

Figure 10.8

Comparative curve of the risk to developed mammary cancer in DMBA treated animals that have been treated with norethynodrel-mestranol (*NM*) or medroxyprogesterone acetate (*MPA*) at low (*LD*) or high dosis (*HD*)

higher risk of breast cancer has been reported in women using progestogen contraceptives before a full-term pregnancy [90], whereas women with anovulatory cycles or late menarche, and therefore exposed for a longer period of their life span to unopposed estrogen stimulation, are at lower risk of developing breast cancer than women with early menarche and rapid establishment of regular cycles [91, 92]. Furthermore, elevated levels of progesterone have been detected in daughters of breast cancer patients [93, 94], observations that challenge the proposed "estrogen window hypothesis" [95] of the etiology of breast cancer.

The realization that mammary gland differentiation can be induced only during a well-defined period in the animal's life span, and that the same hormonal stimulus at the same dose becomes a risk factor when it reaches a less receptive mammary gland, raises a warning in the use of exogenous hormones, not only for the purpose of breast cancer prevention, but also as contraceptive or therapeutic agents, since they may affect secondarily a breast whose potential risk for developing cancer might not have been evaluated or considered when hormones are administered for those purposes. MPA alone has been used for contraception by 11 million women with 100,000 having used this hormone for more than 10 years [96–100]. In addition, it is used for treatment of endometrial carcinoma [101], endometriosis [102], advanced breast cancer [103], and it is administered to treat poor progestational response in pregnant women [104]. It has been administered to lactating women who excrete the hormone in milk, and breast enlargement and feminization in the newborn infant have been reported in breast fed children of mothers taking contraceptives [105].

Observations obtained with the study of this model raised two sets of questions of importance to breast cancer prevention. The first one deals with understanding how the age-dependent response of the mammary gland to contraceptive agent administration is modulated by expression of proliferation versus differentiation in the specific target of the carcinogen that is the TEB. The second and more pressing issue is the atypical response of the mammary gland to the administration of a progestagenic agent, which either induces protection or increases risk, depending upon the age at which it is administered. Therefore, it is required to determine if age-related changes in the mammary epithelium influence its response to exogenous, and probably endogenous, hormonal stimulation. The answers to these questions have to be sought with the realization that the mammary gland does not respond as a unit to either endogenous or exogenous hormonal stimuli, since only specific areas of specific glands are susceptible at a given time.

10.4.4 Role of Pregnancy and Chorionic Gonadotropin in Mammary Gland Differentiation and Cancer Initiation

The direct association of breast cancer risk with the prolongation in the period encompassed between menarche and the first full-term pregnancy, as well as the protection afforded by pregnancy has been partially explained by experimental studies performed in our laboratory [35–38, 47, 53, 61, 62]. We have demonstrated that mammary cancer in rodents can be induced with the polycyclic hydrocarbon 7,12-dimethylbenz(a)anthracene (DMBA) preferentially when the carcinogen is administered to young nulliparous females [38]. Those females that have completed a full term pregnancy prior to carcinogen exposure fail to develop carcinomas [47, 53–56]. We have demonstrated that the inhibitory effect of pregnancy on mammary cancer initiation is mediated by hCG, since virgin rats treated for 21 days with a daily intraperitoneal injection of this hormone prior to carcinogen administration exhibit a dose-related reduction in tumor incidence and number of tumors per animal [35–38, 61, 62]. This phenomenon is in great part mediated by the induction of mammary gland differentiation, inhibition of cell proliferation (Fig. 10.9), increase in the DNA repair capabilities of the mammary epithelium, decrease binding of the carcinogen to the DNA, and activation of genes controlling programmed cell death (PCD) [39–47]. The activation of these genes by hCG is of great relevance because PCD is a physiological and phylogenetically conserved form of active cell death (or apoptosis) that has been

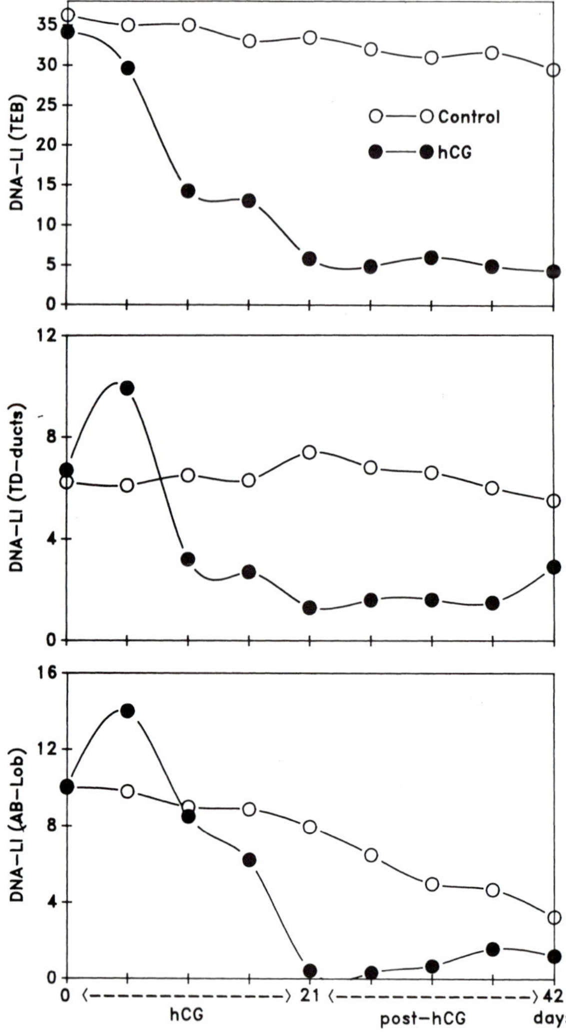

Figure 10.9

The highest DNA labeling index (LI) was observed in the terminal end buds (*TEBs*) of control animals (*upper panel*). DNA-LI was considerably lower in ductal and lobular structures present in the same mammary gland. The response of terminal ducts (*TDs*), ducts (*middle panel*), alveolar buds (*ABs*), and lobules (*lower panel*) to treatment was similar among themselves, and different from that of TEBs; the DNA-LI increased in all of these structures, reaching a peak of maximal activity by the 5th day of injection, then decreased by the 10th day of injection, and more sharply by the 21st day

Figure 10.10 a–j ▶

a Mammary lobule from a 60-day-old untreated virgin female rat immunocytochemically reacted with anti-inhibin antibody. The epithelial cells lining the ductule are completely negative, whereas the surrounding stroma shows a moderate response. Avidin-biotin-peroxidase complex (ABP complex)-DAB-hematoxylin, original magnification ×530. *Bar* = 20 µm. **b** Lobule in the mammary gland of a 60-day-old-virgin female rat treated with hCG for 10 days. The lobules are more developed than those present in the gland of control groups (see **a**). There is positive immunocytochemical reaction (++) in the basal portion of most of the epithelial cells lining the ductules. The secretion within the lumen is negative. ABP complex-DAB-hematoxylin, original magnification ×530. *Bar* = 20 µm. **c** Mammary gland of a 65-day-old untreated virgin female rat showing a poorly developed lobule with negative reaction in the epithelium and slightly positive reaction in the stroma, a pattern of reactivity similar to that shown in **a**. ABP complex-DAB-hematoxylin, original magnification × 530. *Bar* = 20 µm. **d, e** Well-developed lobules present in the mammary gland of a 65-day-old virgin female rat treated with hCG for 15 days. There is a strongly positive (++/+++) immunocytochemical reaction in the lining epithelial cells. The reaction is seen in all the cytoplasm around the clear vacuoles of fat, which are negative. The lumen content, the stroma, and myoepithelial cells are negative. ABP complex-DAB-hematoxylin, original magnification ×530. *Bar* = 20 µm. **f** Mammary ducts in the mammary gland of a 65-day-old rat treated with hCG for 15 days. The ducts are lined by a low columnar epithelium. Neither the lining epithelial cells nor the ductal lumen shows immunoreactivity to inhibin. Compare with **d** and **e**. ABP complex-DAB-hematoxylin, original magnification ×530. *Bar* = 20 µm. **g** Mammary lobule from a 70-day-old untreated virgin female rat immunoreacted with anti-inhibin antibody. Both the epithelium and the stroma are negative. ABP complex-DAB-hematoxylin, original magnification ×800. *Bar* = 10 µm. **h** Mammary gland from a 70-day-old virgin female rat treated with hCG for 20 days. The cytoplasm of epithelial cells lining the ductules shows no inhibin immunoreactivity; it now contains large vacuoles. Occasional cells show a slightly positive reaction. The most remarkable feature at this stage is the appearance of strongly positive immunoreactivity in the intralobular stroma. ABP complex-DAB-hematoxylin, original magnification ×260. *Bar* = 40 µm. **i** Lobule in the mammary gland of a 90-day-old untreated virgin female rat immunocytochemically reacted with anti-inhibin antibody, showing completely negative reaction in the epithelium and stroma. ABP complex-DAB-hematoxylin, original magnification ×800. *Bar* = 10 µm. **j** Mammary gland from a 90-day-old virgin female rat, treated with hCG for 21 days and sacrificed 20 days after termination of treatment. The lobular structures are similar to those of the control group. The immunocytochemical reaction to inhibin is negative. ABP complex-DAB-hematoxylin, Original magnification ×800. *Bar* = 10 μm. Reproduced with permission from: Alvarado, M.E., Russo, J. and Russo, I.H. Immunolocalization of inhibin in the mammary gland of rat treated with hCG. J. Histochem. Cytochem. 41:29–34, 1993

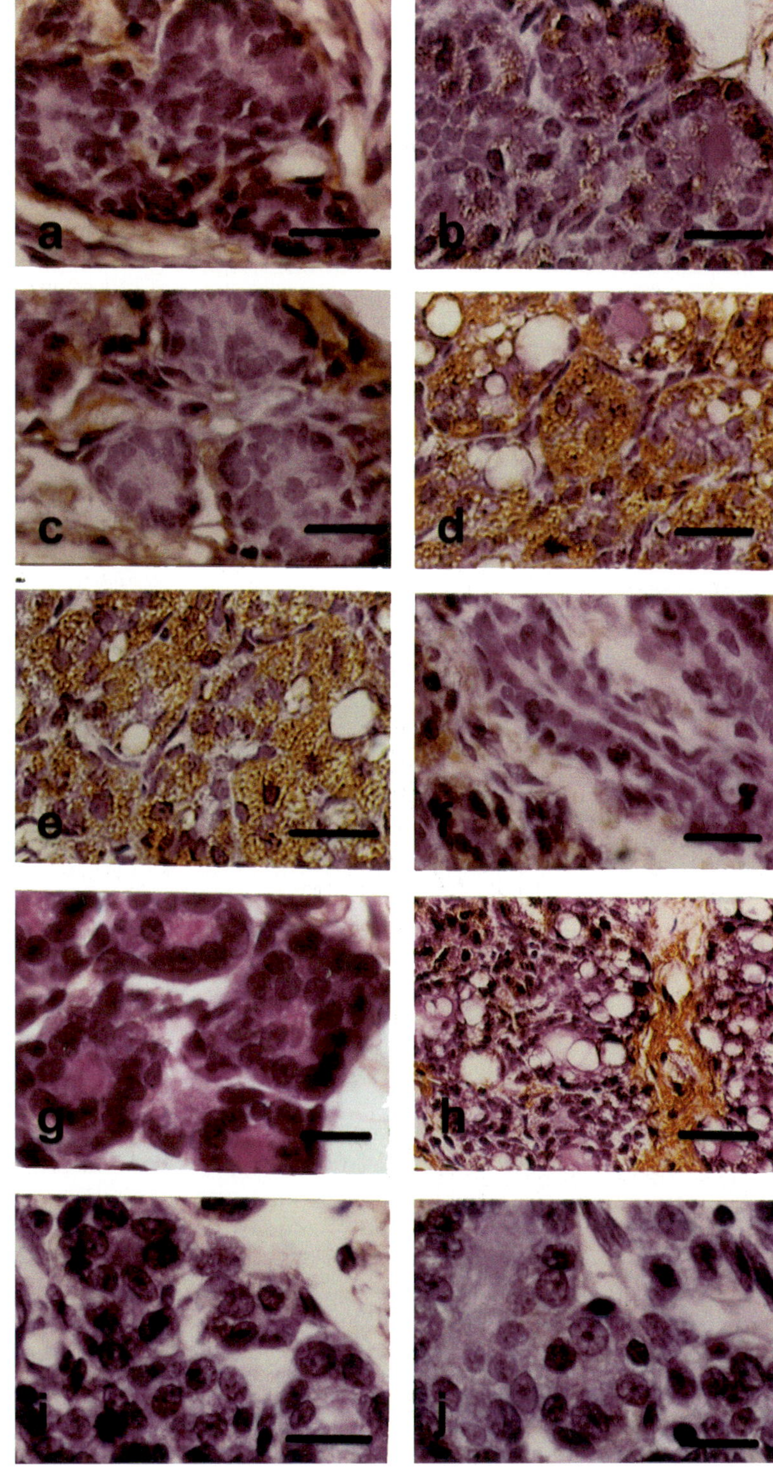

associated with specific phases of development that control cell proliferation and differentiation [44].

A gene product that has been associated with the differentiation of the mammary gland is inhibin. Although the highest concentration of inhibin has been found in testes and ovary, it is also expressed in several nongonadal tissues, including brain, pituitary, placenta, and both human and rat mammary epithelium [46]. The finding of inhibin subunit mRNAs in non-reproductive tissues suggests a role for the inhibin protein outside the reproductive axis as an important regulator of cellular differentiation. The development of gonadal tumors by inhibin-deficient mice homozygous for the null allele identifies a-inhibin as an important negative regulator of cell proliferation.

Since the synthesis of inhibin by the ovary is stimulated by the gonadotropic hormones pregnant mare serum gonadotropin (PMSG) and hCG, hormones known to have a powerful differentiating effect on the mammary gland, our work was designed with the purpose of determining whether inhibin played a role in this process. For this purpose, virgin Sprague-Dawley rats were treated with 100 IU/hCG/day, starting when the animals were 45 days old. Five animals were sacrificed on the first day of injection and additional groups of five animals at 5, 10, 15 and 20 days post-injection. Age-matched animals were used as controls. The mammary glands were removed and processed for light microscopy immunocytochemistry. Immunocytochemical reactions in the control group were essentially negative in the mammary epithelium lining both in ducts and lobular structures (Fig. 10.10). At 5 days of injection the mammary gland of hCG-treated animals exhibited elongation and bifurcation of ducts, which were notable increase in the number of lobular structures, and alveoli per lobule were seen. At this stage the epithelial cells lining the alveoli showed the presence of numerous small vesicles around the nucleus, and the appearance of a moderately inhibin positive (++) immunocytochemical reaction in the cytoplasm. This reaction was circumscribed to the basal portion of the epithelial cells and it was not seen in the adjacent intralobular stroma. At 15 days of treatment a large number of lobules was present; they were lined by cuboi-

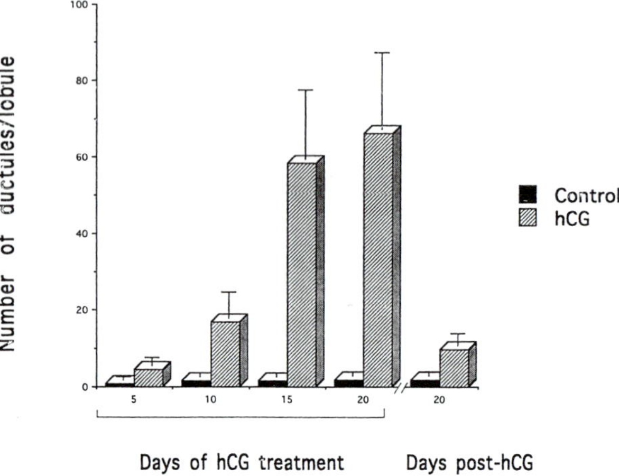

Figure 10.11

Effect of hCG treatment on the lobulo-alveolar development of the mammary gland, measured as the mean ± SD of the number of ductules per lobule counted on 10 slides per gland per animal (ordinate). Days of treatment and post-treatment (abscissa). Reproduced with permission from: Alvarado, M.E., Russo, J. and Russo, I.H. Immunolocalization of inhibin in the mammary gland of rat treated with hCG. J. Histochem. Cytochem. 41:29–34, 1993

dal epithelial cells showing a strong positive (4+) immunocytochemical reaction in greater than 80% of the cells lining the alveoli. The intralobular stroma showed a strong reaction (3+). Ductal cells were lacking in both vacuoles and immunocytochemical reaction. The interlobular and periductal connective tissue were positive, (1-2+), but the reaction was uneven. By the 20th day of hCG treatment, the number of acini per lobule was increased, and the lining epithelial cells showed a moderate (2+) positive reaction, becoming less intense as the size of the vacuoles became larger. The intralobular stroma remained clearly positive. Once hCG treatment was suspended, the lobular structures regressed, however, their number remained slightly higher than in controls. The

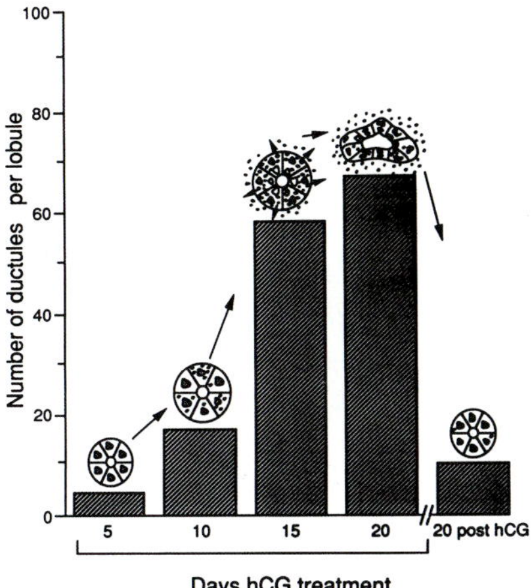

Figure 10.12

Schematic representation depicting inhibin immunoreactivity in the ductular epithelial cell, appearing as perinuclear intracytoplasmic reaction at day 10, filling the cytoplasm and progressing towards the surrounding stroma between days 15 and 20 of treatment and practically disappearing from its intracytoplasmic localization after termination of hCG treatment. It is correlated with lobulo-alveolar development during and after hCG administration, expressed as number of ductules per lobule. Reproduced with permission from: Alvarado, M.E., Russo, J. and Russo, I.H. Immunolocalization of inhibin in the mammary gland of rat treated with hCG. J. Histochem. Cytochem. 41:29–34, 1993

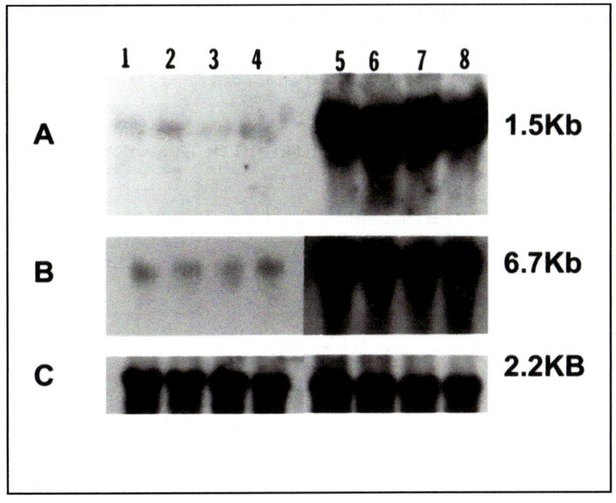

Figure 10.13 a–c

Northern blot analysis of inhibin-α and inhibin-βA subunit mRNA of mammary glands of intact (lanes 1–4) and hCG-treated rats (lanes 5–8). The blot was sequentially hybridized with **a** ^{32}P inhibin α-subunit oligonucleotide, **b** inhibin-βA subunit oligonucleotide, and **c** β-actin cDNA probes. Reprinted with permission from: Alvarado, M.V., Ho, T.Y., Russo, J., and Russo, I.H. Human chorionic gonadotropin regulates the synthesis of inhibin in the ovary and mammary gland of rats. Endocrine 2:1–10, 1994

immunocytochemical reaction to inhibin was markedly reduced or almost negative in both epithelial cells and the surrounding stroma, a reaction similar to that seen in the control group (Figs. 10.11, 10.12). Since maximal immunocytochemical reactivity was observed at the 15th day of treatment, ovaries and mammary glands were collected from these animals for extraction of mRNA for determination of a and BA-inhibin subunit mRNAs. Total RNA from both the ovaries and the mammary glands from hCG-treated and control rats was extracted, fractionated on denaturing agarose gels, and hybridized with ^{32}P-labeled inhibin α-subunit and inhibin BA-subunit oligonucleotide probes. Hybridization of ovarian RNA with the α-subunit probe resulted in a single band of hybridization at about 1.5 kb. The intensity of the hybridization signal was increased up to 10-fold by hCG treatment. Hybridization with the inhibin BA-subunit probe resulted in a predominant signal at 6.7 kb, showing a 7-fold increase after hCG treatment (Fig. 10.13). The total RNA of mammary glands hybridized with the α and B subunits, respectively, showed the same 1.5 and 6.7 kb bands corresponding to the inhibin α and BA-subunit mRNAs present in the ovary. A novel observation was that the basal level of BA-subunit mRNAs in the mammary gland of control animals was higher than in the ovaries of the same group of animals (Fig. 10.14) [71]. Since both pregnancy and hCG treatment induce differentiation of the mammary gland and subsequent protection

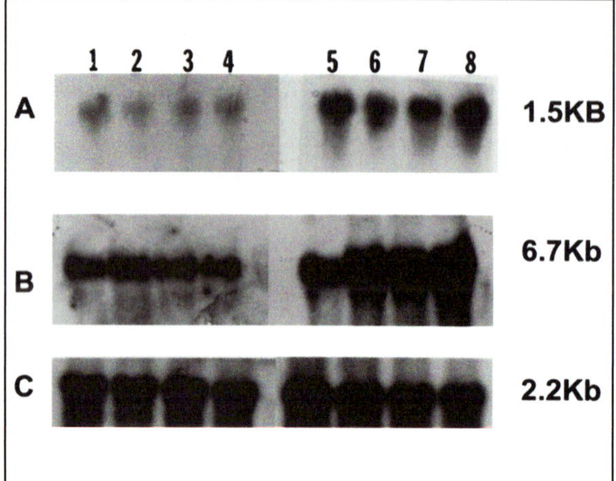

Figure 10.14 a–c

Northern blot analysis of inhibin-α and inhibin-βA-subunit mRNAs in ovary of 65-day-old virgin rats, intact (lanes 1–4) or treated with hCG for 15 days (lanes 5–8). Total RNA was electrophoresed on a l.2%/2.2 M agarose-formaldehyde gel and transferred to a Nytran membrane. The blot was sequentially hybridized with a ^{32}P-labeled inhibin α-subunit oligonucleotide, b inhibin βA-subunit oligonucleotide, and c β-actin cDNA probes. Reprinted with permission from: Alvarado, M.V., Ho, T.Y., Russo, J., and Russo, I.H. Human chorionic gonadotropin regulates the synthesis of inhibin in the ovary and mammary gland of rats. Endocrine 2:1–10, 1994

nective tissue. Following parturition or cessation of hCG treatment, the glands regressed to their initial condition, and inhibin immunoreactivity was seen in the perilobular stroma. mRNA from mammary gland from 10 days hCG treated rats and 10 days of pregnancy clearly shows a significant increase in the level of both inhibins. These results suggest that inhibin mediates the differentiating action of both pregnancy and hCG on the mammary gland, in which it might act as an autocrine and/or paracrine growth regulator [39].

10.5 Role of Human Chorionic Gonadotropin in Breast Cancer Progression

Our studies of the protective effect of hCG-induced differentiation on experimental mammary carcinogenesis led us to postulate the possibility that hCG might be useful in preventing the development of breast cancer in women. The fact that the time of initiation of breast cancer in the female population is not known represented a major drawback for accomplishing the goal of instituting a truly "preventative" hormonal treatment. Thus, It had to be assumed that all women are at risk of being the carriers of "initiated" lesions. This assumption requires that before the hormonal treatment is initiated it has to be proven that it either inhibits the progression of putatively initiated cells, or at least does not to cause tumor progression. Based upon our previous observations that the chemical carcinogen DMBA induces neoplastic transformation in the mammary gland by acting on the highly proliferating TEBs of the virgin animal [40, 47, 53], and that once initiated these structures progress to intraductal proliferations (IDPs) within 3 weeks of exposure to the carcinogen [41, 47], we tested the effect of hCG on tumor progression by administering 8 mg DMBA/100 g body weight to 45-day-old virgin Sprague-Dawley rats. Twenty days later, when IDPs were already evident, the animals were treated with 100 IU/hCG per day for 40 days (DMBA + hCG group). Age matched untreated, hCG-, and DMBA + saline treated rats were used as controls. Tissues were collected at the time of DMBA administration and at 5, 10, 20, and 40 days of hCG injection,

against neoplastic transformation we aimed to determine whether inhibin may mediate the effect in both hCG treated rats and during pregnancy. For this purpose, 50-day-old virgin Sprague-Dawley rats were divided into two groups: one was treated with daily i.p. injections of 100 IU hCG for up to 21 days; the second group of rats was mated. Samples of mammary gland were taken at 7, 10, 15 and 21 days of hCG treatment of pregnancy, respectively, or 20 days treatment/parturition. Inhibin was immunocytochemically detected in mammary gland of both parous and treated rats, increasing progressively up to 15 days of treatment/pregnancy. Thereafter, immunoreactivity decreased in the intracellular compartment and became evident in the surrounding intralobular con-

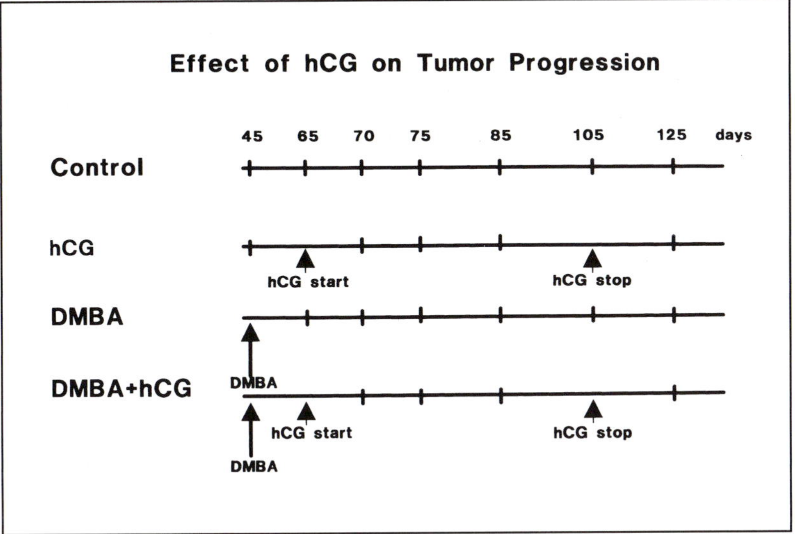

Figure 10.15

Protocol utilized for testing the effect of hCG in the progression of DMBA initiated carcinogenesis

and 20 days post-cessation of treatment (Fig. 10.15) [40, 44].

10.5.1 Mammary Gland Development Under Influence of Human Chorionic Gonadotropin

The development of the mammary gland in the rat requires the evaluation of changes in the parenchyma of the gland, since, unlike women, no significant external changes occur in this organ after puberty [40]. The six pairs of the mammary gland of the young virgin rat is composed of ducts ending in club-shaped terminal end buds (TEBs), which are multilayered structures measuring 100–140 μm in diameter. They are lined by a 3- to 10-layer thick cuboidal epithelium that rests on a discontinuous layer of myoepithelial cells [38, 40, 54]. After the beginning of ovarian function the mammary ducts undergo further longitudinal lengthening and branching with sprouting of a few alveolar buds (ABs) that progressively evolve to lobular structures (Fig. 10.16). The lobules found in the rat mammary gland can be classified according to their degree of development as lobule type 1 (Lob 1), which consists of clusters of approximately 10±4 ductules per unit. Individual ductules are lined by a single layer of cuboidal epithelial cells and few myoepi-

thelial cells. With further growth Lob 1 evolve to lobules type 2 (Lob 2), which are larger, and composed of approximately 40±7 ductules; these progress to lobules type 3 (Lob 3), that contain approximately 60±12 ductules or alveoli per lobule (Fig. 10.16) [37]. The administration of 100 IU/hCG per day for 40 days to young virgin rats deeply affects the development of the mammary gland, modifying profoundly the relative proportions of Lob 1, Lob 2, and Lob 3 (Fig. 10.17). While the concentration of Lob 1 in the mammary gland of untreated or saline-injected control virgin rats decreases slightly as a consequence of aging, in hCG treated animals the number of Lob 1 decreases slightly by the 10th day of hormonal treatment, and even further between the 20th and 40th days (Fig. 10.17). After cessation of treatment their number increases sharply, reaching the same values found in control animals. Lob 2 are practically non-existent in the 45-day-old animals; they became first evident when the animals reach the age of 75 days, and their percentage increases even further in the next 10 days, reaching its peak in the 85-day-old animals, remaining unchanged thereafter (Fig. 10.12). Under hCG treatment the lobules type 2 develop in a biphasic pattern. Their concentration increases progressively from 70 to 85 days of age, decrease significantly by the time the animals reach the age of

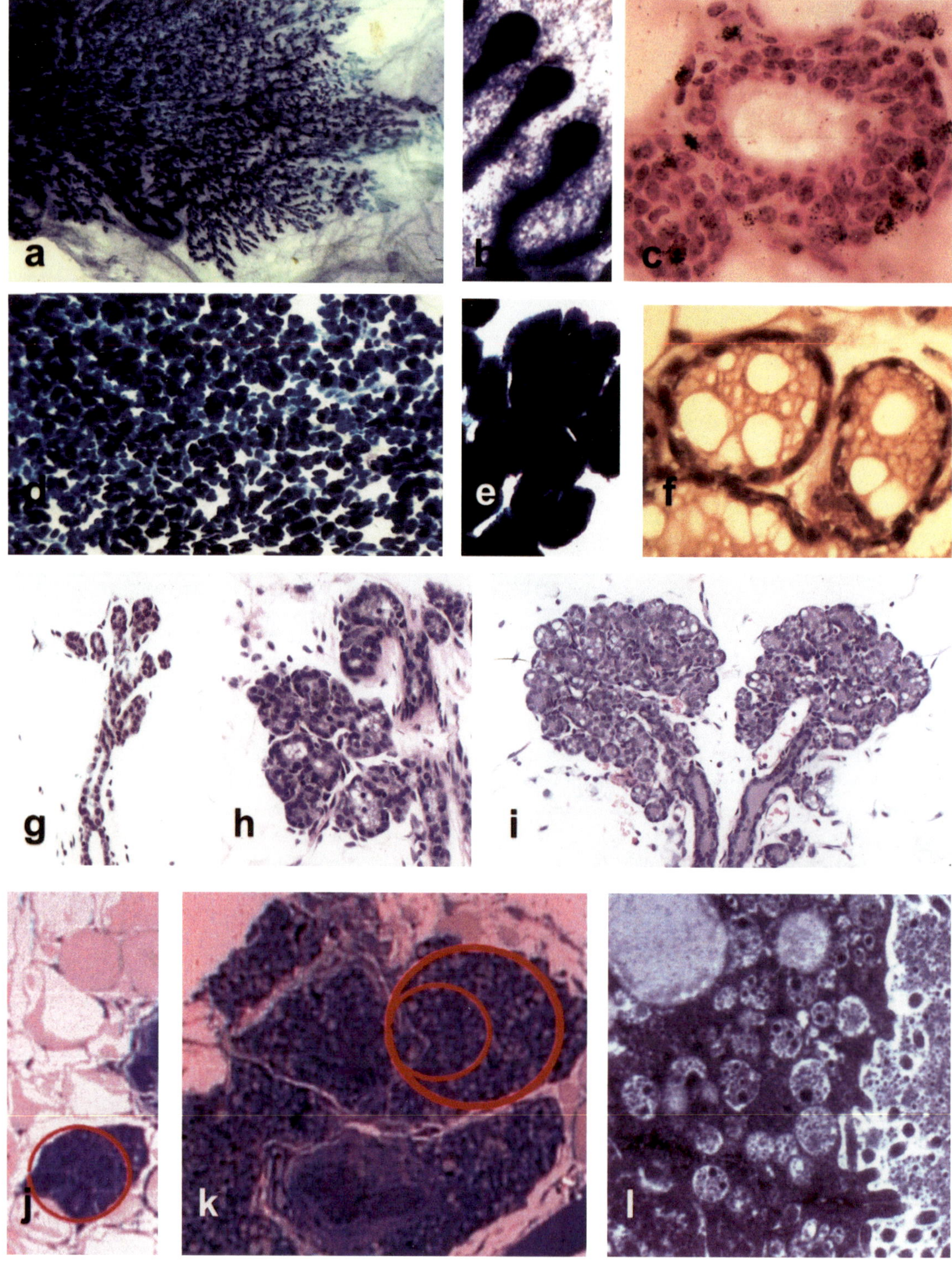

◀ Figure 10.16 a–l

a Whole mount of a virgin rat mammary gland, 55 days of age (toluidine blue, ×2). **b** TEBs (toluidine blue, ×10). **c** TEB is a multilayer structure measuring 100–140 μm in diameter. The TEB is lined by a 3–10 layers thick cuboidal epithelium that rests on a discontinuous layers of myoepithelial cells. **d** Whole mount of a pregnant rat mammary gland, 75 days of age (toluidine blue, ×2). **e** Lobule type 3 (toluidine blue, ×10). **f** Histological section of the ductules of a lobule type 3 containing secretory material (H&E, ×40). **g–i** The lobules found in the rat mammary gland can be classified according to their degree of development as Lob 1, which consists of clusters of approximately 10±4 ductules per unit (**g**). Individual ductules are lined by a single layer of cuboidal epithelial and few myoepithelial cells. With further growth, Lob 1 evolves to Lob 2, which is larger, and composed of approx 40±7 ductules (**h**). Lob 3 contains approx 60±12 ductules or alveoli per lobule (**i**). **j–l** Under the effect of hCG the mammary gland forms lobules type 4 (toluidine blue) (**j**) that are formed by more than 80 ductules per lobular unit containing material in their lumen (**k**), Electron microscopy section in **l**, from area within the *red circle* in **k** shows the proteinaceous and lipid composition of the milk secretion (uranyl acetate and lead nitrate, ×4,000)

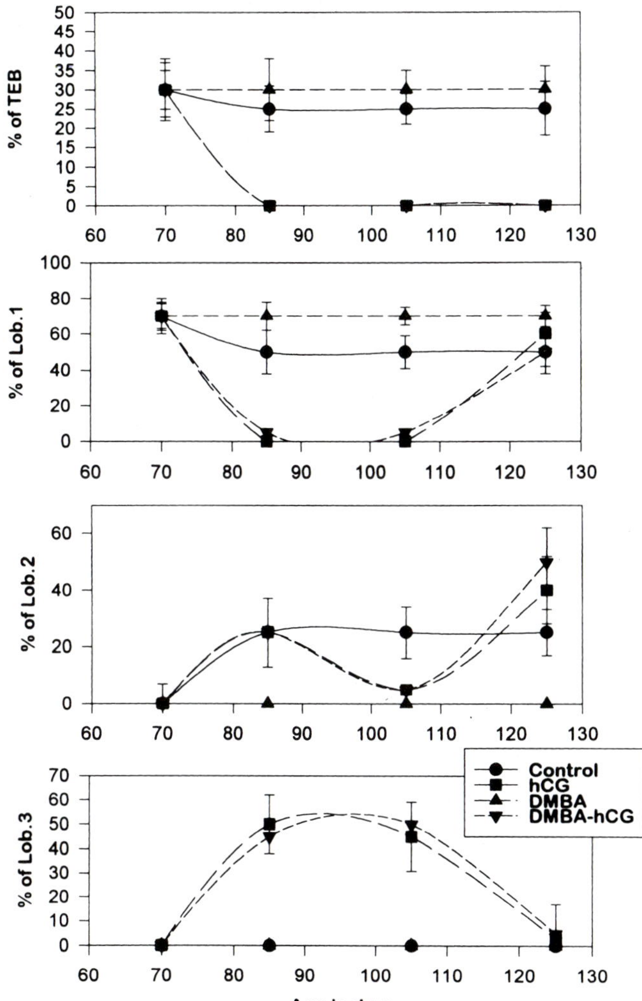

105 days, and increase again after cessation of treatment (Fig. 10.17). Lob 3 formation, on the other hand, starts at the 10th day of treatment, it increases progressively between the 20th and 40th days, decreasing only after cessation of the hormonal treatment due to their regression to Lob 2. The resulting recovery of this type of lobule is absent in control animals (Fig. 10.17).

Figure 10.17

Percentage of TEBs, lobules type 1 (*Lob. 1*), lobules type 2 (*Lob. 2*), and lobules type 3 (*Lob. 3*) in control, *hCG* animals injected daily with 100 IU hCG from 65 to 105 days of age, *DMBA* rats treated with DMBA when they were 45 days old, followed by a daily i.p. saline injection, *DMBA-hCG*, animals treated with DMBA at the age of 45 days and daily with hCG from 65 to 105 days of age. Five animals per group were sacrificed at each one of the age periods indicated

10.5.2 Hormonal Profile Induced by Human Chorionic Gonadotropin

The evaluation of the effect of hCG on the development of the mammary gland requires to assess the effect of this hormone on two important endocrine organs: the ovary and the pituitary gland. The hormonal profile studied at various times during and after hCG treatment comprised the determination of serum levels of the β subunit of the injected hCG, as well as determination of the levels of the ovarian hormones estrogen, progesterone, and inhibin, and the pituitary hormones prolactin, follicle stimulating hormone (FSH) and luteinizing hormone (LH) [42, 43]. The determination of the serum levels of the β subunit of hCG by RIA revealed that this hormone was completely absent at the beginning of treatment and in control animals (Fig. 10.18). By the fifth day of treatment it had reached a level of 2,845±575 mIU/ml. The levels remained elevated until the 20th day, declining rapidly thereafter, despite continuous administration of the hormone for additional 20 days (Fig. 10.18). The progressive increase in hCG serum levels paralleled the increase in ovarian size, which occurred due to the increased number and size of corpora lutea. Ovarian size returned to a normal range after cessation of the hormonal treatment [42].

In the control animals serum estradiol levels ranged from 32.4 pg/ml to 50.2 pg/ml, with no significant variations observed in association with aging. Serum estradiol levels were elevated in hCG treated animals. Maximal values were observed between the 20th and the 40th days of hormonal treatment (Fig. 10.19). The levels of estradiol decreased below those of the controls in the hCG-treated group after the 40th injection, and even further 20 days later [43]. Progesterone levels were significantly elevated in hCG-treated groups in comparison to control animals (Fig. 10.20). The serum levels of progesterone peaked between the 20th and 40th days of hormonal treatment. In the hCG group the serum levels dropped to the levels observed in the controls by the time of the 40th injection and they remained low by 20 days after cessation of treatment [43].

Serum levels of the pituitary hormone LH were similar in all the groups of animal studied, ranging from 3.2 to 8.5 ng/ml. It became evident that hCG treatment had no significant effect on the synthesis and /or secretion of LH because the levels of LH measured in the serum of saline-treated rats were not significantly different from the levels in the hCG-treated groups [43]. Serum FSH levels of female rats were not

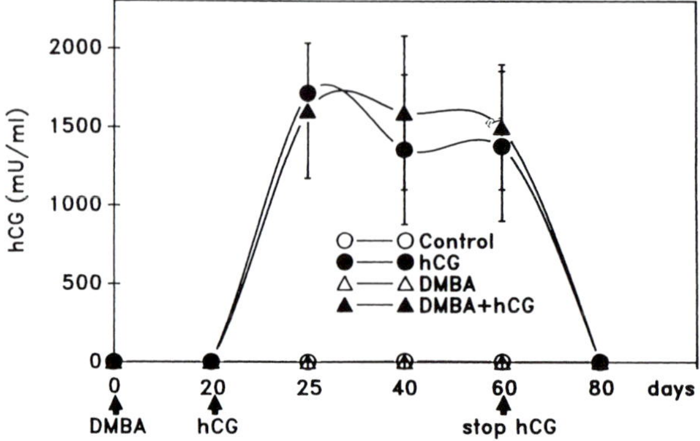

Figure 10.18

β-hCG levels. Mean ± SD of 5–10 animals/ group. Groups as per Fig. 10.15

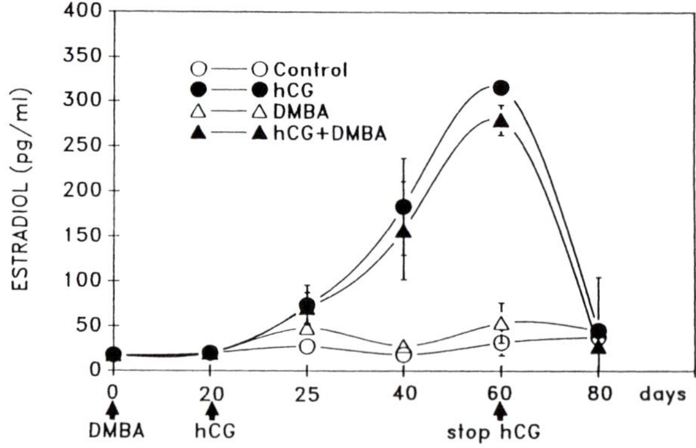

Figure 10.19

Estrogen serum levels. Mean ± SD of 5–10 animals/group. Groups as per Fig. 10.15

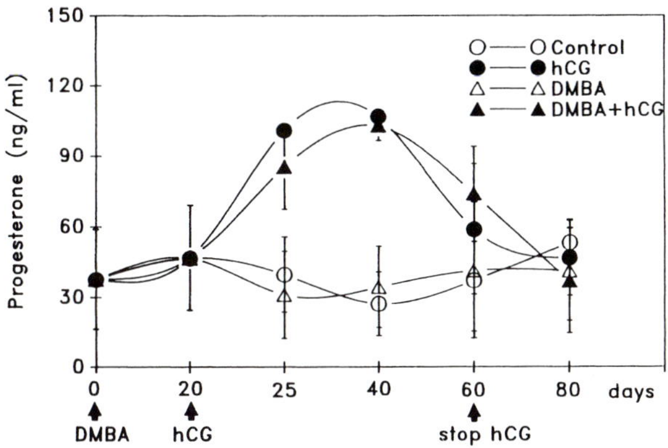

Figure 10.20

Progesterone serum levels. Mean ± SD of 5–10 animals/group. Abbreviations as per Fig. 10.15

10.5.3 Effect of Human Chorionic Gonadotropin on Terminal End Buds, Intraductal Proliferations, and Ductal Carcinomas In Situ

The mammary gland of 45-day-old virgin rats contains the highest number of terminal end buds (TEBs). In animals of the Saline Control group the number of TEBs decreased slightly as a function of age, as it has been previously described, whereas in the DMBA group their number remained constant. In both hCG treated groups a diminution in the relative percentage of TEBs was observed as early as 5 days after the initiation of treatment, and more sharply between the 10th and the 20th days, for reaching a plateau thereafter. The percentage of TEBs in these two groups of animals was significantly lower than the values found in the Saline Control and DMBA

modified by treatment with hCG. All the groups of animals had similar FSH levels and no changes in serum levels were observed with aging. The daily injections of hCG neither stimulated nor inhibited its production [43]. The serum levels of prolactin were not modified by aging. The hormonal treatment moderately affected prolactin levels, since an elevation in serum levels was observed in hCG-treated groups, but the differences with controls were not significant [43].

In summary, administration of hCG to young virgin rats raised the serum levels of estrogen and progesterone, while the levels of prolactin, FSH, LH, and inhibin were not modified significantly by the hormonal treatment [42, 43]. The increment in estrogen and progesterone levels induced by hCG was accompanied by an increase in the size of the ovaries, which was due mainly to the enlargement of the corpora lutea. These effects were transient, since ovarian size regressed to normal values as early as 5 days after cessation of the hormonal treatment. The effect of hCG treatment on the mammary gland, however, persisted even after the cessation of treatment, indicating that the hormonal milieu induced by hCG sufficed for differentiating the mammary epithelium.

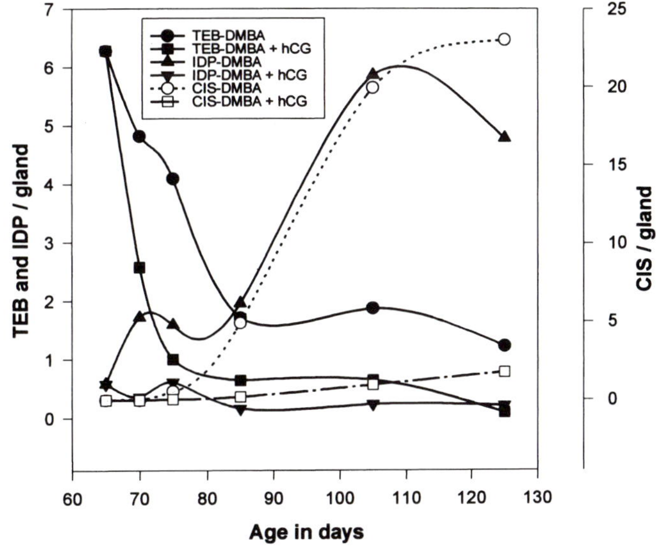

Figure 10.21

Number of TEBs, intraductal proliferations (*IDP*) (*left hand side ordinate*), and carcinoma in situ (*CIS*) (*right hand side ordinate*) in animals treated with DMBA when they were 45 days old, followed by a daily i.p. saline injection (*DMBA*) or hCG from 65 to 105 days of age (*DMBA + hCG*) groups ($p<0.01$) (Fig. 10.21). A more noticeable effect of the hormonal treatment occurred at the level of intraductal proliferations (IDPs) and ductal carcinomas in situ (DCIS) (Fig. 10.21). In DMBA treated animals there were 5.80 IDPs per gland when they reached the age of 105 days, that is, 25-fold higher the values observed in the hCG treated animals, in which there were 0.23 IDP/gland. These differences were still significant in the 125-day-old animals.

The number of DCIS was also higher in the DMBA-treated group, and their number was decreased by 13-fold by hCG treatment. The number of DCIS increased slightly when the animals reached the age of 125 days, averaging 1.76 DCIS/gland, however, it was still significantly lower than that observed in the DMBA group of animals that contained 23 DCIS/gland (Fig. 10.21). Occasional lactating adenomas were observed in both hCG and DMBA + hCG treated animals [44].

10.5.4 Effect of Human Chorionic Gonadotropin Treatment on DMBA-Induced Tumor Progression

While mammary tumors were palpated as early as 25 and 30 days post-carcinogen administration in the DMBA + hCG and DMBA groups respectively, none of the animals in the Saline Control or the hCG-treated groups developed tumors. In the group of animals treated with DMBA the number of palpable tumors continued increasing until the end of the experiment. In the DMBA + hCG group the number of palpable tumors reached a plateau when the animals were 105 days old, and no additional tumors were detected in the 125-day-old animals. The highest total number of tumors and number of tumors per animal were observed in the DMBA group, while the DMBA + hCG group showed a reduction in the total number of palpable tumors and number of tumors per animal at all the time points studied. The histopathological analysis of both palpable tumors and microscopic lesions revealed that most of them were adenocarcinomas with papillary, cribriform or comedo features. Only 3 fibroadenomas developed in the DMBA and 2 in the DMBA + hCG groups respectively. The hormonal

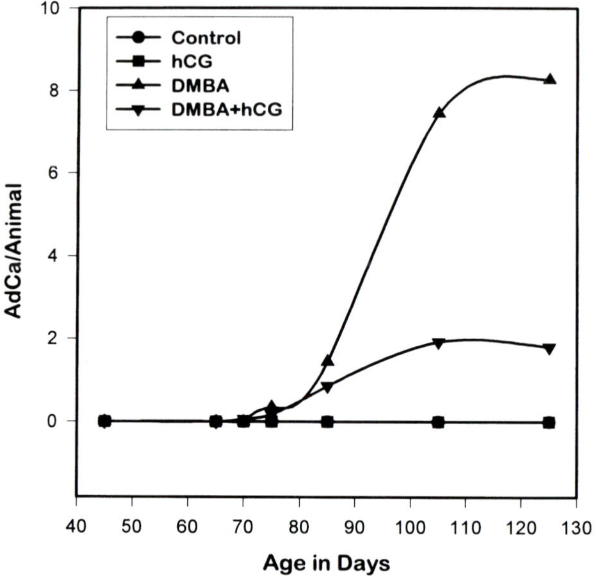

Figure 10.22

Number of adenocarcinomas (AdCa) per animal in rats treated with DMBA when they were 45 days old, followed by a daily i.p. saline injection (*DMBA*) or hCG from 65 to 105 days of age (*DMBA + hCG*)

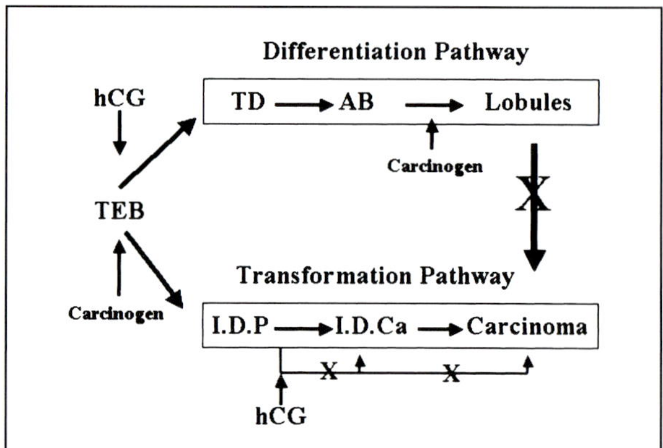

Figure 10.23

hCG plays an important role in the differentiation pathway by eliminating the undifferentiated TEBs and increasing the branching and differentiation to lobule formation. The hormone also is able to affect the transformation pathway by stopping the initiated cells by inhibiting the progression of IDP to CIS and adenocarcinomas (*carcinoma*)

Table 10.3. Effect of hCG treatment on the progression of DMBA-induced mammary tumors. *AD-Ca* adenocarcinoma

Group/treatment	Age/days of treatment[a]	Tumor incidence		Number of tumors per animal/ total number tumors[d]	Number of AD-Ca per animal//total number of AD-Ca[h]
		Number of animals with tumors/ total number of animals[c]	Percentage		
DMBA	70/5	0/11	0.00	0.00/0	0.00/0
DMBA	75/10	4/11	36.36	0.36/4	0.36/4
DMBA	85/20	7/11	63.63	1.45/16	1.45/16
DMBA	105/40	11/11	100.0	7.45/82	7.45/82
DMBA	125/20[b]	11/11	100.0	8.54/94[e]	8.27/91
DMBA+hCG	70/5	1/16	6.25	0.06/1	0.06/1
DMBA+hCG	75/10	3/16	18.75	0.18/3	0.18/3
DMBA+hCG	85/20	8/16	50.00	0.87/14	0.87/14
DMBA+hCG	105/40	13/16	81.25	2.00/32[f]	1.93/31
DMBA+hCG	125/20[b]	13/16	81.25	1.57/30[g]	1.81/29

[a] Age of the animals (in days) at the time of sacrifice/days of treatment with Saline (DMBA) or 100 IU hCG/day (DMBA+hCG)
[b] Twenty days post-termination of the 40-day hCG treatment
[c] Number of animals with tumors/total number of animals per group/treatment and age group
[d] Number of tumors per animal/total number of tumors from each specific group/treatment and animal age group
[e] Three out of 94 tumors were fibroadenomas
[f] One out of 32 tumors was a fibroadenoma
[g] One out of 30 tumors was a fibroadenoma
[h] Number of invasive adenocarcinomas (AD-Ca) per animals/total number of adenocarcinomas per group/treatment and animal age group

treatment reduced more noticeably the incidence of adenocarcinomas, from 8.3 in the DMBA to 1.8 adenocarcinomas per animal in the DMBA + hCG group (Fig. 10.22, Table 10.3) [44].

In summary, hCG treatment inhibited the progression of mammary carcinomas by stopping the development of early lesions, i.e., IDPs and carcinomas in situ (CIS). These findings indicated that hCG has a significant potential as a chemopreventive agent not only before the cell is initiated, but after the carcinogenic process has been initiated and is vigorously progressing. Ours was the first report to indicate that a hormone preventive agent like hCG is able to stop the initiated cells by inhibiting the formation of the intermediate step represented by the CIS, what ultimately results in a lower incidence of invasive tumors (Fig. 10.23) [44].

10.6 Effect of Human Chorionic Gonadotropin on Inhibin Expression and Its Relation with the Activation of Early Response Genes

Our observations that the hCG-induced differentiation of the mammary gland is associated with the synthesis of inhibin, a heterodimeric protein that is structurally related to the transforming growth factor-β (TGF-β) family [45, 46, 106–108], led us to test whether inhibin was also involved in the regression of DMBA-induced rat mammary carcinomas. For these purposes, virgin rats that received 8 mg DMBA /100 g body weight when they were 45 days old; and 20 days later they were injected daily with 100 IU/hCG for 40 days, as described above, with the

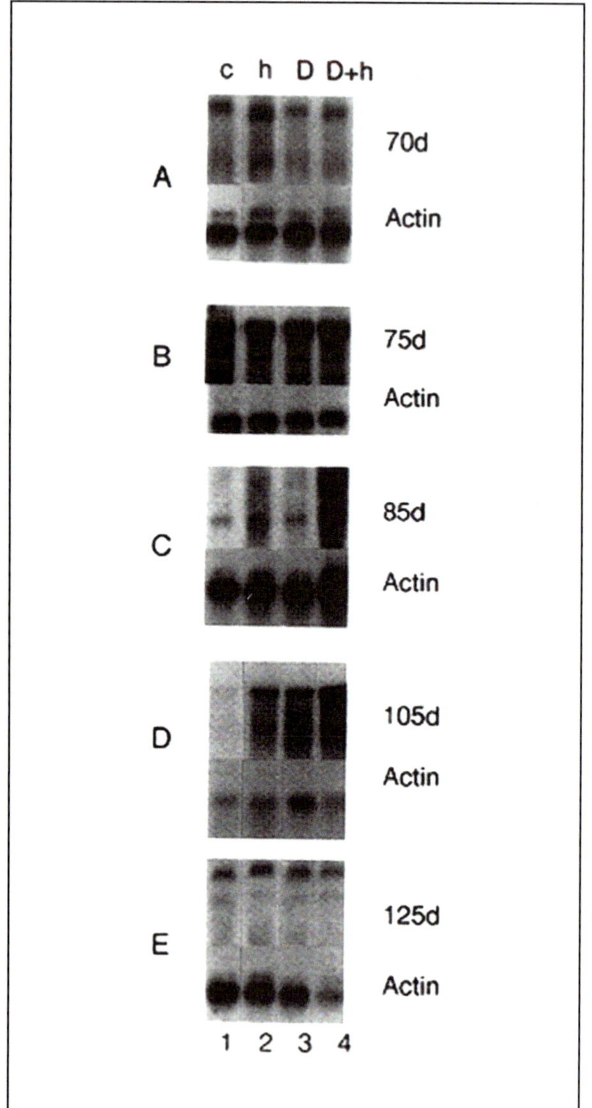

Figure 10.24 a–e

Analysis of inhibin A mRNA levels in the mammary glands of each of the four groups described in Fig. 10.15: control (c), hCG (h), DMBA (D), DMBA + hCG (D+h). Rats were killed at **a** 70, **b** 75, **c** 85, **d** 105, and **e** 125 days of age. β-actin was used to detect the amount of RNA loaded in each lane. The relative levels of transcripts for each experimental group were determined by laser densitometry of autoradiographs and equalized by β-actin, and the statistical significance of differences was determined by Student's *t*-test, The significantly different groups were control and hCG-70d vs. hCG-85d ($p<0.02$) and 105d ($p<0.03$); DMBA-70d vs. DMBA-105d ($p<0.02$); and control and DMBA + hCG-70d vs. DMBA + hCG-85d ($p<001$), 105d ($p<0.008$), and 125d ($p<0.01$). Reprinted with permission from: Srivastava, P., Russo, J., and Russo, I.H. Inhibition of rat mammary tumorigenesis by human chorionic gonadotropin is associated with increased expression of inhibin. Molecular Carcinogenesis, 26:1–10, 1999

corresponding age-matched controls receiving saline, hCG-, or DMBA + saline treatments (Fig. 10.15). Mammary glands and ovaries were collected at the time of DMBA administration and at 5, 10, 20, and 40 days of hCG injection and 20 days post-cessation of treatment. Total and polyadenylated RNAs were probed for inhibin A, B, *c-myc*, *c-fos*, and *c-jun*. The mammary glands of hCG-treated animals exhibited elevated expression of Inhibin A (1.5- to 4.0-fold) and Inhibin B (1.5- to 3.0-fold), from the 5th day of hCG treatment up to 20 days post-treatment. The expression of these genes was also enhanced by hCG in the DMBA treated group, whereas no changes occurred in the animals treated with DMBA alone (Figs. 10.24, 10.25). The hormonal treatment markedly increased the expression of *c-myc* and *c-jun* by 4- to 7-fold and 2- to 3-fold, respectively (Fig. 10.26). No significant changes were found in the levels of *c-fos* expression,

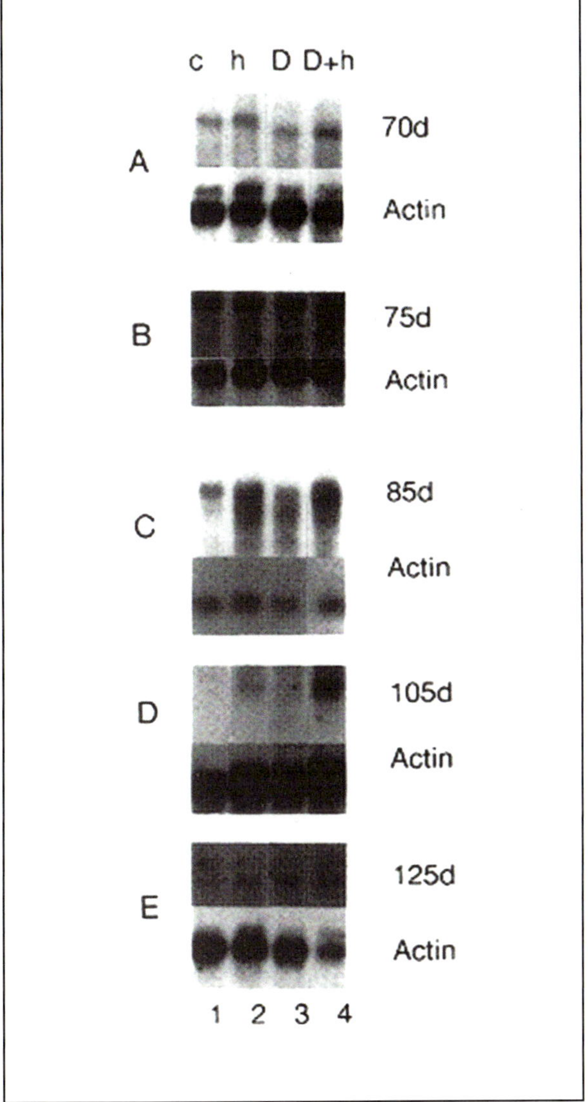

Figure 10.25 a–e

Analysis of inhibin B mRNA in the mammary glands of control and hCG-, DMBA-, and DMBA + hCG-treated rats. Rats were killed at **a** 70, **b** 75, **c** 85, **d** 105, and **e** 125 days of age. The statistical significance of differences was determined by Student's *t*-test. The significantly different groups were control 70d vs. hCG-85d ($p < 0.000001$); control and hCG-105d ($p < 0.01$); control and DMBA + hCG-70d vs. DMBA + hCG-85d ($p < 0.04$), 105d ($p < 0.02$), and 125d ($p < 0.000001$). Reprinted with permission from: Srivastava, P., Russo, J., and Russo, I.H. Inhibition of rat mammary tumorigenesis by human chorionic gonadotropin is associated with increased expression of inhibin. Molecular Carcinogenesis, 26:1–10, 1999

and DMBA treatment alone did not modify the expression of these genes. Immunohistochemical staining showed a very strong immunoreactivity for inhibin α and β subunits in the lobular epithelium. It became evident by the 10th day of treatment, reaching a peak of expression by the 20th day. A similar pattern of reactivity was observed in animals treated with hCG alone or after DMBA (Fig. 10.27). The expression of both inhibin subunits remained elevated up to 20 days post-hormone withdrawal, even though the lobular structures had involuted from the well-developed secretory Lob 3 and Lob 4 to Lob 2 and Lob 1. The finding that *c-myc* and *c-jun* were also elevated at the time of maximal inhibin synthesis indicated that early response genes could be involved in the pathway of hCG-inhibin induced synthesis.

Even though inhibin belongs to the TGF-β family, hCG treatment did not affect the level of expression

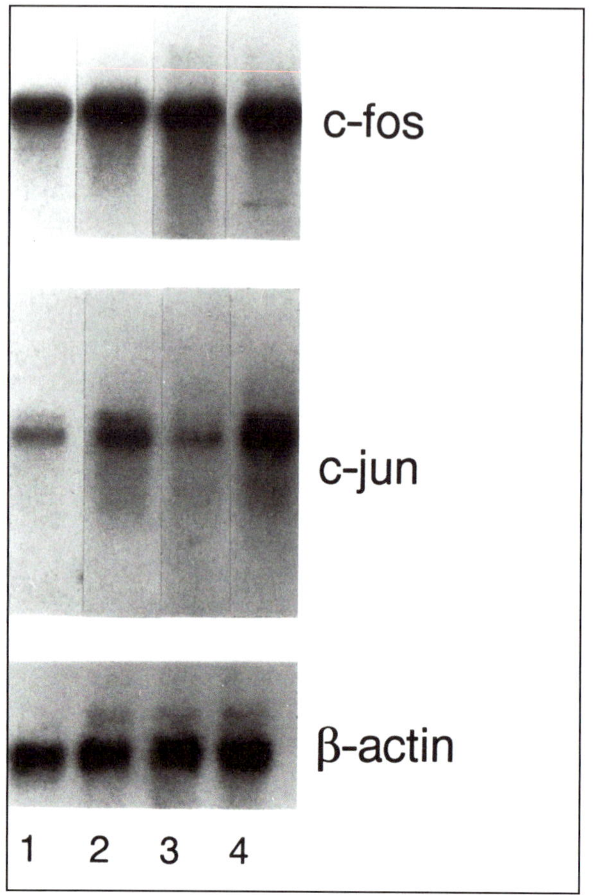

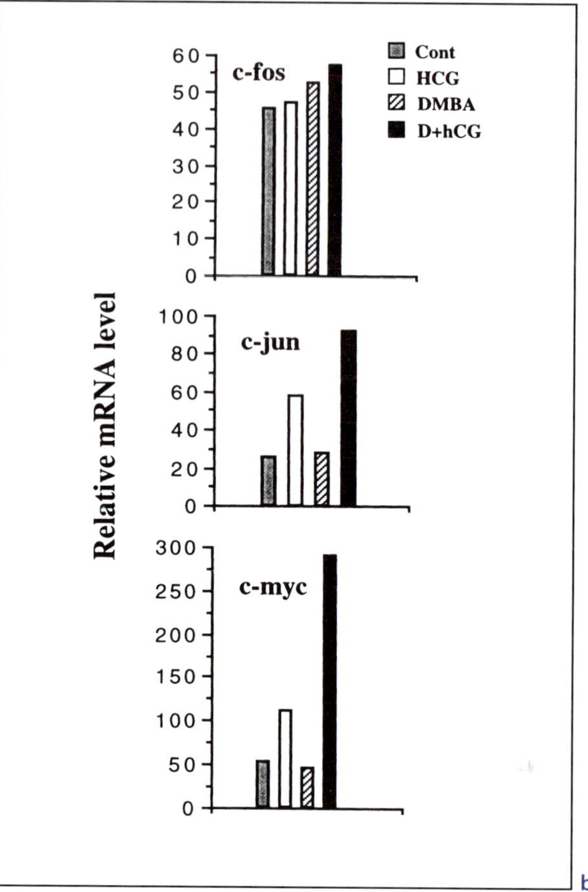

Figure 10.26 a, b

Analysis of *c-fos* and *c-jun* mRNA expression in the Mammary gland. **a** Control (lane 1) and hCG (lane 2), DMBA (lane 3), and DMBA + hCG treated (lane 4) groups of rats killed on day 20 of hCG treatment, when they were 85 days old. Poly(A) + RNA was isolated and hybridized with *c-fos*, *c-jun*, and β-actin. **b** Histogram showing relative *c-myc*, *c-fos* and *c-jun* mRNA expression in the mammary gland of control (*Cont*) and hCG, DMBA, and DMBA + hCG (*D+hCG*) treated animals killed at the time indicated in panel **a**. Relative mRNA contents for each experimental group were determined in autoradiographs by scanning laser densitometry and equalized by detection of β-actin, and the statistical significance of differences was determined by Student's *t*-test. The groups significantly different for *c-jun* were control vs. hCG ($p < 0.04$) and control vs. DMBA + hCG ($p < 0.01$). For *c-myc*, they were control vs. hCG ($p < 0.04$) and control vs. DMBA + hCG ($p < 0.02$). Reprinted with permission from: Srivastava, P., Russo, J., and Russo, I.H. Inhibition of rat mammary tumorigenesis by human chorionic gonadotropin is associated with increased expression of inhibin. Molecular Carcinogenesis, 26:1–10, 1999

Figure 10.27 a–f ▶

Papillary-cribriform adenocarcinomas removed from a DMBA-treated 85-day-old animal and immunohistochemically reacted with **a** pre-immune rabbit serum and **b** rabbit anti-β-inhibin (×10). **c** Well-differentiated adenocarcinoma of a DMBA + hCG treated animal excised at day 20 of hormonal administration (85-day-old animal). **d, e** Sections of adenocarcinoma excised 20 days after cessation of hCG treatment (125-day-old animal) and immunoreacted with rabbit anti-α-inhibin antibody. **f** Sections immunoreacted with rabbit anti-β-inhibin antibody (×40). In all sections, immunostaining was visualized with DAB, the hematoxylin was used as a counterstain. Reprinted with permission from: Srivastava, P., Russo, J., and Russo, I.H. Inhibition of rat mammary tumorigenesis by human chorionic gonadotropin is associated with increased expression of inhibin. Molecular Carcinogenesis, 26:1–10, 1999

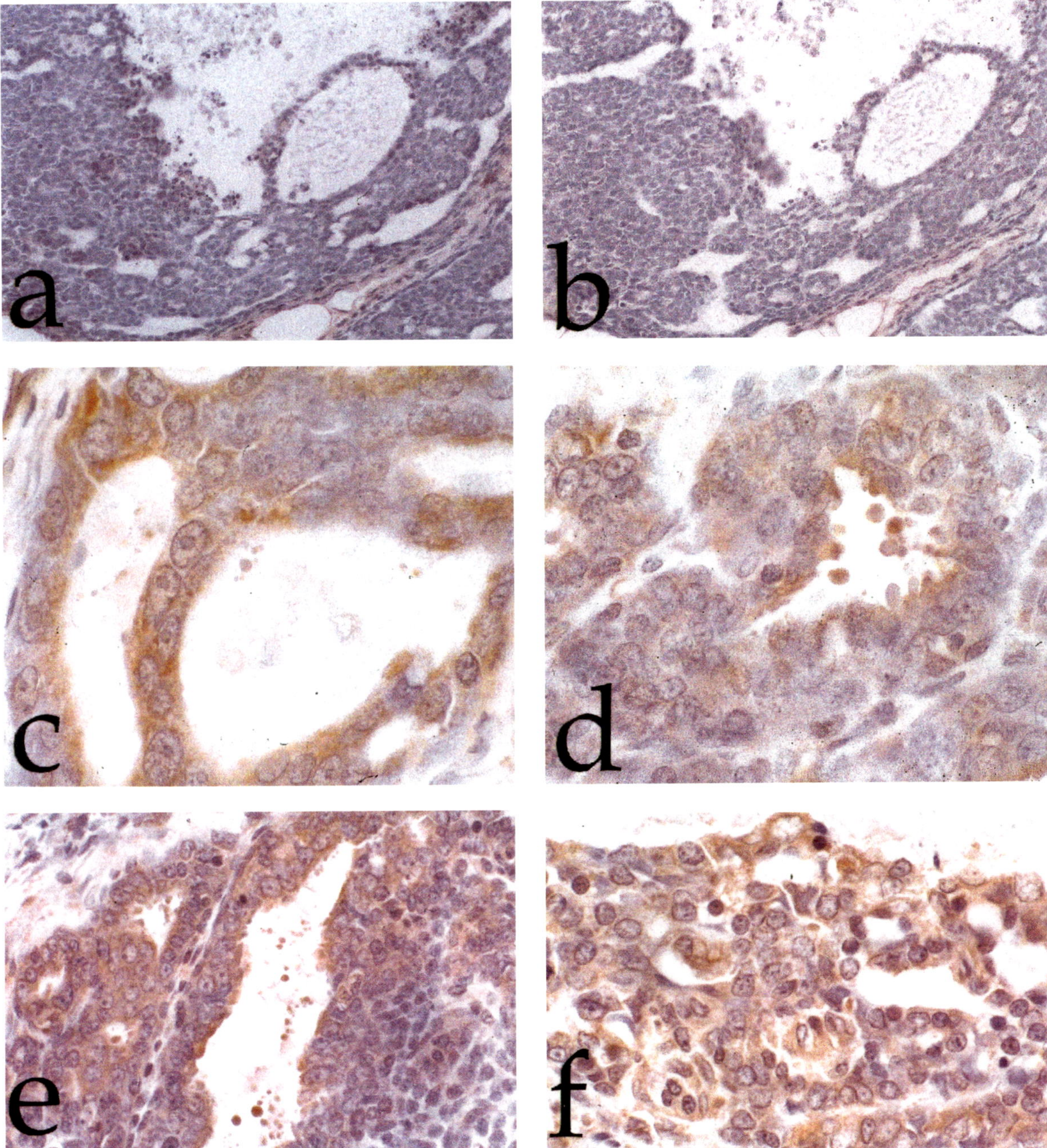

of TGF β or of other members of this family. Our results clearly support the concept that hCG acts as an inducer of inhibin and early response gene expression even in the mammary gland affected by a chemical carcinogen. Although more work needs to be done for understanding the mechanisms mediating hCG's effect on gene activation, our results indicate that both inhibin subunits can be used as intermediate surrogate markers for evaluating the effect of hCG in the mammary gland.

10.7 Effect of Human Chorionic Gonadotropin on Programmed Cell Death Gene Expression

10.7.1 Effect of Human Chorionic Gonadotropin in the Mammary Gland of Animals Treated with DMBA

The mammary glands of hCG and DMBA + hCG groups of animals (Fig. 10.15) showed elevated expression of TRPM2 and ICE transcripts as early as 5 days after initiation of treatment (70-day-old groups); their values remained elevated at all subsequent time points tested, and up to 20 days post-treatment (125-day-old groups) [41]. The hormonal treatment induced an increase of 2.5- to 5.0-fold and 1.5- to 5.0-fold in the expression of TRPM2 and ICE transcripts respectively (Figs. 10.28–10.30). Maximal induction was observed in the animals sacrificed at the ages of 85 and 105 days. DMBA treatment alone, on the other hand, did not modify, or even slightly reduced the expression of TRPM2 and ICE transcripts, since the values found were similar to those of the respective control groups. The product of proto-oncogene bcl2 and one of its family members, bcl-XL, are known to play a role in promoting cell survival and inhibiting apoptosis, while expression of bcl-XS is associated with the induction of apoptosis. We examined by Northern blot analysis the effects of hCG treatment on the mRNA expression of bcl2, bcl-XL and bcl-XS (Figs. 10.31, 10.32). Our results demonstrated that neither DMBA nor hCG treatments had effect on the expression of bcl2 and bcl-XL at any of the time periods tested. Treatment with hCG either alone or after DMBA, on the other hand, induced the

expression of bcl-XS, an effect that was not observed in the DMBA-treated group [41].

In order to determine whether the activation of programmed cell death genes by hCG was dependent on p53 and *c-myc*, we studied their expression at different time periods after the initiation of the hormonal treatment. HCG treatment induced in the mammary gland an increase in the expression of p53 (3- to 5-fold) (Fig. 10.33) and *c-myc* (2- to 4-fold) (Fig. 10.34). This increased expression was maintained from the 5th day of treatment (70-day-old animals) up to 20 days post treatment (125-day-old animals). DMBA treatment did not modify the expression of these genes, whereas in the DMBA + hCG group a dramatic increase in the expression of p53 (10- to 14-fold increase) and *c-myc* (7-fold increase) was noted in the groups of animals sacrificed at the ages of 85 and 105 days. These findings indicated that the induction of programmed cell death observed in the mammary gland of hCG treated animals was dependent on both p53 and *c-myc*. TGF-α and TGF-β genes were normally expressed in the mammary glands of control animals. Administration of hCG, either alone or after DMBA treatment had either very little or almost no effect on the expression of TGF genes [41].

Figure 10.28 a–e ▶

Northern blot analysis of TRPM2 mRNA. Total RNA was obtained from the mammary glands of three animals from each one of the four groups described in Fig. 10.15. Control (*c*; lanes 1–3), hCG (*h*; lanes 4–6), DMBA (*D*; lanes 7–9), DMBA + hCG (*D+h*; lanes 10–12). Rats were sacrificed at **a** 70, **b** 75, **c** 85, **d** 105, and **e** 125 days of age. β-actin was used for detecting the amount of RNA loaded in each lane

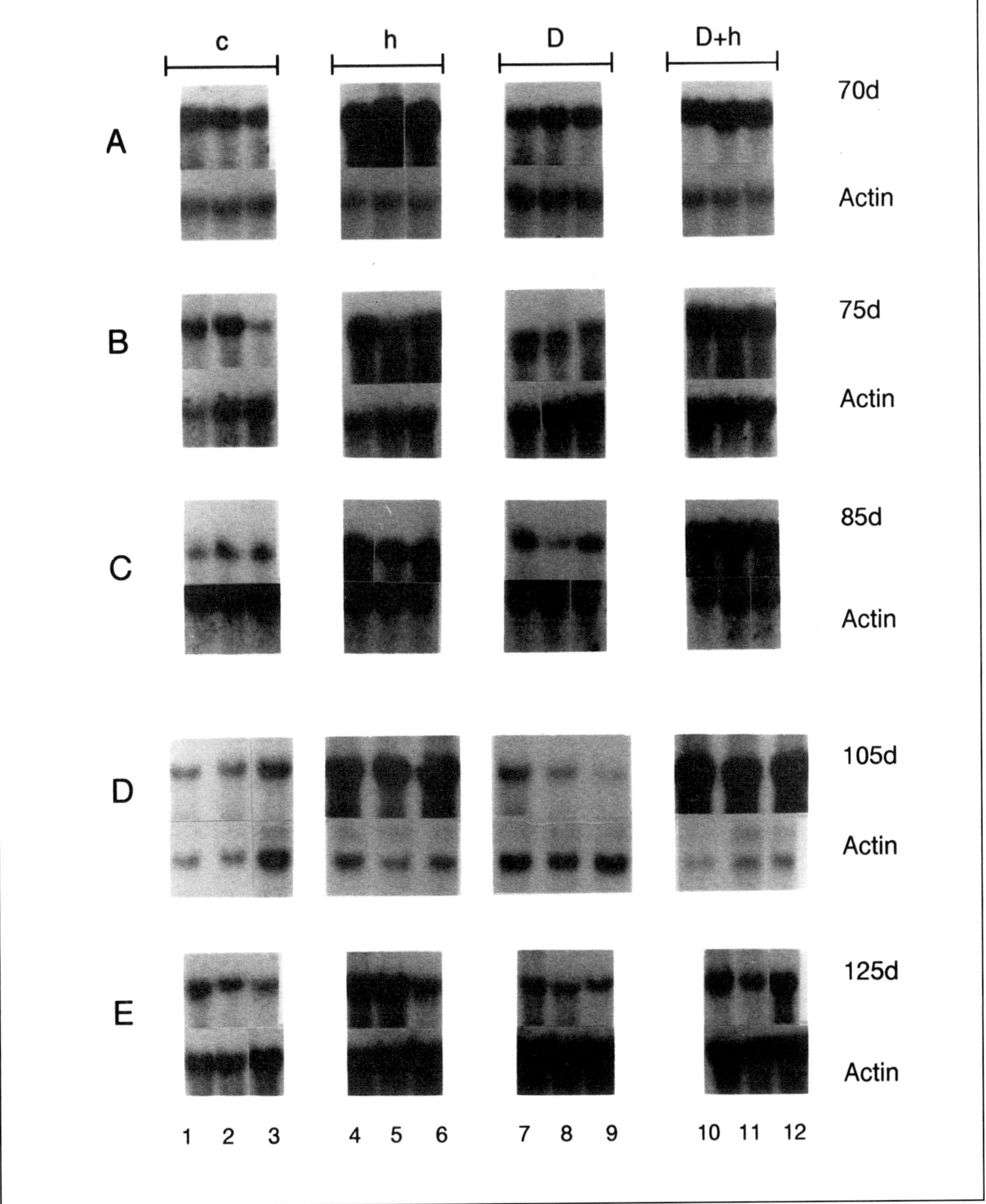
c
h
D
D+h
70d
Actin
75d
Actin
85d
Actin
105d
Actin
125d
Actin
A
B
C
D
E
1 2 3   4 5 6   7 8 9   10 11 12

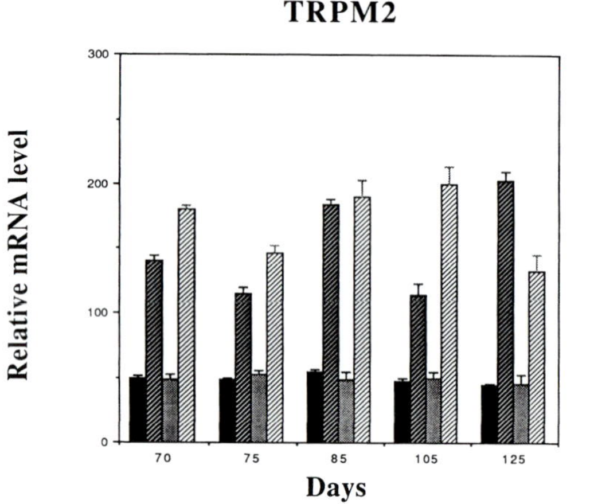

Figure 10.29

Histogram showing the relative expression of TRPM2 mRNA in the mammary gland of control (*Cont*), hCG, DMBA and DMBA + hCG (*D+h*) treated animals sacrificed at the times indicated in the abscissa. The relative level of transcripts for each experimental group was determined by Scanning laser densitometry of autoradiographs, and equalized by detection of β-actin. *Bars* represent the mean ± standard deviation of 5 animals per group. Reprinted with permission from: Srivastava, P., Russo, J. and Russo, I.H. Chorionic gonadotropin inhibits rat mammary carcinogenesis through activation of programmed cell death. Carcinogenesis 18:1799–1808, 1997

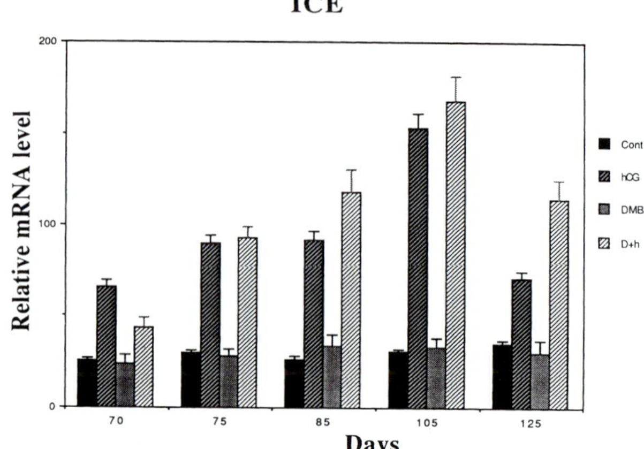

Figure 10.30

Histogram showing relative ICE mRNA expression in the mammary gland of the same groups of animals described in Fig. 10.23. Relative mRNA contents for each experimental group were determined by Scanning laser densitometry of autoradiographs equalized by detection of β-actin. *Bars* represent the mean ± standard deviation of 5 animals per group. Reprinted with permission from: Srivastava, P., Russo, J. and Russo, I.H. Chorionic gonadotropin inhibits rat mammary carcinogenesis through activation of programmed cell death. Carcinogenesis 18:1799–1808, 1997

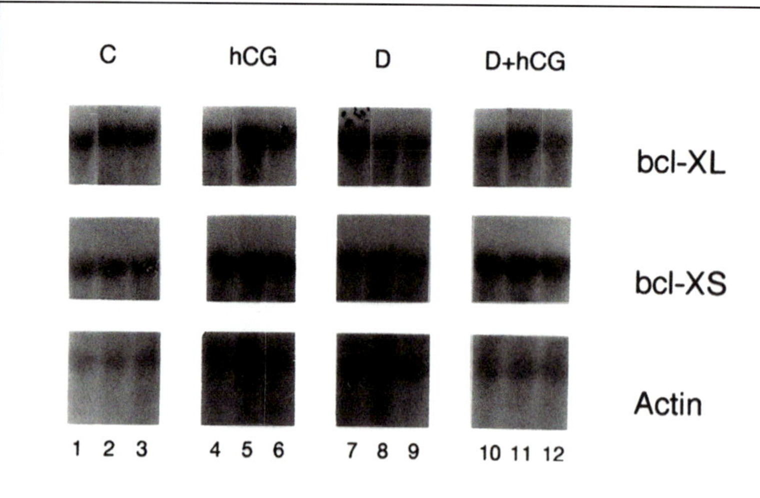

Figure 10.31

Northern blot analysis of bcl2, bcl-XL and bcl-XS in the mammary gland of animals sacrificed at 85 days of age for RNA isolation from frozen mammary glands. Only bcl-XS expression was enhanced by the hCG. Reprinted with permission from: Srivastava, P., Russo, J. and Russo, I.H. Chorionic gonadotropin inhibits rat mammary carcinogenesis through activation of programmed cell death. Carcinogenesis 18:1799–1808, 1997

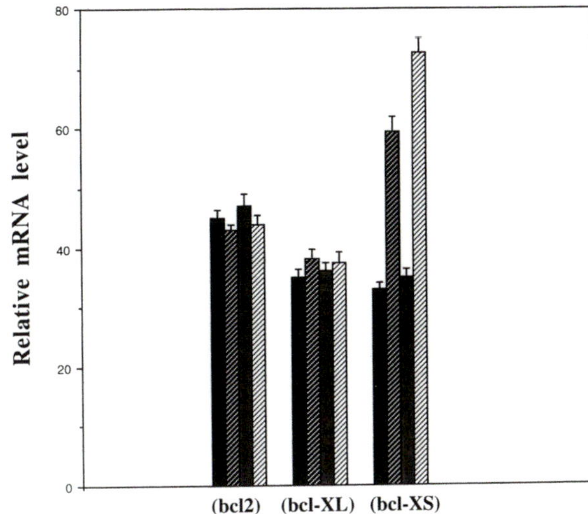

Figure 10.32

Histogram showing relative bcl2, bcl-XL and bcl-XS mRNA expression in the mammary gland of animals sacrificed at 85 days of age for RNA isolation from frozen mammary glands. Only bcl-XS expression was enhanced by the hCG treatment. Relative mRNA contents for each experimental group were determined by Scanning laser densitometry of autoradiographs, and shown as an average. *Bars* represent the mean ± standard deviation of 5 animals per group. Reprinted with permission from: Srivastava, P., Russo, J. and Russo, I.H. Chorionic gonadotropin inhibits rat mammary carcinogenesis through activation of programmed cell death. Carcinogenesis 18:1799–1808, 1997

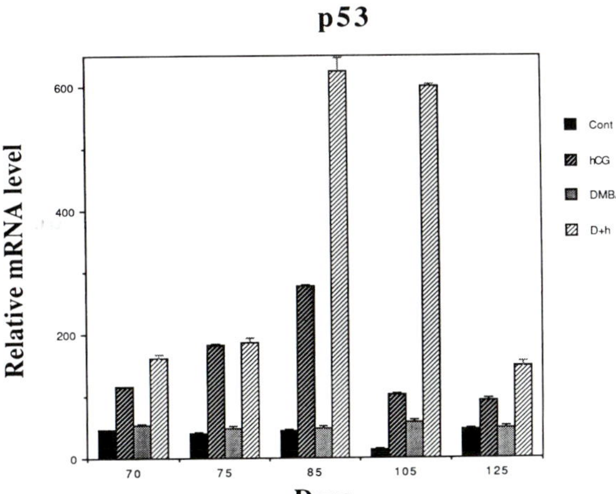

Figure 10.33

Histogram showing relative p53 mRNA expression in the mammary glands of the four groups of animals described in Fig. 10.15. Abbreviations as per Fig. 10.24. Rats were sacrificed at 70, 75, 85, 105, and 125 days of age (abscissa). Relative mRNA contents for each experimental group were determined by Scanning laser densitometry of autoradiographs, and shown as an average. *Bars* represent the mean ± standard deviation of 5 animals per group. Reprinted with permission from: Srivastava, P., Russo, J. and Russo, I.H. Chorionic gonadotropin inhibits rat mammary carcinogenesis through activation of programmed cell death. Carcinogenesis 18: 1799–1808, 1997

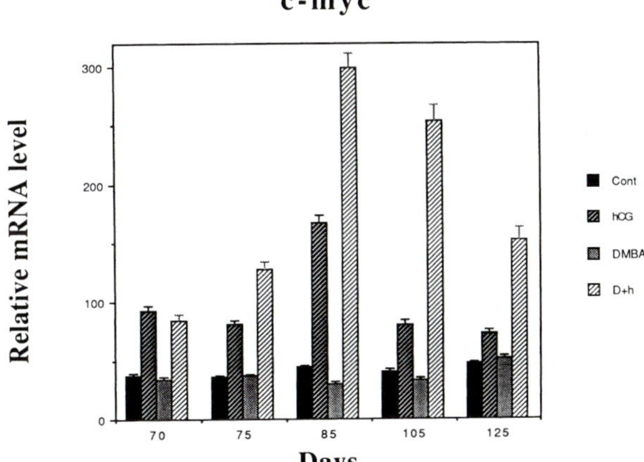

Figure 10.34

Histogram showing relative *c-myc* mRNA expression in the mammary gland of the four groups of animals described in Figs. 10.15 and 10.24. Abbreviations as per Fig. 10.24. Rats were sacrificed at 70, 75, 85, 105, and 125 days of age (abscissa). Relative mRNA contents for each experimental group were determined by Scanning laser densitometry of autoradiographs, and shown as an average. *Bars* represent the mean ± standard deviation of 5 animals per group. Reprinted with permission from: Srivastava, P., Russo, J. and Russo, I.H. Chorionic gonadotropin inhibits rat mammary carcinogenesis through activation of programmed cell death. Carcinogenesis 18:1799–1808, 1997

10.7.2 Effect of Human Chorionic Gonadotropin Treatment on the Expression of Apoptotic Genes in DMBA-Induced Mammary Carcinomas

Mammary adenocarcinomas that reached up to 1.5 cm in diameter from the DMBA and the DMBA + hCG groups were tested for the expression of the same genes described above. In the non-tumoral mammary glands and in the adenocarcinomas developed in those animals treated with DMBA alone the expression of p53, *c-myc*, ICE, bcl2, and TGF-β was not modified in any of the groups studied, whereas in those animals that received hCG after carcinogen treatment the levels of p53, *c-myc*, and ICE were significantly elevated [41] (Figs. 10.35, 10.36). The elevation was more marked in the non-tumoral mammary gland than in the tumors, but the differences with the levels observed in adenocarcinomas developed by the animals treated with DMBA alone were significant. The expression of TRPM2 was significantly elevated in the non-tumoral mammary glands of DMBA + hCG treated animals, whereas it was not modified in any of the tumors. Neither the non-tumoral mammary glands nor the tumors exhibited changes in the expression of bcl2 and TGF-β, or TGF-α as a consequence of the hCG or DMBA treatments (Figs. 10.35, 10.36). These observations indicated that even though in certain animals treated with hCG tumors developed, the hormone was still capable of inducing a certain degree of activation of the apoptotic genes, which might account for the lower overall tumorigenic response in hCG treated animals [41, 109].

10.7.3 Effect of Human Chorionic Gonadotropin Treatment on the Expression of Apoptotic Genes in the Ovary

The specificity of the effect of hCG on the expression of apoptotic genes in the mammary gland was verified by a comparison with the expression of these genes in the ovaries of the same animals. Northern blot analysis revealed that the ovaries of control animals had detectable basal levels of all the apoptotic transcripts tested in the mammary glands, as well as

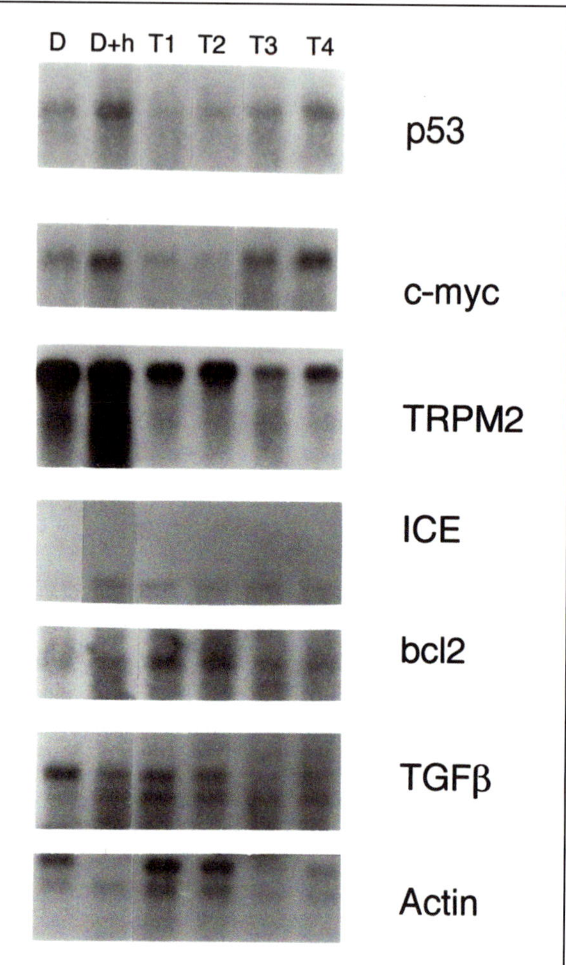

Figure 10.35

Northern blot analysis of p53, *c-myc*, TRPM2, ICE, bcl2, and TGF-β mRNAs. Polyadenylated RNA was isolated from mammary glands of DMBA alone (*D*), and DMBA + hCG (*D+h*) treated animals, and from DMBA-induced mammary adenocarcinomas developed in animals treated with DMBA alone (*T1* and *T2*) or with DMBA+hCG (*T3* and *T4*). β-actin was used for detecting the amount of RNA loaded in each lane. Reprinted with permission from: Srivastava, P., Russo, J. and Russo, I.H. Chorionic gonadotropin inhibits rat mammary carcinogenesis through activation of programmed cell death. Carcinogenesis 18:1799–1808, 1997

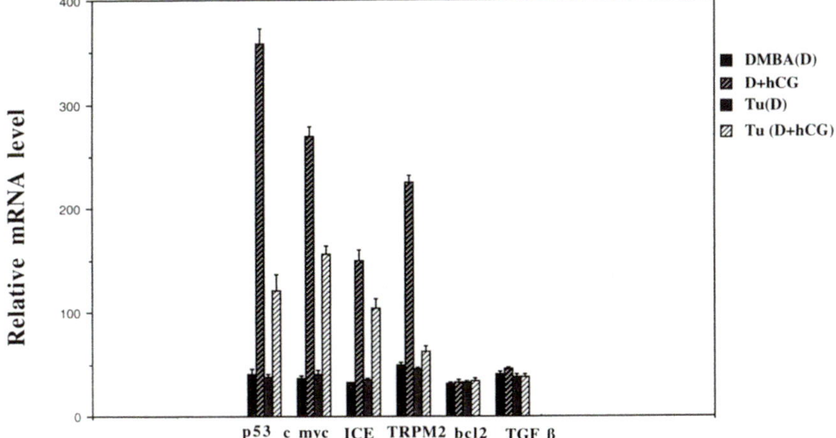

Figure 10.36

Histogram showing relative p53, *c-myc*, ICE, TRPM2, bcl2, and TGF-β mRNA expression in the non-tumoral mammary glands of DMBA (*D*) and DMBA + hCG (*D+hCG*) treated animals, and in DMBA-induced mammary tumors (*Tu*). *Tu (D)* mean values of tumors T1 and T2, shown in Fig. 10.35. *Tu (D+hCG)* mean values of tumors T3 and T4, shown in Fig. 10.35. Reprinted with permission from: Srivastava, P., Russo, J. and Russo, I.H. Chorionic gonadotropin inhibits rat mammary carcinogenesis through activation of programmed cell death. Carcinogenesis 18:1799–1808, 1997

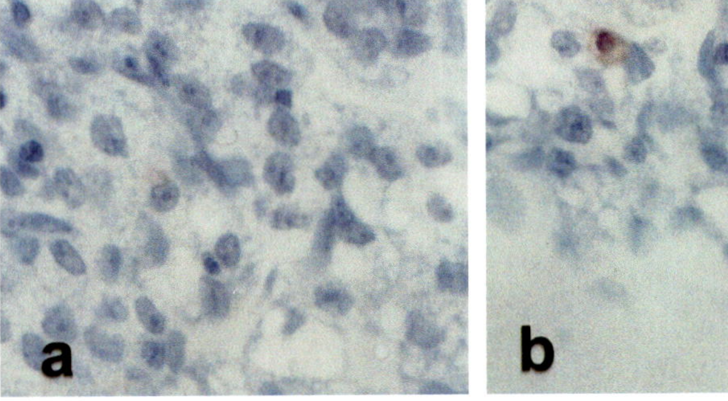

Figure 10.37 a, b

Immunocytochemical detection of apoptotic cells in **a** control and **b** hCG treated mammary gland. In all sections, immunostaining was visualized with DAB, the hematoxylin was used as a counterstain. All photographs were taken at ×40

of TGF-α and TGF-β (Fig. 10.37). No significant alterations in mRNA expression in any of the genes studied were observed to be induced by either hCG or DMBA treatments at any of the time periods tested. These results indicated that the induction of programmed cell death expression by hCG occurred specifically in the mammary gland, but did not modify these parameters in the ovary, despite of being this the target organ of hCG action.

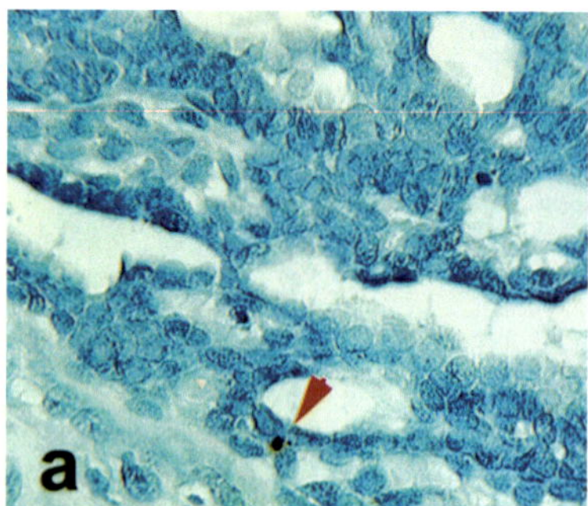
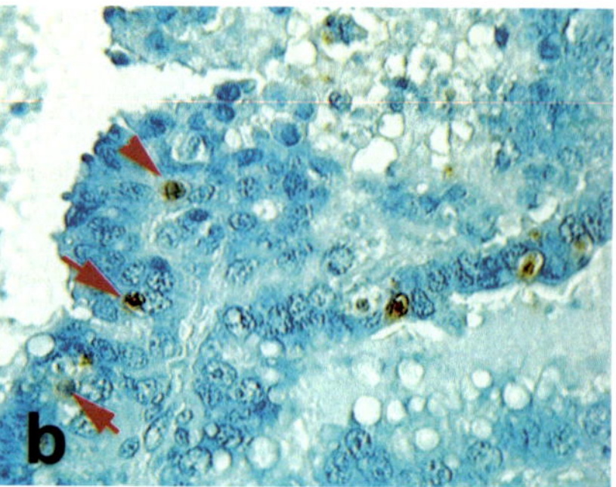

Figure 10.38 a, b

Immunocytochemical detection of apoptotic cells (*arrows*) **a** in a DMBA induced mammary tumor and **b** in a tumor of DMBA + hCG group. In all sections, immunostaining was visualized with DAB, the hematoxylin was used as a counterstain. All photographs were taken at ×40

10.7.4 Effect of Human Chorionic Gonadotropin Treatment on Apoptosis

Apoptosis was detected in 4-µm sections of formalin-fixed, paraffin embedded tissue sections of non-tumoral mammary glands of control, hCG, DMBA and DMBA + hCG treated animals, and in DMBA-induced mammary carcinomas in the two latter groups of animals. Apoptotic cell nuclei were identified using the ApopTag kit (Oncor, Gaithersburg, MD) utilizing standard procedures (Figs. 10.38, 10.39). The number of cells containing apoptotic nuclei was counted in ducts and lobules of non-tumoral mammary glands of animals of the four groups under study, and in three DMBA-induced tumors developed in the DMBA and three in the DMBA + hCG groups of animals. The percentage of positive cells over the total number of cells counted in each specific structure represented the apoptotic index. In the non-tumoral mammary gland the lowest apoptotic index was observed in control animals, and this parameter was not modified by aging. The second lowest index was observed in the DMBA group of animals. Treatment with hCG induced an increase in the apoptotic index which reached its maximum when the animals were 85 days old, and it remained elevated at the same level even after cessation of the hormonal treatment. Administration of hCG after DMBA induced a steady increase in the apoptotic index which reached a peak by the time the animals were 105 days old, but its value decreased sharply after the discontinuation of the hormonal treatment. The apoptotic index of DMBA-induced mammary carcinomas was markedly lower

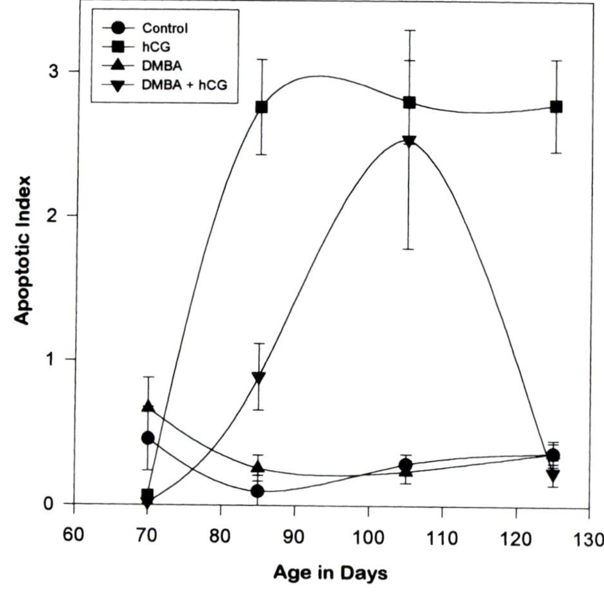

Figure 10.39

Detection of apoptotic cells in non-tumoral mammary glands of the four groups of rats described in Figure 10.15. Results are expressed as the number of immunocytochemically positive cells per total number of cells counted, and expressed as a percentage, or apoptotic index (ordinate). Rats were sacrificed at 70, 85, 105, and 125 days of age (abscissa). *Bars* represent the mean ±standard deviation of 5 animals counted per group and per time point. Reprinted with permission from: Srivastava, P., Russo, J. and Russo, I.H. Chorionic gonadotropin inhibits rat mammary carcinogenesis through activation of programmed cell death. Carcinogenesis 18: 1799–1808, 1997

Table 10.4. Effect of ovariectomy and hCG treatment in DMBA-induced mammary carcinogenesis. *OV* old virgin rats, *EP* estrogen plus progesterone treatment

Group	Number of animals	Number of animals with tumor/number of animals	Percentage	Number of tumors	Tumors/animal
1-DMBA	18	18/18	100	60	3.30
2-DMBA+hCG	20	9/20	45	20	1.00
3-OV+DMBA	18	1/18	6	4	0.22
4-OV+DMBA+hCG	20	0/20	0	0	0.00
5-OV+DMBA+EP	18	6/18	33	8	0.44
6-OV+DMBA+EP+hCG	20	2/20	10	2	0.10

than that of the non-tumoral mammary gland of the animals in the same group. HCG treatment resulted in a marked increase in the apoptotic index of mammary adenocarcinomas with respect to the values found in the tumors of the DMBA group, and also higher than in the non-tumoral mammary gland of the same group of animals (Fig. 10.39, Table 10.5).

The results described above demonstrate that treatment of virgin rats with hCG, in which the mammary carcinogenic process had been initiated with the chemical carcinogen DMBA, induces programmed cell death. We postulate that this effect is *p53* dependent, and is modulated by *c-myc* expression. In addition, the results suggest the possibility of the existence of a cell death program that is dependent on the *bcl2* family because of the potential involvement on *p53*, *bcl-XS* and Bax in apoptosis. The use of agents like hCG, that induce apoptosis, may constitute a useful approach for the prevention and therapy of breast cancer.

10.8 Evidence of a Direct Effect of Human Chorionic Gonadotropin in Mammary Epithelial Cells

10.8.1 Human Chorionic Gonadotropin Has an Inhibitory Effect on DMBA Mammary Carcinogenesis in Ovariectomized Animals

In order to determine if hCG has a direct effect in the mammary gland the experimental protocol depicted in Table 10.4 was utilized. Ovariectomy was performed after DMBA administration (group 3) and compared with intact animals in group 1. As expected the tumor incidence and the number of tumors per animals was significantly reduced by ovarian ablation as well as by hCG (groups 2 and 4). Estrogen supplementation in the ovariectomized animals reestablished the tumor incidence and number of tumors per animals (group 5), however, hCG significantly reduced, in those supplemented animals, the number of tumors per animal as well as the incidence (group 6). These data clearly indicate that hCG has a direct effect on the mammary gland independently of the ovarian function. This also suggests that hCG could be a tumoristatic agent in postmenopausal women, even in presence of hormone replacement therapy (see section 10.10).

10.8.2 Effect of Human Chorionic Gonadotropin in Human Breast Epithelial Cells In Vitro

Treatment of human breast epithelial cells with hCG, inhibits the proliferative activity of the cells and induces activation of apoptotic genes. Inhibition of cell growth was observed only in HBEC, whereas the urothelial cells T24 were not affected by this treatment (Fig. 10.40). MCF-10F cells exhibited activation of the apoptotic genes TRPM2, ICE, TGF-b, p53, bax, and p21$^{WAFI/CIPI}$ (Figs. 10.41, 10.42). BP1-E cells, derived from BP-transformed MCF-10F cells were also growth-inhibited, however the pattern of gene activation differed from that exhibited by the parent cells (Figs. 10.43, 10.44). BP1-E cells exhibited activation of only ICE, bax, and p21$^{WAFI/CIPI}$ and significantly down-regulated bcl2, but did not modify TGF-β, p53 or *c-myc* expression. The urothelial cells did not show activation of any of the apoptotic genes. The lack of activation of the genes that control programmed cell death in these latter cells coincides with the selectivity of hCG in the inhibition of in vitro cell proliferation, which was observed only in HBEC, but not in T24 cells (Fig. 10.45) [43]. This specificity of action might be attributed to a receptor-mediated effect of hCG on human breast epithelial cells, whose presence has been recently reported in rat mammary epithelial cells (see Chapter 3).

Increased expression of TRPM2 and TGF-β genes has been shown during chemotherapeutic regression of a mouse bladder tumor [110], regressing human breast cancer cells and in prostatic tumors after hormone withdrawal [111, 112]. In our experimental model, activation of these genes occurred only in MCF-10F but not in the chemically transformed and T24 cell lines. This observation supports the concept that activation of these, two genes might be dependent on specific cell characteristics. The association between the induction of cell growth inhibition and TRPM2 activation has also been reported to be stimulated in MCF-7 cells by 1,25dihydroxyvitamin D3 [113]. ICE gene expression was increased by hCG treatment in MCF-10F and BPI-E cells by the hormonal treatment. This gene, which belongs to a protease family has been shown to be relevant in the in-

duction of apoptosis (Fig. 10.46) [114–117]. Increases in the levels of ICE (caspase-1) mRNA have been associated with apoptosis in mammary epithelial cells by loss of attachment to extracellular matrix proteins and treatment of some tumor cell lines with chemotherapeutic drugs [118]. Several lines of evidence indicates that the induction of apoptosis can be mediated by both p53 and *c-myc*, which are the major players in the context of growth arrest and apoptosis [119]. We have found that hCG treatment, significantly induced the expression of p53 and p21$^{WAFI/CIPI}$ in MCF-10F cells, observation that suggested that the cell growth arrest was mediated by the tumor suppressor p53 through its downstream target gene p21wAF'/Clp' [119, 120]. Even though BPI-E cells exhibited an inhibition in their in vitro growth, and induced p21$^{WAFI/CIPI}$ mRNA but the expression *c-myc* and p53 genes was not modified by the hormonal treatment. These observations might indicate that cell growth and activation of the apoptotic genes have been independently modulated by other genes and/or other external factors. Recent evidences have shown both p53-dependent and p53-independent apoptosis pathways [121, 122]. Thus, our observation that p53 was significantly activated by hCG treatment in MCF-10F, but not in BP1-E cells led us to postulate that the activation of apoptotic genes might have occurred, through those two different pathways for the inhibition of in vitro cell proliferation (Fig. 10.46). Our observations suggested that in MCF-10F cells hCG arrested the progression of the cell cycle by inducing (probably through its receptor), the CAMP-PKA, and p53, as well as the TGF-β pathways, for acting on their target gene p21$^{WAFI/CIPI}$, proceeding then towards cell cycle arrest and apoptosis (Fig. 10.46). In the case of the chemically transformed cell line, TGF-β, p53, and *c-myc* did not express any changes in their level of expression, although there was a profound induction of p21$^{WAFI/CIPI}$ mRNA, thus suggesting that this gene was induced by hCG independently of p53, probably via transcription factor (TF), differentiation factor (DF) (Fig. 10.46), as it has been shown in other systems [123].

ICE class proteases (caspases) have been shown to play an important role in p53 mediated apoptosis [124], though molecular details are not fully under-

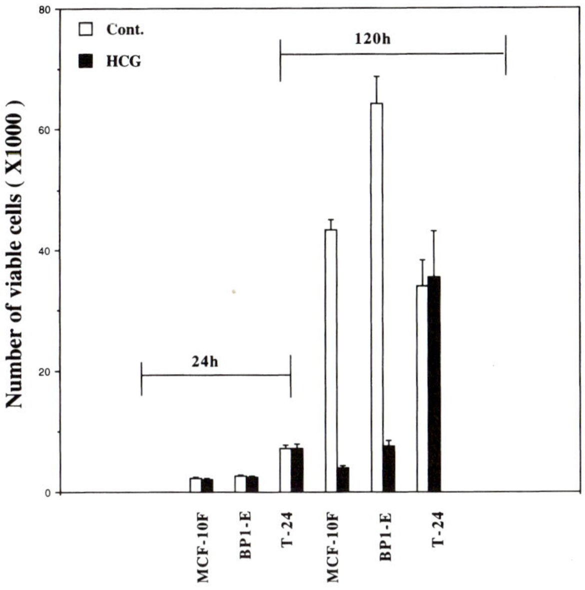

Figure 10.40

Effect of hCG treatment on cell growth. MCF-10F, BPI-E, and T24 cells were treated daily with 100 IU/ml hCG and harvested at 24 and 120 h for cell growth determination by WST-colorimetric assay. Control cells were treated with vehicle only. Values represent the mean number of viable cells ($\times$ 1,000) $\pm$ SD of three wells from two experiments. Reprinted with permission from: Srivastava, P., Russo, J., Mgbonyebi, O.P., and Russo, I.H. Growth inhibition and activation of apoptotic gene expression by human chorionic gonadotropin in human breast epithelial cells. Anticancer Research; 18:4003–4010, 1998

Figure 10.41 ▶

Northern blot analysis of TRPM2, ICE, bcl2, TGF-β, *c-myc*, p53, bax, and p21 gene expression in MCF-10F cells. Polyadenylated RNA was isolated from cells treated daily with 100 IU/ml hCG and harvested at 24 and 120 h. Lanes 1 and 2 represent control cells treated with vehicle solution for 24 and 120 h, while Lanes 3 and 4 represent cells treated with hCG for 24 and 120 h respectively. β-actin was used for detecting the amount of RNA loaded in each lane. Reprinted with permission from: Srivastava, P., Russo, J., Mgbonyebi, O.P., and Russo, I.H. Growth inhibition and activation of apoptotic gene expression by human chorionic gonadotropin in human breast epithelial cells. Anticancer Research; 18:4003–4010, 1998

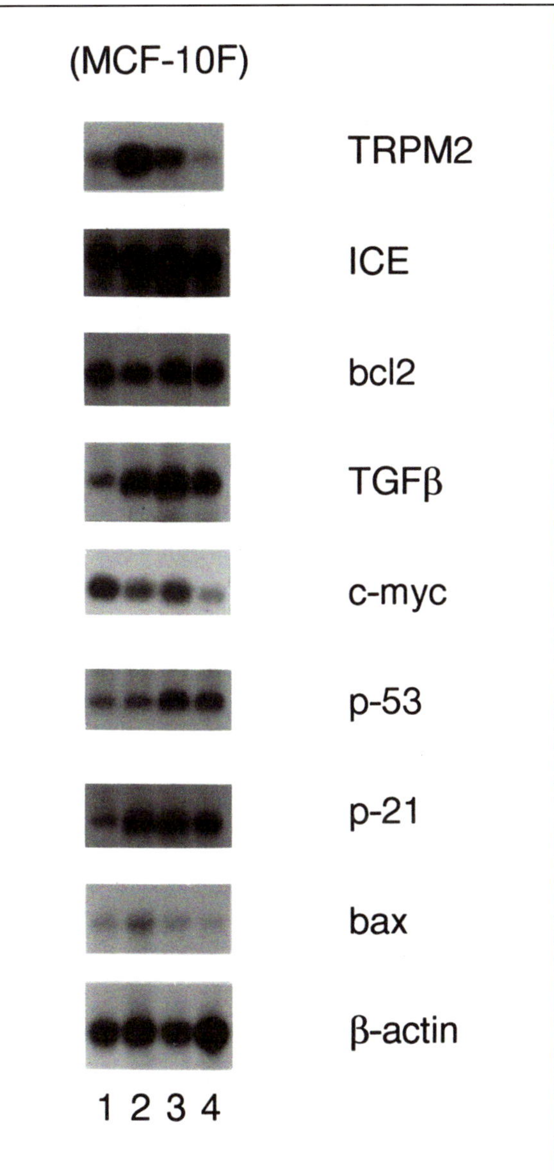

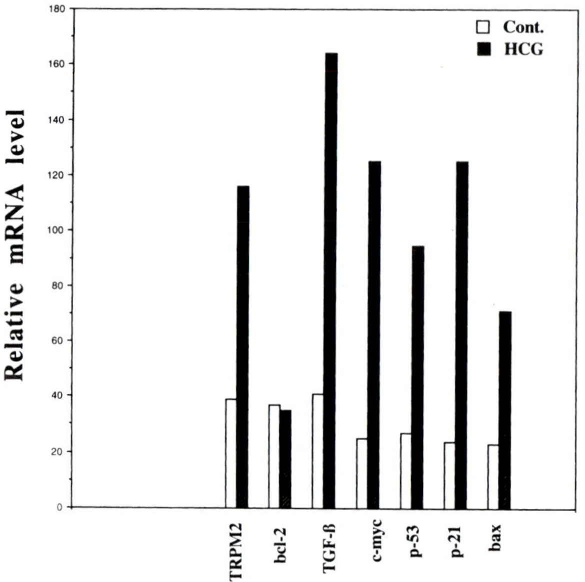

Figure 10.42

Histogram showing the expression of TRPM2, ICE, bcl-2, TGFβ, *c-myc*, p53, bax, and p21 mRNA relative to their respective controls in MCF-10F cells treated with hCG for 24 h. Relative mRNA content was determined by scanning laser densitometry of autoradiographs, and equalized by detection of β-actin. Reprinted with permission from: Srivastava, P., Russo, J., Mgbonyebi, O.P., and Russo, I.H. Growth inhibition and activation of apoptotic gene expression by human chorionic gonadotropin in human breast epithelial cells. Anticancer Research; 18: 4003–4010, 1998

Figure 10.43 ▶

Northern blot analysis of TRPM2, ICE, bcl-2, TGF-β, *c-myc*, p53, bax, and p21 gene expression in BPI-E cells treated with 100 IU hCG/ml. Cells were harvested at 24 and 120 h of treatment for isolation of polyadenylated RNA. Lane identification as per Fig. 10.41. β-actin was used for detecting the amount of RNA loaded in each lane. Reprinted with permission from: Srivastava, P., Russo, J., Mgbonyebi, O.P., and Russo, I.H. Growth inhibition and activation of apoptotic gene expression by human chorionic gonadotropin in human breast epithelial cells. Anticancer Research; 18:4003–4010, 1998

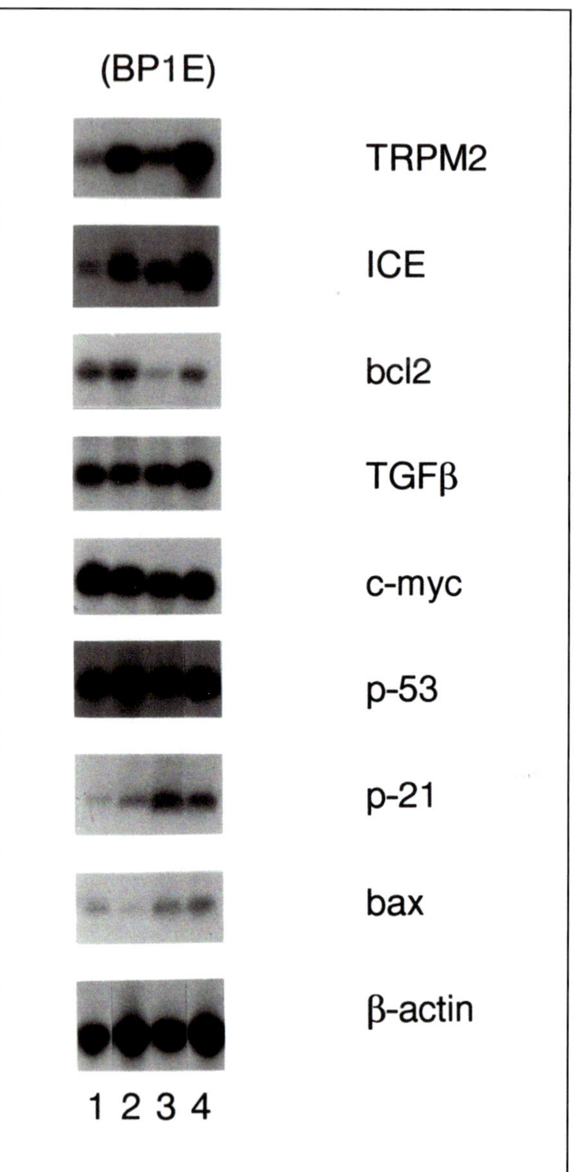

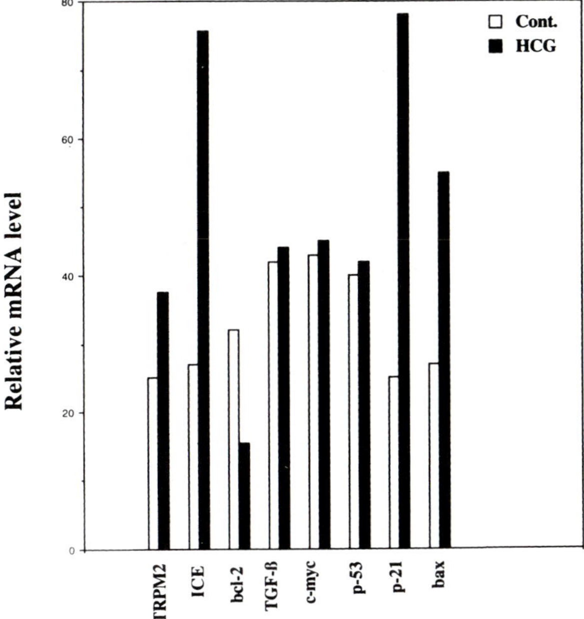

Figure 10.44

Histogram showing the expression of TRPM2, ICE, bcl-2, TGFβ, *c-myc*, p53, bax and p21 MRNA relative to their respective controls in BPI-E cells treated with hCG for 24 h, as described in Fig. 10.43. Relative mRNA content was determined by scanning laser densitometry of autoradiographs, and equalized by detection of β-actin. Reprinted with permission from: Srivastava, P., Russo, J., Mgbonyebi, O.P.; and Russo, I.H. Growth inhibition and activation of apoptotic gene expression by human chorionic gonadotropin in human breast epithelial cells. Anticancer Research; 18:4003–4010, 1998

Figure 10.45 ▶

Northern blot analysis of TRPM2, ICE, bcl-2, TGF-β, *c-myc*, p53, bax, and p21 gene expression in T-24 cells treated with 100 IU hCG/ml. Cells were harvested at 24 and 120 h of treatment for isolation of polyadenylated RNA. Lane identification as per Fig. 10.41. β-actin was used for detecting the amount of RNA loaded in each lane. Reprinted with permission from: Srivastava, P., Russo, J., Mgbonyebi, O.P., and Russo, I.H. Growth inhibition and activation of apoptotic gene expression by human chorionic gonadotropin in human breast epithelial cells. Anticancer Research; 18:4003–4010, 1998

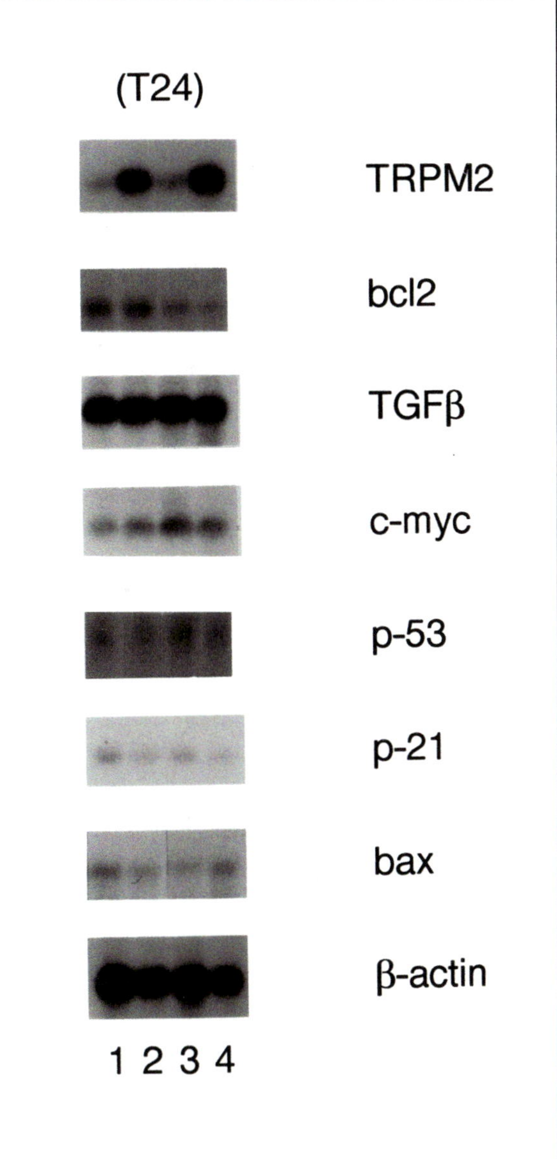

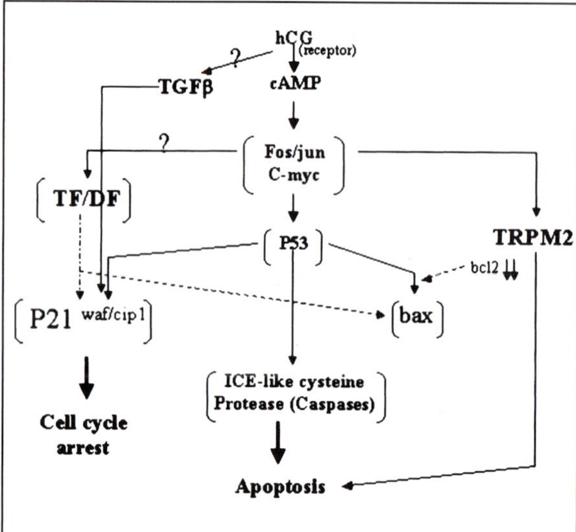

Figure 10.46

Postulated model of hCG-induced cell cycle arrest and apoptosis in human breast epithelial cells. In the presence of hCG for 24 h breast epithelial cells bind the hormone to a putative membrane receptor. This triggers a cascade of programmed cell death gene activation through the cAMP-PKA pathway, as well as through activation of TGF-β. HCG treatment activates (upregulates) TRPM2, ICE, TGF-β, p53, and p21 in MCF-10F cells; in BP1-E cells it activates TRPM2, ICE, p21 and bax, but does not activate TGF-β, *c-myc* or p53, leading us to postulate that p21 and bax activation in these cells proceeds through an alternative pathway, i.e., TF/DF (*broken arrow*). Reprinted with permission from: Srivastava, P., Russo, J., Mgbonyebi, O.P., and Russo, I.H. Growth inhibition and activation of apoptotic gene expression by human chorionic gonadotropin in human breast epithelial cells. Anticancer Research; 18:4003– 4010, 1998

stood. This mechanism is supported by our findings that hCG treatment induces an increase in the expression of both p53 and ICE in MCF-10F cells. Another possible involvement of p53 in apoptosis is the regulation by members of the bcl2 multiprotein family [125, 126]. Some of the members of the bcl2 family such as bcl2 and bcl-XL, are blockers of cell death, while others, i.e., Bax and bcl-XS, are promoters of apoptosis [125, 126]. Recent studies have indicated that bax can be activated by both p53 dependent as well as independent pathways in different system [125]. In the present study, hCG treatment induced bax expression in both MCF-10F and BP1-E cells but it markedly reduced bcl2 expression in BP1-E cells only. The fact that p53, bax and bcl2 expression are differently modulated by the hormonal treatment is a strong indication that alternative pathways might be operational in the activation of apoptotic genes by hCG. In the performance of these studies we observed that control cells exhibited an elevation in the level of expression of apoptotic genes. After 120 h in culture. The level of expression of TRPM2, ICE, TGF-B, bax, and p21$^{\text{WAFI/CIPI}}$ genes was increased in MCF-10F. In BP1-E cells TRPM2, ICE, and p21$^{\text{WAFI/CIPI}}$ were elevated at 120 h in culture in comparison with their levels at 24 h. The similarities in the activation of gene expression between levels in 24-h treated and 120-h controls indicate that hCG accelerates the process of gene activation, a phenomenon that has been reported to be associated with confluence [126].

In conclusion our results demonstrate that the 24-h hCG treatment of immortalized and chemically transformed human breast epithelial cells activates apoptotic genes even before the arrest of cell growth becomes evident. Of relevance is the fact that hCG, that is an inhibitor of in vitro cell proliferation and in vivo acts as a preventive and tumoristatic agent [36, 45], may utilize different pathways for activating apoptotic genes, depending upon the degree of expression of neoplastic phenotypes [127–130]. Taken together, the results of the present study demonstrate that the growth inhibitory effect of hCG is associated with its ability to activate the expression of apoptotic genes. The importance of our present findings lies in the potential use of hCG as a chemopreventive and chemotherapeutic agent in breast cancer.

10.9 Tumoristatic Effect of Human Chorionic Gonadotropin on Malignant Human Breast Epithelial Cells Transplanted in Heterologous Host

The observation that hCG had an inhibitory effect on chemically induced rat mammary carcinomas led us to test whether this hormone had an effect on the in vivo growth of malignant human breast epithelial cells. For these purposes, MCF-7 cells, a cell line derived from a metastatic breast carcinoma, were injected to Balb/c nude mice (nu/nu). The animals were divided into five groups: the animals of four groups had implanted a Silastic tube containing 5 mg 17-β-estradiol in the inter-scapular region 5 days after castration, and one group was castrated but did not receive the estrogen supplementation. The cells were injected in the mammary fat pad of mice in all the groups at a concentration of 1×10^6 cells. HCG was administered to the group of animals that did not receive the estrogen at a dose of 1,000 IU/day, and to the three estrogen-supplemented groups at the doses of 10, 100 or 1,000 IU per day. The animals that received estradiol pellets alone had an incidence of 85% tumor formation. The group of animals injected with hCG alone did not develop tumors (Fig. 10.47). Animals that received estradiol pellets and also hCG exhibited a reduction in both tumor incidence and tumor size which were dose-dependent (Fig. 10.47). These studies led us to conclude that the treatment, with hCG abrogates the effect of the estrogen growth dependency of MCF-7 cells in a heterologous hosts (for more details on MCF7 growth in athymic mice see Chapter 7).

10.10 Effect of Recombinant Human Chorionic Gonadotropin on Primary Breast Cancer

Based on our preclinical data that had demonstrated that r-hCG treatment of virgin rats prevented the initiation and inhibited the progression of DMBA-induced mammary carcinomas, we designed a pilot study for evaluating the effect of r-hCG on primary breast cancer in post-menopausal patients [95]. In a double-blind, placebo-controlled study, 25 post-menopausal women with primary operable breast cancer (T1–T3) whose diagnosis was made by core biopsy performed on day 0, received on alternate days for 2 weeks intramuscular injections of either r-hCG (recombinant hCG) (500 μg); $n=20$) or placebo ($n=5$). Surgery (mastectomy or lumpectomy) was performed on day 15. The tumor tissue obtained in the initial core biopsy and that removed at the time of therapeutic surgery were evaluated to determine the rate of cell proliferation, or proliferative (Ki67) index, inhibin immunoreactivity, and percentage of cells positive for estrogen (ER) and progesterone receptors (PR). The most remarkable effects attributed to this two-week treatment were a significant reduction in Ki67 index from 18% in the initial biopsy to 4% in the mastectomy/lumpectomy specimens ($p < 0.00006$) (Fig. 10.48), and increased synthesis of inhibin.

The percentage of ER and PR positive cells was decreased following the hormonal treatment, changes

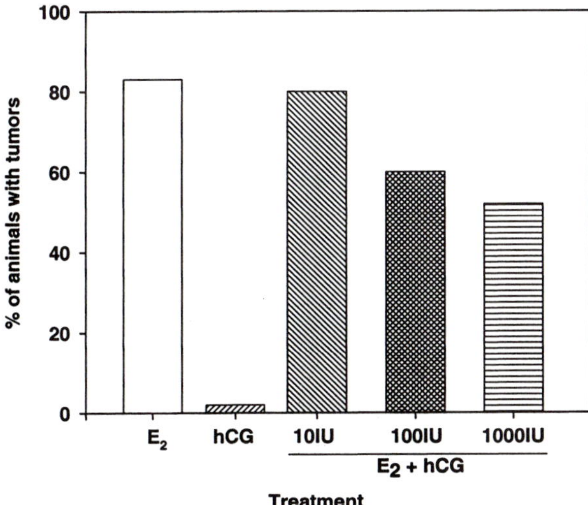

Figure 10.47

Effect of hCG treatment on the growth of tumors formed by MCF-7 cells inoculated in nude mice. *E2* animals treated with pellet of 17-β-estradiol, *hCG* animals treated with hCG alone, *E2+hCG* animals implanted with one pellet of 17-β-estradiol and treated with 10, 100, or 1,000 IU of hCG per day for 50 days

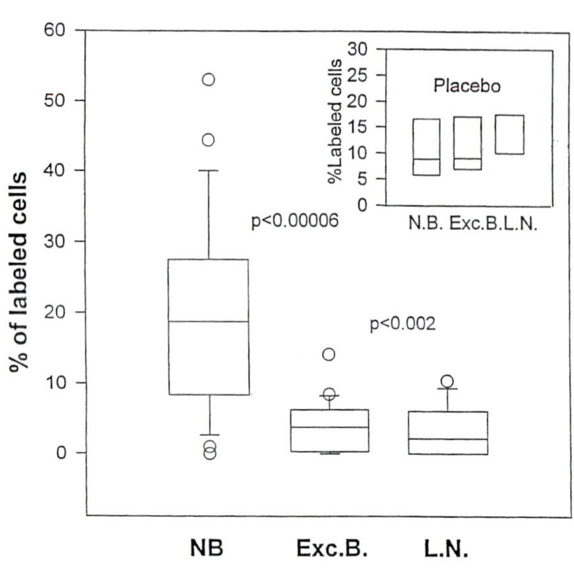

Figure 10.48

Effect of r-hCG in primary breast cancer in postmeno-pausal women. *NB* needle biopsy, *Exc.B* excisional biopsy, *LN* lymph node

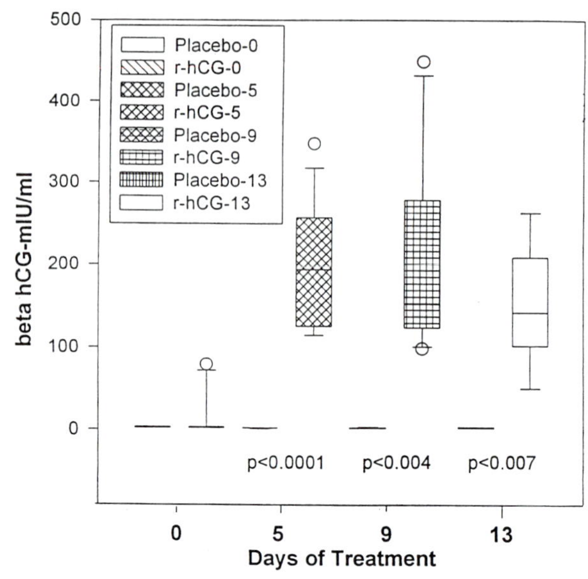

Figure 10.49

Beta hCG serum levels during r-hCG treatment

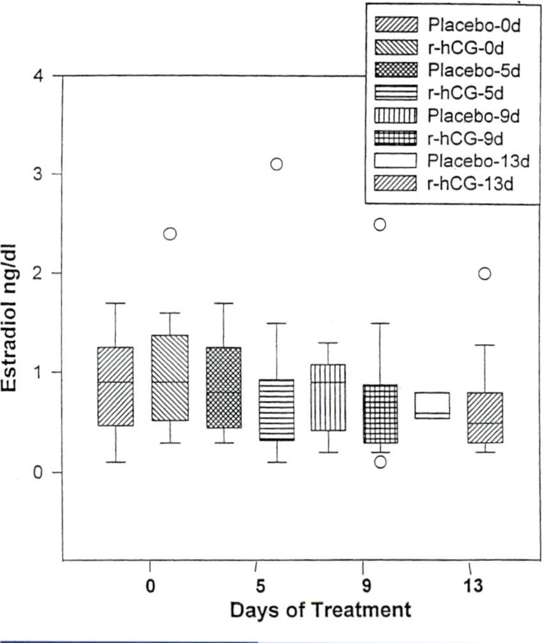

Figure 10.50

Estradiol serum levels during r-hCG treatment

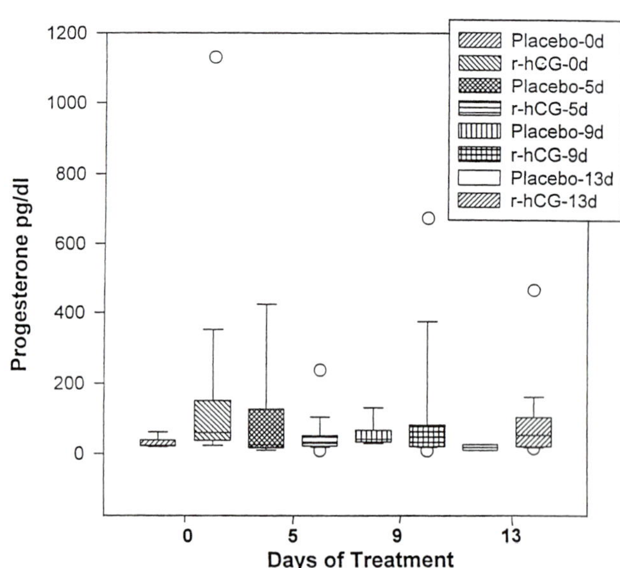

Figure 10.51

Progesterone serum levels during r-hCG treatment

that were not observed in the placebo group. Serum hormonal levels were those characteristics of post-menopausal women, and remained unchanged during and after the treatment, except for elevation in hCG levels during treatment (Fig. 10.49). Serum levels of progesterone (Fig. 10.50), 17-estradiol (Fig. 10.51), SH and LH were not affected by the hormonal treatment. Hormone administration was well tolerated by all patients, and no local or systemic side effects were reported at any time. The data clearly indicates that hCG is an inhibitor of cell proliferation independently of the ovarian function (postmenopausal women) and independent of the estrogen and progesterone receptor status of the host tissue. In addition the data indicates that the recombinant form of this hormone does not affect the hormonal milieu of the patient.

10.11 Isolation and Characterization of New Genes Induced by Human Chorionic Gonadotropin

In addition to the apoptotic pathway modified by hCG, we have postulated that this hormone might also exerts its protective effects on the mammary gland and on HBEC in vitro through activation or downregulation of specific genes. To prove this hypothesis we utilized a differential display (DD) technique for identifying and isolating candidate genes involved in this process and cDNA micro-array that will be discussed in the next section. DD is a powerful technique for identifying genes differentially expressed in normal and cancer cells [131], tumor suppressor genes, such as integrin alpha 6, and genes potentially involved in chemoprevention [132].

10.11.1 Genes Induced by Human Chorionic Gonadotropin in Human Breast Epithelial Cells In Vitro

Differential display was performed with RNA isolated from untreated or control MCF-7 cells and treated with 100 IU of hCG for 24 and 72 h to identify transcriptionally regulated genes potentially involved in

the inhibition of neoplastic cell growth induced by hCG [133]. PCR amplifications were performed using eight primer combinations. Three PCR products that were differentially expressed between control and hCG-treated cells were identified; they were designated bands 19, 29 and 44 (Figs. 10.52). Figure 10.52a and b indicate 2 representative PCR products that were reproducibly downregulated, and Fig. 10.46c shows one fragment that was upregulated by hCG treatment. The two PCR fragments, 19 and 29, were markedly reduced after a 24-h hCG treatment in comparison with their respective controls (Fig. 10.52a, b), and this reduction persisted up to 72 h of treatment. The third PCR fragment was upregulated by the 24-h and the 72-h hCG treatment (Fig. 10.52c). The isolated differentially expressed bands were 265–350 bp in size.

Northern blot analysis using polyadenylated RNA confirmed the differential expression of the bands detected by PCR (Figs. 10.53–10.55). The three PCR bands were cloned and identified as clones 19, 29 and 44. Clone 19 showed two transcripts ranging from 1.2 to 1.8 kb in size (Fig. 10.53a). This suggests that alternate splicing of a common mRNA precursor generated the two mRNAs. Both transcripts were significantly reduced at 24 h after hCG treatment. The 1.2-kb transcript was more significantly reduced than the larger transcript (Fig. 10.53a). Similarly, clone 29 also showed two transcripts (Fig. 10.54a), which ranged from 0.6 to 1.2 kb in size; both transcripts were significantly reduced by hCG treatment for 24 and 72 h. Clone 44 showed an increase in its expression of approximately 4-fold at 24 h of hCG treatment, and it remained elevated up to 72 h (Fig. 10.55).

To date we have found no significant homology with any published genes for the sequences obtained from clones 19 and 29 cDNA fragments, suggesting that they represent previously unknown genes and therefore appears to be novel. Clone 44, that was present in very small amount in control cells, was present in very high amount in cells treated with hCG for both 24 and 72 h (Fig. 10.55). Sequence homology search of this clone showed 98% match with a novel gene expressed in apoptotic T-cell hybridoma cells treated with dexamethasone [134]. In the immune system programmed cell death plays an important

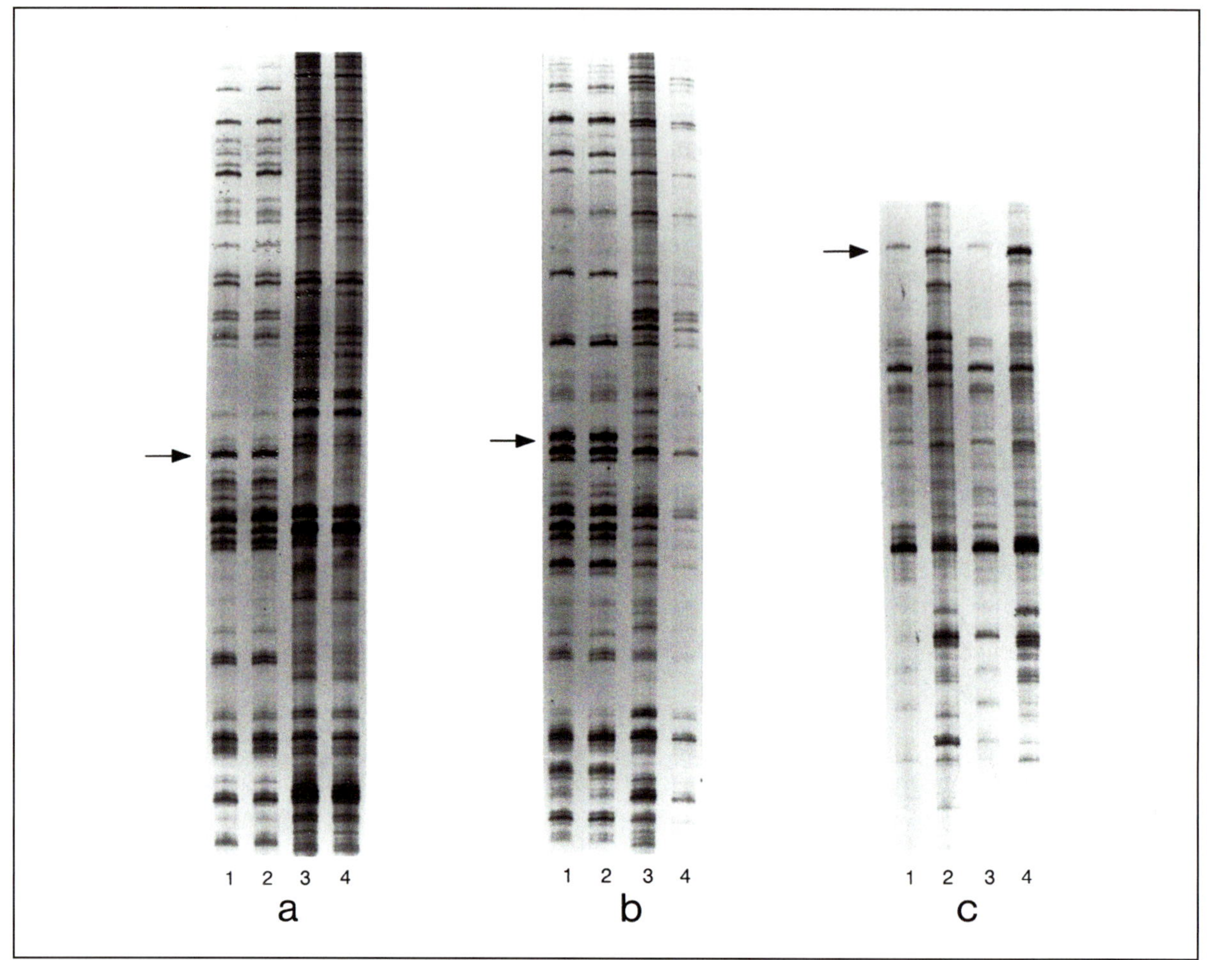

Figure 10.52 a–c

Differential display comparing RNAs from control and hCG-treated MCF-7 cells. **a, b** Autoradiogram of amplified [α-^{33}P]dATP-labeled PCR products are shown for a primer combination that identified two distinct fragments (*arrows*) which were downregulated by hCG treatment. The primer combination included HIIA, G or C and HAP-9. Lanes 1 and 2, MCF-7 control cells; lanes 3 and 4, cells treated with hCG for 24 h. **c** Autoradiogram of amplified [α-^{33}P]dATP-labeled PCR products for the primer combination HI IA, G or C and HAP-1 I that identified one fragment (*arrow*) upregulated by hCG treatment. Lane 1, control; and lane 2, cells treated with hCG for 24 h; lane 3, control; lane 4, cells treated with hCG for 72 h. Reprinted with permission from: Srivastava, P., Silva, I.D.C.G.; Russo, J., Mgbonyebi, O.P.; and Russo, I.H. Identification of genes differentially expressed in breast carcinoma cells treated with chorionic gonadotropin. Int. J. of Oncology 13: 465–469, 1998

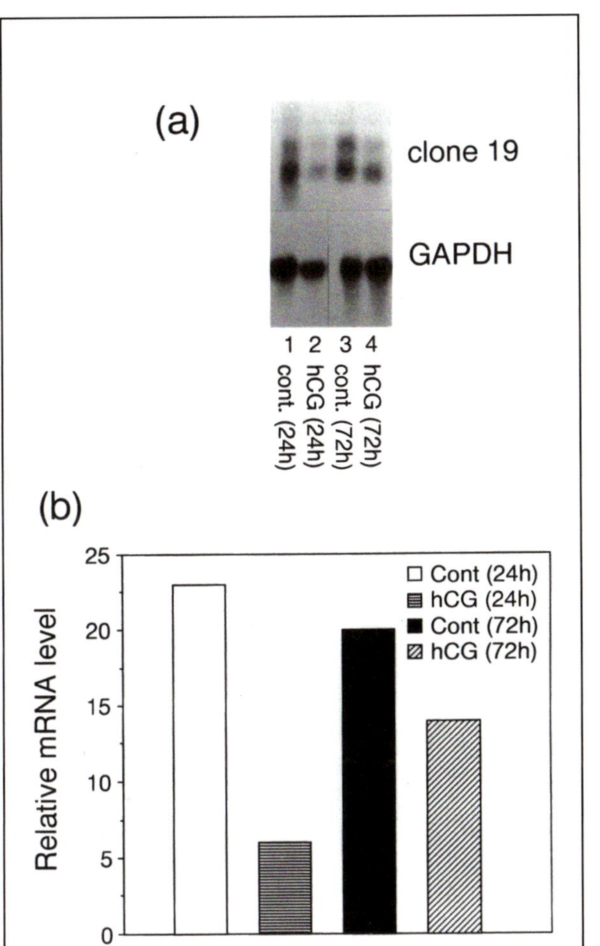

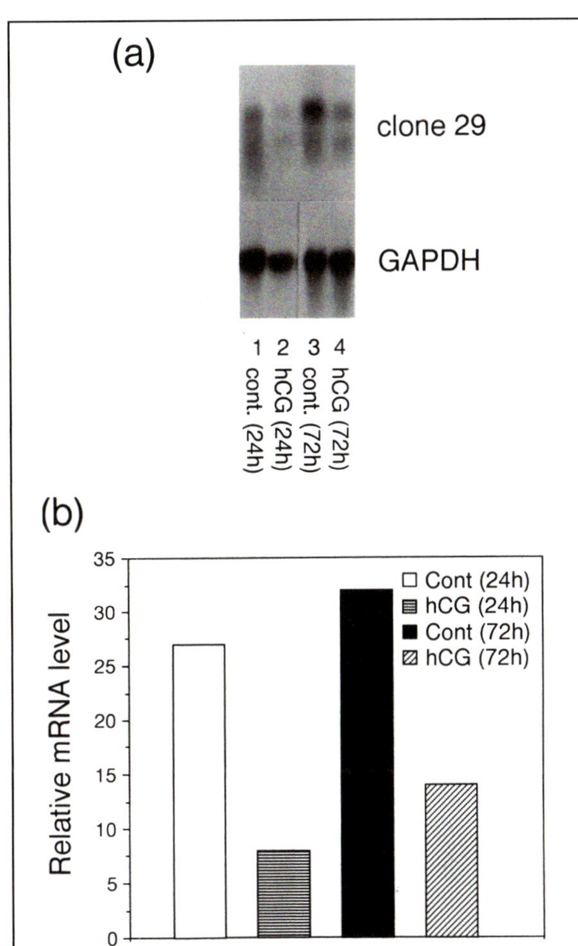

Figure 10.53 a, b

a Northern blot analysis of MCF-7 cells treated with hCG confirming gene expression for differentially displayed bands (clone 19). Probes were generated from the cloned fragments. Glyceraldehyde-3phosphate dehydrogenase (*GAPDH*) mRNA was used as a control for verifying the loading of RNA samples. Lane 1, control cells (*cont.*); lane 2, MCF-7 cells treated with hCG for 24 h; lane 3, 72 h control cells; and lane 4, MCF-7 cells treated with hCG for 72 h. **b** Histogram showing downregulation of mRNA expression of clone 19 by treatment of MCF-7 cells with hCG. Abbreviations as per **a**. Reprinted with permission from: Srivastava, P., Silva, I.D.C.G.; Russo, J., Mgbonyebi, O.P.; and Russo, I.H. Identification of genes differentially expressed in breast carcinoma cells treated with chorionic gonadotropin. Int. J. of Oncology 13: 465–469, 1998

Figure 10.54 a, b

a Northern blot analysis of MCF-7 cells treated with hCG confirming gene expression for differentially displayed bands (clone 29). Probes were generated from the cloned fragments. GAPDH mRNA was used as a control for verifying the loading of RNA samples. **b** Histogram showing downregulation of mRNA expression of clone 29 by treatment of MCF-7 cells with hCG. Abbreviations as per **a**. Reprinted with permission from: Srivastava, P., Silva, I.D.C.G.; Russo, J., Mgbonyebi, O.P.; and Russo, I.H. Identification of genes differentially expressed in breast carcinoma cells treated with chorionic gonadotropin. Int. J. of Oncology 13: 465–469, 1998

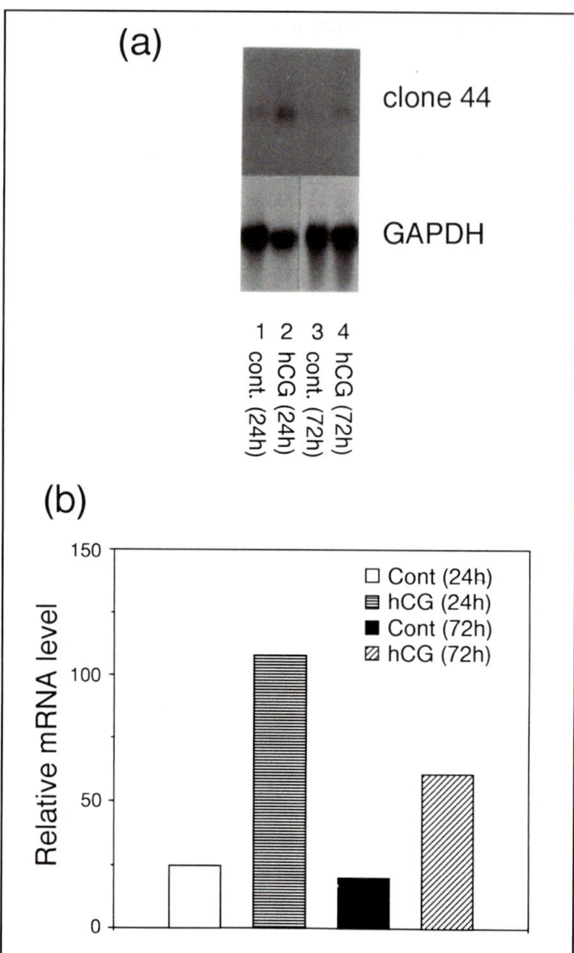

Figure 10.55 a, b

a Northern blot analysis of MCF-7 cells treated with hCG confirming gene expression for differentially displayed bands in treated cells (clone 44). Probes were generated from the cloned fragments. GAPDH mRNA was used as a control for verifying the loading of RNA samples. b Histogram showing increased mRNA expression of clone 44 by treatment of MCF-7 cells with hCG. Abbreviations as per a. Reprinted with permission from: Srivastava, P., Silva, I.D.C.G.; Russo, J., Mgbonyebi, O.P.; and Russo, I.H. Identification of genes differentially expressed in breast carcinoma cells treated with chorionic gonadotropin. Int. J. of Oncology 13: 465–469, 1998

role in the negative selection of immature T-cells [135]. A well-described means of inducing apoptosis in T-cells is their exposure to glucocorticoids. The expression of apoptotic gene(s) is induced in mouse thymocytes and splenocytes cultured with dexamethasone [135]. Our findings indicate that hCG activates in a malignant human breast epithelial cell line the same gene that is activated by glucocorticoids in T-cells. Our results confirm our previous observations that a number of other apoptosis-related genes (e.g., testosterone repressed prostate message 2 [TRPM2], interleukin-lb-converting enzyme [ICE], bcl-Xs, bax, transforming growth factor [TGF]-B, *c-myc* and p53 are also markedly induced by hCG treatment both in vivo and in vitro [41, 109]). The transcriptional activation of apoptotic genes was followed by the detection of fragmented DNA using the Apotag in situ labeling system (Table 10.5). Additionally, we have shown that under in vivo conditions hCG exerts a protective effect on the rat mammary gland from chemically induced carcinogenesis, mainly through the induction of differentiation, inhibition of cell proliferation, and activation of genes controlling programmed cell death leading to apoptosis, as seen in situ in the form of apoptotic bodies. HCG also inhibits the proliferation of other cancer cell lines in vitro through activation of genes controlling DNA repair mechanisms and programmed cell death [44, 56]. Recently it has been also shown that hCG blocks tumorigenesis and metastasis of a neoplastic AIDS-associated Kaposi's sarcoma (KS) cell line in nude mice [130]. Similar hCG preparations have been shown to have antitumor effect on neoplastic cells of various organs, such as prostate, lymphatic and hematopoietic systems (see review [44]).

Nucleotide sequences of two genes (19 and 29 cDNA) showed no homology to published databases, suggesting that they represent previously unknown genes and therefore appeared to be novel. Identification and characterization of these genes are important from a chemotherapeutic point of view. Studies from our laboratory have indicated the possibility that either the up- or downregulation of inhibins, or genes regulating apoptosis and cell cyclins might be involved in the differentiation of the lobular structures of the breast, which in turn, are important mod-

Table 10.5. Apoptotic index of the mammary gland and of DMBA-induced mammary tumors after a 20-day hCG treatment[a]

Group treatment	Number of animals	Tissue	Number of cells counted/labeled	Apoptotic index[e]
Control	5	Mammary gland[b]	7,560/9	0.12±0.11
hCG	5	Mammary gland	12,800/388	3.28±1.00
DMBA	5	Mammary gland	19,270/31	0.25±0.14
DMBA+hCG	5	Mammary gland	39,100/182	0.89±0.20
DMBA	3	Tumor[c]	28,000/18	0.06±0.03
DMBA+hCG	3	Tumor[d]	31,000/360	1.16±0.26

[a] Apoptotic index of the mammary glands of control, hCG, DMBA and DMBA + hCG treated animals and of DMBA-induced mammary tumors, expressed as the mean ± SD

[b] Non-tumoral mammary glands of animals of the four groups under study in which the number of cells containing apoptotic nuclei was counted in ducts and lobules

[c] The apoptotic index was determined in three different tumors developed in DMBA-treated group of animals and in

[d] Three different tumors developed in the DMBA + hCG treated group of animals

[e] Results are expressed as the mean ± SD. Differences were statistically significant in control vs. hCG ($p < 0.0001$), DMBA mammary gland vs. DMBA + hCG mammary gland ($p < 0.002$), and DMBA tumor vs. DMBA + hCG tumor ($p < 0.0001$)

ulators of the susceptibility of this organ to undergo malignant transformation [56]. Our in vivo studies have demonstrated that hCG inhibits tumor progression through the activation or downregulation of the same genes [56], thus indicating that hCG triggers similar responses in both normal and malignant breast epithelial cells from different species. Based upon our recent results we strongly believe that new genes are also involved in the regulation of these complex processes. Our observations indicate that hCG regulates gene expression in breast epithelial cells, thus providing a new tool for determining the precise role of specific genes through the isolation and analysis of their full length cDNAs. Furthermore, these results indicate that induction of apoptosis is an important parameter. Other genes that are affected by this hormonal treatment remain to be identified. These unknown genes might be important in determining the genomic signature needed to identify the chemopreventive effects of hCG.

10.11.2 Genes Induced by Human Chorionic Gonadotropin in the Rat Mammary Gland

For detecting the gene expression profile induced by hCG in the rat mammary gland the protocol depicted in Fig. 10.56 was utilized. Basically there were eight groups:

Group 1: untreated virgin rats sacrificed at the age of 78 days

Group II: untreated virgin rats sacrificed at the age of 126 days

Group III: pregnant rats, sacrificed at 15th day of pregnancy, when they were 86 days old

Group IV: pregnant animals that after completing one pregnancy and delivery breast fed all the litters born for 21 days. Then the litters were separated from the mothers, which were sacrificed 20 days post weaning, when they were 126 days old

Group V: virgin rats treated with 100 IU hCG (Profasi, Serono, Norwell, MA) per day, and sacrificed after the 15th injection, at the age of 86 days

Group VI: virgin rats treated with 100 IU hCG (Profasi) per day for 15 days, and sacrificed 40 days after the last hCG injection, at the age of 126 days

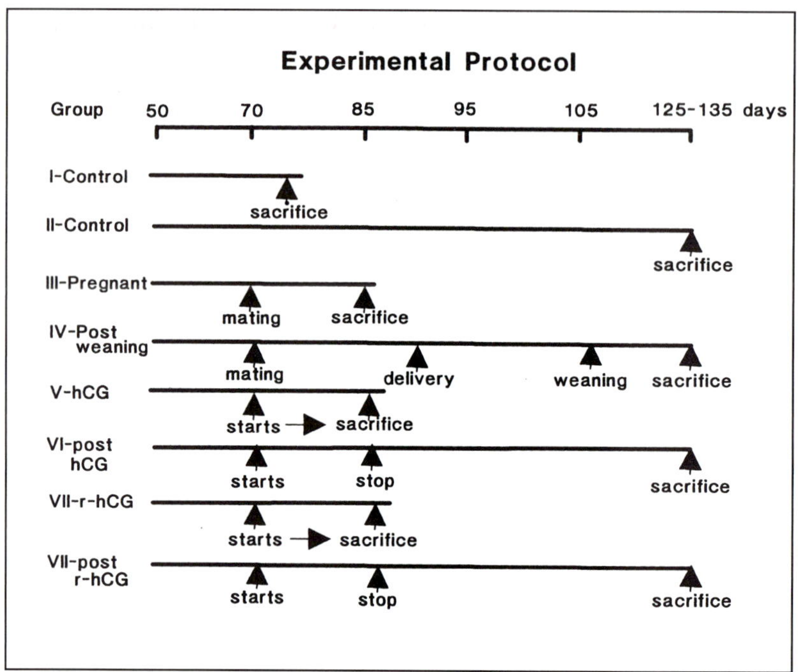

Figure 10.56

Diagram of the experimental protocol designed for testing the effect of pregnancy and hCG treatment on the differentiation and gene expression of the rat mammary gland. Sprague Dawley rats were assigned to one of the following groups: *I-Control* untreated virgin rats sacrificed at the age of 78 days; *II-Control* untreated virgin rats sacrificed at the age of 126 days; *III-Pregnant* rats sacrificed at 15th day of pregnancy (age 86 days old); *IV-Post-weaning* rats sacrificed 20 days post weaning; *V-hCG* virgin rats sacrificed after 15 daily injections of 100 IU hCG (Profasi); *VI-Post-hCG* virgin rats sacrificed 40 days after the last hCG injection; *VII-r-hCG* virgin rats sacrificed after the 15th injection of r-hCG; *VIII-Post-r-hCG* virgin rats sacrificed 40 days after the last r-hCG injection. Animals were sacrificed at each one of the age periods indicated in the *upper line*

Figure 10.57 a–h ▶

Histological sections of thoracic rat mammary glands. **a** Seventy-eight-day-old virgin rat of group I-Control. **b** Fifteenth day of pregnancy (group III-Parous); *inset*, lobules type 3. **c** Virgin rats treated with hCG (Profasi) for 15 days (Group V-hCG). **d** Virgin rats treated with hCG (Profasi) for 15 days (Group V-hCG), which look identical to virgin rats treated with r-hCG for 15 days (not shown); *inset*, lobule type 3 with secretory acini, indicative of progression to lobule type 4. **e** 120-day-old control virgin rat (Group II-Control). **f** Parous rat sacrificed 21 days post-weaning (Group IV-Post-weaning). **g** Mammary glands collected 40 days after the last hCG injection (Group VI-Post-hCG). **h** Mammary glands collected 40 days after the last r-hCG injection (Group VII-Post-r-hCG). All sections were stained with hematoxylin and eosin and photographed at a magnification of ×10, except for *insets* in **b** and **d**, that were photographed at ×40

Group VII: virgin rats treated with 100 IU recombinant hCG (r-hCG) (Serono-Benelux BV, The Hague, The Netherlands) per day, and sacrificed after the 15th injection, at the age of 86 days

Group VIII: virgin rats treated with 100 IU r-hCG per day for 15 days, and sacrificed 40 days after the last r-hCG injection, at the age of 126 days (Fig. 10.56)

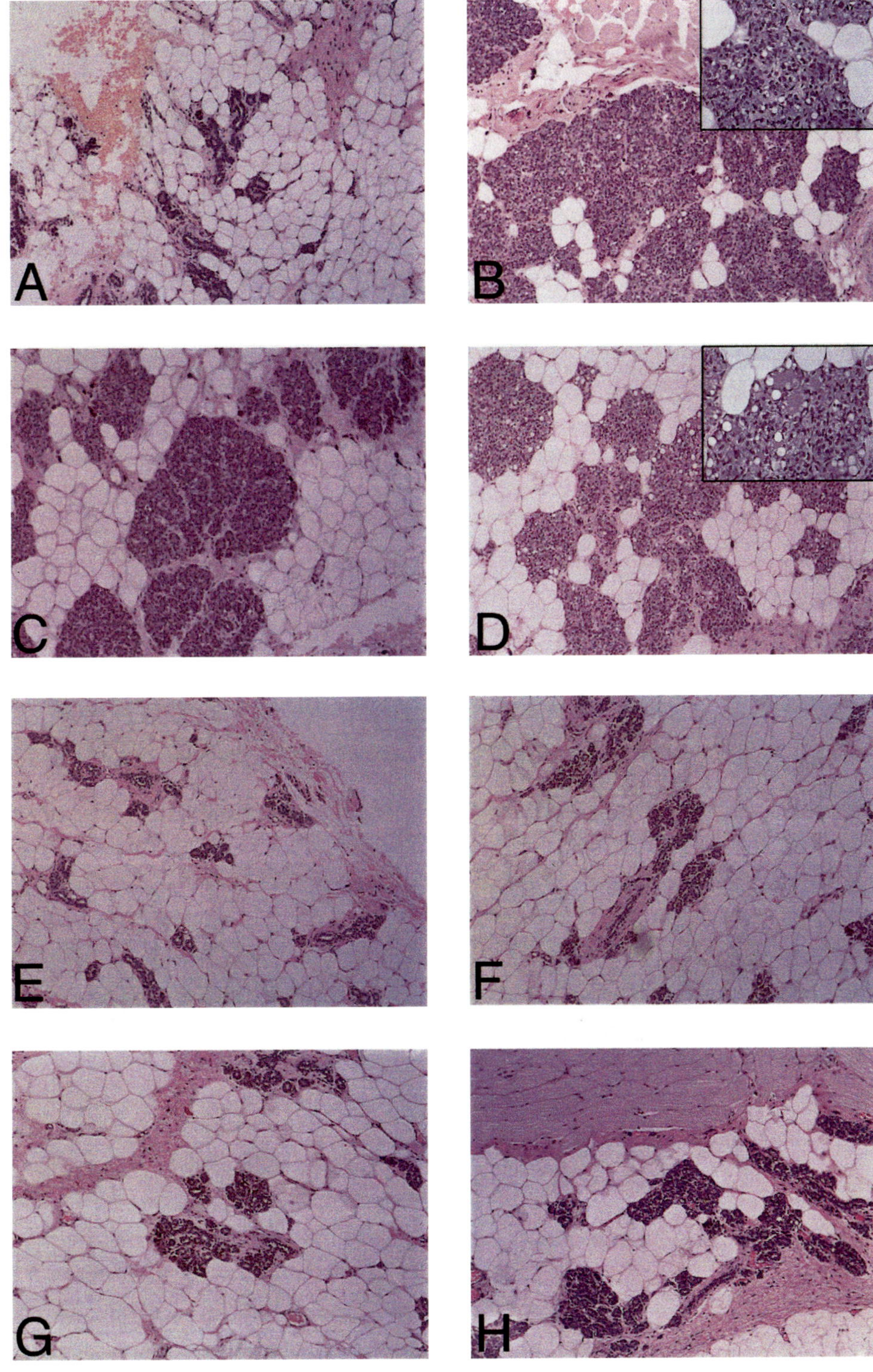

10.11.2.1 Morphological Phenotypes Induced by Urinary and Recombinant Human Chorionic Gonadotropin

The mammary glands of the virgin control rats of group I were composed of ducts ending in terminal end buds (TEB), alveolar buds and ducts (Fig. 10.57a). Pregnancy promoted lobular differentiation by inducing the formation of lobules type 2 and 3. By the 15th day of pregnancy a significant number of lobules type 3 had filled the mammary fat pad. Individual acini were small, containing a moderate amount of secretory material (Fig. 10.57b). Both hCG (Profasi) (Fig. 10.57c) and recombinant hCG (r-hCG) (Fig. 10.57d) induced a pattern of lobular development similar to that observed at 15 days of pregnancy (Fig. 10.57b). In the r-hCG treated group the lobules type 3 were similar in size to those present in the mammary gland of both parous and hCG (Profasi)-treated animals, however, individual acini were more distended, containing more abundant secretion, as commonly seen during lactation in the lobules type 4 (Fig. 10.57d, inset). The mammary gland of parous animals of group IV appeared at 42 days post-lactational involution similar to that of the age-matched virgin controls, since all the secretory lobules type 3–4 had practically disappeared (Fig. 10.57e,f). Some differences, however, persisted, since in the parous animals the mammary glands were slightly more cellular, and contained more lobules type 2 and no TEB were present (Fig. 10.57f). In both hCG treated groups the lobular development had decreased significantly by 42 days post-cessation of treatment (Fig. 10.57g,h). The rate of involution, however, was less pronounced than that observed in the parous animals that had lactated (Fig. 10.57f). Although there were no significant differences between both groups treated with hCG, in the mammary glands of rats treated with the r-hCG persisted more lobules type 2, and occasional small lobules type 3 (Fig. 10.57h).

10.11.2.2 Differential Display and Northern Blot Analysis

Differential display was performed with RNA isolated from the mammary glands of virgin, pregnant, and hCG-treated rats for identifying candidate genes expressed in this organ under the influence of different endocrinological conditions. Using double and single base anchored primer combinations we identified three PCR products that in the mammary glands of virgin controls were expressed differently than in the mammary glands of pregnant, hCG-Profasi and r-hCG-treated virgin rats. These PCR products, designated FH-l, R5C9, and R3A7, that were obtained by

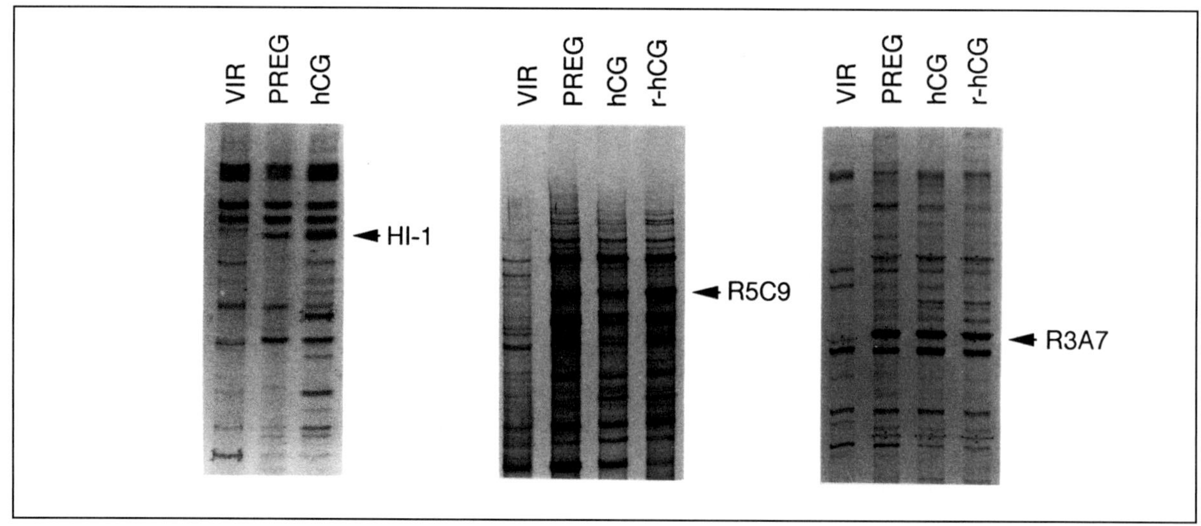

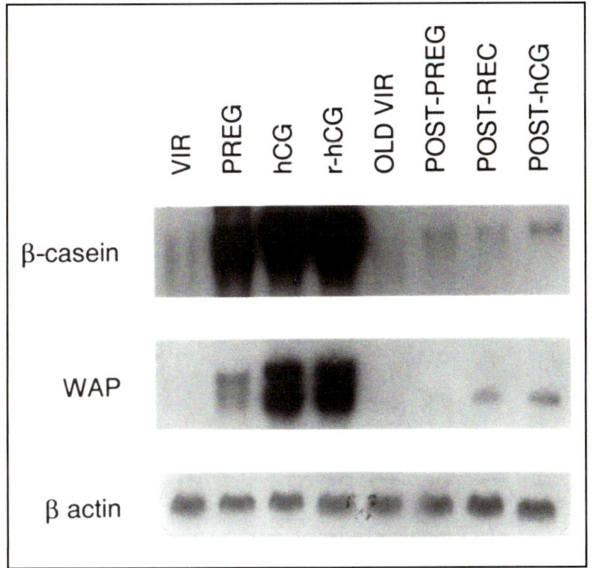

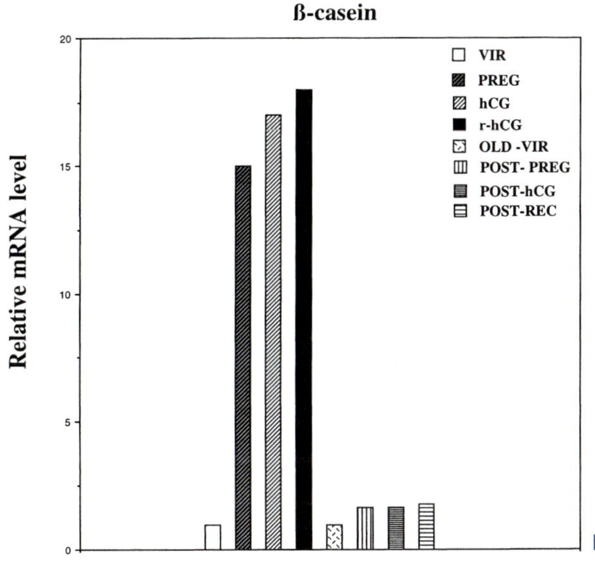

Figure 10.59a–c

a Northern blot hybridization using 30 μg of total RNA obtained from mammary glands of virgin (*VIR*), pregnant (*PREG*), hCG Profasi (*hCG*) and hCG recombinant (*r-hCG*) treated rats. ^{32}P labeled R5C9 and R3A7 cDNAs were used as probes. The R5C9 (β-casein) and R3A7 (WAP) transcripts were found overexpressed in lanes containing RNA from the mammary glands of pregnant, hCG-Profasi and hCG recombinant rats in comparison with the lane from young virgin rat mammary glands. These genes were still over-expressed at post-weaning (*POST-PREG*) and after hCG (Profasi) (*POST-hCG*) and r-hCG (*POST-REC*) withdrawal. **b** Histogram showing relative β-casein expression, which was faint in the virgin rats and increasing from 15-fold in pregnancy to 17- to 18-fold with hCG (Profasi) and r-hCG treatment, respectively. **c** Relative whey acidic protein (WAP) expression, which was faint in virgin animals, increasing by 5-fold by the 15th day of pregnancy, and by 15- to 17-fold under hCG (Profasi) and r-hCG treatments, respectively

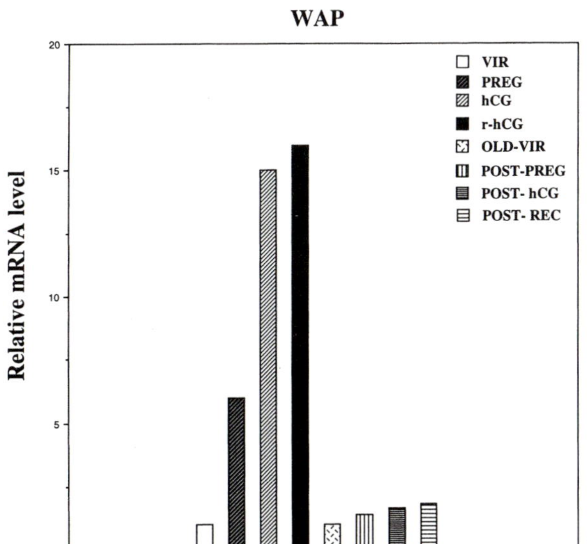

◀ Figure 10.58

Differential display gels of rat mammary gland total RNA. The first gel identifies HI1, which was found to be present in all lanes except in virgin animals; the second gel identifies R5C9, and the third one R3A7, both present in all lanes except in virgin animals. *VIR* virgin rats, *PREG* 15 days pregnant, *hCG* hCG (Profasi) treated virgin rats, *r-hCG* recombinant hCG-treated virgin rats

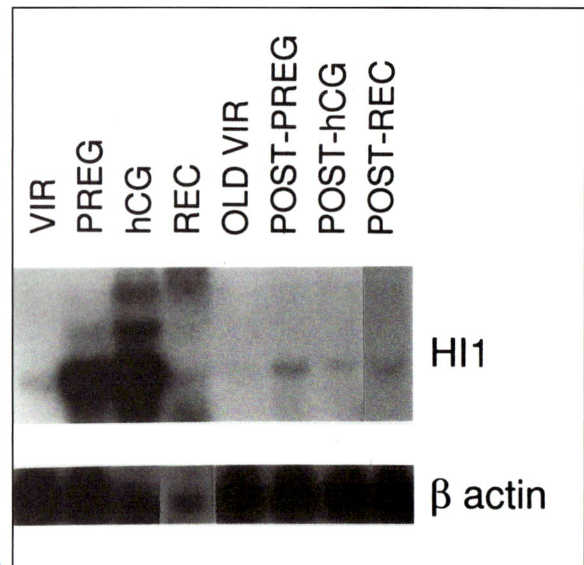

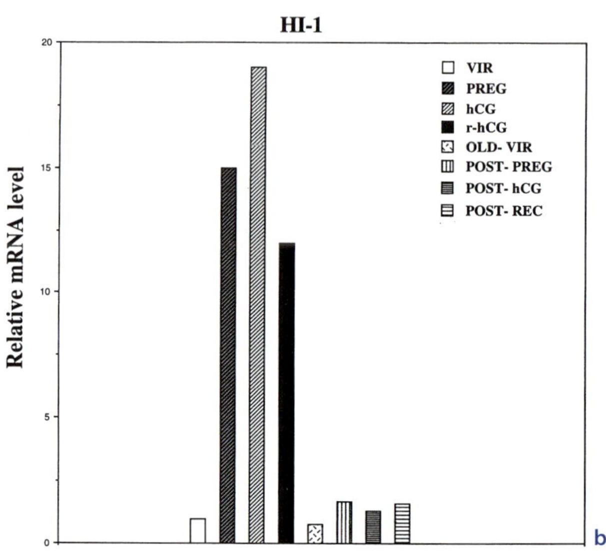

Figure 10.60 a, b

a Northern blot hybridization using 30 µg of total RNA from the mammary glands of the animals described in Fig. 10.56. ^{32}P labeled HI-1 cDNA was used as a probe. The HI-1 transcripts were found to be present, but weakly, in the mammary gland of virgin (*VIR*) rats. Its expression increased by 15-, 19-, and 12-fold in lanes containing RNA from pregnant (*PREG*), hCG-Profasi (*hCG*) and r-hCG treatment (*REC*), respectively. The expression of this gene was still found after delivery and breast feeding (*POST-PREG*) and after hCG Profasi (*POST-hCG*) or r-hCG (*POST-REC*) withdrawal, as shown in **b** the corresponding histogram

three different sets of arbitrary sets of primers are shown in Fig. 10.52. These PCR fragments were found to be reproducible in separate PCR amplifications. All the three PCR fragments were present in a very low amount in the mammary gland of the virgin control rats, but they were significantly upregulated in the pregnant and in both groups of hCG treated rats (Fig. 10.58). These bands ranged from 260 to 625 bp in size. Northern blot analysis using ^{32}P-labeled cloned fragments confirmed the differential expression of the bands detected by PCR (Figs. 10.59, 10.60). A sequence homology search revealed that the DNA sequence of the clones R5C9 and R3 A7 matched with β-casein and whey acidic protein (WAP) in 97% and 98% respectively (Fig. 10.59a, b). Both β-casein and WAP were overexpressed in the mammary glands of pregnant, hCG (Profasi), and r-hCG treated rats (12- to 15-fold induction) (Fig. 10.59a, b). In general, the expression of both genes was downregulated by 42 days post-weaning in the parous animals, or cessation of treatment in hCG treated rats, although the expression remained elevated by 1.7- to 2-fold higher in these groups of animals in comparison with the age-matched virgin controls (Fig. 10.59a, b).

Sequence comparisons of the third cDNA fragment (HI-1) did not show any perfect match with the known genes in the gene bank, and therefore it appeared to be a novel gene. This cDNA was also overexpressed in pregnant and both groups of hCG treated rats (approximately 15- to 17-fold increase) in comparison with the level of expression in the mammary glands of virgin control rats (Fig. 10.60a, b). The expression of this gene was downregulated by 42 days post-weaning in the parous animals, or hormone withdrawal in both groups hCG-treated rats, although its expression remained at least 2-fold elevated in these groups of animals in comparison with the age-matched virgin controls (Fig. 10.60a, b). Interestingly this gene was significantly unregulated in the DMBA induced tumors of animals that have received hCG whereas it was not expressed in the tumors of the untreated animals (Fig. 10.61).

hCG induces a degree of mammary gland differentiation similar to that induced by pregnancy. Furthermore, the lobular development induced by hCG obtained from the urine of pregnant women, such as Profasi, was undistinguishable from that induced by recombinant hCG. Both hCG preparations, like pregnancy, induced the expression of the differentiation genes β-casein and whey acidic protein, as well as the novel gene HI-1. It was also observed that after weaning or after hormone withdrawal the morphology of the mammary gland exhibited a regressed pattern, characterized by the involution of secretary lobules type 4 and lobules type 3 to lobules type 1 or to ducts, with few lobules type 2 present. In addition to the morphological regression of the mammary glands the expression of the differentiation genes induced by both pregnancy and the hormonal treatments was also reduced, although their levels were still higher than those observed in the mammary glands of age-matched virgin controls. Both β-casein and whey acidic proteins are synthesized by the mammary secretory epithelium- they are considered to be two of the major milk proteins found in various species, including mice, rats, cows and humans [136]. About 80% of the milk is composed of caseins, which represent a group of phosphate-containing proteins named α, β and χ casein. Their biological value has been attributed to both their nutritional properties and to the opioid activity of peptides derived by partial enzymatic digestion of caseins [137]. Indeed, casein has a strong antimutagenic activity against several mutagens both in vitro and in vivo [138], and is able to reduce significantly the mutagenic activity of N-methyl-N-nitro-N-nitrosoguanidine (MNNG) in the duodenum, jejunum, ileum and colon of mice [139]. A possible mechanism for these effects is the fact that casein stimulates casein kinase II (CKII) [140], which in turn phosphorylates the tumor suppressor protein p53 [141]. It is possible to postulate that the production of casein under specific endocrinological conditions, such as pregnancy and hCG

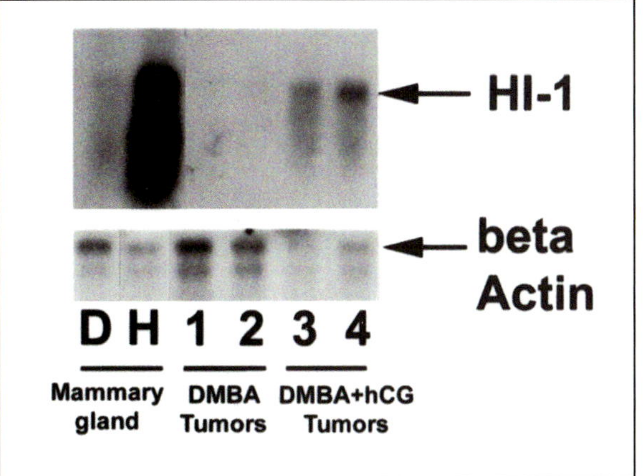

Figure 10.61

Northern blot hybridization using 30 μg of total RNA from mammary gland of DMBA treated animals (*D*), DMBA + hCG (*H*), and adenocarcinomas from the DMBA group (1 and 2) and DMBA + hCG group (3 and 4) as described in protocol of Fig. 10.15. ^{32}P labeled HI-1 cDNA was used as a probe. The HI-1 transcripts were found to be weak or negative in the mammary gland of DMBA groups and were significantly over-expressed in the mammary glands and carcinomas of the DMBA + hCG group

treatment, might result in subsequent p53 activation, resulting in an inhibition of both tumor initiation and promotion [41]. Recent studies have shown that β and α casomorphins, which are opioids produced by enzymatic degradation of β and α casein respectively, are both able to significantly reduce the proliferative activity of the breast cancer cell line T47D [142]. These opioids, which can be produced in vivo and in vitro, exert their inhibitory action on the proliferation of the breast cancer cell lines T47D and MCF7 very likely through interactions with somatostatin receptors [143, 144], known to be implicated in the control of tumor growth in different organs, including breast [145–147].

Whey proteins consist of α-lactalbumin, β-lactoglobulin, immunoglobulins, lactoferrin, transferrin, serum albumin and the proteose-peptone fraction [136]. Whey proteins are cysteine-rich polypeptides that appear to exert an inhibitory effect on both the initiation and progression of dimethylhydrazine induced malignancies [148], and have shown promissory results as anticancer substances in phase I–II clinical trials, since in tumor tissues they downregulate glutathione production, the major cellular antioxidant and detoxifying agent which is usually overexpressed in tumors [145]. Alpha-lactalbumin is able to induce apoptosis in transformed and embryonic cells, but not in mature epithelial elements [144].

The third isolated cDNA fragment named HI-1 is expressed according to the same pattern observed for β-casein and whey acidic protein, and therefore it might, as well, play roles in the differentiation of the mammary gland and its protection against cancer. In conclusion, these results indicate that it is hCG itself the hormone responsible for the differentiation of the rat mammary gland. This phenomenon encompasses various aspects, from the morphological changes in lobular pattern to the enhanced synthesis of β casein, whey acidic proteins, and the novel gene HI-1. The long lasting effect of these three genes in the genomic signature of the mammary epithelium and in conferring refractoriness to neoplastic transformation is less clear and probably are markers of transient functional differentiation.

10.12 Genomic Signature Induced by Human Chorionic Gonadotropin and Pregnancy

RNA was obtained from mammary glands of rats in their 15th and 21st day pregnancy or hCG treatment, and 21 and 42 days post-partum or treatment, respectively. RNAs were analyzed utilizing two membranes for each animal and compared with mRNA of age-matched virgin control rats. RNAs were hybridized to cDNA array membranes that contained 5,800 rat genes (Research Genetics, Alabama). Cluster analysis was performed using the Jaidexp (Java Analysis Information and Data Exploration) specific program version 1:0 and statistically analyzed. Four clusters of genes were identified (Fig. 10.62): *Cluster A* shows genes that were over expressed (3-fold at 15 and 21 days of pregnancy/hCG treatment, but decreased

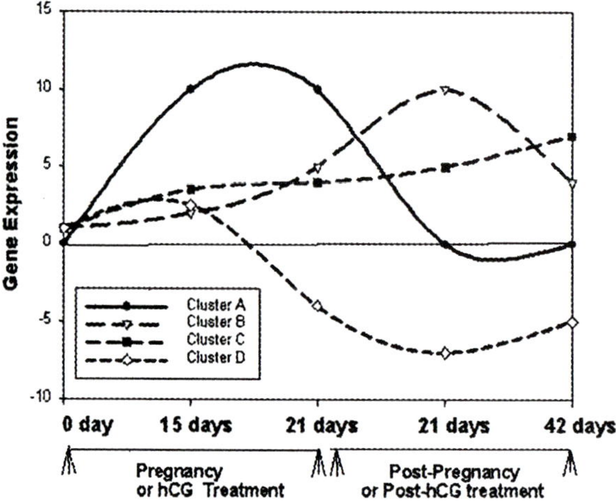

Figure 10.62

Cluster analysis of rat mammary gland gene expression during and after pregnancy and hCG treatment

to control values after 21 and 42 days post-partum or treatment, respectively. These genes, which included beta casein and alpha lactalbumin, are related to the secretory properties of the mammary epithelium [149]. Similar genes were identified suing the DD technique as explained above. *Cluster B* was composed of genes that were (3-fold increased at 21 days of pregnancy/treatment and continued rising, reaching the highest peak at 21 days, decreasing by 42 days post-partum/hCG treatment. Among these genes were the fatty acid binding protein, the EST Rn.37635 with high homology to BCL7B gene, catechol-O-methyltransferase, and the EST genes Rn. 5953, Rn. 22912 and Rn. 4339 [149]. The upregulation of catechol-O-methyltransferase is significant because it can be involved in the conjugation of estradiol and catechol estrogens, reducing the carcinogenic effect of these hormones. Genes related to the apoptotic pathways, such as testosterone repressed prostate message 2 (TRPM2), interleukin 1β-converting enzyme (ICE), bcl2, bcl-XL, bcl-XS, p53, p21, and *c-myc* were also up regulated from 3- to 5-fold [149] (Fig. 10.62). We have shown that the activation of programmed cell death genes occurred through a p53-dependent process, modulated by *c-myc* and with partial dependence on the bcl2-family related genes [41, 44, 150]. In this cluster were also included inhibins A and B, heterodimeric non-steroidal secreted glycoproteins with tumor suppressor activity [99, 100]. We have found that inhibins are not present in the normal resting mammary gland, but are induced by pregnancy or hCG treatment [45, 46]. We have also shown that hCG has an autocrine or paracrine effect on mammary epithelial cells [44]. HCG also activates the cluster B of genes in DMBA-induced mammary tumors, indicating that this hormone acts through the same pathways for exerting its preventative and therapeutic effects (Fig. 10.62). *Cluster C* (Fig. 10.62) represents genes whose level of expression progressively increased with time of pregnancy or hCG treatment, reaching their highest levels between 21 and 42 days post-partum or end of treatment. Among these were known genes such as those coding for a fragment of glycogen phosphorylase, AMP-activated kinase, bone morphogenetic protein 4 and vesicle-associated protein 1 [149]. G/T mismatch-specific thymine DNA glycosylase gene, which was observed to be upregulated in the Lob 3 of the human breast, was also increased 5-fold in this model. These data indicate that the activation of genes involved in the DNA repair process is part of the signature induced in the mammary gland by either pregnancy or hCG treatment of virgin animals. These observations confirm our previous findings that in vivo the ability of the cells to repair carcinogen-induced damage by unscheduled DNA synthesis and adduct removal is more efficient in the parous and in the hCG treated virgin than in the untreated virgin animal mammary gland (Fig. 10.2) [47, 68–71]. Therefore, a principal mechanism mediating the protection from mammary carcinogenesis conferred by either full term pregnancy or hCG treatment is the enhancement of the ability of the cells to repair DNA damage, which is in turn the determinant of the lower susceptibility to carcinogenesis. *Cluster D* consists of genes coding for pro-alpha collagen III, pro collagen II alpha 1, BTG1 and thymosin beta 4, which were upregulated more than (3-fold at the 15th day of pregnancy or hCG treatment, downregulated at the

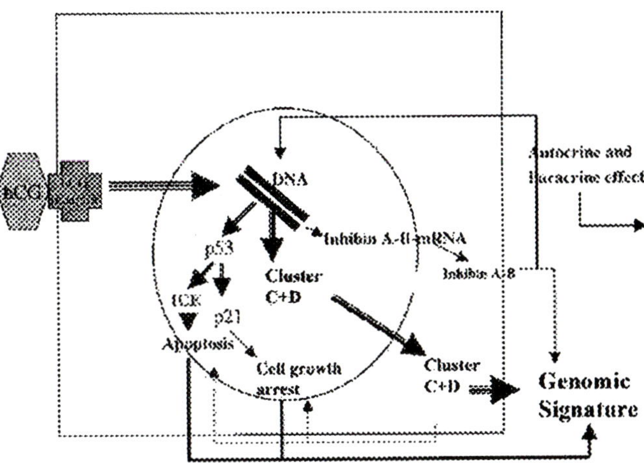

Figure 10.63

Postulated mechanism of action of hCG. The hormone binds to a specific membrane receptor, activating genes identified to be specific for pregnancy or hCG-induced differentiation, and that have been found to be correlated with the lobular development of the mammary tissue. Thus, a pathway of activation of p53 and ICE may lead to apoptosis or through p21 to cell growth arrest. Activation of inhibin A and B may lead to differentiation through autocrine or paracrine mechanisms. The activation of genes (clusters C and D are responsible for the refractoriness of the gland to carcinogenesis

21st day in both pregnant and hCG treated animals, and remained downregulated up to 42nd days (Fig. 10.62) [149]. Cluster D, in combination with Cluster C, is a component of the signature induced by hCG in the mammary gland (Fig. 10.63).

These data demonstrate that the genomic signature of the mammary gland induced in virgin animals by exogenous administration of hCG is similar to that induced by pregnancy, and that specific genomic profiles are still manifested by 42 days post termination of treatment. The importance of these specific signatures is highlighted by the fact that administration of carcinogen to hCG-treated or control virgin rats whose mammary glands appear morphologically similar will induce a markedly different tumorigenic response, supporting the concept that the differentiation in-

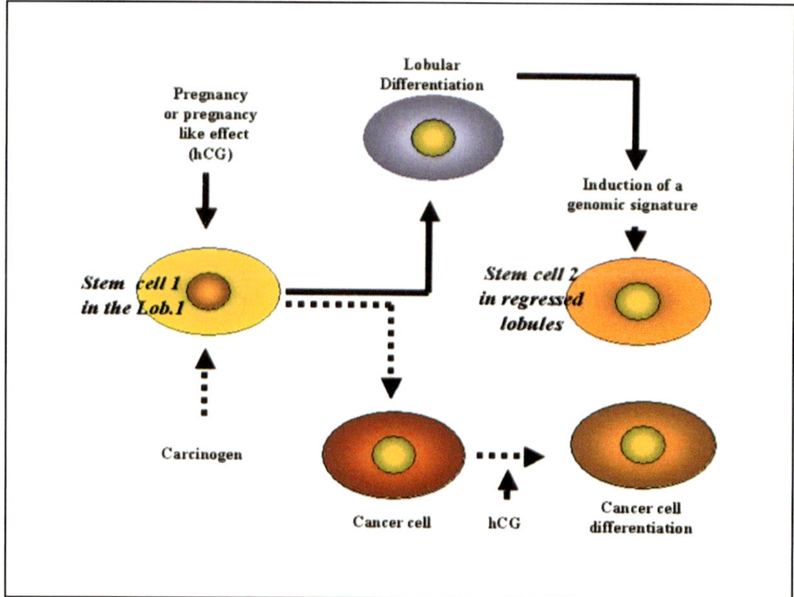

Figure 10.64

Differentiation induces a shift of the stem cell 1 to a stem cell 2 that is refractory to carcinogenesis (Adapted from Russo J and Russo IH, Endocrine Related Cancer 4:7–21,1997)

duced by hCG is expressed at genomic level, and results in a shift of the susceptible stem cell 1 to a refractory stem cell 2 (see Fig. 10.64). The permanence of these changes, in turn, makes them ideal surrogate markers for the evaluation of hCG effect as a breast cancer preventive agent.

10.13 Unifying Concepts

Breast cancer originates in the undifferentiated terminal duct of the Lob 1 that contains stem cells (Stem cell 1) the site of origin of ductal carcinomas. The susceptibility of Lob 1 to undergo neoplastic transformation has been attributed to its high rates of cell proliferation and of carcinogen binding to the DNA and low reparative activity [151–153]. The hormonal milieu of an early full term pregnancy or hCG treatment induces lobular development, completing the cycle of differentiation of the breast. This process induces a specific genomic signature in the mammary gland that is represented by the Stem cell 2 (Fig. 10.64). Even though differentiation significantly reduces cell proliferation in the mammary gland, the mammary epithelium remains capable of responding with proliferation to given stimuli, such as a new pregnancy. The stem cell 2 is able to metabolize the carcinogen and repair the induced DNA damage more efficiently than the stem cell 1, as it has been demonstrated in the rodent experimental system [47, 68–71]. We also have evidence that hCG has an effect in the cancer cell by further the differentiation pattern (Fig. 10.23) [127]. The finding that differentiation is a powerful inhibitor of cancer initiation provides a strong rationale for identifying the genes that control this process. The basic biological concept is that pregnancy or hCG shifts the stem cell 1 to the stem cell 2 that is refractory to carcinogenesis. This concept is supported by the laboratory findings described in the previous sections and summarized below:

1. Based in our knowledge of the pathogenesis of mammary cancer we have tested the effect of hCG hormone on the early phases of tumor progression, namely from TEBs damaged by DMBA to IDPs, in situ carcinomas and invasive carcinomas and demonstrate that this hormone inhibits the progression of 7,12-dimethylbenz(a)anthracene (DMBA)-induced mammary tumors

2. Treatment of young virgin rats with hCG induced a profuse lobular development of the mammary gland, practically eliminating the highly proliferating TEBs, with overall reduction in the proliferative activity of the mammary epithelium, and induction of the synthesis of inhibin, a secreted protein with tumor-suppressor activity

3. The hormonal treatment induced differentiation of the mammary gland, which was manifested at morphological, cell kinetic and functional levels. The morphological changes consisted of progressive branching of the mammary parenchyma and lobule formation. They were accompanied by reduction in the rate of cell proliferation

4. The functional changes comprised increased synthesis of inhibin, β-casein and other milk-related bioactive peptides. In addition, hCG also increased the expression of the programmed cell death TRPM2, ICE, p53, *c-myc*, and bcl-XS, inducing as well apoptosis, and down regulation of cyclins. Programmed cell death genes were activated through a p53-dependent process, modulated by *c-myc*, and with partial dependence on the bcl-2 family-related genes

5. hCG action treatment activates known and new genes. For this purpose we have used a differential display technique that allowed us to identify a series of new genes, among them the gene 19, 29 and 44 in the hCG treated MCF-7 cells and the hormone-Induced-1 (HI-1) in the rat mammary gland of animals treated with hCG. HI-1 might be of potential for clarifying the mechanisms through which hCG inhibits the initiation and progression of mammary cancer. Of relevance was the observation that lobular development, which reached its maximal expression after the 15th day of hCG treatment, regressing after hormone withdrawal, was preceded by activation of genes associated with the expression of programmed cell death, and furthermore, that the expression of these genes, including the newly identified gene HI-1, was still elevated 20 days post-cessation of treatment

6. Data generated with the new tools provided by the cDNA micro array techniques have allowed to demonstrated that while lobular development regressed after the cessation of hormone adminis-

tration, programmed cell death genes remained activated, but more importantly a new set of genes (Cluster D) reached the maximum expression whereas other (Cluster C) are downregulated. Those genes in Clusters C and D are the one that are providing the genomic signature that is specific for hCG and pregnancy

7. The genomic signature is specific for pregnancy and hCG and significantly different than the one induced by other hormones such as estrogen and progesterone

These mechanisms play a role in the protection exerted by hCG from chemically induced carcinogenesis, and might be even involved in the life-time reduction in breast cancer risk induced in women by full-term and multiple pregnancies. *The implications of these observations are 2-fold: on one hand, they indicate that hCG, as pregnancy, may induce early genomic changes that control the progression of the differentiation pathway* (Fig. 10.23), *and that these changes are permanently imprinted in the genome, regulating the long-lasting refractoriness to carcinogenesis* (Figs. 10.6, 10.64). *The permanence of these changes, in turn, makes them ideal surrogate markers of hCG effect in the evaluation of this hormone as a breast cancer preventive agent.*

References

1. Greenlee, R.T., Hill-Harmon, M.B., Murray, T., Thun, M. Cancer Statistics, 2001. CA Cancer J Clin. 51:15–36, 2001.

2. Jemal, A., Thomas, A., Murray, T., Thun, M. Cancer Statistics, 2002, CA Cancer J Clin., 52:23–47, 2002.

3. Forbes, J.F. The incidence of breast cancer: the global burden, public health considerations. Semin Oncol. 24 (1 Suppl 1):S1–20-S1–35, 1997.

4. Howe, H.L., Wingo, P.A., Thun, M.J., Ries, L.A., Rosenberg, H.M., Feigal, E.G., Edwards BK. Annual report to the nation on the status of cancer (1973 through 1998), featuring cancers with recent increasing trends. J. Natl. Cancer Inst., 93: 824–842. 2001.

5. Chang, J., Elledge, R.M. Clinical management of women with genomic BRCA1 and BRCA2 mutations. Breast Cancer Res Treat. 69:101–113, 2001.

6. Mirza, A.N., Mirza, N.Q., Vlastos, G., Singletary, S.E. Prognostic factors in node-negative breast cancer: a review of

studies with sample size more than 200 and follow-up more than 5 years. Ann. Surg. 235:10–26, 2002.

7. Hoffmann, D., Hoffmann, I., El-Bayoumy, K. The less harmful cigarette: a controversial issue. a tribute to Ernst L. Wynder. Chem Res Toxicol., 14:767–90, 2001.

8. Matsumoto, H., Yamane, T. Green Tea and Cancer Prevention. J. Women's Cancer, 2: 153–158, 2000.

9. Dunn, B.K., McCaskill-Stevens, W., Kramer, B., Ford, L.G. Chemoprevention of breast cancer: The NSABP's breast cancer prevention trial. J. Women's Cancer, 2: 177–191, 2000.

10. King, M.C., Wieand, S., Hale, K., Lee, M., Walsh, T., Owens, K., Tait, J., Ford, L., Dunn, B.K., Costantino, J., Wickerham, L., Wolmark, N., Fisher, B. Tamoxifen and breast cancer incidence among women with inherited mutations in BRCA1 and BRCA2: National Surgical Adjuvant Breast and Bowel Project (NSABP-P1) Breast Cancer Prevention Trial. JAMA, 286:2251–2256, 2001.

11. Lynch, H.T., Casey, M.J. Current status of prophylactic surgery for hereditary breast and gynecologic cancers. Curr. Opin. Obstet. Gynecol., 13:25–30, 2001.

12. Narod, S.A., Brunet, J.S., Ghadirian, P., Robson, M., Heimdal, K., Neuhausen, S.L., Stoppa-Lyonnet, D., Lerman, C., Pasini, B., de los Rios, P., Weber, B., Lynch, H. Tamoxifen and risk of contralateral breast cancer in BRCA1 and BRCA2 mutation carriers: a case-control study. Hereditary Breast Cancer Clinical Study Group. Lancet, 356:1876–1881, 2000.

13. Khurana, K.K., Loosmann, A., Numann, P.J., Khan, S.A. Prophylactic mastectomy – Pathologic findings in high-risk patients. Arch. Pathol. Lab. Med., 124:378–381, 2000.

14. Narod, S. Prophylactic mastectomy in carriers of BRCA mutations. N. Engl. J. Med., 345:1498; 2001.

15. Riggs, T. Prophylactic mastectomy in carriers of BRCA mutations. N Engl J Med., 345: 1499–500, 2001.

16. Stoutjesdijk, M.J., Barentsz, J.O. Prophylactic mastectomy in carriers of BRCA mutations. N. Engl. J. Med., 345:1499, 2001.

17. Hartmann, L.C., Sellers, T.A., Schaid, D.J., Frank, T.S., Soderberg, C.L., Sitta, D.L., Frost MH, Grant, C.S., Donohue, J.H., Woods, J.E., McDonnell, S.K., Vockley, C.W., Deffenbaugh, A., Couch, F.J., Jenkins, R.B. Efficacy of bilateral prophylactic mastectomy in BRCA1 and BRCA2 gene mutation carriers. J. Natl. Cancer Inst., 93:1633–1637, 2001.

18. McGregor, D.H., Land, C.E., Choi, K., Tokuoka, S., Liu, P.I., Wakabayashi, I., Beebe, G.W. Breast cancer incidence among atomic bomb survivors, Hiroshima and Nagasaki 1950–1989. J. Natl. Cancer Inst. 59:799–811, 1977.

19. Boice JD Jr, Preston D, Davis FG, Monson RR. Frequent chest X-ray fluoroscopy and breast cancer incidence among tuberculosis patients in Massachusetts. Radiation Research. 125: 214–222, 1991.

20. Clemons M, Loijens L, Goss P. Breast cancer risk following irradiation for Hodgkin's disease. Cancer Treat Rev. 26(4): 291–302, 2000.

21. Cutuli, B., Borel, C., Dhermain, F., Magrini, S.M., Wasserman, T.H., Bogart, J.A., Provencio, M., de Lafontan, B., de la Rochefordiere, A., Cellai, E., Graic, Y., Kerbrat, P., Alzieu, C., Teissier, E., Dilhuydy, J., Mignotte, H., Velten, M. Breast cancer occurred after treatment for Hodgkin's disease: analysis of 133 cases. Radiother Oncol 59(3):247–255, 2001.

22. Janov, A.J., Tulecke, M., O'Neill, A., Lester, S., Mauch, P.M., Harris, J., Schnitt, S.J., Shapiro, C.L. Clinical and Pathologic Features of Breast Cancers in Women Treated for Hodgkin's Disease: A Case-Control Study. Breast J. 7:46–52, 2001.

23. Tymchuk, CN., Tessler, S.B., Barnard, R.J. Changes in sex hormone-binding globulin, insulin, and serum lipids in postmenopausal women on a low-fat, high-fiber diet combined with exercise. Nutr. Cancer, 38:158–62, 2000.

24. Baum, M. The ATAC (Arimidex, Tamoxifen, Alone or in Combination) adjuvant breast cancer trial in post-menopausal women. Breast Cancer Research and Treatment 69(3): 210, 2001.

25. Mouridsen, H., Gershanovich, M., Sun, Y., Perez-Carrion, R., Boni, C., Monnier, A., Apffelstaedt, J., Smith, R., Sleeboom, H.P., Janicke, F., Pluzanska, A., Dank, M., Becquart, D., Bapsy, P.P., Salminen, E., Snyder, R., Lassus, M., Verbeek, J.A., Staffler, B., Chaudri-Ross H.A., Dugan, M. Superior efficacy of letrozole versus tamoxifen as first-line therapy for postmenopausal women with advanced breast cancer: results of a phase III study of the International Letrozole Breast Cancer Group. J Clin Oncol., 19: 2596–2606, 2001.

26. Robertson, J.F., Nicholson, R.I., Bundred, N.J., Anderson, E., Rayter, Z., Dowsett, M., Fox, J.N., Gee, J.M., Webster, A., Wakeling, A.E., Morris, C., and Dixon, M. Comparison of the short-term biological effects of 7alpha-[9-(4,4,5,5,5-pentafluoropentylsulfinyl)-nonyl-estra-1,3,5, (10)-triene-3,17beta-diol (Faslodex) versus tamoxifen in postmenopausal women with primary breast cancer. Cancer Res. 61: 6739–46, 2001.

27. Gail, M.H., Brinton, L.A., Byar, D.P., Corle, D.K., Breen, S.B., Schairer, C., Mulvihill, J.J. Projecting individualized probabilities of developing breast cancer for white females who are being examined annually. J. Natl. Cancer Inst., 81: 1879–1886, 1989.

28. Trapido, E.J. Age at first birth, parity and breast cancer risk Cancer 51:946–948, 1983.

29. MacMahon, B., Cole, P., Lin, T.M. Age at first birth and breast cancer risk. Bull. Nat'l. Hlth. Org. 43:209,1970.

30. Chie, W.C., Hsieh, C., Newcomb, P.A., Longnecker, M.P., Mittendorf, R., Greenberg, E.R., Clapp, R.W., Burke, K.P., Titus-Ernstoff, L., Trentham-Dietz, A., MacMahon, B. Age at any full-term pregnancy and breast cancer risk. Am J Epidemiol. 151:715–722, 2000.

31. Holmberg, E., Holm, L.E., Lundell, M., Mattsson, A., Wallgren, A., Karlsson, P. Excess breast cancer risk and the role of parity, age at first childbirth and exposure to radiation in infancy. Br. J. Cancer 85:362–366, 2001.

32. Vessey, M.D., McPherson, K., Roberts, M.M., Neil, A. and Jones, L. Fertility and the risk of breast cancer. Br. J. Cancer 52:625–628, 1985.

33. Kelsey, J.L. and Horn-Ross, P.L. Breast Cancer: Magnitude of the problem and descriptive epidemiology. Epidemiologic Reviews, 15: 7–16, 1993.

34. Lambe, M., Hsieh, C.C., Chan, H.W., Ekbom, A., Trichopoulos, D. and Adami, H. O. Parity, age at first and last birth, and risk of breast cancer: A population based study in Sweden. Breast Cancer Res. Treat. 38: 305–311, 1996.

35. Russo, I.H. and Russo, J. Chorionic Gonadotropin: A Tumoristatic and Preventive Agent in Breast Cancer, in Drug Resistance in Oncology (Teicher, B.A., ed.), Marcel Dekker, Inc. 1993,pp. 537–560.

36. Russo, I.H., Koszalka, M. and Russo, J. Human chorionic gonadotropin and rat mammary cancer prevention. J. Natl. Cancer Inst. 82: 1286–1289, 1990.

37. Russo, I.H., Koszalka, M., and Russo, J. Effect of human chorionic gonadotropin on mammary gland differentiation and carcinogenesis. Carcinogenesis 11: 1849–1855, 1990.

38. Russo, J., Saby, J., Isenberg, W. and Russo, I.H. Pathogenesis of mammary carcinoma induced in rats by 7,12-dimethylbenz(a)anthracene. J. Natl. Cancer Inst. 59: 435–445,1977.

39. Russo, I.H. and Russo, J. Role of hCG and inhibin in breast cancer (Review). Int. J. Oncol. 4: 297–306, 1994.

40. Russo, I.H. and Russo, J. Mammary gland neoplasia in long-term rodent studies. Environmental Health Perspectives 104: 938–967,1996.

41. Srivastava, P., Russo, J. and Russo, I.H. Chorionic gonadotropin inhibits rat mammary carcinogenesis through activation of programmed cell death. Carcinogenesis 18: 1799–1808, 1998.

42. Mgbonyebi, O. P., Tahin, Q., Russo, J. and Russo, I.H. Serum levels of chorionic gonadotropin in treated female rats during the progression of DMBA-induced tumorigenesis. Proc. Am. Assoc. Cancer Res. 37: 1564a, 1996.

43. Tahin, Q., Mgbonyebi, O. P., Russo, J. and Russo, I.H. Influence of hormonal changes induced by the placental hormone chorionic gonadotropin on the progression of mammary tumorigenesis. Proc. Am. Assoc. Cancer Res. 37: 1622a, 1996.

44. Russo, J and Russo, I.H. Human Chorionic Gonadotropin in Breast Cancer Prevention In: "Endocrine Oncology, (S.P. Ethier, editor), Humana Press Inc., Totowa, NJ. 2000, pp 121–136.

45. Alvarado, M.E., Alvarado, N.E., Russo, J. and Russo, I.H. Human chorionic gonadotropin inhibits proliferation and induces expression of inhibin in human breast epithelial cells in vitro. In Vitro 30A: 4–8, 1994.

46. Alvarado, M.V., Russo, J. and Russo, I.H. Immunolocalization of inhibin in the mammary gland of rats treated with hCG. J. Histochem. and Cytochem. 41: 29–34, 1993.

47. Russo, J., Tay, L.K., and Russo, I.H. Differentiation of the mammary gland and susceptibility to carcinogenesis. Breast Cancer Res. Treat. 2: 5–37, 1982.

48. Rao, D.N., Ganesh, B., and Desai, P.B. Role of reproductive factors in breast cancer in a low-risk area: a case-control study. Br. J. Cancer, 70: 129–152,1994.

49. Coe, K. Breast cancer in Hispanic women. Women and Cancer, 1: 38–43,1998.

50. Gaudette, L.A., Silberberg, C., Altmayer, C.A., and Gao, R.N. Trends in breast cancer incidence and mortality. Health Reports. 8: 29–40, 1996.

51. Apter, D. Hormonal events during female puberty in relation to breast cancer risk. Europ. J. Cancer Prev. 5: 476–482, 1996.

52. Shivvers, S.A., Miller, D.S. Preinvasive and invasive breast and cervical cancer prior to or during pregnancy. [Review]. Clinics in Perinatology, 24: 369–389,1997.

53. Russo, J., Wilgus, G. and Russo, I.H. Susceptibility of the mammary gland to carcinogenesis. I. Differentiation of the mammary gland as determinant of tumor incidence and type of lesion. Am. J. Pathol. 96: 721–734,1979.

54. Russo, J. and Russo, I.H. Influence of differentiation and cell kinetics on the susceptibility of the mammary gland to carcinogenesis. Cancer Res. 40: 2677–2687, 1980.

55. Russo, J. and Russo, I.H. Susceptibility of the mammary gland to carcinogenesis. II. Pregnancy interruption as a risk factor in tumor incidence. Am. J. Pathol. 100:497–512, 1980.

56. Russo, J. and Russo, I.H. Toward a physiological approach to breast cancer prevention. Cancer Epidemiol. Biomarkers & Prev. 3:353–364, 1994.

57. Russo, J., Rivera, R., and Russo, I.H. Influence of age and parity on the development of the human breast. Breast Cancer Res. and Treat. 23: 211–218, 1992.

58. Russo, J. and Russo, I.H. Developmental pattern of the human breast and susceptibility to carcinogenesis. European J. of Cancer Prevention 2: 85–100, 1993.

59. Nandi, S., Guzman, R.C., and Yang, J. Hormones and mammary carcinogenesis in mice, rats and humans: a unifying hypothesis. Proc. Natl. Acad., Sc. USA, 92: 3650–3657,1995.

60. Sinha, D.K., Patzik, J.E., and Dao, T.L. Progression of rat mammary development with age and its relationship to carcinogenesis by a chemical carcinogen. Int. J. Cancer, 31:321–327, 1983.

61. Russo, I.H., Koszalka, M., and Russo, J. Comparative study of the influence of pregnancy and hormonal treatment on mammary carcinogenesis. Brit. J. Cancer, 64: 481–484, 1991.

62. Russo, I.H. and Russo, J. Role of pregnancy and chorionic gonadotropin in breast cancer prevention, in Proc. IV. European Congress on Menopause. (M.H. Birkhauser and H. Rozenbaum, eds.) Editions ESKA, Paris, 1998. pp. 133–142.

63. Russo, I.H., Russo, J. Developmental stage of the rat mammary gland as determinant of its susceptibility to 7,12-dimethylbenz[a] anthracene. J. Natl. Cancer Inst. 61:1439, 1978.

64. Russo, J., Russo, I.H. DNA-labeling index and structure of the rat mammary gland as determinants of its susceptibility to carcinogenesis. J Natl Cancer Inst 61:1451. 1978.

65. Dao, T.L, Bock, F.G., Greiner, M.J. Mammary carcinogenesis by 3-methylcholanthrene: inhibitory effect of pregnancy and lactation on tumor induction. J. Natl. Cancer Inst. 25:991, 1960.

66. Huggins, C., Grand, L.C., Brillantes, F. Critical significances of breast structure in the induction of mammary cancer in the rat. Proc. Natl. Acad. Sci. 45:1294, 1959.

67. Ciocca, D.R., Parente, A., Russo, J. Endocrinologic milieu and susceptibility of the rat mammary gland to carcinogenesis. Am. J. Pathol. 109:74, 1982.

68. Tay, L.K. and Russo, J. Metabolism of 7,12-Dimethyl-benz(a)anthracene by Rat Mammary Epithelial Cells in Culture. Carcinogenesis 4:733–738, 1983.

69. Russo, J., Tay, L.K., Russo, I.H. Differentiation of the mammary gland and susceptibility to carcinogenesis. Breast Cancer Res. Treat. 2:5–75, 1982.

70. Tay, L.K., Russo, J. 7,12-dimethylbenz [a] anthracene-induced DNA binding and repair synthesis in susceptible and non-susceptible mammary epithelial cells in culture. J. Natl. Cancer Inst. 67:155, 1981.

71. Tay, L.K., Russo, J. Formation and removal of 7,12-dimethyl-benz [a] anthracene-nucleic acid adducts in rat mammary epithelial cells with different susceptibility to carcinogenesis. Carcinogenesis 2:1327–1332, 1981.

72. Russo, I.H and Russo, J. Atlas and histologic classification of tumors of the rat mammary gland. Mammary Gland Biology and Neoplasia 5:187–200, 2000.

73. Russo, J. and Russo, I.H. Susceptibility of the mammary gland to carcinogenesis. II. Pregnancy interruption as a risk factor in tumor incidence. Am J. Pathology, 100:497–512, 1980.

74. Russo, J. Basis of cellular autonomy in susceptibility to carcinogenesis. Toxicol. Pathol. 11:149–155, 1983.

75. Russo, J., Miller, J., Russo, I.H. Hormonal treatment prevents DMBA-induced rat mammary carcinoma. Proc. Am. Assoc. Cancer Res. 23:348a, 1982.

76. Russo, I.H., Pokorzynski, T., Russo, J. Contraceptives as hormone-preventive agents in mammary carcinogenesis. Proc. Am. Assoc. Cancer Res. 27:912a, 1986.

77. Dao, T.L. Carcinogenesis of mammary gland in rat. Prog. Exp. Tumor Res .5:157,1964.

78. Russo, I.H., Al-Rayess, M., Russo, J. Role of contraceptive agents in breast cancer prevention. Proc. Biennial International Breast Cancer Research Conference, London, United Kingdom, March 24 to 28, 1985, p 87.

79. Russo, I.H., Al-Rayess, M., Sabharwal, S. Effect of contraceptive agents on mammary gland structure and susceptibility to carcinogenesis. Proc. Am. Assoc. Cancer Res. 26:460a, 1985.

80. The Centers for Disease Control Cancer and Steroid Hormone Study. Long term oral contraceptives use and the risk of breast cancer. JAMA 249:1591, 1983

81. Edgren, R.A. The biology of steroidal contraceptives. In: Contraception: Chemical Control of Fertility, edited by Lednicer D, New York, Marcel Dekker, 1969, p23.

82. Gurpide, E., Tseng, L., Gusberg, S.B. Estrogen metabolism in normal and neoplastic endometrium. Am. J. Obstet. Gynecol. 129:809, 1977.

83. Rall, H.H., Soto-Ferreira, J., Janssens, K.Y. Effect of medro-xyprogesterone acetate contraception on cytoplasmic estrogen receptor content of the human cervix uteri. Int. J. Fertil. 23:41, 1978.

84. Russo, I.H., Gimotty, P., Dupuis, M. and Russo, J. Effect of Medroxyprogesterone Acetate on the Response of the Rat Mammary Gland to Carcinogenesis. British J. of Cancer 59:210–216,1989.

85. Russo, I.H., and Russo, J. Hormone prevention of mammary carcinogenesis by norethynodrel-mestranol. Breast Cancer Res. Treat. 14:43–56,1989.

86. Coleman, M.E., Murchison, T.E., Frank, D. Mammary nodules in dogs receiving Depo-Provera and progesterone: an interim progress report. Toxicol. Appl. Pharmacol. 37:213a, 1976.

87. Wazeter, F.X., Geil, R.G., Cookson, K.M., Berliner, V.R., Lamar, J.K. Seven years progress report on long term oral contraceptive studies in female dogs and monkeys. Toxicol. Appl. Pharmacol. 37:208a, 1976.

88. Finkel, M.J., Berliner, V.R. The extrapolation of experimental findings (animal to man):the dilemma of the systemically administered contraceptives. Bull. Sco. Pharmacol. Environ. Pathol. 4:13, 1973.

89. Fowler, E.H., Vaughan, T., Gotezik, F., Reichart, P., Reed, C. Pathologic changes in mammary glands and uteri from beagle bitches receiving low levels of medroxyprogesterone acetate: an overview of research in progress. In Pharmacology of Steroid Contraceptive Drugs, edited by Garattini S, Berendes HW, New York, Raven Press, 1977, p 185.

90. Pike, M.C., Henderson, B.E., Krailo, M.D. Breast cancer in young women and use of oral contraceptives: possible modifying effect of formulation and age at use. Lancet 11:926, 1983

91. Henderson, B.E., Koss, R.K., Judd, H.L., Krailo, M.S., Pike, M.C. Do regular ovulatory cycles increase breast cancer risk? Cancer 56:1206, 1985.

92. MacMahon, B., Trichopoulos, D., Brown, J. Age at menarche: probability of ovulation and breast cancer risk. Int. J. Cancer 29:13, 1982.

93. Henderson, B.E., Berkins, V., Rosario, L., Casagrande, J., Pike, M.C. Elevated serum levels of estrogen and prolactin in daughters of patients with breast cancer. N. Engl. J. Med. 293:790, 1975.

94. Trichopoulos, D., Brown, J.B., Garas, J., Papionnaou, A., Mac-Mahon, B: Elevated urine estrogen and pregnanediol levels in daughters of breast cancer patients. J Natl. Cancer Inst. 67:603, 1981.

95. Korenman, S.G. Oestrogen window hypothesis of the aetiology of breast cancer. Lancet 1:700, 1980.

96. Bloch, B., Davies, A.H. Evaluation of a combined oestrogen-progestogen injectable contraceptive. S. Afr. Med. J. 53:846, 1978.

97. Jeppsson, S., Gerghagen, S., Hohansson, E.D., Rannevik, G. Plasma levels of medroxyprogesterone acetate (MPA), sex-hormone binding globulin, gonadal steroids, gonadotropins and prolactin in women during long-term use of depo-

MPA (Depo-Provera) as a contraceptive agent. Acta Endocrinol. (Copenh) 99:339, 1982.

98. Johansson, E.D.B. Depression of the progesterone levels in women treated with synthetic gestagens after ovulation. Acta Endocrinol. 68:771, 1971

99. Sun, M. Panel says Depo-Provera not proved safe. Science 226:950, 1984.

100. Vermeulen, A., Dhnodt, M., Their, Y.K., Van Der Kerckhove, D. Plasma sex steroid and gonadotropin levels in control and silastic vaginal medroxyprogesterone acetate-impregnated ring cycles. Fertil. Steril. 27:773, 1976.

101. Bonte, J., Decoster, J.M., Ide, P. Vaginal cytologic evaluation as a practical link between hormone blood levels and tumor hormone dependency in exclusive medroxyprogesterone treatment of recurrent or metastatic endometrial adenocarcinoma. Acta Cytol. 21:218, 1977.

102. Venter, P.F., Anderson, J.D., Van-Veldon. D.J.J. Postmenopausal endometriosis: a case report. S. Afr. Med. J. 56:1136, 1979.

103. Geschikter, C.H. Diseases of the Breast, Philadelphia, Lippincott Co, 1948. p 1.

104. Dubin, N.H., Moszkowski, E.F., Kavoussi, K.N., Ward, M.M., Ances, J.G. Serum progesterone and estradiol in pregnant women selected for progestogen treatment. Int. J. Fertil. 24:86, 1979.

105. Curtis, E.M. Oral contraceptive-feminization of a normal infant: report of a case. Obstet. Gynecol. 23:295, 1964.

106. Woodruff, T.K. and Mayo, K.E. Regulation of inhibin synthesis in the rat ovary. Annu. Rev. Physiol. 52, 807–827, 1990.

107. Meunier, H., Rivier, C., Evans, R., Vale, W. Gonadal and extragonadal expression of inhibin α-, βA-, and βB-subunits in various tissues predicts diverse functions. Proc Natl Acad Sci USA; 85: 247–251, 1988.

108. Matzuk, M.M., Finegold, M.J., Su, J-G., Hsueh, A.J.W., Bradley, E. β-Inhibin is a tumour-suppressor gene with gonadal specificity in mice. Nature, 360: 313–319, 1992.

109. Russo, I.H., Srivastava, P., Mgbonyebi, O.P., and Russo, J. Activation of Programmed Cell Death by Human Chorionic Gonadotropin in Breast Cancer Therapy. Acta Haematologica, 98 (S1): 16, 1997.

110. Buttyan, R., Olsson, C.A., Pintar, J., Chang, C., Bandyk, Ng, P, and Sawczuk, I.S. Induction of the TRPM2 gene in cells undergoing program-ed cell death. Mol Cell Biol 9:3473–3481, 1989.

111. Armstrong, D.K., Issacs, J.T., Ottaviano, Y.L. and Davidson, N.E. Programmed cell death in an estrogen-independent human breast cancer cell line, MDA-MB-468. Cancer Res. 52:3418–3424, 1992.

112. Kyprianou, N., English, H.F., Davidson, N.E. and Issacs, J.T. Programmed cell death during regression of MCF-7 human breast cancer following estrogen ablation. Cancer Res 51: 162–166, 1991.

113. Simboli-Campbell, M., Narvaez, C.J., Tenniswood, M. and Welsh, J.E. 1,25- Dihydroxyvitamin D3 induces morphological and biochemical markers of apoptosis in MCF-7 breast cancer cells. J. Steroid Biochem. Molec. Biol. 58:367–376, 1996.

114. Tewari, M., Quan, L.T., O'Rourke, A., Desnoyers, S., Zeng, Z., Beidler, D.R., Poirier, G.G., Salvesen, G.S. and Dixit, V.M. Yama/CPP32, a mammalian homolog of CED-3, is a Crm A-inhibitable protease that cleaves the death substrate poly(ADP-Ribose) polymerase. Cell 81: 801–809, 1995.

115. Fernandes-Ainemri, T., Takashi, A., Armstrong, R., Krebs, J., Fritz, L., Tommaselli, K.J., Wang, L., Yu, Z., Croce, C. M., Saiveson, G., Earnshaw, W. C., Litwack, G., and Alnemri, E.S. Mch3, a novel human apoptotic cysteine protease highly related to CPP32. Cancer Res. 55: 6045–6052, 1995.

116. Femandes-Alnemri, T., Litwack, G., and Alnemri, E.S. Mch2, a new member of the apoptotic ced-3/ice cysteine protease gene family. Cancer Res. 55:2737–2742, 1995.

117. Harvey, K.J. Blomquist, J.F.I. and Ucker, D.S. Commitment and effector phases of the physiological cell death pathway elucidated with respect to Bcl-2 caspase, and cyclin-dependent kinase activities. Molecular & Cellular Biology 18: 2912–2922,1998.

118. Boudrau, N., Sympson, C.J., Werb, Z. and Bissell, M.J. Suppression of ICE and apoptosis in mammary epithelial cells by extracellular matrix. Science 267:891–893, 1995.

119. Evan, G.I. and Littlewood, T.D. The role of c-myc in cell growth. Current Opinions in Genetics & Development 3: 44–49, 1993.

120. El-Deiry, W., Tokino, T., Velculescu, V.E., Levy, D.B., Parsons, R., Trent, J.M., Lin, D., Mercer, W.E., Kinzler, K.W. and Vogelstein, B. WAF1, a potential mediator of p53 tumor suppression. Cell 75:817–825, 1993.

121. Sakamuro, D., Eviner, V., Elliott, K.J., Showe, L., White, E., and Prendergast, G.C. C-myc induces apoptosis in epithelial cells by both p-53 dependent and p53 independent mechanisms. Oncogene 11:2411–2418,1995.

122. Ronen, D., Schwartz, D., Teitz, Y., Goldfinger, N. and Rotter, V. Induction of HL-60 cells to undergo apoptosis is determined by high levels of wild type p-53 protein whereas differentiation of the cells is mediated by lower p53 levels. Cell growth & Differentiation 7:21–30, 1996.

123. Johnson, M., Dimitrov, D., Vojta, P.J., Barrett, J.C., Noda, A., Pereira-Smith, O.M., and Smith, J.R. Evidence for a p53-independent pathway for upregulation of SDI/CIPI/WAFI/p21 RNA in human cells. Mol. Carcinog. 1: 59–64, 1994.

124. Harris, C.C. Structure and function of the p53 tumor suppressor gene: clues for rational cancer therapeutic strategies. J. Natl. Cancer Inst. 88:1442–1455, 1996.

125. Strobel, T., Swanson, L., Korsmeyer, S. and Cannistra, S.A. Bax enhances pacitaxel-induced apoptosis through a p53-independent pathway. Proc. Natl. Acad. Sciences 93: 14094–14099, 1996.

126. Merlo, G.R., Cella, N., and Hynes, N. Apoptosis is accompanied by changes in Bcl-2 and Bax expression, induced by loss of attachment, and inhibited by specific extracellular matrix proteins in mammary epithelial cells. Cell Growth & Differentiation 8:251–260, 1997.

127. Russo, J., Janssens, J. and Russo, I.H. Recombinant human chorionic gonadotropin (r-hCG) significantly reduces primary tumor cell proliferation in patients with breast cancer. Breast Cancer Research and Treatment. 64:161a, 2001.

128. Calaf, G., and Russo, J. Transformation of human breast epithelial cells by chemical carcinogens. Carcinogenesis 14:483–492, 1993.

129. Mgbonyebi, O.P., Russo, J., and Russo, I.H. Induction of reversible growth arrest of immortal and neoplastic human breast epithelial cells by human chorionic gonadotropin (hCG). Proc. Am. Assoc. Cancer Res. 38:294–295, 1997.

130. Albini, A., Pagliefi, L., Orengo, G., Carlene, S., Aluigi, M., De Maachi, R., Matteucci, C., Mantovani, A., Carozzi, S., and Benelli, R. The B-core fragment of human chorionic gonadotropin inhibits growth of Kaposi's sarcoma derived cells and a new immortalized Kaposi's sarcoma cell line. AIDS 11: 713–721, 1997.

131. Liang, P. and Pardee, A.B. Differential display of eukaryotic mRNA by means of the polymerase chain reaction. Science 257:967–971, 1992.

132. Sager, R., and Anisowicz, A. Identification by differential display of alpha 6 integrin as a candidate tumor suppressor gene. FASEB J 7: 964–970, 1993.

133. Srivastava, P., Silva, I.D.C.G.; Russo, J., Mgbonyebi, O.P., and Russo, I.H. Identification of genes differentially expressed in breast carcinoma cells treated with chorionic gonadotropin. Int. J. of Oncology 13: 465–469, 1998.

134. Sakazume, S., Kimura, M. and Katagiri, M. Analysis of a novel gene expressed in apoptotic T-cell hybridoma treated with dexamethasone. Hokkaido lgaku Zasshi 71: 33–44, 1996.

135. Zacharchuk, C.M., Mercep, M., Chakraborti, P.K., Simons, S.S. and Ashwell, J.D. Programmed T lymphocyte death. Cell activation and steroid induced pathways are mutually antagonistic. J. Immunol 145: 4037–4045, 1990.

136. Hennighausen, L.G. and Sippel, A.E. Comparative sequence analysis of the MRNA s coding of mouse and rat whey proteins Nucleic Acid. Res. 10: 3733–3744, 1982.

137. Schlimme, E., and Meisel, H. Bioactive peptides derived from milk proteins. Structural, physiological and analytical aspects. Die Nahrung, 39: 1–20, 1995.

138. Jongen, W.M.F., van Boekel, M.A.J.S., and van Brockhoven, L.W. Inhibitory effect of cheese and some food constituents on mutagenicity generated in Vicia faba after treatment with nitride. Food Chem. Toxicol. 25: 141–145, 1987.

139. van Boekel, M.A.J.S., Goeptar, A.R., Alink, G.M. Antimutagenic activity of casein against MNNG in the E.coli repair host mediated assay. Cancer Lett. 114:85–87,1997.

140. Meek, D.W., Simon, S., Kikkawa, U. and Eckhart, W. The p53 tumor suppressor protein is phosphorylated at serine 389 by casein kinase 11. EMBO J. 9: 3253–3260, 1990.

141. Edelman, A.M., Blumental, D.K., Krebs, E.G. Protein Serine/ Threonine Kinases. Annu. Rev. Biochem. 56: 567–613, 1987.

142. Hatzoglow, A., Bakogeorgou, E., Hatzoglow, C., Marti, P.M., and Castanas, E. Antiproliferative and receptor bindings properties of (α and β- casomorphins in the T47D human breast cancer cell line. Eur. J. Pharmacol. 310: 217–223, 1996.

143. Hatzoglow, A., Ouafik, L., Bakogeorgou, E., Thermos, K., and Castanas, E. Morphine cross-reacts with somatostatin receptors SSTR2 in the T47D human breast cancer cell line and decreases cell growth. Cancer Res. 55: 5632–5636, 1995.

144. Maneckjee, R., Biswas, R., and Vonderhaas, B.K. Binding of opioids to human MCF-7 breast cancer cells and their effects on growth. Cancer Res. 50: 2234–2238, 1990.

145. Seytono-Han, B., Henkelman, M.S., Foeckens, J.A., and Klijn, J.G. Direct inhibitory effects of somatostatin [analogues] on the growth of human breast cancer cells. Cancer Res. 47:1566–1570, 1987.

146. Reubi, J. C., Maurer, R., von Werder, K., Torhorst, J., Klijn, J. G. M., Lamberts, S. W. J. Somatostatin receptors in human endocrine tumors. Cancer Res. 47: 551–558, 1987.

147. Hatzoglow, A., Ouafik, L., Bakogeorgou, E., Thermos, K., and Castanas, E. Morphine cross reacts with somatostatin receptor SSTR2 in the T47D human breast cancer cell line and decreases cell growth. Cancer Res.55: 5632–5636, 1995.

148. Bounous, G., Papemburg, R., Kongshavn, P.A.L., Gold, P., Fleisze, D. Dietary whey protein inhibits the development of dimethylhydrazyne induced malignancy. Clin. Invest. Med. 11:213–217, 1988.

149. Mailo, D., Russo, J., Sheriff, F., Hu, YF., Tahin, Q., Mihaila, D., Balogh G and Russo, I.H.. Genomic signature induced by differentiation in the rat mammary gland. Proc. Am. Assoc. Cancer Res. 43: 5368a, 2002

150. Srivastava, P., Russo, J. and Russo, I.H. Inhibition of rat mammary tumorigenesis by human chorionic gonadotropin is associated with increased expression of inhibin. Mol. Carcinog. 26: 10–19, 1999.

151. Russo, J. and Russo, I.H. Differentiation and Breast Cancer Development. In:" Advances in Oncobiology. Vol. 2 (Heppner, G. Ed), JAI. Press, Inc. 1998, pp. 1–10.

152. Russo, J. Tahin, Q., Lareef, H.M., Hu, YF. Russo, I.H. Neoplastic transformation of human breast epithelial cells by estrogens and chemical carcinogens. Environmental and Molecular Mutagenesis. 39: 254–263, 2002.

153. Russo, J. and Russo, I.H. Role of differentiation in the pathogenesis and prevention of breast cancer. Endocrine Related Cancer 4:7–21,1997.

Subject Index